BEING NO ONE

BEING NO ONE
The Self-Model Theory of Subjectivity

Thomas Metzinger

A Bradford Book
The MIT Press
Cambridge, Massachusetts
London, England

First MIT Press paperback edition, 2004

This book was set in Times Roman by SNP Best-set Typesetter Ltd., Hong Kong and was printed and bound in the United States of America.

Library of Congress Cataloging-in-Publication Data

Metzinger, Thomas, 1958–
  Being no one: the self-model theory of subjectivity / Thomas Metzinger.
    p. cm.
  "A Bradford book."
  Includes bibliographical references and index.
  ISBN 978-0-262-13417-0 (hc.: alk. paper)—978-0-262-63308-6 (pbk.: alk. paper)
  1. Consciousness. 2. Cognitive neuroscience. 3. Self psychology. I. Title.

QP411 .M485   2003
153—dc21   2002071759

To Anja and my parents

Contents

Acknowledgments

This book has a long history. Many people and a number of academic institutions have supported me along the way.

The introspectively accessible partition of my phenomenal self-model has it that I first became infected with the notion of a "self-model" when reading Philip Johnson-Laird's book *Mental Models*—but doubtlessly its real roots run much deeper. An early precursor of the current work was handed in as my *Habilitationsschrift* at the Center for Philosophy and Foundations of Science at the Justus Liebig-Universität Giessen in September 1991. The first German book version appeared in 1993, with a slightly revised second printing following in 1999. Soon after this monograph appeared, various friends and researchers started urging me to bring out an English edition so that people in other countries could read it as well. However, given my situation then, I never found the time to actually sit down and start writing. A first and very important step was my appointment as the first Fellow ever of the newly founded Hanse Institute of Advanced Studies in Bremen-Delmenhorst. I am very grateful to its director, Prof. Dr. Dr. Gerhard Roth, for providing me with excellent working conditions from April 1997 to September 1998 and for actively supporting me in numerous other ways. Patricia Churchland, however, deserves the credit for making me finally sit down and write this revised and expanded version of my work by inviting me over to the philosophy department at UCSD for a year. Pat and Paul have been the most wonderful hosts anyone could have had, and I greatly profited from the stimulating and highly professional environment I encountered in San Diego. My wife and I still often think of the dolphins and the silence of Californian desert nights. All this would not have been possible without an extended research grant by the German Research Foundation (Me 888/4-1/2). During this period, The MIT Press also contributed to the success of the project by a generous grant. After my return, important further support came from the McDonnell Project in Philosophy and the Neurosciences. I am greatly indebted to Kathleen Akins and the James S. McDonnell Foundation—not only for funding, but also for bringing together the most superb group of young researchers in the field I have seen so far.

In terms of individuals, my special thanks go to Sara Meirowitz and Katherine Almeida at The MIT Press, who, professionally and with great patience, have guided me through a long process that was not always easy. Over the years so many philosophers and scientists have helped me in discussions and with their valuable criticism that it is impossible to name them all—I hope that those not explicitly mentioned will understand and forgive me. In particular, I am grateful to Ralph Adolphs, Peter Brugger, Jonathan Cole, Antonio Damasio, Chris Eliasmith, Andreas Engel, Chris Frith, Vittorio Gallese, Andreas Kleinschmidt, Marc Jeannerod, Markus Knauff, Christof Koch, Ina Leiß, Toemme Noesselt, Wolf Singer, Francisco Varela, Bettina Walde, and Thalia Wheatley. At the University of Essen, I am grateful to Beate Mrugalla and Isabelle Rox, who gave me technical help with the manuscript. In Mainz, Saku Hara, Stephan Schleim, and Olav Wiegand have supported me. And, as with a number of previous enterprises of this kind, the one person in the background who was and is *most* important, has been, as always, my wife, Anja.

BEING NO ONE

1 Questions

1.1 Consciousness, the Phenomenal Self, and the First-Person Perspective

This is a book about consciousness, the phenomenal self, and the first-person perspective. Its main thesis is that no such things as selves exist in the world: Nobody ever *was* or *had* a self. All that ever existed were conscious self-models that could not be recognized *as* models. The phenomenal self is not a thing, but a process—and the subjective experience of *being someone* emerges if a conscious information-processing system operates under a transparent self-model. You are such a system right now, as you read these sentences. Because you cannot recognize your self-model *as* a model, it is transparent: you look right through it. You don't see it. But you see *with* it. In other, more metaphorical, words, the central claim of this book is that as you read these lines you constantly *confuse* yourself with the content of the self-model currently activated by your brain.

This is not your fault. Evolution has made you this way. On the contrary. Arguably, until now, the conscious self-model of human beings is the best invention Mother Nature has made. It is a wonderfully efficient two-way window that allows an organism to conceive of itself *as a whole*, and thereby to causally interact with its inner and outer environment in an entirely new, integrated, and intelligent manner. Consciousness, the phenomenal self, and the first-person perspective are fascinating *representational* phenomena that have a long evolutionary history, a history which eventually led to the formation of complex societies and a cultural embedding of conscious experience itself. For many researchers in the cognitive neurosciences it is now clear that the first-person perspective somehow must have been the decisive link in this transition from biological to cultural evolution. In philosophical quarters, on the other hand, it is popular to say things like "The first-person perspective cannot be reduced to the third-person perspective!" or to develop complex technical arguments showing that some kinds of irreducible first-person facts exist. But nobody ever asks what a first-person perspective *is* in the first place. This is what I will do. I will offer a representationalist and a functionalist analysis of what a consciously experienced first-person perspective is.

This book is also, and in a number of ways, an experiment. You will find conceptual tool kits and new metaphors, case studies of unusual states of mind, as well as multilevel constraints for a comprehensive theory of consciousness. You will find many well-known questions and some preliminary, perhaps even some new answers. On the following pages, I try to build a better bridge—a bridge connecting the humanities and the empirical sciences of the mind more directly. The tool kits and the metaphors, the case studies and the constraints are the very first building blocks for this bridge. What I am interested in is finding conceptually convincing links between subpersonal and personal levels of description, links that at the same time are empirically plausible. What *precisely* is the point at which objective, third-person approaches to the human mind can be integrated with first-person, subjective, and purely theoretical approaches? How *exactly* does strong, consciously experienced subjectivity emerge out of objective events in the natural world? Today, I believe, this is what we need to know more than anything else.

The epistemic goal of this book consists in finding out whether conscious experience, in particular the experience of *being someone*, resulting from the emergence of a phenomenal self, can be convincingly analyzed on subpersonal levels of description. A related second goal consists in finding out if, and how, our Cartesian intuitions—those deeply entrenched intuitions that tell us that the above-mentioned experience of being a subject and a rational individual can *never* be naturalized or reductively explained—are ultimately rooted in the deeper representational structure of our conscious minds. Intuitions have to be taken seriously. But it is also possible that our best theories about our own minds will turn out to be radically counterintuitive, that they will present us with a new kind of self-knowledge that most of us just cannot believe. Yes, one can certainly look at the current explosion in the mind sciences as a new and breathtaking phase in the pursuit of an old philosophical ideal, the ideal of self-knowledge (see Metzinger, 2000b, p. 6*ff.*). And yes, nobody ever said that a fundamental expansion of knowledge about ourselves necessarily has to be *intuitively* plausible. But if we want it to be a philosophically interesting growth of knowledge, and one that can also be culturally integrated, then we should at least demand an understanding of *why* inevitably it is counterintuitive in some of its aspects. And this problem cannot be solved by any single discipline alone. In order to make progress with regard to the two general epistemic goals just named, we need a better bridge between the humanities and cognitive neuroscience. This is one reason why this book is an experiment, an experiment in *interdisciplinary* philosophy.

In the now flowering interdisciplinary field of research on consciousness there are two rather extreme ways of avoiding the problem. One is the attempt to proceed in a highly pragmatic way, simply generating empirical data without ever getting clear about what the *explanandum* of such an enterprise actually is. The explanandum is that which is to be explained. To give an example, in an important and now classic paper, Francis Crick and Christof Koch introduced the idea of a "neural correlate of consciousness" (Crick and Koch 1990; for further discussion, see Metzinger 2000a). They wrote:

Everyone has a rough idea of what is meant by consciousness. We feel that it is better to avoid a precise definition of consciousness because of the dangers of premature definition. Until we understand the problem much better, any attempt at a formal definition is likely to be either misleading or overly restrictive, or both. (Crick and Koch 1990, p. 264)

There certainly are a number of good points behind this strategy. In complex domains, as historical experience shows, scientific breakthroughs are frequently achieved simply by stumbling onto highly relevant data, rather than by carrying out rigorously systematized research programs. Insight often comes as a surprise. From a purely heuristic perspective, narrowing down the scope of one's search too early certainly is dangerous, for instance, by making attempts at excessive, but not yet data-driven formal modeling. A certain degree of open-mindedness is necessary. On the other hand, it is simply not true that everyone has a rough idea of what the term "consciousness" refers to. In my own experience, for example, the most frequent misunderstanding lies in confusing phenomenal experience as such with what philosophers call "reflexive self-consciousness," the actualized capacity to cognitively refer to yourself, using some sort of concept-like or quasi-linguistic kind of mental structure. According to this definition hardly anything on this planet, including many humans during most of their day, is ever conscious at all. Second, in many languages on this planet we do not even find an adequate counterpart for the English term "consciousness" (Wilkes 1988b). Why did all these linguistic communities obviously not see the need for developing a unitary concept of their own? Is it possible that the *phenomenon* did not exist for these communities? And third, it should simply be embarrassing for any scientist to not be able to clearly state *what* it is that she is trying to explain (Bieri 1995). What is the *explanandum*? What are the actual entities between which an explanatory relationship is to be established? Especially when pressed by the humanities, hard scientists should at least be able to state clearly what it is they want to know, what the target of their research is, and what, from their perspective, would count as a successful explanation.

The other extreme is something that is frequently found in philosophy, particularly in the best of philosophy of mind. I call it "analytical scholasticism." It consists in an equally dangerous tendency toward arrogant armchair theorizing, at the same time ignoring first-person phenomenological as well as third-person empirical constraints in the formation of one's basic conceptual tools. In extreme cases, the target domain is treated as if it consisted only of *analysanda*, and not of explananda *and* analysanda. What is an analysandum? An analysandum is a certain way of speaking about a phenomenon, a way that creates logical and intuitive problems. If consciousness and subjectivity were only analysanda, then we could solve all the philosophical puzzles related to consciousness, the phenomenal self, and the first-person perspective by changing the way we talk. We would have to do to modal logic and formal semantics, and not cognitive neuroscience. Philosophy would be a fundamentalist discipline that could decide on the truth and falsity of empirical statements by logical argument alone. I just cannot believe that this should be so.

Certainly by far the best contributions to philosophy of mind in the last century have come from analytical philosophers, philosophers in the tradition of Frege and Wittgenstein. Because many such philosophers are superb at analyzing the deeper structure of language, they often fall into the trap of analyzing the conscious mind as if it were *itself* a linguistic entity, based not on dynamical self-organization in the human brain, but on a disembodied system of rule-based information processing. At least they frequently assume that there is a "content level" in the human mind that can be investigated without knowing anything about "vehicle properties," about properties of the actual physical carriers of conscious content. The vehicle-content distinction for mental representations certainly is a powerful tool in many theoretical contexts. But our best and empirically plausible theories of representation, those now so successfully employed in connectionist and dynamicist models of cognitive functioning, show that any philosophical theory of mind treating vehicle and content as anything more than two strongly interrelated aspects of one and the same phenomenon simply deprives itself of much of its explanatory power, if not of its realism and epistemological rationality. The resulting terminologies then are of little relevance to researchers in other fields, as some of their basic assumptions immediately appear ridiculously implausible from an empirical point of view. Because many analytical philosophers are excellent logicians, they also have a tendency to get technical even if there is not yet a point to it—even if there are not yet any data to fill their conceptual structures with content and anchor them in the real-world growth of knowledge. Epistemic progress in the real world is something that is achieved by all disciplines *together*. However, the deeper motive behind falling into the other extreme, the isolationist extreme of sterility and scholasticism, may really be something else. Frequently it may actually be an unacknowledged respect for the rigor, the seriousness, and the true intellectual substance perceived in the hard sciences of the mind. Interestingly, in speaking and listening not only to philosophers but to a number of eminent neuroscientists as well, I have often discovered a "motivational mirror image." As it turns out, many neuroscientists are actually much more philosophers than they would like to admit. The same motivational structure, the same sense of respect exists in empirical investigators avoiding precise definitions: They know too well that deeper methodological and metatheoretical issues exist, and that these issues are important and extremely difficult at the same time. The lesson to be drawn from this situation seems to be simple and clear: somehow the good aspects of both extremes have to be united. And because there already is a deep (if sometimes unadmitted) mutual respect between the disciplines, between the hard sciences of the mind and the humanities, I believe that the chances for building more direct bridges are actually better than some of us think.

As many authors have noted, what is needed is a *middle course* of a yet-to-be-discovered nature. I have tried to steer such a middle course in this book—and I have paid a high price for it, as readers will soon begin to notice. The treatment of philosophical issues will strike all philosophers as much too brief and quite superficial. On the other hand, my selection of empirical constraints, of case studies, and of isolated data points must strike neuro- and cognitive scientists alike as often highly idiosyncratic and quite badly informed. Yet bridges begin with small stones, and there are only so many stones an individual person can carry. My goal, therefore, is rather modest: If at least *some* of the bits and pieces here assembled are useful to *some* of my readers, then this will be enough.

As everybody knows the problem of consciousness has gained the increasing attention of philosophers (see, e.g., Metzinger 1995a), as well as researchers working in the neuro- and cognitive sciences (see, e.g., Metzinger 2000a), during the last three decades of the twentieth century. We have witnessed a true renaissance. As many have argued, consciousness is the most fascinating research target conceivable, the greatest remaining challenge to the scientific worldview as well as the centerpiece of any philosophical theory of mind. What is it that makes consciousness such a special target phenomenon? In conscious experience *a reality is present*. But what does it mean to say that, for all beings enjoying conscious experience, necessarily *a world appears*? It means at least three different things: In conscious experience there is a world, there is a self, and there is a relation between both—because in an interesting sense this world appears *to* the experiencing self. We can therefore distinguish three different aspects of our original question. The first set of questions is about what it means that a reality *appears*. The second set is about how it can be that this reality appears to *someone*, to a subject of experience. The third set is about how this subject becomes the center of its own world, how it transforms the appearance of a reality into a truly *subjective* phenomenon by tying it to an individual first-person perspective.

I have said a lot about what the problem of consciousness as such amounts to elsewhere (e.g., Metzinger 1995e). The deeper and more specific problem of how one's own personal *identity* appears in conscious experience and how one develops an inward, subjective *perspective* not only toward the external world as such but also to other persons in it and the ongoing internal process of experience itself is what concerns us here. Let us therefore look at the second set of issues. For human beings, during the ongoing process of conscious experience characterizing their waking and dreaming life, *a self is present*. Human beings consciously experience themselves as *being someone*. The conscious experience of being someone, however, has many different aspects—bodily, emotional, and cognitive. In philosophy, as well as in cognitive neuroscience, we have recently witnessed a lot of excellent work focusing on bodily self-experience (see, e.g., Bermúdez, Marcel, and Eilan 1995), on emotional self-consciousness (see, e.g., Damasio 1994, 2000), and on the intricacies involved in cognitive self-reference and the conscious experience of being an embodied *thinking self* (see, e.g., Nagel 1986, Bermúdez 1998). What does it mean to say that, for conscious human beings, *a self is present*? How are the different layers of the embodied, the emotional, and the thinking self connected to each other? How do they influence each other? I prepare some new answers in the second half of this book.

This book, however, is not only about consciousness and self-consciousness. The yet deeper question behind the phenomenal appearance of a world and of a self is connected to the notion of a consciously experienced "first-person perspective": what precisely makes consciousness a *subjective* phenomenon? This is the second half of my first epistemic target. The issue is not only how a phenomenal self per se can arise but how beings like ourselves come to use this phenomenal self as a tool for experiencing themselves as subjects. We need interdisciplinary answers to questions like these: What does it mean that in conscious experience we are not only *related to the world*, but related to it *as knowing selves*? What, exactly, does it mean that a phenomenal self typically is not only present in an experiential reality but that at the same time it forms the *center* of this reality? How do we come to think and speak about ourselves as *first persons*? After first having developed in chapters 2, 3, and 4 some simple tools that help us understand how, more generally, a reality can appear, I proceed to tackle these questions from the second half of chapter 6 onward. More about the architecture of what follows in section 1.3.

1.2   Questions

In this section I want to develop a small and concise set of questions, in order to guide us through the complex theoretical landscape associated with the phenomenon of subjective experience. I promise that in the final chapter of this book I will return to each one of these questions, by giving brief, condensed answers to each of them. The *longer* answers, however, can only be found in the middle chapters of this book. This book is written for readers, and one function of the following minimal catalogue of philosophical problems consists in increasing its usability. However, this small checklist could also function as a starting point for a minimal set of criteria for judging the current status of competing approaches, including the one presented here. How many of these questions can it answer in a satisfactory way? Let us look at them. A first, and basic, group of questions concerns the meaning of some of the explanatory core concepts already introduced above:

What does it mean to say of a mental state that it is conscious?

Alternatively, what does it mean of a conscious system—a person, a biological organism, or an artificial system—if taken as a whole to say that it is conscious?

What does it mean to say of a mental state that it is a part of a given system's self-consciousness?

What does it mean for any conscious system to possess a phenomenal self? Is selfless consciousness possible?

What does it mean to say of a mental state that it is a subjective state?

What does it mean to speak of whole systems as "subjects of experience?"

What is a phenomenal first-person perspective, for example, as opposed to a linguistic, cognitive, or epistemic first-person perspective? Is there anything like aperspectival consciousness or even self-consciousness?

Next there is a range of questions concerning ontological, logical-semantic, and epistemological issues. They do not form the focus of this investigation, but they are of great relevance to the bigger picture that could eventually emerge from an empirically based philosophical theory of self-consciousness.

Is the notion of a "subject" logically primitive? Does its existence have to be assumed a priori? Ontologically speaking, does what we refer to by "subject" belong to the basic constituents of reality, or is it an entity that could in principle be eliminated in the course of scientific progress?

In particular, the semantics of the indexical word *I* needs further clarification. What is needed is a better understanding of a certain class of sentences, namely, those in which the word *I* is used in the autophenomenological self-ascription of phenomenal properties (as in "I am feeling a toothache right now").

What are the truth-conditions for sentences of this type?

Would the elimination of the subject use of I *leave a gap in our understanding of ourselves?*

Is subjectivity an epistemic relation? Do phenomenal states possess truth-values? Do consciousness, the phenomenal self, and the first-person perspective supply us with a specific kind of information or knowledge, not to be gained by any other means?

Does the incorrigibility of self-ascriptions of psychological properties imply their infallibility?

Are there any irreducible facts concerning the subjectivity of mental states that can only be grasped under a phenomenal first-person perspective or only be expressed in the first person singular?

Can the thesis that the scientific worldview must in principle *remain incomplete be derived from the subjectivity of the mental? Can subjectivity, in its full content, be naturalized?*

Does anything like "first-person data" exist? Can introspective reports compete with statements originating from scientific theories of the mind?

The true focus of the current proposal, however, is phenomenal content, the way certain representational states *feel* from the first-person perspective. Of particular importance are attempts to shed light on the historical roots of certain philosophical intuitions—like, for instance, the Cartesian intuition that *I could always have been someone else*; or that my own consciousness necessarily forms a single, unified whole; or that phenomenal experience actually brings us in direct and immediate contact with ourselves and the world around us. Philosophical problems can frequently be solved by conceptual analysis or by transforming them into more differentiated versions. However, an additional and interesting strategy consists in attempting to also uncover their introspective roots. A careful inspection of these roots may help us to understand the *intuitive force* behind many bad arguments, a force that typically survives their rebuttal. I will therefore supplement my discussion by taking a closer look at the genetic conditions for certain introspective certainties.

What is the "phenomenal content" of mental states, as opposed to their representational or "intentional content?" Are there examples of mentality exhibiting one without the other? Do double dissociations exist?

How do Cartesian intuitions—like the contingency intuition, the indivisibility intuition, or the intuition of epistemic immediacy—emerge?

Arguably, the human variety of conscious subjectivity is unique on this planet, namely, in that it is culturally embedded, in that it allows not only for introspective but also for linguistic access, and in that the contents of our phenomenal states can also become the target of exclusively internal cognitive self-reference. In particular, it forms the basis of *intersubjective* achievements. The interesting question is how the actual contents of experience *change* through this constant integration into other representational media, and how specific contents may genetically depend on social factors.

Which new phenomenal properties emerge through cognitive and linguistic forms of self-reference? In humans, are there necessary social correlates for certain kinds of phenomenal content?

A final set of phenomenological questions concerns the internal web of relations between certain phenomenal state classes or global phenomenal properties. Here is a brief selection:

What is the most simple form of phenomenal content? Are there anything like "qualia" in the classic sense of the word?

What is the minimal set of constraints that have to be satisfied for conscious experience to emerge at all? For instance, could qualia exist without the global property of consciousness, or is a qualia-free form of consciousness conceivable?

What is phenomenal selfhood? What, precisely, is the nonconceptual sense of ownership that goes along with the phenomenal experience of selfhood or of "being someone?"

How is the experience of agency *related to the experience of ownership? Can both forms of phenomenal content be dissociated?*

Can phenomenal selfhood be instantiated without qualia? Is embodiment necessary for selfhood?

What is a phenomenally represented first-person perspective? How does it contribute to other notions of perspectivalness, for example, logical or epistemic subjectivity?

Can one have a conscious first-person perspective without having a conscious self? Can one have a conscious self without having a conscious first-person perspective?

In what way does a phenomenal first-person perspective contribute to the emergence of a second-person perspective and to the emergence of a first-person plural perspective? What forms of social cognition are inevitably mediated by phenomenal self-awareness? Which are not?

Finally, one last question concerns the status of *phenomenal universals*: Can we define a notion of consciousness and subjectivity that is hardware- and species-independent? This issue amounts to an attempt to give an analysis of consciousness, the phenomenal self, and the first-person perspective that operates on the representational and functional levels of description alone, aiming at liberation from any kind of physical domain-specificity. Can there be a *universal* theory of consciousness? In other words:

Is artificial *subjectivity possible? Could there be nonbiological phenomenal selves?*

1.3 Overview: The Architecture of the Book

In this book you will find twelve new conceptual instruments, two new theoretical entities, a double set of neurophenomenological case studies, and some heuristic metaphors. Perhaps most important, I introduce two new theoretical entities: the "phenomenal self-model" (PSM; see section 6.1) and the "phenomenal model of the intentionality relation" (PMIR; see section 6.5). I contend that these entities are *distinct* theoretical entities and argue that they may form the decisive conceptual link between first-person and third-person approaches to the conscious mind. I also claim that they are distinct in terms of relating to clearly isolable and correlated phenomena on the phenomenological, the representationalist, the functionalist, and the neurobiological levels of description. A PSM and a PMIR are something to be *found* by empirical research in the mind sciences. Second, these two hypothetical entities are helpful on the level of conceptual analysis as well. They may form the decisive conceptual link between consciousness research in the humanities and consciousness research in the sciences. For philosophy of mind, they serve as important conceptual links between personal and subpersonal levels of description for conscious systems. Apart from the necessary normative context, what makes a nonperson a person is a very special sort of PSM, plus a PMIR: You *become* a person by possessing a transparent self-model plus a conscious model of the "arrow of intentionality" linking you to the world. In addition, the two new hypothetical entities can further support us in developing an extended representationalist framework for intersubjectivity and social cognition, because they allow us to understand the *second*-person perspective—the consciously experienced *you*—as well. Third, if we want to get a better grasp on the transition from biological to cultural evolution, both entities are likely to constitute important aspects of the actual linkage to be described. And finally, they will also prove to be fruitful in developing a metatheoretical account about what actually it *is* that theories in the neuro- and cognitive sciences are talking about.

As can be seen from what has just been said, chapter 6 is in some ways the most important part of this book, because it explains what a phenomenal self-model and the phenomenal model of the intentionality relation actually are. However, to create some common ground I will start by first introducing some simple tools in the following chapter. In chapter 2 I explain what mental representation is, as opposed to mental *simulation* and mental *presentation*—and what it means that all three phenomena can exist in an unconscious and a conscious form. This chapter is mirrored in chapter 5, which reapplies the new conceptual distinctions to *self*-representation, *self*-simulation, and *self*-presentation. As chapter 2 is of a more introductory character, it also is much longer than chapter 5. Chapter 3 investigates more closely the transition from unconscious information processing in the brain to full-blown phenomenal experience. There, you will find a set of ten constraints, which any mental representation has to satisfy if its content wants to count as *conscious* content. However, as you will discover, some of these constraints are domain-specific, and not all of them form strictly necessary conditions: there are *degrees* of phenomenality. Neither consciousness nor self-consciousness is an all-or-nothing affair. In addition, these constraints are also "multilevel" constraints in that they make an attempt to take the first-person phenomenology, the representational and functional architecture, and the neuroscience of consciousness seriously at the same time. Chapter 3 is mirrored in the first part of chapter 6, namely, in applying these constraints to the special case of self-consciousness. Chapter 4 presents a brief set of neurophenomenological case studies. We take a closer look at interesting clinical phenomena such as agnosia, neglect, blindsight, and hallucinations, and also at ordinary forms of what I call "deviant phenomenal models of reality," for example, dreams. One function of these case studies is to show us what is *not necessary* in the deep structure of conscious experience, and to prevent us from drawing false conclusions on the conceptual level. They also function as a harsh reality test for the philosophical instruments developed in both of the preceding chapters. Chapter 4 is mirrored again in chapter 7. Chapter 7 expands on chapter 4. Because self-consciousness and the first-person perspective constitute the true thematic focus of this book, our reality test has to be much more extensive in its second half, and harsher too. In particular, we have to see if not only our new set of concepts and constraints but the two central theoretical entities—the PSM and the PMIR, as introduced in chapter 6—actually have a chance to survive any such reality test. Finally, chapter 8 makes an attempt to draw the different threads together in a more general and illustrative manner. It also offers minianswers to the questions listed in the preceding section of this chapter, and some brief concluding remarks about potential future directions.

This book was written for readers, and I have tried to make it as easy to use as possible. Different readers will take different paths. If you have no time to read the entire book, skip to chapter 8 and work your way back where necessary. If you are a philosopher interested in neurophenomenological case studies that challenge traditional theories of the conscious mind, go to chapters 4 and 7. If you are an empirical scientist *or* a philosopher mainly interested in constraints on the notion of conscious representation, go to chapter 3 and then on to sections 6.1 and 6.2 to learn more about the specific application of these constraints in developing a theory of the phenomenal self. If your focus is on the heart of the theory, on the two new theoretical entities called the PSM and the PMIR, then you should simply try to read chapter 6 first. But if you are interested in learning why qualia don't exist, what the actual items in our basic conceptual tool kit are, and why all of this is primarily a *representationalist* theory of consciousness, the phenomenal self, and the first-person perspective, then simply turn this page and go on.

2   Tools I

2.1   Overview: Mental Representation and Phenomenal States

On the following pages I take a fresh look at problems traditionally associated with phenomenal experience and the subjectivity of the mental by analyzing them from the perspective of a naturalist theory of mental representation. In this first step, I develop a clearly structured and maximally simple set of conceptual instruments, to achieve the epistemic goal of this book. This goal consists in discovering the foundations for a general theory of the phenomenal first-person perspective, one that is not only conceptually convincing but also empirically plausible. Therefore, the conceptual instruments used in pursuing this goal have to be, at the same time, open to semantic differentiations and to continuous enrichment by empirical data. In particular, since the general project of developing a comprehensive theory of consciousness, the phenomenal self, and the first-person perspective is clearly an enterprise in which many different disciplines have to participate, I will try to keep things simple. My aim is not to maximize the degree of conceptual precision and differentiation, but to generate a theoretical framework which does not exclude researchers from outside of philosophy of mind. In particular, my goal is *not* to develop a full-blown (or even a sketchy) theory of mental representation. However, two simple conceptual tool kits will have to be introduced in chapters 2 and 5. We will put the new working concepts contained in them to work in subsequent chapters, when looking at the representational deep structure of the phenomenal experience of the world and ourselves and when interpreting a series of neurophenomenological case studies.

In a second step, I attempt to develop a theoretical prototype for the content as well as for the "vehicles"[1] of phenomenal representation, on different levels of description. With regard to our own case, it has to be plausible phenomenologically, as well as from the

---

1. Regarding the conceptual distinction between "vehicle" and "content" for representations, see, for example, Dretske 1988. I frequently use a closely related distinction between *phenomenal* content (or "character") and its vehicle, in terms of the *representatum*, that is, the concrete internal state functioning as carrier or medium for this content. As I explain below, two aspects are important in employing these traditional conceptual instruments carefully. First, for phenomenal content the "principle of local supervenience" holds: *phenomenal* content is determined by internal and contemporaneous properties of the conscious system, for example, by properties of its brain. For *intentional* content (i.e., *representational* content as more traditionally conceived) this does not have to be true: *What* and *if* it actually represents may change with what actually exists in the environment. At the same time the phenomenal content, how things subjectively *feel* to you, may stay invariant, as does your brain state. Second, the limitations and dangers of the original conceptual distinction must be clearly seen. As I briefly point out in chapter 3, the vehicle-content distinction is a highly useful conceptual instrument, but it contains subtle residues of Cartesian dualism. It tempts us to reify the vehicle and the content, conceiving of them as ontologically distinct, independent entities. A more empirically plausible model of representational content will have to describe it as an aspect of an ongoing *process* and not as some kind of abstract object. However, as long as ontological atomism and naive realism are avoided, the vehicle-content distinction will prove to be highly useful in many contexts. I will frequently remind readers of potential difficulties by putting "vehicle" in quotation marks.

third-person perspective of the neuro- and cognitive sciences. That will happen in the second half of chapter 2, and in chapter 3 in particular. In chapter 4, I use a first series of short neurophenomenological case studies to critically assess this first set of conceptual tools, as well as the concrete model of a representational vehicle: Can these instruments be employed in successfully analyzing those phenomena which typically constitute inexplicable mysteries for classic theories of mind? Do they really do justice to all the colors, the subtleness, and the richness of conscious experience? I like to think of this procedure (which will be repeated in chapter 7) as a "neuropsychological reality test." This reality test will be carried out by having a closer look at a number of special configurations underlying unusual forms of phenomenal experience that we frequently confront in clinical neuropsychology, and sometimes in ordinary life as well. However, everywhere in this book where I am not explicitly concerned with this type of reality test, the following background assumption will always be made: the intended class of systems is being formed by human beings in nonpathological waking states. The primary target of the current investigation, therefore, is ordinary humans in ordinary phases of their waking life, presumably just like you, the reader of this book. I am fully aware that this is a vague characterization of the intended class of systems—but as readers will note in the course of this book, as a general default assumption it fully suffices for my present purposes.

In this chapter I start by first offering a number of general considerations concerning the question of how parts of the world are internally represented by mental states. These considerations will lead to a reconstruction of mental representation as a special case of a more comprehensive process—mental *simulation*. Two further concepts will naturally flow from this, and they can later be used to answer the question of what the most simple and what the most comprehensive forms of phenomenal content actually are. Those are the concepts of "mental presentation" and of "global metarepresentation" respectively of a "global model of reality" (see sections 2.4 and 3.2.3). Both concepts will help to develop demarcation criteria for genuinely conscious, phenomenal processes of representation as opposed to merely *mental* processes of representation. In chapter 3, I attempt to give a closer description of the concrete vehicles of representation underlying the flow of subjective experience, by introducing the working concept of a "phenomenal mental model." This is in preparation for the steps taken in the second half of the book (chapters 5 through 7), trying to answer questions like these: What exactly is "perspectivalness," the dominant structural feature of our phenomenal space? How do some information-processing systems achieve generating complex internal representations of *themselves*, using them in coordinating their external behavior? How is a phenomenal, a consciously experienced *first-person perspective* constituted? Against the background of my general thesis, which claims that a very specific form of mental self-modeling is the key to understanding the perspectivalness of phenomenal states, at the end of this book (chapter 8) I try to give some new answers to the philosophical questions formulated in chapter 1.

2.2   From Mental to Phenomenal Representation: Information Processing, Intentional Content, and Conscious Experience

Mental representation is a process by which some biosystems generate an internal depiction of parts of reality.[2] The states generated in the course of this process are *internal* representations, because their content is only—if at all—accessible in a very special way to the respective system, by means of a process, which, today, we call "phenomenal experience." Possibly this process itself is another representational process, a higher-order process, which only operates on internal properties of the system. However, it is important for us, right from the beginning, to clearly separate three levels of conceptual analysis: internality can be described as a phenomenal, a functional, or as a physical property of certain system states. Particularly from a phenomenological perspective, internality is a highly salient, global feature of the contents of conscious self-awareness. These contents are continuously accompanied by the *phenomenal* quality of internality in a "prereflexive" manner, that is, permanently and independently of all cognitive operations.

Phenomenal self-consciousness generates "inwardness." In chapters 5 and 6 we take a very careful look at this special phenomenal property. On the functional level of description, one discovers a second kind of "inwardness." The content of mental representations is the content of *internal* states because the causal properties making it available for conscious experience are only realized by a single person and by physical properties, which are mostly internally exemplified, realized within the body of this person. This observation leads us to the third possible level of analysis: mental representations are *individual* states, which are internal system states in a simple, physical-spatial sense. On this most trivial reading we look only at the carriers or vehicles of representational content themselves. However, even this first conceptual interpretation of the internality of the mental as a physical type of internality is more than problematic, and for many good reasons.

Obviously, it is the case that frequently the representations of this first order are in their content determined by certain facts, which are external facts, lying outside the system in a very simple and straightforward sense. If your current mental book representation really

---

2. "Representation" and "depiction" are used here in a loose and nontechnical sense, and do not refer to the generation of symbolic or propositionally structured representations. As will become clear in the following sections, internal structures generated by the process of phenomenal representation differ from descriptions with the help of internal sentence analogues (e.g., in a *lingua mentis*; see Fodor 1975) by the fact that they do not aim at truth, but at similarity and viability. Viability is *functional adequacy*.

has the content "book" in a strong sense depends on whether there really *is* a book in your hands right now. Is it a representation or a misrepresentation? This is the classic problem of the intentionality of the mental: mental states seem to be always directed at an *object*, they are states *about* something, because they "intentionally" contain an object *within themselves*. (Brentano 1874, II, 1: §5). Treating intentional systems as information-processing systems, we can today develop a much clearer understanding of Brentano's mysterious and never defined notion of *intentionale Inexistenz* by, as empirical psychologists, speaking of "virtual object emulators" and the like (see chapter 3). The most fundamental level on which mental states can be individuated, however, is not their intentional content or the causal role that they play in generating internal and external behavior. It is constituted by their *phenomenal* content, by the way in which they are experienced from an inward perspective. In our context, phenomenal content is what stays the same irrespective of whether something is a representation or a misrepresentation.

Of course, our views about what truly is "most fundamental" in grasping the true nature of mental states may soon undergo a dramatic change. However, the first-person approach certainly was *historically* fundamental. Long before human beings constructed theories about intentional content or the causal role of mental representations, a folk-psychological taxonomy of the mental was already in existence. Folk psychology naively, successfully, and consequently operates from the first-person perspective: a mental state simply is what I subjectively *experience* as a mental state. Only later did it become apparent that not all mental, object-directed states are also conscious states in the sense of actual phenomenal experience. Only later did it become apparent how theoretical approaches to the mental, still intuitively rooted in folk psychology, have generated very little growth of knowledge in the last twenty-five centuries (P. M. Churchland 1981). That is one of the reasons why today those properties, which the mental representation of a part of reality has to possess in order to become a phenomenally experienced representation, are the focus of philosophical debates: What sense of internality is it that truly allows us to differentiate between mental and phenomenal representations? Is it phenomenal, functional, or physical internality?

At the outset we are faced with the following situation: representations of parts of the world are traditionally described as mental states if they possess a further functional property. This functional property is a *dispositional* property; as possible contents of consciousness, they can in principle be turned into subjective experiences. The contents of our subjective experience in this way are the results of an unknown representational achievement. It is brought about by our brains in interaction with the environment. If we are successful in developing a more precise analysis of this representational achievement and the functional properties underlying it, then this analysis will supply us with defining characteristics for the concept of consciousness.

However, the generation of mental states itself is only a special case of biological information processing: The large majority of cases in which properties of the world are represented by generating specific internal states, in principle, take place without any instantiation of phenomenal qualities or subjective awareness. Many of those complicated processes of internal information processing which, for instance, are necessary for regulating our heart rate or the activity of our immune system, seldom reach the level of explicit[3] conscious representation (Damasio, 1999; Metzinger, 2000a,b; for a concrete example of a possible molecular-level correlate in terms of a cholinergic component of conscious experience, see Perry, Walker, Grace, and Perry 1999).[4] Such purely biological processes of an elementary self-regulatory kind certainly carry information, but this information is not *mental* information. They bring about and then stabilize a large number of internal system states, which can never become contents of subjective, phenomenal consciousness. These processes, as well, generate relationships of similarity, isomorphisms; they track and covary with certain states of affairs in the body, and thereby create representations of facts—at least in a certain, weak sense of object-directedness. These states are states which carry information about subpersonal properties of the system. Their informational content is used by the system to achieve its own survival. It is important to note how such processes are only internal representations in a purely physical sense; they are not *mental* representations in the sense just mentioned, because they cannot, in principle, become the content of phenomenal states, the objects of conscious experience. They lack those functional properties which make them *inner* states in a phenomenological sense. Obviously, there are a number of unusual situations—for instance, in hypnotic states, during somnambulism, or in epileptic absence automatisms—in which functionally active and very complex representations of the environment plus of an agent *in* this environment

3. I treat an *explicit* representation as one in which changes in the representandum invariably lead to a change on the content level of the respective medium. *Implicit* representation will only change functional properties of the medium—for instance, by changing synaptic weights and moving a connectionist system to another position in weight space. Conscious content will generally be explicit content in that it is globally available (see section 3.2.1) and, in perception, directly covaries with its object. This does not, of course, mean that it has to be linguistic or *conceptually* explicit content.

4. Not all relevant processes of biological information processing in individual organisms are processes of *neural* information processing. The immune system is an excellent example of a functional mechanism that constitutes a self–world border *within* the system, while itself only possessing a highly distributed localization, hence there may exist physical correlates of conscious experience, even of self-consciousness, that are not *neural* correlates in a narrow sense. There is a whole range of only weakly localized informational systems in human beings, like neurotransmitters or certain hormones. Obviously, the properties of such weakly localized functional modules can strongly determine the content of certain classes of mental states (e.g., of emotions). This is one reason why neural nets may still be biologically rather unrealistic theoretical models. It is also conceivable that those functional properties necessary to fully determine the actual content of conscious experience will eventually have to be specified not on a cellular, but on a *molecular* level of description for neural correlates of consciousness.

are activated without phenomenal consciousness or memories being generated at the same time (We return to such cases in chapter 7.) Such states have a rich informational content, but they are not yet tied to the perspective of a conscious, experiencing self.

The first question in relation to the phenomenon of mental representation, therefore, is: What makes an internal representation a *mental* representation; what transforms it into a process which can, at least in principle, possess a phenomenal kind of "inwardness?" The obvious fact that biological nervous systems are able to generate representations of the world and its causal matrix by forming internal states which then function as internal representations of this causal matrix is something that I will not discuss further in this book. Our problem is not intentional, but *phenomenal* content. Intentionality does exist, and there now is a whole range of promising approaches to naturalizing intentional, representational content. Conscious intentional content is the deeper problem. Could it be possible to analyze phenomenal representation as a convolved, a nested and complex variant of *intentional* representation? Many philosophers today pursue a strategy of intentionalizing phenomenal consciousness: for them, phenomenal content is a higher-order form of representational content, which is intricately interwoven with itself. Many of the representational processes underlying conscious experience seem to be isomorphy-preserving processes; they systematically covary with properties of the world and they actively conserve this covariance. The covariance generated in this way is embedded into a causal-teleological context, because it possesses a long biological history and is used by individual systems in achieving certain goals (see Millikan 1984, 1993; Papineau 1987, 1993; Dretske 1988; and section 3.2.11). The *intentional* content of the states generated in this way then plays a central role in explaining external behavior, as well as the persistent internal reconfiguration of the system.

However, the astonishing fact that such internal representations of parts of the world can, besides their intentional content, also turn into the experiences of systems described as *persons*, directs our attention to one of the central constraints of any theory of subjectivity, namely, addressing the incompatibility of personal and subpersonal levels of description.[5] This further aspect simultaneously confronts us with a new variant of the mind-body problem: It seems to be, in principle, impossible to describe causal links

---

5. It is one of the many achievements of Daniel Dennett to have so clearly highlighted this point in his analyses. See, for example, Dennett 1969, p. 93 *ff*.; 1978b, p. 267 *ff*.; 1987b, p. 57 *ff*. The fact that we have to predicate differing logical subjects (persons and subpersonal entities like brains or states of brains) is one of the major problems dominating the modern discussion of the mind-body problem. It has been introduced into the debate under the heading "nomological incommensurability of the mental" by authors like Donald Davidson and Jaegwon Kim and has led to numerous attempts to develop a nonreductive version of materialism. (Cf. Davidson 1970; Horgan 1983; Kim 1978, 1979, 1982, 1984, 1985; for the persisting difficulties of this project, see Kim's presidential address to the American Psychological Ascociation [reprinted in Kim 1993]; Stephan 1999; and Heil and Mele 1993.)

between events on personal and subpersonal levels of analysis and then proceed to describe these links in an ever more fine-grained manner (Davidson 1970). This new variant in turn leads to considerable complications for any naturalist analysis of conscious experience. It emerges through the fact that, from the third-person perspective, we are describing the subjective character of mental states under the aspect of information processing carried out by subpersonal modules: What is the relationship of complex information-processing events—for instance, in human brains—to simultaneously evolving phenomenal episodes, which are then, by the systems themselves, described as *their own* subjective experiences when using external codes of representation? How was it possible for this sense of personal-level ownership to appear? How can we adequately conceive of representational states in the brain as being, at the same time, object-directed and subject-related? How can there be subpersonal and personal states at the same time?

The explosive growth of knowledge in the neuro- and cognitive sciences has made it very obvious that the occurrence as well as the content of phenomenal episodes is, in a very strong way, determined by properties of the information flow in the human brain. Cognitive neuropsychology, in particular, has demonstrated that there is not only a strong correlation but also a strong bottom-up dependence between the neural and informational properties of the brain and the structure and specific contents of conscious experience (see Metzinger 2000a). This is one of the reasons why it is promising to not only analyze mental states in general with the help of conceptual tools developed on a level of description that looks at objects with psychological properties as information-processing systems but also at the additional bundle of problematic properties possessed by such states that are frequently alluded to by key philosophical concepts like "experience," "perspectivalness," and "phenomenal content." The central category on this theoretical level today is no doubt formed by the concept of "representation." In our time, "representation" has, through its semantic coupling with the concept of information, been transposed to the domain of mathematical precision and subsequently achieved empirical anchorage. This development has made it an interesting tool for naturalistic analyses of cognitive phenomena in general, but more and more for the investigation of *phenomenal* states as well. In artificial intelligence research, in cognitive science, and in many neuroscientific subdisciplines, the concept of representation today plays a central role in theory formation. One must not, however, overlook the fact that this development has led to a semantic inflation of the term, which is more than problematic.[6] Also, we must not ignore the fact of "information," the very concept which has made this development toward bridging the gap between the natural sciences and the humanities possible in the first place, being by far the younger category

---

6. Useful conceptual clarifications and references with regard to different theories of mental representation can be found in S. E. Palmer 1978; see also Cummins 1989, Stich, 1992; von Eckardt 1993.

of both.[7] "Representation" is a traditional topos of Occidental philosophy. And a look at the many centuries over which this concept evolved can prevent many reinventions of the wheel and theoretical cul-de-sacs.

At the end of the twentieth century in particular, the concept of representation migrated out of philosophy and came to be used in a number of, frequently very young, disciplines. In itself, this is a positive development. However, it has also caused the semantic inflation just mentioned. In order to escape the vagueness and the lack of precision that can be found in many aspects of the current debate, we have to first take a look at the logical structure of the representational relation itself. This is important if we are to arrive at a consistent working concept of the epistemic and phenomenal processes in which we are interested. The primary goal of the following considerations consists in generating a clear and maximally simple set of conceptual instruments, with the help of which subjective experience—that is, the dynamics of exclusively *phenomenal* representational processes— can step by step and with increasing precision be described as a special case of *mental* representation. After this has been achieved, I offer some ideas about how the concrete structures, to which our conceptual instruments refer, could look.

The concept of "mental representation" can be analyzed as a three-place relationship between representanda and representata with regard to an individual system: Representation is a process which achieves the internal depiction of a representandum by generating an internal state, which functions as a representatum (Herrmann 1988). The representandum is the *object* of representation. The representatum is the concrete internal *state* carrying information related to this object. Representation is the *process* by which the system as a whole generates this state. Because of the representatum, the vehicle of representation, being a physical part of the respective system, this system continuously changes itself in the course of the process of internal representation; it generates new physical properties within itself in order to track or grasp properties of the world, attempting to "contain" these properties in Brentano's original sense. Of course, this is already the place where we have to apply a first caveat: If we presuppose an externalist theory of meaning and the first insights of dynamicist cognitive science (see Smith and Thelen 1993; Thelen and Smith 1994; Kelso 1995; Port and van Gelder 1995; Clark 1997b; for reviews, see Clark

---

7. The first safely documented occurrence of the concept in the Western history of ideas can be found in Cicero, who uses *repraesentatio* predominantly in his letters and speeches and less in his philosophical writings. A Greek prototype of the Latin concept of *repraesentatio*, which could be clearly denoted, does not exist. However, it seems as if all current semantic elements of "representation" already appear in its Latin version. For the Romans *repraesentare*, in a very literal sense, meant to bring something back into the present that had previously been absent. In the early Middle Ages, the concept predominantly referred to concrete objects and actions. The semantic element of "taking the place of" has already been documented in a legal text stemming from the fourth century (Podlech 1984, p. 510*ff.*). For an excellent description of the long and detailed history of the concept of representation, see Scheerer 1990a,b; Scholz 1991b; see also Metzinger 1993, p. 49*f.*, 5n.

1997a, 1999; and Beer 2000; Thompson and Varela 2001), then the physical representatum, the actual "vehicle" of representation, does not necessarily have its boundaries at our
skin. For instance, perceptual representational processes can then be conceived of as highly
complex dynamical interactions within a sensorimotor loop activated by the system and
sustained for a certain time. In other words, we are systems which generate the intentional
content of their overall representational state by pulsating into their causal interaction
space by, as it were, transgressing their physical boundaries and, in doing so, extracting
information from the environment. We could conceptually analyze this situation as the
activation of a new system state functioning as a representatum by being a *functionally*
internal event (because it rests on a transient change in the functional properties of the
system), but which has to utilize resources that are *physically* external for their concrete
realization. The direction in which this process is being optimized points toward a functional optimization of behavioral patterns and not necessarily toward the perfectioning of
a structure-preserving kind of representation. From a theoretical third-person perspective,
however, we can best understand the *success* of this process by describing it as a representational process that was optimized under an evolutionary development and by making
the background assumption of realism. Let us now look at the first simple conceptual
instrument in our tool kit (box 2.1).

Let me now offer two explanatory comments and a number of remarks clarifying the
defining characteristics with regard to this first concept. The first comment: Because
conceptually "phenomenality" is a very problematic property of the results of internal

Box 2.1

Mental Representation: Rep$_M$ (S, X, Y)

· S is an individual information-processing system.

· Y is an aspect of the current state of the world.

· X represents Y *for* S.

· X is a functionally internal system state.

· The intentional content of X can become available for introspective attention. It possesses
the potential of itself becoming the representandum of *subsymbolic* higher-order representational processes.

· The intentional content of X can become available for cognitive reference. It can in turn
become the representandum of *symbolic* higher-order representational processes.

· The intentional content of X can become globally available for the selective control of
action.

information processing, which, however, will have to be at the heart of any naturalist theory of subjective experience, it is very important to first of all clearly separate *processes* and *results* on the analytical level. The reason we have to do this is to prevent certain equivocations and phenomenological fallacies. As a matter of fact, large portions of the current discussion suffer from the fact that a clear distinction between "representation" and "representatum" is often not made. A representatum is a theoretical fiction, a *time slice* of an ongoing representational process, viewed under the aspect of its content. What does this mean?

As long as we choose to operate on the representational level of description, it is not the basic neural process as such that is mental or that becomes the content of consciousness, it is a specific subset of likely more abstract properties of specific internal activation states, neurally realized "data structures," which are generated by this process. The phenomenal content, the experiential character of these activation states, is generated by a certain subset of the functional and computational properties of the underlying physiological dynamics. Phenomenology supervenes on internally realized functional properties. If you now look at the book in your hands, you are not aware of the highly complex *neural* process in your visual cortex, but of the content of a phenomenal mental model (for the concept of a phenomenal mental model, see section 3.3 in chapter 3), which is first of all generated by this process within you. If, at the same time, you introspectively observe the mental states evoked in you by reading this—maybe boredom, emotional resistance, or sudden interest—then the contents of your consciousness are mental representata and not the neural process of construction itself. There is a content-vehicle distinction. In short, if we talk about the contents of subjective experience, we do not talk about the underlying process *under a neuroscientific description.* What we talk about are phenomenal "content properties," abstract features of concrete states in the head. At least under a classic conception of representation there is a difference between vehicle properties and content properties.

A second aspect is important. In doing this, we almost always forget about or abstract from the temporal dynamics of this process and treat individual time slices *as objects*—particularly if their content properties show some invariance over time. I call this the "error of phenomenological reification." There exists a corresponding and notorious grammatical mistake inherent to folk psychology, which, as a *logical* error, possesses a long philosophical tradition. In analytical philosophy of mind, it is known as the "phenomenological fallacy."[8] However, one has to differentiate between two levels on which this unnoticed

---

8. Cf. an early formulation by Place 1956, section V: "This logical mistake, which I shall refer to as the 'phenomenological fallacy,' is the mistake of supposing that when the subject describes his experience, when he describes how things look sound, smell, taste or feel to him, he is describing the literal properties of objects and

transition from a mental process to an individual, from an innocent sequence of events to an indivisible mental object, can take place. The first level of representation is constituted by *linguistic* reference to phenomenal states. The second level of representation is constituted by phenomenal experience *itself*. The second can occur without the first, and this fact has frequently been overlooked. My thesis is that there is an intimate connection between those two levels of representation and that philosophy of mind should not confine itself to an investigation of the first level of representation alone. Why? The grammatical mistake inherent to the descriptions of folk psychology is ultimately rooted in the functional architecture of our nervous system; the logical structure of linguistic reference to mental states is intimately connected with the deep representational structure of our phenomenal space. What do I mean by saying this?

Phenomenality is a property of a certain class of mental representata. Among other features, this class of representata is characterized by the fact that it is being activated within a certain time window (see, e.g., Metzinger 1995b, the references given there and section 3.2.2 of chapter 3). This time window always is larger than that of the underlying neuronal processes, which, for instance, leads to the activation of a coherent phenomenal object (e.g., the perceived book in your hands). In this elementary process of object formation, as many empirical data show, a large portion of the fundamental processuality on the physical level is being, as it were, "swallowed up" by the system. In other words, what you subjectively experience as an integrated object possessing a transtemporal identity (e.g., the book you are holding in your hand) is being constituted by an ongoing process, which constitutes a stable, coherent content and, in doing so, systematically deletes its own temporality. The illusion of substantiality arises only from the first-person perspective. It is the persistent activity of an *object emulator*, which leads to the phenomenal experience of a robust object. More about this later (for further details and references, see Metzinger 1995b; Singer 2000).

It is important to note how on a second level the way we refer to phenomenal contents in public language once again deletes the underlying dynamics of information processing. If we speak of *a* "content of consciousness" or *a* content of *a single* phenomenal "representation," we reify the experiential content of a continuous representational process. In this way the process becomes an object; we automatically generate a phenomenal individual and are in danger of repeating the classic phenomenological fallacy. This fallacy consists in the unjustified use of an existential quantifier within a psychological operator: If I look into a red flash, close my eyes, and then experience a green afterimage, this does not mean that a nonphysical object possessing the property of "greenness" has

---

events on a peculiar sort of internal cinema or television screen, usually referred to in the modern psychological literature as the 'phenomenal field'."

emerged. If one talks like this, one very soon will not be able to understand what the relationship between such phenomenal individuals and physical individuals could have been in the first place. The only thing we can legitimately say is that we are currently in a state which *under normal conditions* is being triggered by the visual presence of objects, which in such standard situations we describe as "green." As a matter of fact, such descriptions do not refer to a phenomenal individual, but only to an introspectively accessible time slice of the actual process of representation, that is, to a content property of this process at *t*. The physical carrier of this content marked out by a temporal indicator is what I will henceforth refer to as the "representatum." So much for my second preliminary comment.

Let us now proceed by clarifying the concept of "mental representation" and let us first turn to those relata which fix the intentional content of mental representations: those facts in the world which function as representanda in our ternary relation. Representanda are the *objects* of representation. Representanda can be external facts like the presence of a natural enemy, a source of food, or a sexual partner, but also symbols, arguments, or theories about the subjectivity of mental states. Internal facts, like our current blood sugar level, the shape of our hormonal landscape, or the existence of infectious microorganisms, can also turn into representanda by modulating the activity of the central nervous system and in this way changing its internal information flow. Properties or relations too can be objects of the representational process and serve as starting points for higher cognitive operations. Such relations, for instance, could be the distance toward a certain goal state, which is also internally represented. We can also mentally represent classes, for instance, of prototypical sets of behavior producing pleasure or pain.[9] Of particular importance in the context of phenomenal experience is the fact that the system *as a whole*, with all its internal, public, and relational, properties, can also become a representandum (see chapter 6). Representanda, therefore, can be external as well as internal parts of the world, and global properties of the system play a special role in the present theoretical context. The system *S* itself, obviously, forms the first and most invariant relatum in our three-place representational relationship. By specifying *S* as an *individual* information-processing system I want to exclude more specific applications of the concept of a "representational system," for instance, to ant colonies, Chinese nations (Block 1978),

---

9. The theoretical framework of connectionism offers mathematically precise criteria for the similarity and identity of the content of internal representations within a network. If one assumes that such systems, for example, real-world neural nets, generate internal representations as activation vectors, which can be described as states within an n-dimensional vector space, then one can analyze the similarity ("the distance") between two representata as the *angle* between two activation vectors. For a philosophical naturalization of epistemology, this fact can hardly be underestimated as to its importance. About connectionist *identity criteria* for content, see also P. M. Churchland 1998, unpublished manuscript; Laakso and Cottrell 1998.

scientific communities, or intelligent stellar clouds. Again, if nothing else is explicitly stated, individual members of *Homo sapiens* always form the target class of systems.

The representandum, *Y*, is being formed by an *actual* state of the world. At this point, a particularly difficult problem arises: What, precisely, is "actuality?" Once again, we discover that one always has to presuppose a certain temporal frame of reference in order to be able to speak of a representation in "real time" at all. Without specifying this temporal framework, expressions like "representation of the system's environment in real time" or "actual state of the world" are contentless expressions. Let me explain.

Conscious angels, just like ant colonies or intelligent stellar clouds, do not belong to our intended class of explanatory targets—but for a different reason: because they possess only mental, but no physical properties. For physical individuals, absolute instantaneousness, unfortunately, presents an impossibility. Of course, all physically realized processes of information conduction and processing take time. For this reason, the information available in the nervous system in a certain, very radical sense never is *actual* information: the simple fact alone that the trans- and conduction velocities of different sensory modules differ leads to the necessity of the system defining elementary ordering thresholds and "windows of simultaneity" for itself. Within such windows of simultaneity it can, for instance, integrate visual and haptic information into a multimodal object representation— an object that we can consciously see and feel at the same time.[10] This simple insight is the first one that possesses a genuinely philosophical flavor; the "sameness" and the temporality in an expression like "at the same time" already refer to a *phenomenal* "now," to the way in which things *appear* to us. The "nowness" of the book in your hands is itself an internally constructed kind of representational content; it is not actuality *simpliciter*, but actuality *as represented*. Many empirical data show that our consciously experienced present, in a specific and unambiguous sense, is a remembered present (I return to this point at length in section 3.2.2).[11] The phenomenal now is itself a representational construct, a *virtual* presence. After one has discovered this point, one can for the first time start to grasp the fact of what it means to say that phenomenal space is a virtual space; its content is a *possible* reality.[12] This is an issue to which we shall return a number of times during the course of this book: the realism of phenomenal experience is generated by a representational process which, for each individual system and in an untranscendable way,

10. For the importance of an "ordering threshold" and a "window of simultaneity" in the generation of phenomenal time experience, see, for example, Pöppel 1978, 1988, 1994; see also Ruhnau 1995.

11. Edelman 1989, of course, first introduced this idea; see also Edelman and Tononi 2000b, chapter 9.

12. My own ideas in this respect have, for a number of years, strongly converged with those of Antti Revonsuo: Virtual reality currently is the best *technological* metaphor we possess for phenomenal consciousness. See, for instance, Revonsuo, 1995, 2000a; Metzinger 1993; and section 8.1 in chapter 8.

depicts a possibility as a reality. The simple fact that the actuality of the phenomenal "now" is a virtual form of actuality also possesses relevance in analyzing a particularly interesting, higher-order phenomenological property, the property of you as a subject being consciously *present* within a multimodal scene or a world. I return therefore to the concept of virtual representation in chapters 6 (sections 6.2.2 and 6.5.2) and 8. At this point the following comment will suffice: Mental representation is a process, whose function *for* the system consists in representing actual physical reality within a certain, narrowly defined temporal framework and with a sufficient degree of functionally adequate precision. In short, no such thing as absolute actuality exists on the level of real-world information flow in the brain, but possibly there exist compensatory mechanisms on the level of the temporal *content* activated through this process (for an interesting empirical example, see Nijhawan and Khurana 2000). If we say that the representandum, Y, is formed by an *actual* state of the world, we are never talking about absolute actuality or temporal immediacy in a strictly physical sense but about a frame of reference that proved to be adaptive for certain organisms operating under the selective pressure of a highly specific biological environment.

What does it mean if we say that a state described as a representational state fulfills a function *for* a system? In the definition of the representational relationship Rep$_M$, which I have just offered, representata have been specified by an additional *teleological* criterion: an internal state X represents a part of the world Y *for* a system S. This means that the respective physical state within the system only possesses its representational content in the context of the history, the goals, and the behavioral possibilities of this particular system. This context, for instance, can be of a social or evolutionary nature. Mental states possess causal properties, which, in a certain group of persons or under the selective pressure of a particular biological environment, can be more or less adequate. For example, they can make successful cooperation with other human beings and purely genetic reproductive success more or less likely. It is for this reason that we can always look at mental states with representational content as instruments or as weapons. If one analyzes active mental representata as internal tools, which are currently used by certain systems in order to achieve certain goals, then one has become a teleofunctionalist or a teleorepresentationalist.[13] I do not explicitly argue for teleofunctionalism in this book, but I will make it one of my implicit background assumptions from now on.

---

13. Teleofunctionalism is the most influential current attempt to develop an answer to a number of problems which first surfaced in the context of classic machine functionalism (H. Putnam 1975; Block 1978; Block and Fodor 1972) as a strategy to integrate functional- and intentional-level explanations of actions (Beckermann 1977, 1979). William Lycan, in particular (see, e.g., Lycan 1987, chapter 5), has emphasized that the functionalistic strategy of explanation must not be restricted to a two-level functionalism, which would possess no neurobiological plausibility, because, in reality, there is a *continuity* of levels of explanation. He writes:

The explanatory principle of teleofunctionalism can easily be illustrated by considering the logical difference between artificial and biological systems of representation (see section 3.2.11). Artificial systems—as we knew them in the last century—do not possess any interests. Their internal states do not fulfill a *function for* the system itself, but only for the larger unit of the man-machine system. This is why those states do not *represent* anything in the sense that is here intended. On the other hand, one has to clearly see that today the traditional, conceptual difference between artificial and natural systems is not an exclusive and exhaustive distinction anymore. Empirical evidence can be found in recent advances of new disciplines like artificial life research or hybrid biorobotics. *Postbiotic* systems will use biomorphous architectures and sociomorphous selection mechanisms to generate nonbiological forms of intelligence. However, those forms of intelligence are then only nonbiological with regard to the form of their physical realization. One philosophically interesting question, of course, is if only intelligence, or even subjective experience, is a *medium-invariant* phenomenon in this sense of the word. Does consciousness supervene on properties which have to be individuated in a more universal teleofunctionalist manner, or only on classic biological properties as exemplified on this planet?

The introduction of teleofunctionalist constraints tries to answer a theoretical problem, which has traditionally confronted all isomorphist theories of representation. Isomorphist theories assume a form of similarity between image and object which rests on a partial conservation of *structural* features of the object in the image. The fundamental problem on the formal level for such theories consists in the fact of the representational relation as a *two-place* relation between pairs of complexes and as a simple structure-preserving projection being easy targets for certain trivialization arguments. In particular, structure-preserving isomorphisms do not uniquely mark out the representational relation we are looking for here. Introducing the system as a whole as a third relatum solves this problem by embedding the overall process in a causal-teleological context. Technically speaking, it helps to eliminate the reflexivity and the symmetry of a simple similarity relationship.[14]

"Neither living things nor even computers themselves are split into a purely 'structural'-level of biological/physiochemical description and any one 'abstract' computational level of machine/psychological description. Rather, they are all hierarchically organized at many levels, each level 'abstract' with respect to those beneath it but 'structural' or concrete as it realizes those levels above it. The 'functional'/'structural' or 'software'/'hardware' distinction is entirely relative to one's chosen level of organization" (Lycan 1990, p. 60). This insight possesses great relevance, especially in the context of the debate about connectionism, dynamicist cognitive science, and the theoretical modeling of neural nets. Teleofunctionalism, at the same time, is an attempt to sharpen the concept of "realization" used by early machine functionalism, by introducing teleonomical criteria relative to a given class of systems and thereby adding biological realism and domain-specificity. See also Dennett 1969, 1995; Millikan 1984, 1989, 1993; and Putnam 1991; additional references may be found in Lycan 1990, p. 59.
14. Oliver Scholz has pointed out all these aspects in a remarkably clear way, in particular with regard to the difficulties of traditional attempts to arrive at a clearer definition of the philosophical concept of "similarity."

It is important to note how a three-place relationship can be logically decomposed into three two-place relations. First, we might look at the relationship between system and representandum, for example, the relationship which you, as a system as a whole, have to the book in your hands, the perceptually given representandum. Let us call this the relation of *experience*: you consciously experience the book in your hands and, if you are not hallucinating, this experience relation is a *knowledge* relation at the same time. Misrepresentation is possible at any time, while the phenomenal character of your overall state (its *phenomenal* content) may stay the same. Second, we might want to look at the relationship between system and representatum. It is the relationship between the system as a whole and a subsystemic *part* of it, possessing adaptive value and functioning as an epistemic tool. This two-place relation might be the relation between you, as the system as a whole, and the particular activation pattern in your brain now determining the phenomenal content of your conscious experience of the book in your hand. Third, embedded in the overall three-place relation is the relationship between this brain state and the actual book "driving" its activity by first activating certain sensory surfaces. Embedded in the three-place relationship between system, object, and representing internal state, we find a two-place relation, holding between representandum and representatum. It is a subpersonal relation, not yet involving any reference to the system as a whole. This two-place relationship between representandum and representatum has to be an *asymmetrical* relationship. I will call all relations asymmetrical that fulfill the following three criteria: First, the possibility of an identity of image and object is excluded (irreflexivity). Second, for both relations forming the major semantic elements of the concept of "representation," namely, the relation of "*a* depicts or describes *b*" and the relation "*a* functions as a placeholder or as an internal functional substitute of *b*," it has to be true that they are not identical with their converse relations. Third, representation in this sense is an intransitive relation. Those cases we have to grasp in a conceptually precise manner, therefore, are exactly those cases in which one individual state generated by the system functions as an internal "description" and as an internal functional substitute of a part of the world—but not the other way around. In real-world physical systems representanda and representata always have to be thought of as *distinct* entities. This step is important as soon as we

---

Scholz writes: "Structural similarity—just as similarity—is a reflexive and symmetrical relation. (In addition, structural similarity is transitive.) Because this is not true of the representational relation, it cannot simply consist in an isomorphic relation . . ." (Scholz 1991a, p. 58). In my brief introduction to the concept of mental representation given in the main text, the additional teleological constraint also plays a role in setting off isomorphism theory against "trivialization arguments." "The difficulty, therefore, is not that image and object are not isomorphic, but that this feature does not yet differentiate them from other complexes. The purely formal or logical concept of isomorphy has to be strengthened by empirical constraints, if it is supposed to differentiate image/object pairs from others" (Scholz 1991a, p. 60). In short, an isomorphism can only generate mental content for an organism if it is embedded in a causal-teleological context in being *used* by this organism.

extend our concept to the special case of phenomenal *self*-representation (see section 5.2), because it avoids the logical problems of classical idealist theories of consciousness, as well as a host of nonsensical questions ubiquitous in popular debates, such as "How could consciousness ever understand itself?" or "How can a conscious self be subject and object at the same time?"

Teleofunctionalism solves this fundamental problem by transforming the two-place representational relationship into a three-place relation: if something possesses representational content simply depends on how it is being *used* by a certain system. The system as a whole becomes the third relatum, anchoring the representational relation in a causal context. Disambiguating it in this way, we can eliminate the symmetry, the reflexivity, and the transitivity of the isomorphy relationship. One then arrives at a concept of representation, which is, at the same time, attractive by being perfectly plausible from an evolutionary perspective. Teleofunctionalism, as noted above, will be my first background assumption. Undoubtedly it is very strong because it presupposes the truth of evolutionary theory as a whole and integrates the overall biological history of the representational system on our planet into the explanatory basis of phenomenal consciousness. Nevertheless, as teleofunctionalism has now proved to be one of the most successful research programs in philosophy of mind, as evolutionary theory is one of the most successful empirical theories mankind ever discovered, and as my primary goals in this book are different, I will not explicitly argue for this assumption here.

The next defining characteristic of mental representational processes is their *internality*. I have already pointed out how this claim has to be taken with great care, because in many cases the intentional content of a mental representatum has to be externalistically individuated. If it is true that many forms of content are only fixed if, for example, the physical properties of complicated sensorimotor loops are fixed, then it will be spatially external events which help to fix the mental content in question (see, e.g., Grush 1997, 1998; Clark and Chalmers 1998). On the other hand, it seems safe to say that, in terms of their content properties, mental representational states in the sense here intended are *temporarily* internal states; they exclusively represent actual states of the system's environment. They do so within a window of presence that has been functionally developed by the system itself, that is, within a temporal frame of reference that has been defined *as* the present. In this sense the content of consciously experienced mental representata is temporally internal content, not in a strictly physical, but only in a functional sense. As soon as one has grasped this point, an interesting extended hypothesis emerges: *phenomenal* processes of representation could be exactly those processes which also supervene on internally realized functional properties of the system, this time in a spatial respect. Internality could be interpreted not only as a temporal content property but as a spatial vehicle property as well. The spatial frame of reference would here be constituted by the physical boundaries of the individual organism (this is one reason why we had to exclude ant colonies as target systems). I will, for now, accept this assumption as a working hypothesis without giving any further argument. It forms my second conceptual background assumption: if all spatially internal properties (in the sense given above) of a given system are fixed, the phenomenal content of its representational state (i.e., what it "makes present") is fixed as well. In other words, what the system consciously experiences locally supervenes on its physical properties with nomological necessity. Among philosophers today, this is a widely accepted assumption. It implies that active processes of mental representation can only be internally accessed on the level of conscious experience, and this manner of access must be a very specific one. If one looks at consciousness in this way, one could, for example, say that phenomenal processing represents certain properties of simultaneously active and exclusively internal states of the system in a way that is aimed at making their intentional content globally available for attention, cognition, and flexible action control. What does it mean to say that these target states are exclusively internal? Once again, three different interpretations of "internality" have to be kept apart: physical internality, functional internality, and the phenomenal qualities of subjectively experienced "nowness" and "inwardness." Interestingly, there are three corresponding interpretations of concepts like "system-world border." At a later stage, I attempt to offer a clearer conception of the relationship between those two conceptual assumptions.

Let us briefly take stock. Mental states are *internal* states in a special sense of functional internality: their intentional content—which can be constituted by facts spatially external in a physical sense—can be made globally available within an individually realized window of presence. (I explain the nature of such windows of presence in section 3.2.2.) It thereby has the potential to become transformed into *phenomenal* content. For an intentional content to be transformed in this way means for it to be put into a new context, the context of a lived present. It may be conceivable that representational content is embedded into a new temporal context by an exclusively internal mechanism, but what precisely is "global availability?" Is this second constraint one that has to be satisfied either by the vehicles or rather by the contents of conscious experience?

This question leads us back to our starting point, to the core problem: What are the defining characteristics marking out a subset of active representata in our brain's *mental* states as possessing the disposition of being transformed into *subjective* experiences? On what levels of description are they to be found? What we are looking for is a domain-specific set of phenomenological, representational, functional, and neuroscientific constraints, which can serve to reliably mark out the class of *phenomenal* representata for human beings.

I give a set of new answers to this core question by constructing such a catalogue of constraints in the next chapter. Here, I will use only *one* of these constraints as a "default definiens," as a preliminary instrument employed *pars pro toto*—for now taking the place of the more detailed set of constraints yet to come. Please note that introducing this default-defining characteristic only serves as an illustration at this point. In chapter 3 (sections 3.2.1 and 3.2.3) we shall see how this very first example is only a restricted version of a much more comprehensive multilevel constraint. The reason for choosing this particular example as a single representative for a whole set of possible constraints to be imposed on the initial concept of mental representation is very simple: it is highly intuitive, and it has been already introduced to the current debate. The particular notion I am referring to was first developed by Bernard Baars (1988, 1997) and David Chalmers (1997): *global availability*.

The concept of global availability is an interesting example of a first possible criterion by which we can demarcate phenomenal information on the functional level of description. It will, however, be necessary to further differentiate this criterion right at the beginning. As the case studies to be presented in chapters 4 and 7 illustrate, neuropsychological data make such a conceptual differentiation necessary. The idea runs as follows. Phenomenally represented information is exactly that subset of currently active information in the system which possesses one or more of the following three dispositional properties:

• availability for *guided attention* (i.e., availability for introspection; for nonconceptual mental metarepresentation);

• availability for *cognitive processing* (i.e., availability for thought; i.e., for mental concept formation);

• availability for *behavioral control* (i.e., availability for motor selection; volitional availability).

It must be noted that this differentiation, although adequate for the present purpose, is somewhat of a crude fiction from an empirical point of view. For instance, there is more than one kind of attention (e.g., deliberately initiated, focused high-level attention, and automatic low-level attention). There are certainly different styles of thought, some more pictorial, some more abstract, and the *behavioral* control exerted by a (nevertheless conscious) animal may turn out to be something entirely different from rationally guided human *action* control. In particular, as we shall see, there are a number of atypical situations in which less than three of these subconstraints are satisfied, but in which phenomenal experience is, arguably, still present. Let us first look at what is likely to be the most fundamental and almost invariable characteristic of all conscious representations.

2.2.1   Introspectability as Attentional Availability

Mental states are all those states which can in principle become available for introspection. All states that are available, and particularly those that are *actually* being introspected, are phenomenal states. This means that they can become objects of a voluntarily initiated and goal-directed process of internal attention (see also section 6.4.3). Mental states possess a certain functional property: they are attentionally accessible. Another way of putting this is by saying that mental states are *introspectively penetrable*. "Voluntarily" at this stage only means that the process of introspection is itself typically being accompanied by a particular higher-order type of phenomenal content, namely, a subjectively experienced quality of agency (see sections 6.4.3, 6.4.4, and 6.4.5). This quality is what German philosopher, psychiatrist, and theologian Karl Jaspers called *Vollzugsbewusstsein*, "executive" consciousness, the untranscendable experience of the fact that the initiation, the directedness, and the constant sustaining of attention is an inner kind of *action*, an activity that is steered by the phenomenal subject itself. However, internal attention must not be interpreted as the activity of a homunculus directing the beam of a flashlight consisting of his already existing consciousness toward different internal objects and thereby transforming them into phenomenal individuals (cf. Lycan 1987; chapter 8). Rather, introspection is a subpersonal process of representational resource allocation taking place in some information-processing systems. It is a special variant of exactly the same processes that forms the topic of our current concept formation: introspection is the internal[15] representation of active mental representata. Introspection is metarepresentation. Obviously, the interesting class of representata are marked out by being operated on by a subsymbolic, nonconceptual form of metarepresentation, which turns them into the content of higher-order representata. At this stage, "subsymbolic," for introspective processing means "using a nonlinguistic format" and "not approximating syntacticity." A more precise demarcation of this class is an empirical matter, about which hope for epistemic progress in the near future is justified. Those functional properties which transform some internal representata into potential representanda of global mental representational processes, and thereby into introspectable states, it can be safely assumed, will be described in a more precise manner by future computational neuroscientists. It may be some time before we discover the actual algorithm, but let me give an example of a simple, coarse-grained functional analysis, making it possible to research the neural correlates of introspection.

---

15. It only is an internal representational process (but not a *mental* representational process), because even in standard situations it does not possess the potential to become a content of consciousness itself, for example, through a higher-order process of mental representation. Outside of the information-processing approach, related issues are discussed by David Rosenthal in his higher-order thought theory (cf., e.g., Rosenthal, 1986, 2003), internally by Ray Jackendoff in his "intermediate-level theory" of consciousness; see Jackendoff 1987.

Attention is a process that episodically increases the capacity for information processing in a certain partition of representational space. Functionally speaking, attention is internal *resource allocation*. Attention, as it were, is a representational type of zooming in, serving for a local elevation of resolution and richness in detail within an overall representation. If this is true, phenomenal representata are those structures which, independently of their causal history, that is, independently if they are primarily transporting visual, auditory, or cognitive content, are currently making the information they represent *available* for operations of this type.

Availability for introspection in this sense is a characteristic feature of conscious information processing and it reappears on the phenomenological level of description. Sometimes, for purely pragmatic reasons, we are interested in endowing internal states with precisely this property. Many forms of psychotherapy attempt to transform pathological mental structures into introspectable states by a variety of different methods. They do so because they work under a very strong assumption, which is usually not justified in any theoretical or argumentative way. This assumption amounts to the idea that pathological structures can, simply by gaining the property of introspective availability, be dissolved, transformed, or influenced in their undesirable effects on the subjective experience of the patient by a magical and never-explained kind of "top-down causation." However, theoretically naive as many such approaches are, there may be more than a grain of truth in the overall idea; by introspectively attending to "conflict-generating" (i.e., functionally incoherent) parts of one's internal self-representation, additional processing resources are automatically allocated to this part and may thereby support a positive (i.e., integrative) development. We all use different variants of introspection in nontherapeutic, everyday situations: when trying to enjoy our sexual arousal, when concentrating, when trying to remember something important, when trying to find out what it *really* is that we desire, or, simply, when we are asked how we are today. Furthermore, there are passive, not goal- but process-oriented types of introspection like daydreaming, or different types of meditation. The interesting feature of this subclass of states is that it lacks the executive consciousness mentioned above. The wandering or heightening of attention in these phenomenological state classes seems to take place in a spontaneous manner, not involving subjective agency. There is no *necessary* connection between personal-level agency and introspection in terms of low-level attention. What is common to all the states of phenomenal consciousness just mentioned is the fact that the representational content of already active mental states has been turned into the object of inner attention.[16] The

16. There are forms of phenomenal experience—for instance, the states of infants, dreamers, or certain types of intoxication—in which the criterion of "attentional availability" is, in principle, not fulfilled, because something like controllable attention does not exist in these states. However, please recall that, at this level of our

introspective availability of these states is being utilized in order to episodically move them into the focus of subjective experience. Phenomenal experience possesses a variable focus; by moving this focus, the amount of extractable information can episodically be maximized (see also section 6.5).

Now we can already start to see how availability for introspective attention marks out conscious processing: Representational content active in our brains but principally unavailable for attention will never be *conscious* content. Before we can proceed to take a closer look at the second and third subconstraints—availability for cognition and availability for behavioral control—we need to take a quick detour. The problem is this: What does it actually mean to speak about *intro*spection? Introspection seems to be a necessary phenomenological constraint in understanding how internal system states can become mental states and in trying to develop a conceptual analysis of this process. However, phenomenology is not enough for a modern theory of mind. Phenomenological "introspective availability under standard conditions" does not supply us with a satisfactory working concept of the mental, because it cannot fixate the sufficient conditions for its application. We all know conscious contents—namely, phenomenal models of distal objects in our environment (i.e., active data structures coded *as* external objects, the "object emulators" mentioned above)—that, under standard conditions, we never experience as introspectively available. Recent progress in cognitive neuroscience, however, has made it more than a rational assumption that these types of phenomenal contents as well are fully determined by internal properties of the brain: all of them will obviously possess a *minimally sufficient neural correlate*, on which they supervene (Chalmers 2000). Many types of hallucinations, agnosia, and neglect clearly demonstrate how narrow and how strict correlations between neural and phenomenal states actually are, and how strong their determination "from below" (see the relevant sections in chapters 4 and 7; see also Metzinger 2000a). These data are, as such, independent of any theoretical position one might take toward the mind-body problem in general. For instance, there are perceptual experiences of external objects, the subjective character of which we would never describe as "mental" or "introspective" on the level of our prereflexive subjective experience. However, scientific research shows that even those states can, under differing conditions, become experienced *as* mental, inner, or introspectively available states.[17] This leads to a simple, but important conclusion: the process of mental representation, in many cases, generates phenomenal states which are being experienced as mental from the first-person perspective and

---

investigation, the intended class of systems is only formed by adult human beings in nonpathological waking states. This is the reason why I do not yet offer an answer to the question of whether attentional availability really constitutes a *necessary* condition in the ascription of phenomenal states at this point. See also section 6.4.3.

17. This can, for instance, be the case in schizophrenia, mania, or during religious experiences. See chapter 7 for some related case studies.

which are experienced as potential objects of introspection and *inward* attention. It also generates representata that are being experienced as nonmental and as external states. The kind of attention we direct toward those states is then described as *external* attention, phenomenologically as well on the level of folk psychology. So mental representation, as a process analyzed from a cognitive science third-person perspective, does not exclusively lead to mental states, which are being *experienced* as subjective or internal on the phenomenal level of representation.[18] The internality as well as the externality of attentional objects seems to be a kind of representational content itself. One of the main interests of this work consists in developing an understanding of what it means that information processing in the central nervous system phenomenally represents some internal states *as* internal, as bodily or mental states, whereas it does not do so for others.[19]

Our ontological working hypothesis says that the phenomenal model of reality exclusively supervenes on internal system properties. Therefore, we now have to separate two different meanings of "introspection" and "subjective." The ambiguities to which I have just pointed are generated by the fact that phenomenal introspection, as well as phenomenal extrospection, is, on the level of functional analysis, a type of representation of the content properties of currently active internal states. In both cases, their content emerges because the system accesses an already active internal representation a second time and thereby makes it globally available for attention, cognition, and control of action.

It will be helpful to distinguish four different notions of introspection, as there are two types of internal metarepresentation, a subsymbolic, attentional kind (which only "highlights" its object, but does not form a mental concept), and a cognitive type (which forms or applies an enduring mental "category" or prototype of its object).

18. This thought expresses one of the many possibilities in which a modern "informationalistic" theory of mind can integrate and conserve the essential insights of classic idealistic, as well as materialistic, philosophies of consciousness. In a certain respect, everything (*as phenomenally represented* in this way) is "within consciousness"—"the objective" as well as the "resistance of the world." However, at the same time, the underlying functions of information processing are exclusively realized by internal physical states.

19. Our illusion of the *substantiality*, the object character, or "thingness" of perceptual objects emerging on the level of subjective consciousness can, under the information-processing approach, be explained by the assumption that for certain sets of data the brain stops iterating its basic representational activity after the first mental representational step. The deeper theoretical problem in the background is that *iterative* processes—like recursive mental representation or self-modeling (see chapters 5, 6, and 7)—possess an infinite logical structure, which can in principle not be realized by finite physical systems. As we will see in chapter 3, biologically successful representata must never lead a system operating with limited neurocomputational resources into infinite regressions, endless internal loops, and so on, if they do not want to endanger the survival of the system. One possible solution is that the brain has developed a functional architecture which stops iterative but computationally necessary processes like recurrent mental representation and self-modeling by *object formations*. We find formal analogies for such phenomena in logic (Blau 1986) and in the differentiation between object and metalanguage.

1. *Introspection₁* ("external attention"). Introspection₁ is subsymbolic metarepresentation operating on a preexisting, coherent world-model. This type of introspection is a phenomenal process of attentionally representing certain aspects of an internal system state, the intentional content of which is constituted by a part of the world depicted *as external*. The accompanying phenomenology is what we ordinarily describe as attention or the subjective experience of attending to some object in our environment. Introspection₁ corresponds to the *folk-psychological* notion of attention.

2. *Introspection₂* ("consciously experienced cognitive reference"). This second concept refers to a conceptual (or quasi-conceptual) form of metarepresentation, operating on a preexisting, coherent model of the world. This kind of introspection is brought about by a process of phenomenally representing cognitive reference to certain aspects of an internal system state, the intentional content of which is constituted by a part of the world depicted *as external*.

Phenomenologically, this class of state is constituted by all experiences of attending to an object in our environment, while simultaneously *recognizing* it or forming a new mental concept of it; it is the conscious experience of cognitive reference. A good example is what Fred Dretske (1969) called "epistemic seeing."

3. *Introspection₃* ("inward attention" and "inner perception"). This is a subsymbolic metarepresentation operating on a preexisting, coherent *self*-model (for the notion of a "self-model" see Metzinger 1993/1999, 2000c). This type of introspective experience is generated by processes of phenomenal representation, which direct attention toward certain aspects of an internal system state, the intentional content of which is being constituted by a part of the world depicted *as internal*.

The phenomenology of this class of states is what in everyday life we call "inward-directed attention." On the level of philosophical theory it is this kind of phenomenally experienced introspection that underlies classical theories of *inner perception*, for example, in John Locke or Franz Brentano (see Güzeldere 1995 for a recent critical discussion).

4. *Introspection₄* ("consciously experienced cognitive self-reference"). This type of introspection is a conceptual (or quasi-conceptual) kind of metarepresentation, again operating on a preexisting, coherent self-model. Phenomenal representational processes of this type generate conceptual forms of self-knowledge, by directing cognitive processes toward certain aspects of internal system states, the intentional content of which is being constituted by a part of the world depicted *as internal*.

The general phenomenology associated with this type of representational activity includes all situations in which we consciously think about ourselves *as* ourselves (i.e., when we think what some philosophers call I*-thoughts; for an example see Baker 1998, and section 6.4.4). On a theoretical level, this last type of introspective experience clearly constitutes the case in which philosophers of mind have traditionally been most interested: the phenomenon of *cognitive self-reference* as exhibited in reflexive self-consciousness.

Obviously the first two notions of introspection, respectively, introspective availability, are rather trivial, because they define the internality of potential objects of introspection entirely by means of a simple physical concept of internality. In the present context, internality *as phenomenally experienced* is of greater relevance. We now have a clearer understanding of what it means to define phenomenal states as making information globally available for a system, in particular of the notion of *attentional* availability. It is interesting to note how this simple conceptual categorization already throws light on the issue of what it actually means to say that conscious experience is a *subjective* process.

What does it mean to say that conscious experience is *subjective* experience? It is interesting to note how the step just taken helps us to keep apart a number of possible answers to the question of what actually constitutes the subjectivity of subjective experience. Let us here construe subjectivity as a property not of representational content, but of information. First, there is a rather trivial understanding of subjectivity, amounting to the fact that information has been integrated into an exclusively internal model of reality, active within an individual system and, therefore, giving this particular system a kind of privileged introspective access to this information in terms of *uniquely direct causal links* between this information and higher-order attentional or cognitive processes operating on it. Call this "functional subjectivity."

A much more relevant notion is "phenomenal subjectivity." Phenomenally subjective information has the property of being integrated into the system's current conscious self-representation; therefore, it contributes to the content of its *self-consciousness*. Of course, phenomenally subjective information creates new functional properties as well, for instance, by making system-related information available to a whole range of processes, not only for attention but also for motor control or autobiographical memory. In any case, introspection$_3$ and introspection$_4$ are those representational processes making information *phenomenally* subjective (for a more detailed analysis, see sections 3.2.6 and 6.5).

Given the distinctions introduced above, one can easily see that there is a third interpretation of the subjectivity of conscious experience, flowing naturally from what has just been said. This is *epistemic* subjectivity. Corresponding to the different functional modes of presentation, in which information can be available within an individual system, there are types of epistemic access, types of knowledge about world and self accompanying the process of conscious experience. For instance, information can be subjective by contributing to nonconceptual or to conceptual knowledge. In the first case we have epistemic access generated by introspection$_1$ and introspection$_3$: functional and phenomenal ways in which information is *attentionally* available through the process of subsymbolic resource allocation described above. *Cognitive* availability seems to generate a much stronger kind of knowledge. Under the third, epistemological reading, subjectivity only is a property of precisely that subset of information within the system which directly contributes to consciously experienced processes of conceptual reference and self-reference, corresponding to the functional and the phenomenal processes of introspection$_2$ and introspection$_4$. Only information that is in principle categorizable is cognitively available information (see section 2.4.4). After this detour, let us now return to our analysis of the concept of "global availability." In the way I am developing this concept, it possesses two additional semantic elements.

2.2.2 Availability for Cognitive Processing

I can only deliberately think about those things I also consciously experience. Only phenomenally represented information can become the object of cognitive reference, thereby entering into thought processes which have been voluntarily initiated. Let us call this the "principle of phenomenal reference" from now on. The most interesting fact in this context is that the second constraint has only a limited range of application: there exists a fundamental level of sensory consciousness, on which cognitive reference inevitably fails. For most of the most simple contents of sensory consciousness (e.g., for the most subtle nuances within subjective color experiences), it is true that, because of a limitation of our perceptual memory, we are not able to construct a *conceptual* form of knowledge with regard to their content. The reason for this consists in introspection not supplying us with transtemporal and, a fortiori, with logical identity criteria for these states. Nevertheless, those strictly stimulus-correlated forms of simple phenomenal content are globally available for external actions founded on discriminatory achievements (like pointing movements) and for noncognitive forms of mental representation (like focused attention). In sections 2.4.1 though 2.4.4, I take a closer look at this relationship. I introduce a new concept in an attempt to do justice to the situation just mentioned. This concept will be called "phenomenal presentation" (see also Metzinger 1997).

Phenomenally *re*presented information, however, can be categorized and, in principle, be memorized: it is *recognizable* information, which can be classified and saved. The general trend of empirical research has, for a long period of time now, pointed toward the fact that, as cognitive subjects, we are not carrying out anything even remotely resembling rule-based symbol processing in the narrow sense of employing a mental language of thought (Fodor 1975). However, one can still say the following: In some forms of cognitive operation, we *approximate* syntactically structured forms of mental representation so successfully that it is possible to describe us as cognitive agents in the sense of the classic approach. We are beings capable of mentally simulating logical operations to a sufficient degree of precision. Obviously, most forms of thought are much more of a pictorial and sensory, perception-emulating, movement-emulating, and sensorimotor loop–emulating character than of a strictly logical nature. Of course, the underlying dynamics of cognition is of a fundamentally subsymbolic nature. Still, our first general criterion for the demarcation of mental and phenomenal representations holds: phenomenal information (with the exceptions to be explained at the end of this chapter) is precisely information that enables thought processes that are deliberately initiated thought processes. The principle of phenomenal reference states that self-initiated, explicit cognition always operates on the content of phenomenal representata only. In daydreaming or while freely associating, conscious thoughts may be triggered by unconscious information causally active in the system. The same is true of low-level attention. Thinking in the more narrow and philosophically interesting sense, however, underlies what could also be termed the "phenomenal boundary principle." This principle is a relative of the principle of phenomenal reference, as applied to *cognitive* reference: We can only form conscious thoughts about something that has been an element of our phenomenal model of reality before (introspection$_{2/4}$). There is an interesting application of this principle to the case of cognitive self-reference (see section 6.4.4). We are beings which, in principle, can only form thoughts about those aspects of *themselves* that in some way or another have already been available on the level of conscious experience. The notion of introspection$_4$ as introduced above is guided by this principle.

2.2.3   Availability for the Control of Action

Phenomenally represented information is characterized by exclusively enabling the initiation of a certain class of actions: *selective* actions, which are directed toward the content of this information. Actions, by being highly selective and being accompanied by the phenomenal experience of agency, are a particularly flexible and quickly adaptable form of behavior. At this point, it may be helpful to take a first look at a concrete example.

A blindsight patient, suffering from life-threatening thirst while unconsciously perceiving a glass of water within his scotoma, that is, within his experiential "blind spot," is not able to initiate a grasping or reaching movement directed toward the glass (for further details, see section 4.2.3). In a forced-choice situation, however, he will in very many cases correctly guess what type of object it is that he is confronted with. This means that information about the identity of the object in question is already functionally active in the system; it was first extracted on the usual path using the usual sensory organs, and under special conditions it can again be made explicit. Nevertheless, this information is not phenomenally represented and, therefore, is not available for the control of action. Unconscious motion perception and wavelength sensitivity are well-documented phenomena in blindsight, and it is well conceivable that a cortically blind patient might to a certain degree be able to use visual information about local object features to execute well-formed grasping movements (see section 4.2.3). But what makes such a selectively generated movement an *action*?

Actions are voluntarily guided body movements. "Voluntarily" here only means that the process of initiating an action is itself accompanied by a higher-order form of phenomenal content. Again, this is the conscious experience of agency, executive consciousness, the untranscendable experience of the fact that the initiation, the fixation of the fulfillment conditions, and the persisting pursuit of the action is an activity directed by the phenomenal subject itself. Just as in introducing the notion of "introspective availability," we again run the risk of being accused of circularity, because a higher-order form of phenomenal content remains as an unanalyzed rest. In other words, our overall project has become enriched. It now contains the following question: What precisely is phenomenal agency? At this point I will not offer an answer to the question of what functional properties within the system are correlated with the activation of this form of phenomenal content. However, we return to this question in section 6.4.5.

One thing that can be safely said at the present stage is that "availability for control of action" obviously has a lot to do with sensorimotor integration, as well as with a flexible and intelligent decoupling of sensorimotor loops. If one assumes that every action has to be preceded by the activation of certain "motoric" representata, then phenomenal representata are those which enable an important form of sensorimotor integration: The information made internally available by phenomenal representata is that kind of information which can be *directly* fed into the activation mechanism for motor representata.

Basic actions are always physical actions, bodily motions, which require an adequate internal representation of the body. For this reason phenomenal information must be functionally characterized by the fact that it can be directly fed and integrated into a dynamical representation of one's own body as a currently acting system, as an agent, in a particularly easy and effective way. This agent, however, is an *autonomous* agent: willed actions (within certain limits) enable the system to perform a *veto*. In principle, they can be interrupted anytime. This fast and flexible possibility of decoupling motor and sensory information processing is a third functional property associated with phenomenal experience. If freedom is the opposite of functional rigidity, then it is exactly conscious experience which turns us into free agents.[20]

---

20. I am indebted to Franz Mechsner, from whom I learned a lot in mutual discussions, for this particular thought. The core idea is, in discussions of freedom of the will, to escape from the dilemma of having to choose between a strong deterministic thesis and a strong, but empirically implausible thesis of the causal indeterminacy of mental states by moving from a modular, subpersonal level of analysis to the global, personal level of description while simultaneously introducing the notion of "degrees of flexibility." We are now not discussing the causally

Let us now briefly return to our example of the thirsty blindsight patient. He is not a free agent. With regard to a certain element of reality—the glass of water in front of him that could save his life—he is not capable of initiating, correcting, or terminating a grasping movement. His domain of flexible interaction has shrunken. Although the relevant information has already been extracted from the environment by the early stages of his sensory processing mechanisms, he is functionally rigid with respect to this information, as if he were a "null Turing machine" consistently generating zero output. Only consciously experienced information is available for the fast and flexible control of action. Therefore, in developing conceptual constraints for the notions of exclusively internal representation, mental representation, and phenomenal representation, "availability for action control" is a third important example.

In conscious memory or future planning, the object of a mental representation can be available for attention and cognition, but not for selective action. In the conscious perception of subtle shades of color, information may be internally represented in a way that makes it available for attention and fine-grained discriminative actions, but not for concept formation and cognitive processing. Attentional availability, however, seems to be the most basic component of global availability; there seem to be no situations in which we can choose to cognitively process and behaviorally respond to information that is not, in principle, available for attention at the same time. I return to this issue in chapter 3.

The exceptions mentioned above demonstrate how rich and complex a domain phenomenal experience is. It is of maximal importance to do phenomenological justice to this fact by taking into account exceptional cases or impoverished versions like the two examples briefly mentioned above as we go along, continuously enriching our concept of consciousness. A whole series of additional constraints are presented in the chapter 3; and further investigations of exceptional cases in chapters 4 and 7 will help to determine how wide the scope of such constraints actually is. However, it must be noted that under standard conditions phenomenal representations are interestingly marked out by the feature of *simultaneously* making their contents globally available for attention, cognition, and action control.

Now, after having used this very first and slightly differentiated version of the global availability constraint, originally introduced by Baars and Chalmers, plus the

---

determined nature of individual subsystemic states anymore, but the impressive degree of flexibility exhibited *by the system as a whole*. I believe it would be interesting and rewarding to spell out this notion further, in terms of behavioral, attentional, and cognitive flexibility, with the general philosophical intuition guiding the investigation being what I would term the "principle of phenomenal flexibility": *the more conscious you are*, the more flexible you are as an agent, as an attentional subject, and as a thinker. I will not pursue this line of thought here (but see sections 6.4.5 and 7.2.3.3 in particular). For a neurophilosophical introduction to problems of free will, see Walter 2001.

presentationality constraint based on the notion of a "virtual window of presence" defining certain information as the *Now* of the organism, we are for the first time in a position to offer a very rudimentary and simple concept of *phenomenal* representation (box 2.2).

Utilizing the distinctions now introduced, we can further distinguish between three different kinds of representation. *Internal* representations are isomorphy-preserving structures in the brain which, although usually possessing a true teleofunctionalist analysis by fulfilling a function *for* the system as a whole, in principle, can never be elevated to the level of global availability for purely functional reasons. Such representational states are always unconscious. They possess intentional content, but no qualitative character or phenomenal content. *Mental* representations are those states possessing the dispositional property of episodically *becoming* globally available for attention, cognition, and action control in the window of presence defined by the system. Sometimes they are conscious, sometimes they are unconscious. They possess intentional content, but they are only accompanied by phenomenal character if certain additional criteria are met. *Phenomenal* representations, finally, are all those mental representations currently satisfying a yet to-be-determined set of multilevel constraints. Conscious representations, for example, are all those which are *actually* an element of the organism's short-term memory or those to which it *potentially* attends.

It is of vital importance to always keep in mind that the two additional constraints of temporal internality and global availability (in its new, differentiated version), which have now been imposed on the concept of mental representation, only function as *examples* of possible conceptual constraints on the functional level of analysis. In order to arrive at a

Box 2.2

Phenomenal Representation: Rep$_P$ (S, X, Y)

· S is an individual information-processing system.

· Y is the intentional content of an actual system state.

· X phenomenally represents Y *for* S.

· X is a physically internal system state, which has functionally been defined as temporally internal.

· The intentional content of X *is* currently introspectively$_1$ available; that is, it is disposed to become the representandum of *subsymbolic* higher-order representational processes.

· The intentional content of X *is* currently introspectively$_2$ available for cognitive reference; it can in turn become the representandum of *symbolic* higher-order representational processes.

· The intentional content of X *is* currently available for the selective control of action.

---

truly rich and informative concept of subjective experience, a whole set of additional constraints on the phenomenological, representationalist, functional, and neuroscientific levels of description will eventually have to be added. This will happen in chapter 3. Here, the purely functional properties of global availability and integration into the window of presence only function as preliminary placeholders that serve to demonstrate how the transition from *mental* representation to *phenomenal* representation can be carried out. Please note how this transition will be a gradual one, and not an all-or-nothing affair. The representationalist level of description for conscious systems is the decisive level of description, because it is on this conceptual niveau that the integration of first-person and third-person insights can and must be achieved. Much work remains to be done. In particular, representation as so far described is not the basic, most fundamental phenomenon underlying conscious experience. For this reason, our initial concept will have to be developed further in two different directions in the following two sections.

2.3   From Mental to Phenomenal Simulation: The Generation of Virtual Experiential Worlds through Dreaming, Imagination, and Planning

Mental representata are instruments used by brains. These instruments are employed by biological systems to process as much information relevant to survival as fast as possible and as effectively as possible. I have analyzed the process by which they are generated as a three-place relationship between them, a system and external or internal representanda. In our own case, one immediately notices that there are many cases in which this analysis is obviously false. One of the most important characteristics of human phenomenal experience is that mental representata are frequently activated and integrated with each other in situations where those states of the world forming their content are not actual states: human brains can generate phenomenal models of *possible* worlds.[21]

Those representational processes underlying the emergence of possible phenomenal worlds are "virtual" representational processes. They generate subjective experiences, which only partially reflect the actual state of the world, typically by emulating aspects of real-life perceptual processing or motor behavior. Examples of such "as-if" states are spontaneous fantasies, inner monologues, daydreams, hallucinations, and nocturnal dreams. However, they also comprise deliberately initiated cognitive operations: the planning of possible actions, the analysis of future goal states, the voluntary "*re*presentation" of past perceptual and mental states, and so on. Obviously, this phenomenological state class does not present us with a case of mental representation, because the respective representanda

---

21. "Possible world" is used here in a nontechnical sense, to describe an ecologically valid, adaptationally relevant proper subset of nomologically possible worlds.

Box 2.3

Mental Simulation: Sim$_M$ (S, X, Y)

· S is an individual information-processing system.

· Y is a counterfactual situation, relative to the system's representational architecture.

· X simulates Y *for* S.

· X is a physically internal system state.

· The intentional content of X can become available for introspective attention. It possesses the potential of itself becoming the representandum of *subsymbolic* higher-order representational processes.

· The intentional content of X can become available for cognitive reference. It can in turn become the representandum of *symbolic* higher-order representational processes.

· The intentional content of X can become globally available for the selective control of action.

---

are only partially given as elements of the actual environment of the system, even when presupposing its own temporal frame of reference. Seemingly, the function of those states is to make information about *potential* environments of the system globally available. Frequently this also includes possible states of the system itself (see section 5.2).

The first conclusion that can be drawn from this observation is as follows: Those representata taking part in the mental operations in question are not activated by ordinary sensory input. It may be that those processes are being induced or triggered by external stimuli, but they are not stimulus-correlated processes in a strict sense. Interestingly, we frequently experience the phenomena just mentioned when the processing capacity of our brains is not particularly challenged because there are no new, difficult, or pressing practical problems to be solved (e.g., during routine activities, e.g., when we are caught in a traffic jam) or because the amount of incoming information from the environment is drastically decreasing (during resting phases, while falling asleep). There may, therefore, be a more or less nonspecific internal activation mechanism which creates the necessary boundary conditions for such states.[22] I will henceforth call all mental states coming about by a representation of counterfactual situations mental *simulations* (box 2.3).

---

22. On a global level, of course, a candidate for such an unspecific activation system is the oldest part of our brain: the formatio reticularis, the core of the brainstem. It is able to activate and desynchronize electrical cortical rhythms while severe damage and lesions in this area lead to irreversible coma. For the wider context, that is, the function of the brainstem in anchoring the phenomenal self, see Parvizi and Damasio 2001 and section 5.4.

Let me again offer a number of explanatory comments to clarify this third new concept. "Elementary" qualities of sensory awareness, like redness or painfulness in general, cannot be transferred into simulata (at the end of this chapter I introduce a third basic concept specifically for such states: the concept of "presentata").[23] The reason for this is that in their physical boundary conditions, they are bound to a constant flow of input, driving, as it were, their content—they cannot be *re*presented. It is therefore plausible to assume that they cannot be integrated into ongoing simulations, because systems like ourselves are not able to internally emulate the full flow of input that would be necessary to bring about the maximally determinate and concrete character of this special form of content. A plausible prediction following from this assumption is that in all those situations in which the general level of arousal is far above average (e. g., in the dream state or in disinhibited configurations occurring under the influence of hallucinogenic agents) so that an actual internal emulation of the full impact of external input does become possible, the border between perception and imagination will become blurred on the level of phenomenology. In other words, there are certain types of phenomenal content that are strictly stimulus-correlated, causally anchoring the organism in the present. Again, there are a number of exceptions—for instance, in so-called eidetic imagers. These people have an extremely accurate and vivid form of visual memory, being able to consciously experience eidetic images of nonexistent, but full-blown visual scenes, including full color, saturation, and brightness. Interestingly, such eidetic images can be scanned and are typically consciously experienced as being outside of the head, in the external environment (Palmer 1999, p. 593*ff.*). However, eidetic imagery is a very rare phenomenon. It is more common in children than in adults, but only 7% of children are full eidetic imagers. For them, there may not yet be a difference between imagination and perception (however, see section 3.2.7); for them, imagining a bright-red strawberry with the eyes closed may *not* make a big difference to afterward opening their eyes and looking at the strawberry on a plate in front of them— for instance, in terms of the richness, crispness, and ultimately realistic character of the sensory quality of "redness" involved. The phenomenal states of eidetic children, hallucinogen users, and dreamers provide an excellent example of the enormous richness and complexity of conscious experience. No simplistic conceptual schematism will ever be able to do justice to the complex landscape of this target domain. As we will discover many times in the course of this book, for every rule at least one exception exists.

Nonsensory aspects of the content of mental representata can also be activated in nonstandard stimulus situations and be employed in mental operations: they lose their

---

23. Exceptions are formed by all those situations in which the system is confronted with an *internal* stimulus of sufficient strength, for instance, in dreams or during hallucinations. See sections 4.2.4 and 4.2.5.

original intentional content,[24] but retain a large part of their phenomenal character and thereby become mental *simulata*. If this is correct, then imaginary representata—for instance, pictorial mental imagery—have to lack the qualitative "signal aspect," which characterizes presentata. This signal aspect is exactly that component of the content of mental representata which is strictly stimulus-correlated: if one subtracts this aspect, then one gets exactly the information that is also available for the system in an *offline* situation. As a matter of phenomenological fact, for most of us deliberately imagined pain is not truly painful and imagined strawberries are not truly red.[25] They are less determinate, greatly impoverished versions of nociception and vision. Exceptions are found in persons who are able to internally emulate a sensory stimulation to its full extent; for instance, some people are eidetics by birth or have trained their brain by visualization exercises. From a phenomenological point of view, it is interesting to note that in deliberately initiated mental simulations, the higher-order phenomenal qualities of "immediacy," "givenness," and "instantaneousness" are generated to a much weaker degree. In particular, the fact *that* they are simulations is available to the subject of experience. We return to this issue in section 3.2.7.

Organisms unable to recognize simulata as such and taking them to be representata (or *presentata*) dream or hallucinate. As a matter of fact, many of the relevant types of mental states are frequently caused by an unspecific disinhibition of certain brain regions, calling into existence strong internal sources of signals. It seems that in such situations the human brain is not capable of representing the causal history of those stimuli *as internal*. This is one of the reasons why in dreams, during psychotic episodes, or under the influence of certain psychoactive substances, we sometimes *really* are afraid. For the subject of experience, an alternate reality has come into existence. An interesting further exception is formed by those states in which the system manages to classify simulata as such, but the global state persists. Examples of such representational situations in which knowledge about the type of global state is available, although the system is flooded by artifacts, are pseudohallucinations (see section 4.2.4) and lucid dreams (see section 7.2.4). There are also global state classes in which *all* representata subjectively appear to be normal *simulata* and any attempt to differentiate between the phenomenal inner and the phenomenal outer disappears in another way. Such phenomenological state classes can, for instance, be found in mania or in certain types of religious experiences. Obviously,

---

24. They do not represent the *real* world *for* the system anymore. However, if our ontology allows for complex abstracta (e.g., possible worlds) then, given a plausible teleofunctional story, we may keep on speaking about a real representational relation, and not only of an internally simulated *model* of the intentionality relation. For the concept of an internally simulated model of ongoing subject-object relations, see section 6.5.

25. Possibly a good way to put the point runs like this: "Emulated," that is, imagined, pain experiences and memorized red experiences are, respectively, underdetermined and *incompletely individuated* phenomenal states.

any serious and rigorous philosophical theory of mind will have to take all such exceptional cases into account and draw conceptual lessons from their existence. They demonstrate which conjunctions of phenomenological constraints are not *necessary* conjunctions.

Second, it is important to clearly separate the genetic and logical dimensions of the phenomenon of mental simulation. The developmental history of mental states, leading from rudimentary, archaic forms of sensory microstates to more and more complex and flexible macrorepresentata, the activation of which then brings about the instantiation of ever new and richer psychological properties, was primarily a *biological* history. It was under the selection pressure of biological and social environments that new and ever more successful forms of mental content were generated.[26] Maybe the genetic history of complex mental representata could be interestingly described as a biological history of certain internal states, which in the course of time have acquired an increasing degree of relationality and autonomy in the sense of functional complexity and input independence, thereby facilitating their *own* survival within the brains of the species in which they emerge (see section 3.2.11).

The first kind of complex stimulus processing and explicitly intelligent interaction with the environment may have been the reflex arc: a hard-wired path, leading from a stimulus to a rigid motor reaction without generating a specific and stable internal state. The next step may have been the mental presentatum (see section 2.4.4). Color vision is the standard example. It is already characterized by a more or less marked *output decoupling*. This is to say the following: mental presentata are specific inner states, indicating the actual presence of a certain state of affairs with regard to the world or the system itself. Their content is indexical, nonconceptual, and context dependent. They point to a specific stimulus source in the current environment of the system, but do so without automatically leading to a fixed pattern of motor output. They are new mental instruments, for the first time enabling an organism to internally present information without being forced to react to it in a predetermined manner. Presentata increase selectivity. Their disadvantage is constituted by their input dependence; because their content can only be sustained by a continuous flow of input, they can merely depict the actual presence of a stimulus source. Their advantage, obviously, is greater speed. Pain, for instance, has to be *fast* to fulfill its

---

26. Many authors have emphasized the biological functionality of mental content. Colin McGinn points out that what he, in alluding to Ruth Millikan, calls the "relational proper function" of representational mental states coincides with their intrinsically individuated content (e.g., McGinn 1989a, p. 147), that is, the relationality of mental content reflects the relational profile of the accompanying biological state. All these ways of looking at the problem are closely related to the perspective that I am, more or less implicitly, in this chapter and in chapter 3, developing of phenomenal mental models as a type of abstract organ. See also McGinn 1989a; P. S. Churchland 1986; Dretske 1986; Fodor 1984; Millikan 1984, 1989, 1993; Papineau 1987; Stich 1992.

biological function.[27] To once again return to the classic example: a conscious pain experience presents tissue damage or another type of bodily lesion to the subject of experience. To a certain degree of intensity of what I have called the "signal aspect," the subject is not forced to react with external behavior at all. Even if, by sheer strength of the pure presentational aspect, she is forced to react, she now is able to choose from a larger range of possible behaviors. The disadvantage of pain is that we can only in a very incomplete way *re*present its full experiential profile after it has vanished. The informational content of such states is online content only.

The essential transition in generating a genuine inner reality may then have consisted in the additional achievement of *input decoupling* for certain states. Now relations (e.g., causal relations) between representanda could be internally represented, even when those representanda were only partially given in the form of typical stimulus sources. Let us think of this process as a higher-order form of pattern completion. In this way, for the first time, the possibility was created to process abstract information and develop cognitive states in a more narrow sense. Simulata, therefore, must correspondingly possess different subjective properties as presentata, namely, because they have run through a different causal history. They can be embedded in more comprehensive representata, and they can also be activated if their representandum is not given by the flow of input but only through the relational structure of other representata (or currently active simulata). This is an important point: simulata can mutually activate each other, because they are causally linked through their physical boundary conditions (see section 3.2.4).[28] In this way it becomes conceivable how higher-order mental structures were first generated, the representational content of which was not, or only partially, constituted by external facts, which were actually given at the moment of their internal emergence. Those higher-order mental structures can probably be best understood by their function: they enable an organism to carry out internal simulations of complex, counterfactual sequences of events. Thereby new cognitive achievements like memory and strategic planning become possible. The new instruments with which such achievements are brought about are mental simulations—chains of internal states making use of the relational network holding between all

---

27. As a matter of fact, the majority of primary nociceptive afferents are unmyelinated C fibers and conduct comparatively slowly (about 1 m/s), whereas some primary nociceptive afferents, A fibers, conduct nerve impulses at a speed of about 20 m/s due to the presence of a myelin sheath. In this sense the biological function mentioned above itself possesses a fine-grained internal structure: Whereas C fibers are involved in slower signaling processes (e.g., the control of local blood vessels, sensitivity changes, and the perception of a delayed "second pain"), A fibers are involved in motor reflexes and fast behavioral responses. Cf. Treede 2001.

28. Within connectionist systems such an associative coupling of internal representata can be explained by their causal similarity or their corresponding position in an internal "energy landscape" formed by the system. *Representational* similarity of activation vectors also finds its physical expression in the probability of two stable activation states of the system occurring simultaneously.

mental representata in order to activate comprehensive internal structures independently of current external input. The theory of connectionist networks has given us a host of ideas about how such features can be achieved on the implementational level. However, I will not go into any technical details at this point.

Simulations are important, because they can be compared to goal-representing states. What precisely does this mean? The first function of biological nervous systems was generating coherent, global patterns of motor behavior and integrating sensory perception with such behavioral patterns. For this reason, I like to look at the emergence of mental, and eventually of subjectively experienced, conscious content as a process of behavioral evolution: mental simulation is a new form of internalized *motor behavior*. For my present purpose it suffices to differentiate between three different stages of this process. Presentata, through their output decoupling, enable the system to develop a larger behavioral repertoire relative to a given stimulus situation. Representata integrate those basic forms of sensory-driven content into full-blown models of the current state of the external world. Advanced representata, through input decoupling, then allow a system to develop a larger *inner* behavioral repertoire, if they are activated by internal causes—that is, *as simulata*. Differently put, mental simulation is a new form of behavior, in some cases even of inner action.[29] As opposed to stimulus-correlated or "cued" representational activity, this is a "detached" activity (Brinck and Gärdenfors 1999, p. 90*ff.*). It may be dependent on an internal context, but with regard to the current environment of the organism it is context-independent. The generation of complex mental simulata, which are to a certain degree independent of the stream of actual input and do not by necessity lead to overt motoric "macrobehavior," is one precondition for this new form of behavior. Very roughly, this could have been the biological history of complex internal states, which ultimately integrated the properties of representationality and functionality in an adaptive way. However, mental simulation proves to be a highly interesting phenomenon on the level of its conceptual interpretation as well.

Perhaps the philosophically most interesting point consists of mental representation being a *special case* of mental simulation: Simulations are internal representations of properties of the world, which are not *actual* properties of the environment as given through

---

29. Higher cognitive achievements like the formation of theories or the planning of goal-directed behavior are for this reason only possible with those inner tools which do *not* covary with actual properties of the environment. The content and success of cognitive models cannot be explained by covariance theory alone. "But in order to model possible worlds, we must have cognitive models able to break away from covariance with the actual world. If we are going to treat all cases of non-covarying representation as cases of 'mis'representation, then it seems that misrepresentation is by no means sub-optimal, but is in fact a necessary and integral part of cognition" (cf. Kukla 1992, p. 222).

the senses. Representations, however, are internal representations of states of the world which have functionally already been *defined* as actual by the system.

To get a better grasp of this interesting relationship, one has to differentiate between a teleofunctionalist, an epistemological, and a phenomenological interpretation of the concepts of "representation" and "simulation." Let us recall: at the very beginning we had discovered that, under an analysis operating from the objective, third-person perspective of science, information available in the central nervous system never truly is *actual* information. However, because the system defines ordering thresholds within sensory modalities and supramodal windows of simultaneity, it generates a temporal frame of reference *for itself* which fixes what is to be treated as its own present (for details, see section 3.2.2). Metaphorically speaking, it owns reality by simulating a Now, a fictitious kind of temporal internality. Therefore, even this kind of presence is a virtual presence; it results from a *constructive* representational process. My teleofunctionalist background assumption now says that this was a process which proved to be adaptive: it possesses a biological proper function and for this reason has been successful in the course of evolutionary history. Its function consists in representing environmental dynamics with a sufficient degree of precision and within a certain, narrowly defined temporal frame of reference. The adaptive function of mental simulation, however, consists in adequately grasping relevant aspects of reality *outside* of this self-defined temporal frame of reference. Talking in this manner, one operates on the teleofunctionalist level of description.

One interesting aspect of this way of talking is that it clearly demonstrates—from the objective third-person perspective taken by natural science—in which way every phenomenal *representation* is a *simulation* as well. If one analyzes the representational dynamics of our system under the temporal frame of reference given by physics, all mental activities are *simulational* activities. If one then interprets "representation" and "simulation" as epistemological terms, it becomes obvious that we are never in any direct epistemic contact with the world surrounding us, even while *phenomenally* experiencing an immediate contact (see sections 3.2.7, 5.4, and 6.2.6). On the third, the phenomenological level of description, simulata and representata are two distinct state classes that conceptually cannot be reduced to each other. Perception never is the same experience as memory. Thinking differs from sensing. However, from an epistemological point of view we have to admit that every representation is also a simulation. What it simulates is a "Now."

Idealistic philosophers have traditionally very clearly seen this fundamental situation under different epistemological assumptions. However, describing it in the way just sketched also enables us to generate a whole new range of phenomenological metaphors. If the typical state classes for the process of mental simulation are being formed by conceptual thought, pictorial imagery, dreams, and hallucinations, then *all* mental dynamics within phenomenal space as a whole can metaphorically always be described as a specific form of thought, of pictorial imagination, of dreaming, and of hallucinating. As we will soon see, such metaphors are today, when facing a flood of new empirical data, again characterized by great heuristic fertility.

Let me give you a prime example of such a new metaphor to illustrate this point: Phenomenal experience during the waking state is an *online* hallucination. This hallucination is *online* because the autonomous activity of the system is permanently being modulated by the information flow from the sensory organs; it is a hallucination because it depicts a possible reality as an actual reality. Phenomenal experience during the dream state, however, is just a complex *offline* hallucination. We must imagine the brain as a system that constantly directs questions at the world and selects appropriate answers. Normally, questions and answers go hand in hand, swiftly and elegantly producing our everyday conscious experience. But sometimes unbalanced situations occur where, for instance, the automatic questioning process becomes too dominant. The interesting point is that what we have just termed "mental simulation," as an unconscious process of simulating possible situations, may actually be an *autonomous* process that is incessantly active.

As a matter of fact, some of the best current work in neuroscience (W. Singer, personal communication, 2000; see also Leopold and Logothetis 1999) suggests a view of the human brain as a system that *constantly* simulates possible realities, generates internal expectations and hypotheses in a top-down fashion, while being constrained in this activity by what I have called mental presentation, constituting a constant stimulus-correlated bottom-up stream of information, which then finally helps the system to select one of an almost infinitely large number of internal possibilities and turning it into phenomenal reality, now explicitly expressed as the content of a conscious *representation*. More precisely, plausibly a lot of the spontaneous brain activity that usually was just interpreted as noise could actually contribute to the feature-binding operations required for perceptual grouping and scene segmentation through a topological specificity of its own (Fries, Neuenschwander, Engel, Goebel, and Singer 2001). Recent evidence points to the fact that background fluctuations in the gamma frequency range are not only chaotic fluctuations but contain information—philosophically speaking, information about what is *possible*. This information—for example, certain grouping rules, residing in fixed network properties like the functional architecture of corticocortical connections—is structurally laid-down information about what was possible and likely in the past of the system and its ancestors. Certain types of ongoing background activity could therefore just be the continuous process of hypothesis generation mentioned above. Not being chaotic at all, it might be an important step in translating structurally laid-down information about what was possible in the past history of the organism into those transient, dynamical elements of the processing that are right now actually contributing to the content of conscious experience. For instance, it could contribute to sensory grouping, making it faster and more efficient (see Fries et al. 2001, p. 199 for details). Not only fixed network properties could in this indirect way shape what in the end we actually *see* and consciously experience, but if the autonomous background process of thousands of hypotheses continuously chattering away can be modulated by true top-down processing, then even specific *expectations* and focal *attention* could generate precise correlational patterns in peripheral processing structures, patterns serving to compare and match actually incoming sensory signals. That is, in the terminology here proposed, not only unconscious *mental* simulation but also deliberately intended high-level *phenomenal* simulations, conscious thoughts, personal-level memories, and so on can modulate unconscious, subpersonal matching processes. In this way for the first time it becomes plausible how exactly personal-level expectations can, via unconscious dynamic coding processes chattering away in the background, shape and add further meaning to what is then actually experienced consciously.

If this general picture is correct, there are basically two kinds of hallucinations. First, sensory hallucinations may be those in which the bottom-up process gets out of control, is disinhibited, or in other ways too dominant, and therefore floods the system with pre-sentational artifacts. A second way in which a system can become overwhelmed by an unbalanced form of conscious reality-modeling would become manifest in all those situations in which top-down, hypothesis-generating processes of simulation have become too dominant and are underconstrained by current input. For instance, if the process of autonomous, but topologically specific background fluctuation mentioned above is derailed, then self-generated patterns can propagate downward into primary sensory areas. The switching of a Necker cube and a whole range of multistable phenomena (Leopold and Logothetis 1999) are further examples of situations where "expectations become reality." In our present context, a fruitful way of looking at the human brain, therefore, is as a system which, even in ordinary waking states, constantly hallucinates at the world, as a system that constantly lets its internal autonomous simulational dynamics collide with the ongoing flow of sensory input, vigorously dreaming at the world and thereby generating the content of phenomenal experience.

One interesting conceptual complication when looking at things this way consists in the fact that there are also phenomenal simulations, that is, mental simulations, which are *experienced* by the system itself within its narrow temporal framework as not referring to actual reality. Of course, the classic examples are cognitive processes, deliberately initiated, conscious thought processes. Even such phenomenal simulations can be described as hallucinations, because a virtual cognitive subject is phenomenally depicted as real while cognitive activity unfolds (see section 6.4.4). We will learn more about global *offline* hallucinations, which phenomenally are depicted as simulations, in section 7.2.5.

Let us return to the concept of mental simulation. What precisely does it mean when we say that Sim_M is not a case of Rep_M? What precisely does it mean to say that the process of mental simulation represents counterfactual situations for a system? Mental representation can be reconstructed as a special case of mental simulation, namely, as exactly that case of mental simulation in which, first, the simulandum (within the temporal frame of reference defined by the system for itself) is given as a *representandum*, that is, as a component of that partition of the world which it functionally treats as its present; and second, the simulandum causes the activation of the simulatum by means of the standard causal chains, that is, through the sensory organs. In addition to this functional characterization, we may also use a difference in intentional content as a further definiens, with representation targeting a very special possible world, namely, the *actual* world (box 2.4). According to this scheme, every representation also is a simulation, because—with the real world—there always exists one possible world in which the representandum constitutes an actual state of affairs. The content of mental simulata consists of states of affairs in possible worlds. From the point of view of its logical structure, therefore, simulation is the more comprehensive phenomenon and representation is a restricted special case: Representata are those simulata whose function *for* the system consists in depicting states of affairs in the *real* world with a sufficient degree of temporal precision. However, from a genetic perspective, the phenomenon of representation clearly is the earlier kind of phenomenon. Only by perceiving the environment have organisms developed those modules in their functional architecture, which later they could use for a nonrepresentational activation of mental states. We first developed these modules, and then we learned to take them offline. Perception preceded cognition, perceptual phenomenal models are the precursors of phenomenal discourse models (see chapter 3), and the acquisition of reliable representational resources was the condition of possibility for the

Box 2.4

Mental Simulation: Sim'_M (W, S, X, Y)

· There is a possible world W, so that Sim_M (S, X, Y), where Y is a fulfilled fact in W.

Mental Representation: Rep_M (S, X, Y) $\leftrightarrow$ Sim'_M (W_0, S, X, Y)

· There is a real world W_0.

· Y is a fulfilled fact in W_0.

· Y causes X by means of the standard causal chains.

· X is functionally integrated into the window of presence constituted by S.

---

occurrence of reliable mental simulation. In other words, only those who can see can also dream.[30]

Importantly, we now have to introduce a further conceptual difference. It is of great philosophical interest because it pertains to the concept of possibility. Without going into any technical issues at all, I want to briefly differentiate between three possible interpretations: logical possibility, mental possibility, and phenomenal possibility.

• *Logical possibility.* Logically possible states of affairs or worlds are those which can be coherently described in an external medium. This is to say that at least one formally consistent *propositional* representation of such states or worlds exists. This concept of possibility always is relative to a particular set of theoretical background assumptions, for instance, to a certain system of modal logic.

• *Mental possibility.* Mental possibility is a property of all those states of affairs or worlds which we can, in principle, think about or imagine: all states of affairs or worlds which can be *mentally simulated.* Hence, there is at least one internal, coherent mental simulation of these states of affairs or worlds. This concept of possibility is always relative to a certain class of concrete representational systems, all of which possess a specific functional profile and a particular representational architecture. It is important to note that the mechanisms of generating and evaluating representational coherence employed by such systems have been optimized with regard to their biological or social functionality, and do *not* have to be subject to classic criteria of adequacy, rationality, or epistemic justification in the narrow sense of philosophical epistemology. Second, the operation of such mechanisms does not have to be conscious.

• *Phenomenal possibility.* Phenomenal possibility is a property of all states of affairs or worlds which, as a matter of fact, we can actually *consciously* imagine or conceive of: all those states of affairs or worlds which can enter into conscious thought experiments, into cognitive operations, or explicit planning processes, but also those which could constitute the content of dreams and hallucinations. Again, what is phenomenally possible is always relative to a certain class of concrete conscious systems, to their specific functional profile, and to the deep representational structure underlying their specific form of phenomenal experience.

---

30. This may be true of language and thought as well. Possibly we first had to learn the manipulation of discrete symbol tokens in an external environment (by operating with internal physical symbols like signs or self-generated sounds) before being able to mentally simulate them. There are some arguments in favor of this intuition which are related to the stability of conceptual structures and the simulation of speech processing in connectionist systems, and which are also supported by empirical data. See McClelland, Rumelhart, and the PDP Research Group 1986; Goschke and Koppelberg 1990, p. 267; Helm 1991, chapter 6; Johnson-Laird 1990; Bechtel and Abrahamsen 1991. In particular, see the work of Giacomo Rizzolatti and Vittorio Gallese, as referred to in section 6.3.3.

Why is it that the difference, in particular that between logical and phenomenal possibility, is of philosophical relevance? First, it is interesting to note how it is precisely those states of affairs and worlds just characterized as phenomenally possible which appear as *intuitively plausible* to us: We can define intuitive plausibility as a property of every thought or idea which we can successfully transform into the content of a coherent *phenomenal simulation*. In doing so, the internal coherence of a conscious simulation may vary greatly. The result of a certain thought experiment, say, of Swampman traveling to Inverted Earth (Tye 1998) may intuitively appear as plausible to us, whereas a dream, in retrospect, may look bizarre. Of course, the reverse is possible as well. Again, it is true that phenomenal possibility is always relative to a certain class of concrete representational systems and that the mechanisms of generating and evaluating coherence employed by those systems may have been optimized toward functional adequacy and not subject to any criteria of epistemic justification in the classic epistemological sense of the word.[31] In passing, let me briefly point to a second, more general issue, which has generated considerable confusion in many current debates in philosophy of mind. Of course, from phenomenal possibility (or necessity), neither nomological nor logical possibility (or necessity) will follow. The statement that all of us are purportedly able to coherently conceive of or imagine a certain situation—for instance, an *imitation man* (K. K. Campbell 1971, p. 120) or a *zombie* (see Chalmers 1996, p. 94 *ff*.)—is rather trivial from a philosophical point of view because ultimately it is just an empirical claim about the history of the human brain and its functional architecture. It is a statement about a world that is a phenomenally possible world for human beings. It is not a statement about the modal strength of the relationship between physical and phenomenal properties; logical possibility (or necessity) is not implied by phenomenal possibility (or necessity). From the simple fact that beings like ourselves are able to phenomenally simulate a certain *apparently* possible world, it does not follow that a consistent or even only an empirically plausible description of this world exists. On the contrary, the fact that such descriptions can be generated today shows how devoid of empirical content our current concept of consciousness still is (P. M. Churchland 1996).

A second problem may be even more fundamental. Many of the best current philosophical discussions of the notion of "conceivability" construe conceivability as a property of statements. However, there are no entailment relations between nonpropositional forms of mental or conscious content and statements. And our best current theories about the real representational dynamics unfolding in human brains (for instance, connectionist models of human cognition or current theories in dynamicist cognitive science) all have

31. For instance, for neural nets, the functional correlate of intuitive plausibility as represented on the phenomenal level could consist in the *goodness of fit* of the respective, currently simulated state.

one crucial property in common: the forms of content generated by those neurocomputational processes very likely underlying our conscious thoughts while, for instance, we imagine an *imitation man* or a *zombie* do not possess a critical feature which in philosophy of mind is termed "propositional modularity" (see Stich 1983, p. 237*ff.*). Propositional modularity is a classic way of thinking about propositional attitudes as states of a representational system; they are functionally discrete, they process a semantic interpretation, and they play a distinct causal role with regard to other propositional attitudes and behavioral patterns. In terms of the most rational and empirically plausible theory about the real representational dynamics underlying conscious thought—for example, about a philosopher engaging in *zombie* thought experiments and investigations of consciousness, conceivability, and possibility—is that the most interesting class of connectionist models will be nonlocalistic, representing these cognitive contents in a distributed fashion. There will be no obvious symbolic interpretation for single hidden units, while at the same time such models are genuinely cognitive models and not only implementations of cognitive models. As Ramsey, Stich, and Garon (1991) have shown, propositional modularity is not given for such models, because it is impossible to localize discrete propositional representata beyond the input layer. The most rational assumption today is that no singular hidden unit possesses a propositional interpretation (as a "mental statement" which could possess the property of conceivability), but that instead a whole *set* of propositions is coded in a holistic fashion. Classicist cognitive models compete with connectionist models on the same explanatory level; the latter are more parsimonious, integrate much more empirical data in an explanatory fashion, but do not generate *propositional* cognitive content in a classic sense. Therefore, if *phenomenal* possibility (the conscious experience of conceivability) is likely to be realized in a medium that only approximates propositional modularity, but never fully realizes it, nothing in terms of *logical* conceivability or possibility is entailed. Strictly speaking, even conscious thought is not a propositional form of mental content, although we certainly are systems that sometimes approximate the property of propositional modularity to a considerable degree. There simply are no entailment relations between nonpropositional, holistic *conscious* contents and statements we can make in an external, linguistic medium, be they conceivable or not. However, two further thoughts about the phenomenon of mental simulation may be more interesting. They too can be formulated in a clearer fashion with the conceptual instruments just introduced.

First, every phenomenal representation, as we have seen, is also a simulation; in a specific functional sense, its content is always formed by a *possible* actual world. Therefore, it is true to say that the fundamental intentional content of conscious experience in standard situations is *hypothetical* content: a hypothesis about the actual state of the world and the self in it, given all constraints available to the system. However, in our own case, this process is tied into a fundamental architectural structure, which from now on, I will call *autoepistemic closure*. We return to this structure at length in the next chapter when discussing the transparency constraint for phenomenal mental models (see section 3.2.7). What is autoepistemic closure?

"Autoepistemic closure" is an epistemological, and not (at least not primarily) a phenomenological concept. It refers to an "inbuilt blind spot," a structurally anchored deficit in the capacity to gain knowledge about oneself. It is important to understand that autoepistemic closure as used in this book does not refer to *cognitive* closure (McGinn 1989b, 1991) or epistemic "boundedness" (Fodor 1983) in terms of the unavailability of *theoretical*, propositionally structured self-knowledge. Rather, it refers to a closure or boundedness of attentional processing with regard to one's own internal representational dynamics. Autoepistemic closure consists in human beings in ordinary waking states, using their internal representational resources—that is, by introspectively guiding *attention*—not being able to realize what I have just explained: the simple fact that the content of their subjective experiences always is counterfactual content, because it rests on a temporal fiction. Here, "realize" means "phenomenally represent." On the *phenomenal level* we are not able to represent this common feature of representation and simulation. We are systems, which are not able to consciously experience the fact that they are never in contact with the actual present, that even what we experience as the phenomenal "Now" is a constructive hypothesis, a *simulated* Now. From this, the following picture emerges: Phenomenal representation is that form of mental simulation, the proper function[32] of which consists in grasping the actual state of the world with a sufficient degree of accuracy. In most cases this goal is achieved, and that is why phenomenal representation is a functionally adequate process. However, from an epistemological perspective, it is obvious that the phenomenal "presence" of conscious representational content is a fiction, which could at any time turn out to be false. Autoepistemic closure is a highly interesting feature of the human mind, because it possesses a higher-order variant.

Second, all those phenomenal states, in which—as during thought, planning, or pictorial imagination—we additionally experience ourselves as subjects deliberately simulating mentally possible worlds, are obviously being experienced as states which are unfolding *right now*. Leaving aside special cases like lucid dreams, the following principle seems to be valid: Simulations are always embedded in a global representational context, and this context is to a large extent constituted by a transparent representation of temporal internality (see section 3.2.7 for the notion of "phenomenal transparency"). They take place against the background of a phenomenal present that is defined as real. Call this the "background principle." Temporal internality, this arguably most fundamental

---

32. For the concept of a proper function, see Millikan 1989.

structural feature of our conscious minds, is defined as real, in a manner that is experientially untranscendable for the system itself. Most importantly, phenomenal simulations are always "owned" by a subject also being experienced as real, by a person who experiences himself as *present* in the world. However, the considerations just offered lead us to the thought that even such higher-order operations could take place under the conditions of autoepistemic closure: the presence of the phenomenal subject itself, against the background of which the internal dynamics of its phenomenal simulations unfolds, would then again be a functionally adequate, but epistemically unjustified representational fiction. This fiction might precisely be what Kant thought of as the transcendental unity of apperception, as a condition of possibility for the emergence of a phenomenal first-person perspective: the "I think," the certainty that *I myself am the thinker*, which can in principle accompany every single cognitive episode. The *cognitive* first-person perspective would in this way be anchored in the *phenomenal* first-person perspective, a major constitutive element of which is autoepistemic closure. I return to this point in chapters 6 and 8. However, before we can discuss the process of conscious self-simulation (see section 5.3), we have first to introduce a working concept of phenomenal simulation (box 2.5).

Systems possessing mental states open an immensely high-dimensional mental space of possibility. This space contains everything which can, in principle, be simulated by those systems. Corresponding to this space of possibility there is a mental *state space*, a description of those concrete mental states which can result from a realization of such possibilities. Systems additionally possessing phenomenal states open a *phenomenal* possibility space, forming a subregion within the first space. Individual states, which can be

Box 2.5

Phenomenal Simulation: Sim$_P$ (S, X, Y)

· S is an individual information-processing system.

· Y is a possible state of the world, relative to the system's representational architecture.

· X phenomenally simulates Y *for* S.

· X is a physically internal system state, the content of which has functionally been defined as temporally external.

· The intentional content of X *is* currently introspectively$_1$ available; that is, it is disposed to become the representandum of *subsymbolic* higher-order representational processes.

· The intentional content of X *is* currently introspectively$_2$ available for cognitive reference; it can in turn become the representandum of *symbolic* higher-order representational processes.

· The intentional content of X *is* currently available for the selective control of action.

---

described as concrete realizations of points within this phenomenal space of possibility, are what today we call conscious experiences: transient, complex combinations of actual values in a very large number of dimensions. What William James described as the stream of consciousness under this description becomes a trajectory through this space. However, to live your life as a genuine phenomenal subject does not only mean to episodically follow a trajectory through the space of possible states of consciousness. It also means to actively *change* properties of the space itself—for instance, its volume, its dimensionality, or the inner landscape, making some states within the space of consciousness more probable than others. Physicalism with regard to phenomenal experience is represented by the thesis that the phenomenal state space of a system always constitutes a subspace of its *physical* state space. Note that it is still true that the content of a conscious experience always is the content of a phenomenal simulation. However, we can now categorize simulations under a number of new aspects.

In those cases in which the intentional content of such a simulation is being depicted as temporally external, that is, as not actually being positioned within the functional window of presence constituted by the system, it will be experienced as a simulation. In all other cases, it will be experienced as a representation. This is true because there is not only a functionalist but an epistemological and phenomenological interpretation of the concept of "simulation." What, with regard to the first of these two additional aspects, *always* is a simulation, subjectively appears as a representation in one situation and as a simulation in another, namely, with respect to the third, the phenomenological reading. From an epistemological perspective, we see that our phenomenal states at no point in time establish a direct and immediate contact with the world for us. Knowledge by simulation always is approximative knowledge, leaving behind the real temporal dynamics of its objects for principled reasons. However, on the level of a phenomenal representation of this knowledge, this fact is systematically suppressed; at least the contents of noncognitive consciousness are therefore characterized by an additional quality, the phenomenal quality of *givenness*. The conceptual instruments of "representation" and "simulation" now available allow us to avoid the typical phenomenological fallacy from phenomenal to epistemic givenness, by differentiating between a purely descriptive and an epistemological context in the use of both concepts.

Interesting new aspects can also be discovered when applying a teleofunctionalist analysis to the concept of phenomenal simulation. The internal causal structure, the topology of our phenomenal space, has been adapted to the nomological space of possibilities governing middle-sized objects on the surface of this planet over millions of years. Points within this space represent what was relevant, on the surface of our planet, in our behavioral space in particular, to the maximization of our genetic fitness. It is represented in a way that makes it available for fast and flexible control of action. Therefore, we can today more easily imagine and simulate those types of situations, which possess great relevance to our survival. For example, sexual and violent fantasies are much easier and more readily accessible to us than the mental simulation of theoretical operations on syntactically specified symbol structures. They represent possible situations characterized by a much higher *adaptive value*. From an evolutionary perspective, we have only started to develop phenomenal simulations of complex symbolic operations a very short time ago. Such *cognitive* simulations were the dawning of theoretical awareness.

There are at least three different kinds of phenomenal simulations: those, the proper function of which consists in generating representations of the *actual* world which are nomologically possible and possess a sufficient degree of probability (e.g., *perceptual* phenomenal representation); those, the proper function of which consists in generating general overall models of the world that are nomologically possible and biologically relevant (e.g., pictorial mental imagery and spatial cognitive operations in planning goal-directed actions); and—in very rare cases—phenomenal simulations, the primary goal of which consists in generating quasi-symbolic representations of *logically* possible worlds that can be fed into truly propositional, linguistic, and external representations. Only the last class of conscious simulations constitutes genuinely theoretical operations; only they constitute what may be called the beginning of philosophical thought. This type of thought has evolved out of a long biological history; on the level of the individual, it uses representational instruments, which originally were used to secure survival. Cognitive processes clearly possess interesting biohistorical roots in spatial perception and the planning of physical actions.

Precisely what function could be fulfilled for a biological system by the internal simulation of a possible world? Which biological proper function could consist in making nonexisting worlds the object of mental operations? A selective advantage can probably only be achieved if the system manages to extract a subset of biologically realistic worlds from the infinity of possible worlds. It has to possess a general heuristics, which compresses the vastness of logical space to two essential classes of "intended realities," that is, those worlds that are causally conducive and relevant to the selection process. The first class will have to be constituted by all desirable worlds, that is, all those worlds in which the system is enjoying optimal external conditions, many descendants, and a high social status. Those worlds are interesting simulanda when concerned with mental *future planning*. On the other hand, all those possible and probable worlds are interesting simulanda in which the system and its offspring have died or have, in another way, been impeded in their reproductive success. Those worlds are intended simulanda when mentally assessing the *risk* of certain behavioral patterns.

Hence, if conscious mental simulations are supposed to be successful instruments, there must be a possibility of ascribing different probabilities to different internally generated macrosimulata. Let us call such global simulational macrostructures "possible phenomenal worlds." A possible phenomenal world is a world that *could* be consciously experienced. Assessing probabilities consists in measuring the distance from possible worlds to the real world. *Mental* assessment of probabilities therefore can only consist in measuring the distance between a mental macrosimulatum that has just been activated to an already existing mental macro*representatum*. Given that this process has been deliberately initiated and therefore takes place consciously, a possible phenomenal world has to be compared with a model of the world as *real*—a world that *could* be "the" world with a world that *is* "the" world. This is to say that, in many cognitive operations, complex internal system states have to be compared with each other. In order to do so, an internal metric must be available, with the help of which such a comparison can be carried out. The representationalist analysis of neural nets from the third-person perspective has already supplied us with a precise set of conceptual tools to achieve this goal: in a connectionist system, one can represent internal states as sets of subsymbols, or as activation vectors. The similarity of two activation vectors can be mathematically described in a precise way; for instance, by the angle they form in vector space (see, e.g., P. M. Churchland 1989; Helm 1991). Internalist criteria for the identity of content (and phenomenal content *is* internal in that it supervenes locally) can be derived from the relative distances between prototype points in state space (P. M. Churchland 1998). Without pursuing these technical issues any further, I want to emphasize that the adaptive value of possessing a function to assess the *distance* between two models of the world can play a decisive explanatory role in answering the question, why something like phenomenal consciousness exists *at all*.

In the course of this book, I offer a series of more or less speculative hypotheses about possible adaptive functions of conscious experience. Here is the first one. I call this hypothesis the "world zero hypothesis." What precisely does it claim? There has to exist a global representational *medium*, in which the mental assessment of probabilities just mentioned could take place. In order to do so, an overarching context has to be created, forming the background against which the distance between differing models of the world can be analyzed and possible paths from one world to the other can be searched, evaluated, and compared. This context, I claim, can only be generated by a globalized version of the phenomenal variant of mental representation; in order to be biologically adaptive (assuming the simplest case of only two integrated macrostructures being compared), one of both world-models has to be defined as the *actual* one for the system. One of both simulations has to be represented as the *real* world, in a way that is functionally nontranscendable for the system itself. One of both models has to become indexed as the *reference model*, by being internally defined as real, that is, as *given* and not as constructed. And it is easy to see why.

Simulations can only be successful if they do not lead the system into parallel dream worlds, but enable it to simultaneously generate a sufficiently accurate representation of the actual world, which can serve as a representational anchor and *evaluative context* for the content of this simulation. In order to achieve this goal, a functional mechanism has to be developed which makes sure that the current active model of the actual world can also, in the future, constantly be recognized as such. This mechanism would then also be the functional basis for the mysterious phenomenal quality of *presence*. Without such a mechanism, and on the level of subjective experience, it would not be possible to differentiate between dream and reality, between plan and current situation. Only if this foundation exists would it become possible, in a third step, to evaluate phenomenal simulations and make the result available for the future planning of actions. In other words, by generating a suitable and further inner system state, a higher-order metarepresentatum has to be generated, which once again mentally depicts the "probability distance" between simulatum and representatum (this is what, e.g., from the third-person perspective of computational neuroscience could be described as the angle between two activation vectors), thereby making it globally available. The two most fundamental phenomenological constraints of any concept of consciousness are globality and presence (see chapter 3), the requirement that there is an untranscendable *presence of a world*.[33] I propose that this kind of phenomenal content—a reality reliably depicted as an *actual* reality—had to evolve, because it is a central (possibly *the* central) necessary condition for the development of future planning, memory, flexible and intelligent behavioral responses, and for genuinely cognitive activity, for example, the mental formation of concept-like structures. What all these processing capacities have in common is that their results can only be successfully evaluated against a firm background that reliably functions as the reference model. If what I have presented here as the world zero hypothesis for the function of conscious experience points in the right direction, then we are immediately led to another highly interesting question: How precisely is it possible for the content of phenomenal representata—as opposed to the content of phenomenal simulata—to be depicted as *present*?

2.4 From Mental to Phenomenal Presentation: Qualia

Perhaps the most fundamental epistemic goal in forming a representationalist theory of phenomenal experience consists in first isolating the most simple elements within the target domain. One has to ask questions like these: What, first of all, are the most *simple* forms

---

33. I return to this point at the end of section 3.2.7. The phenomenological notion of the "presence of a world" results from the second, third, and seventh constraints developed in chapter 3 and can be described as what I call *minimal* consciousness.

of phenomenal content? Do something like "phenomenal primitives" exist? Do *atoms* of subjective experience exist, elementary contents of consciousness, resisting any further analysis? Can such primitive contents of experience at all be isolated and described in a precise, conceptually convincing manner?

The traditional philosophical answer to these types of questions runs like this: "Yes, primitive elements of phenomenal space do exist. The name for these elements is 'qualia,' and their paradigmatic expression can be found in the simple qualities of sensory awareness: in a visual experience of redness, in bodily sensations like pain, or in the subjective experience of smell caused by sandalwood." Qualia in this sense of the word are interesting for many reasons. For example, they simultaneously exemplify those higher-order phenomenal qualities of presence and immediacy, which were mentioned at the end of the last section, and they do so in an equally paradigmatic manner. Nothing could be more *present* than sensory qualities like redness or painfulness. And nothing in the domain of conscious experience gives us a stronger sense of direct, *unmediated* contact to reality as such, be it the reality of our visual environment or the reality of the bodily self. Qualia are maximally concrete. In order to understand how a possibility can be experienced as a reality, and in order to understand how abstract intentional content can go along with concrete *phenomenal* character, it may, therefore, be fruitful to develop a representational analysis of qualia. As a matter of fact, a number of very precise and interesting representational theories of qualia have recently been developed,[34] but as it turns out, many of these theories face technical difficulties, for example, concerning the notion of higher-order misrepresentation (e.g., see Neander 1998). Hence, a natural question is if *nonrepresentational* phenomenal qualities exist. In the following sections, I try to steer a middle course between the two alternatives of representational and nonrepresentational theories of qualia, thereby hoping to avoid the difficulties of both and shed some new light on this old issue. Again, I shall introduce a number of simple but, I hope, helpful conceptual distinctions.

One provisional result of the considerations so far offered is this: For conscious experience, the concept of "representation," in its teleofunctionalist and in epistemological uses, can be reduced to the concept of "simulation." Phenomenal representations are a subclass of simulations. However, when trying to develop further constraints on the phenomenological level of description, this connection seems to be much more ambiguous. Phenomenal representations form a distinct class of experiential states, opposed to simulations.

In terms of phenomenal content, perceptions of the actual environment and of one's own body are completely different from daydreams, motor imagery, or philosophical

34. See Austen Clark 1993, 2000; Lycan 1987, 1996; Tye, 1995, 1998, 2000.

thought experiments. The connecting element between both classes of experiences seems to be the fact that a stable phenomenal self exists in both of them. Even if we have episodically lost the explicit phenomenal self, perhaps when becoming fully absorbed in a daydream or a philosophical thought experiment, there exists at least a mental representation of the self which is at any time *available*—and it is the paradigm example of a representation which at no point in time is ever completely experienced as a simulation.[35] What separates both classes are those elementary sensory components, which, in their very specific *qualitative* expressions, only result from direct sensory contact with the world. Imagined strawberries are never *truly* red, and the awfulness of mentally simulated pain is a much weaker and fainter copy of the original online event. An analysis of simple qualitative content, therefore, has to provide us with an answer to the question of what precisely the differences between the intentional content of representational processes and simulational processes actually are.

In order to do so, I have to invite readers to join me in taking a second detour. If, as a first step, one wants to offer a list of defining characteristics for the canonical concept of a "quale," one soon realizes that there is no answer which would even be shared by a simple majority of theoreticians working in this area of philosophy or relevant subdisciplines within the cognitive neurosciences. Today, there is no agreed-on set of necessary or sufficient conditions for anything to fall under the concept of a "quale." Leading researchers in the neurosciences simply perceive the philosophical concept of a quale as ill-defined, and therefore think it is best ignored by anyone interested in rigorous research programs. When asking what the most *simple* forms of consciousness actually are (e.g., in terms of possible explananda for interdisciplinary cooperation) it is usually very hard to even arrive at a very basic consensus. On the other hand, excellent approaches to developing the necessary successor concepts are already in existence (for a recent example, see Clark 2000).

In the following four sections, I first argue that qualia, in terms of an analytically strict definition—as the simplest form of conscious experience in the sense of first-order phenomenal properties—do not exist.[36] Rather, simple empirical considerations already show that we do not possess introspective identity criteria for many simple forms of sensory contents. We are not able to *recognize* the vast majority of them, and, therefore, we can neither cognitively nor linguistically grasp them in their full content. We cannot form a concept of them, because they are ineffable. Using our new conceptual tools, we can now say: Simple qualitative information, in almost all cases, is only attentionally and discrim-

---

35. I return to this point at great length in chapter 6, section 6.2.6.

36. In what follows I draw on previous ideas only published in German, mainly developed in Metzinger 1997. But see also Metzinger and Walde 2000.

inatively available information. If this empirical premise is correct, it means that subjective experience *itself* does not provide us with transtemporal identity criteria for the most simple forms of phenomenal content. However, on our way toward a conceptually convincing theory of phenomenal consciousness, which at the same time is empirically anchored, a clear interpretation of those most simple forms of phenomenal content is absolutely indispensable.

Conceptual progress could only be achieved by developing precise *logical* identity criteria for those concepts by which we publicly refer to such private and primitive contents of consciousness. Those identity criteria for phenomenological concepts would then have to be systematically differentiated, for instance, by using data from psychophysics. In section 2.4.2, therefore, I investigate the relationship between transtemporal and logical criteria of identity. However, the following introductory section will proceed by offering a short argument for the *elimination* of the classic concept of a quale. The first question is, What actually are we talking about, when speaking about the most *simple* contents of phenomenal experience?

First-order phenomenal properties, up to now, have been the canonical candidates for those smallest "building blocks of consciousness." First-order properties are phenomenal primitives, because using the representational instruments available for the respective system does not permit them to be further analyzed. Simplicity is *representational atomism* (see Jakab 2000 for an interesting discussion). Atomism is relative to a certain set of tools. In the case of human beings, the "representational instruments" just mentioned are the capacities corresponding to the notions of introspection$_1$, introspection$_2$, introspection$_3$, and introspection$_4$: As it were, we simply "discover" the impenetrable phenomenal primitives at issue by letting higher-order capacities like attention and cognition wander around in our phenomenal model of the world or by directing these processes toward our currently conscious self-representation. In most animals, which do not possess genuinely cognitive capacities, it will only be the process of *attending* to their ongoing sensory experience, which reveals elementary contents to these animals. They will in turn be forced to experience them as givens, as elementary aspects of their world. However, *conceptually* grasping such properties within and with the aid of the epistemic resources of a specific representational system always presupposes that the system will later be able to *re*identify the properties it has grasped. Interestingly, human beings don't seem to belong to this class of systems: phenomenal properties in *this* sense do *not* constitute the lowest level of reality, as it is being standardly represented by the human nervous system operating on the phenomenal level of organization (with regard to the concept of conscious experience as a "level of organization," see Revonsuo 2000a). There is something that is simpler, but still conscious. For this reason, we have to eliminate the theoretical entity in question (i.e., simple "qualitative" content and those first-order phenomenal property predicates corresponding to it), while simultaneously developing a set of plausible successor predicates. Those successor predicates for the most simple forms of phenomenal content should at least preserve the original descriptive potential and, on an empirical level, enable us to proceed further in isolating the minimally sufficient neural and "functional" correlates of the most simple forms of conscious experience (for the notion of a "minimally sufficient neural correlate," see Chalmers 2000). Therefore, in section 2.4.4, I offer a successor concept for qualia in the sense of the most *simple* form of phenomenal content and argue that the logical identity criteria for *this* concept cannot be found in introspection, but only through neuroscientific research. Those readers who are only interested in the two concepts of "mental presentation" and "phenomenal presentation," therefore, can skip the next three sections.

2.4.1   What Is a Quale?

During the past two decades, the purely philosophical discussion of qualia has been greatly intensified and extended, and has transgressed the boundaries of the discipline.[37] This positive development, however, has simultaneously led to a situation in which the concept of a "quale" has suffered from semantic inflation. It is more and more often used in too vague a manner, thereby becoming the source of misunderstandings not only between the disciplines but even within philosophy of mind itself (for a classic frontal attack, see Dennett 1988). Also, during the course of the history of ideas in philosophy, from Aristotle to Peirce, a great variety of different meanings and semantic precursors appeared.[38] This already existing net of implicit theoretical connotations, in turn, influences the current debate and, again, frequently leads to further confusion in the way the concept is being used. For this reason, it has today become important to be clear about what one actually discusses, when speaking of qualia. The classic locus for the discussion of the twentieth century can be found in Clarence Irving Lewis. For Lewis, qualia were *subjective universals*:

There *are* recognizable qualitative characters of the given, which may be repeated in different experiences, and are thus sort of universals; I call these "qualia." But although such qualia are universals, in the sense of being recognized from one to another experience, they must be distinguished from the properties of objects. . . . The quale is directly intuited, given, and is not the subject of any possible error because it is purely subjective. The property of an object is objective; the ascription

37. Extensive references can be found in sections 1.1, 3.7, 3.8, and 3.9 of Metzinger and Chalmers 1995; see also the updated electronic version of Metzinger 2000d.

38. Peter Lanz gives an overview of different philosophical conceptions of "secondary qualities" in Galileo. Hobbes, Descartes, Newton, Boyle, and Locke, and the classic figures of argumentation tied to them and their systematic connections (Lanz 1996, chapter 3). Nick Humphrey develops a number of interesting considerations starting from Thomas Reid's differentiation between perception and sensation (Humphrey 1992, chapter 4).

of it is a judgment, which may be mistaken; and what the predication of it asserts is something which transcends what could be given in any single experience. (C. I. Lewis 1929, p. 121)

For Lewis it is clear, right from the beginning, that we possess introspective identity criteria for qualia: they can be *recognized* from one experiential episode to the next. Also, qualia form the intrinsic core of all subjective states. This core is inaccessible to any relational analysis. It is therefore also ineffable, because its phenomenal content cannot be transported to the space of public systems of communication. Only statements about objective properties can be falsified. Qualia, however, are phenomenal, that is, *subjective* properties:

Qualia are subjective; they have no names in ordinary discourse but are indicated by some circumlocution such as "looks like"; they are ineffable, since they might be different in two minds with no possibility of discovering that fact and no necessary inconvenience to our knowledge of objects or their properties. All that can be done to designate a quale is, so to speak, to locate it in experience, that is, to designate the conditions of its recurrence or other relations of it. Such location does not touch the quale itself; if one such could be lifted out of the network of *its* relations, in the total experience of the individual, and replaced by another, no social interest or interest of action would be affected by such substitution. What is essential for understanding and for communication is not the quale as such but that pattern of its stable relations in experience which is implicitly predicated when it is taken as the sign of an objective property. (C. I. Lewis 1929, p. 124*ff.*)

In this sense, a quale is a first-order property, as grasped from the first-person perspective, in subjective experience itself. A first-order property is a simple object property, and not a higher-order construct, like, for instance, a property of another *property*. The fact of Lewis himself being primarily interested in the most simple form of phenomenal content can also be seen from the examples he used.[39] We can, therefore, say: The canonical definition of a quale is that of a "first-order property" as phenomenally represented.[40] From this narrow definition, it immediately follows that the instantiation of

39. For example, "In any presentation, this content is either a specific quale (such as the immediacy of redness or loudness) or something analyzable into a complex of such" (cf. Lewis 1929, p. 60).

40. By choosing this formulation, I am following a strategy that has been called the "hegemony of representation" by Bill Lycan. This strategy consists in a weak variant of Franz Brentano's intentionalism. The explanatory base for *all* mental properties is formed by a certain, exhaustive set of functional and representational properties of the system in question (cf. Lycan 1996, p. 11). Lycan, as well, opposes any softening of the concept of a quale and pleads for a strict definition in terms of a first-order phenomenal property (see, e.g., Lycan 1996, p. 69*f.*, n. 3, p. 99*f.*). One important characteristic of Lycan's use of the term is an empirically very plausible claim, namely, that simple sensory content can also be causally activated and causally active *without* an accompanying episode of conscious experience corresponding to it. The logical subjects for the ascription of first-order phenomenal properties are, for Lycan, intentionally inexistents in a Brentanoian sense. My own intuition is that, strictly speaking, neither phenomenal properties nor phenomenal individuals—if real or intentionally inexistent—exist. What do exist are holistic, functionally integrated complexions of subcategorical content, active feature detectors episodically bound into a coherent microfunctional whole through synchronization processes in the brain. I have called such integrated wholes "phenomenal holons" (Metzinger 1995b). In describing them

such a property is always relative to a certain class of representational systems: Bats construct their phenomenal model of reality from different basic properties than human beings because they embody a different representational architecture. Only systems possessing an identical architecture can, through their sensory perceptions, exemplify identical qualities and are then able to introspectively access them as primitive elements of their subjective experience. Second, from an epistemological point of view, we see that phenomenal properties are something very different from physical properties. There is no one-to-one mapping. This point was of great importance for Lewis:

The identifiable character of presented qualia is *necessary to* the predication of objective properties and to the recognition of objects, but it is not *sufficient for* the verification of what such predication and recognition implicitly assert, both because what is thus asserted transcends the given and has the significance of the prediction of further possible experience, and because the *same* property may be validly predicated on the basis of *different* presented qualia, and *different* properties may be signalized by the *same* presented quale. (C. I. Lewis 1929, p. 131; emphasis in original)

In sum, in this canonical sense, the classic concept of a quale refers to a special form of mental content, for which it is true that

1. Subjective identity criteria are available, by which we can introspectively recognize their transtemporal identity;

2. It is a maximally simple, and experientially concrete (i.e., maximally *determinate*) form of content, without any inner structural features;

3. It brings about the instantiation of a first-order nonphysical property, a *phenomenal* property;

4. There is no systematic one-to-one mapping of those subjective properties to objective properties;

5. It is being grasped directly, intuitively, and in an epistemically immediate manner;

6. It is subjective in being grasped "from the first-person perspective";

7. It possesses an intrinsic phenomenal core, which, analytically, cannot be dissolved into a network of relations; and

8. Judgments about this form of mental content cannot be false.

---

as individuals and by then "attaching" properties to them we import the ontology underlying the grammar of natural language into another, and much older, representational system. For this reason, it might be possible that no form of abstract analysis which decomposes phenomenal content into an individual component (the logical subject) and the property component (the phenomenal properties ascribed to this logical subject) can really do justice to the enormous subtlety of our target phenomenon. Possibly the grammar of natural languages just cannot be mapped onto the representational deep structure of phenomenal consciousness. All we currently know about the representational dynamics of human brains points to an "internal ontology" that does not know anything like fixed, substantial individuals or invariant, intrinsic properties. Here, however, I only investigate this possibility with regard to the most *simple* forms of phenomenal content.

Of course, there will be only a few philosophers who agree with precisely this concept of a quale. On the other hand, within the recent debate, no version of the qualia concept can, from a systematic point of view, count as its *paradigmatic* expression. For this reason, from now on, I will take Lewis's concept to be the canonical concept and as my starting point in the following. I do this purely for pragmatic reasons, only to create a solid base for the current investigation. Please note that for this limited enterprise, it is only the first two defining characteristics of the concept (the existence of transtemporal identity criteria plus maximal simplicity), which are of particular relevance. However, I briefly return to the concept as a whole at the end of section 2.4.4.

2.4.2   Why Qualia Don't Exist

Under the assumption of qualitative content being the most *simple* form of content, one can now claim that qualia (as originally conceived of by Clarence Irving Lewis) do not exist. The theoretical entity introduced by what I have called the "canonical concept of a quale" can safely be eliminated. In short, qualia *in this sense* do not exist and never have existed. Large portions of the philosophical debate have overlooked a simple, empirical fact: the fact that for almost all of the most simple forms of qualitative content, we do not possess any introspective identity criteria, in terms of the notion of introspection$_2$, that is, in terms of cognitively referring to elementary features of an internal model of reality. Diana Raffman has clearly worked this out. She writes:

It is a truism of perceptual psychology and psychophysics that, with rare exceptions [Footnote: The exceptions are cases of so-called categorical perception; see Repp 1984 and Harnad 1987 for details], discrimination along perceptual dimensions surpasses identification. In other words, our ability to judge whether two or more stimuli are the same or different in some perceptual respect (pitch or color, say) far surpasses our ability to type-identify them. As Burns and Ward explain, "[s]ubjects can typically discriminate many more stimuli than they can categorize on an absolute basis, and the discrimination functions are smooth and monotonic" (see Burns and Ward 1977, p. 457). For instance, whereas normal listeners can discriminate about 1400 steps of pitch difference across the audible frequency range (Seashore 1967, p. 60), they can type-identify or recognize pitches as instances of only about eighty pitch categories (constructed from a basic set of twelve). [Footnote: Burns and Ward 1977, 1982; Siegel and Siegel 1977a, b, for example. Strictly speaking, only listeners with so-called perfect pitch can identify pitches per se; listeners (most of us) with relative pitch can learn to identify musical *intervals* if certain cues are provided. This complication touches nothing in the present story.] In the visual domain, Leo Hurvich observes that "there are many fewer absolutely identifiable [hues] than there are discriminable ones. Only a dozen or so hues can be used in practical situations where absolute identification is required" (Hurvich 1981, p. 2). Hurvich cites Halsey and Chapanis in this regard:

. . . the number of spectral [hues] which can be easily identified is very small indeed compared to the number that can be discriminated 50 percent of the time under ideal laboratory conditions. In the range from 430 to 650 [nm], Wright estimates that there are upwards of 150 discriminable wavelengths. Our experiments show that less than one-tenth this number of hues can be distinguished when observers are required to identify the hues singly and with nearly perfect accuracy. (Halsey and Chapanis 1951: 1058)

The point is clear: we are much better at discriminating perceptual values (i.e., making same/ different judgments) than we are at identifying or recognizing them. Consider for example two just noticeably different shades of red—red_{31} and red_{32}, as we might call them. *Ex hypothesis* we can tell them apart in a context of pairwise comparison, but we cannot recognize them—cannot identify them as red_{31} and red_{32}, respectively—when we see them. (Raffman 1995, p. 294*ff.*)

In what follows, I base my considerations on Diana Raffman's representation and her interpretation of the empirical data, explicitly referring readers to the text just mentioned and the sources given there. If parts of the data or parts of her interpretation should prove to be incorrect, this will be true for the corresponding parts of my argument. Also, for the sake of simplicity, I limit my discussion to human beings in standard situations and to the phenomenal primitives activated within the visual modality, and to color vision in particular. In other words, let us for now restrict the discussion to the *chromatic* primitives contributing to the phenomenal experience of standard observers. Raffman's contribution is important, partly because it directs our attention to the limitations of perceptual memory—*the memory constraint.* The notion of a "memory constraint" introduced by Raffman possesses high relevance for understanding the difference between the attentional and cognitive variants of introspection already introduced. What Raffman has shown is the existence of a shallow level in subjective experience that is so subtle and fine-grained that—although we can *attend* to informational content presented on this level—it is neither available for memory nor for cognitive access in general. Outside of the phenomenal "Now" there is no type of subjective access to this level of content. However, we are, nevertheless, confronted with a disambiguated and maximally determinate form of phenomenal content. We cannot—this seems to be the central insight—achieve any epistemic progress with regard to this most subtle level of phenomenal nuances, by persistently extending the classic strategy of analytical philosophy into the domain of mental states, stubbornly claiming that basically there must be some form of linguistic content as well, and even analyzing phenomenal content *itself* as if it were a type of conceptual or syntactically structured content—for instance, as if the subjective states in question were brought about by predications or demonstrations directed to a first-order perceptual state from the first-person perspective.[41] The value of Raffman's argument consists in precisely

41. Cf. Lycan, 1990; 1996; Loar 1990; and Raffman's critique of these strategies, especially in sections 2, 4, and 5 of Raffman 1995. What George Rey has called CRTQ, the *c*omputational *r*epresentational *t*heory of *t*hought and *q*ualitative states, is a further example of essentially the same strategy. Sensory content is here "intentionalized" in accordance with Brentano and on a theoretical level being assimilated into a certain class of propositional attitudes. However, if one follows this line, one cannot understand anymore what a sensory predication, according to Rey, would be, the output of which would, for principled reasons, not be available anymore to a

marking the point at which the classic, analytical strategy is confronted with a principled obstacle. In other words, either we succeed at this point in handing the qualia problem over to the empirical sciences, or the project of a naturalist theory of consciousness faces major difficulties.

Why is this so? There are three basic kinds of properties by which we can conceptually grasp mental states: their representational or intentional content; their functional role as defined by their causal relations to input, output, and to other internal states; and by their phenomenal or experiential content. The central characteristic feature in individuating mental states is their phenomenal content: the way in which they *feel* from a first-person perspective. Long before Brentano ([1874] 1973) clearly formulated the problem of intentionality, long before Turing (1950) and Putnam (1967) introduced functionalism as a philosophical theory of mind, human beings successfully communicated about their mental states. In particular, generations of philosophers theorized about the mind without making use of the conceptual distinction between intentional and phenomenal content. From a genetic perspective, phenomenal content is the more fundamental notion. But even today, dreams and hallucinations, that is, states that arguably possess no intentional content, can reliably be individuated by their phenomenal content. Therefore, for the project of a naturalist theory of mind, it is decisive to first of all analyze the most *simple* forms of this special form of mental content, in order to then be capable of a step-by-step construction and understanding of more complex combinations of such elementary forms. The most simple forms of phenomenal content themselves, however, cannot be *introspectively*$_2$ individuated, because, for these forms of content, beings like ourselves do not possess any transtemporal identity criteria. A fortiori we cannot form any logical identity criteria which could be anchored in introspective experience itself and enable us to form the corresponding phenomenal concepts. Neither introspective experience, nor cognitive processes operating on the output of perceptual memory, nor philosophical, conceptual analysis taking place within intersubjective space seems to enable a retrospective epistemic access to these most simple forms of content once they have disappeared from the conscious present. The primitives of the phenomenal system of representation are epistemically unavailable to the cognitive subject of consciousness (see also section 6.4.4). I will soon offer some further comments about the difference between transtemporal and logical identity criteria for phenomenal states and concepts. Before doing so, let us prevent a first possible misunderstanding.

---

computationally modeled type of cognition (the *comp-thinking system*) or to a computationally interpreted judgment system (*comp-judged*). But it is exactly that kind of state, which, as the empirical material now shows, really forms the target of our enterprise. Cf. George Rey's contribution in Esken and Heckmann 1998, section 2, in particular.

Of course, something like schemata, temporarily stable psychological structures generating phenomenal types, *do* exist, and thereby make categorical color information available for thought and language. Human beings certainly possess color schemata. However, the point at issue is not the ineffability of phenomenal types. This was the central point in Thomas Nagel's early work (Nagel 1974). Also, the crucial point is not the *particularity* of the most simple forms of phenomenal content; the current point is not about what philosophers call *tropes*.[42] The core issue is the ineffability, the introspective and cognitive impenetrability of phenomenal *tokens*. We do not—this is Raffman's terminology— possess phenomenal *concepts* for the most subtle nuances of phenomenal content: we possess a phenomenal concept of red, but no phenomenal concept of red_{32}, a phenomenal concept of turquoise, but not of $turquoise_{57}$. Therefore, we are not able to carry out a mental type identification for these most simple forms of sensory concepts. This kind of type identification, however, is precisely the capacity underlying the *cognitive* variants of introspection, namely $introspection_2$ and $introspection_4$. Introspective cognition directed at a currently active content of one's conscious color experience must be a way of mentally forming concepts. Concepts are always something under which multiple elements can be subsumed. Multiple, temporarily separated tokenings of $turquoise_{57}$, however, due to the limitation of our perceptual memory, cannot, in principle, be conceptually grasped and integrated into cognitive space. In its subtlety, the pure "suchness" of the finest shades of conscious color experience is only accessible to attention, but not to cognition. In other words, we are not able to phenomenally *re*present such states *as such*. So the problem precisely does not consist in that the very special content of those states, as experienced from the first-person perspective, cannot find a suitable expression in a certain natural language. It is not the unavailability of external color predicates. The problem consists in the fact of beings with our psychological structure and in most perceptual contexts not being able to recognize this content *at all*. In particular, the empirical evidence demonstrates that the classic interpretation of simple phenomenal content as an instantiation of phenomenal properties, a background assumption based on a careless conceptual interpretation of introspective experience, has been false. To every property at least one concept, one predicate on a certain level of description, corresponds. If a physical concept successfully grasps a certain property, this property is a physical property. If a phenomenological concept successfully grasps a certain property, this property is a *phenomenal* property. Of course, something can be the instantiation of a physical and a phenomenal property at the same time, as multiple descriptions on different levels may all be true of one and the same target

---

42. Tropes are particularized properties which (as opposed to universals) cannot be instantiated in multiple individuals at the same time. Tropes can be used in defining individuals, but just like them, only exist as particulars.

property (see chapter 3). However, if, relative to a certain class of systems, a certain phenomenological concept of a certain target property can *in principle* never be formed, this property is not a phenomenal property.

A property is a cognitive construct, which only emerges as the result of an achievement of successful recall and categorization, transcending perceptual memory. *Qualia* in this sense of a *phenomenal* property are cognitive structures reconstructed from memory and, for this reason, can be functionally individuated. Of course, the activation of a color schema, itself, will also become phenomenally represented and will constitute a separate form of phenomenal content, which we might want to call "categorical perceptual content." If, however, we point to an object experienced as colored and say, "This piece of cloth is dark indigo!," then we refer to an aspect of our subjective experience, which precisely is *not* a phenomenal property for us, because we cannot remember it. Whatever this aspect is, it is only a content of the capacity introduced as introspection$_1$, not a possible object of introspection$_2$.

The internal target state, it seems safe to say, certainly possesses *informational* content. The information carried by it is available for attention and online motor control, but it is not available for cognition. It can be functionally individuated, but not introspectively. For this reason, we have to semantically differentiate our "canonical" concept of qualia. We need a theory about *two*—as we will see, maybe even more—forms of sensory phenomenal content. One form is *categorizable* sensory content, as, for instance, represented by pure phenomenal colors like yellow, green, red, and blue; the second form is subcategorical sensory content, as formed by all *other* color nuances. The beauty and the relevance of this second form lie in that it is so subtle, so volatile as it were, that it evades cognitive access in principle. It is nonconceptual content.

What precisely does it mean to say that one type of sensory content is more "simple" than another one? There must be at least one constraint which it doesn't satisfy. Recall that my argument is restricted to the chromatic primitives of color vision, and that it aims at maximally determinate forms of color experience, not at any abstract features, but at the glorious concreteness of these states as such. It is also important to note how this argument is limited in its scope, even for simple color experience: in normal observers, the pure colors of red, yellow, green, and blue *can*, as a matter of fact, be conceptually grasped and recognized; the absolutely pure versions of chromatic primitives *are* cognitively available. If "simplicity" is interpreted as the conjunction of "maximal determinacy" and "lack of attentionally available internal structure," all conscious colors are the same. Obviously, on the level of content, we encounter the same concreteness and the same structureless "density" (in philosophy, this is called the "grain problem"; see Sellars 1963; Metzinger 1995b, p. 430*ff.*; and section 3.2.10) in both forms. What unitary hues and ineffable shades differ in can now be spelled out with the help of the very first conceptual constraint for the ascription of conscious experience which I offered at the beginning of this chapter: it is the *degree of global availability*. The lower the degree of constraint satisfaction, the higher the simplicity as here intended.

We can imagine simple forms of sensory content—and this would correspond to the classic Lewisian concept of qualia, which are globally available for attention, mental concept formation, and different types of motor behavior such as speech production and pointing movements. Let us call all maximally determinate sensory content on the three-constraint level "Lewis qualia" from now on. A more simple form would be the same content which just possesses *two* out of these three functional properties—for instance, it could be attentionally available, and available for motor behavior in discrimination tasks, like pointing to a color sample, but not available for cognition. Let us call this type "Raffman qualia" from now on. It is the most interesting type on the two-constraint level, and part of the relevance and merit of Raffman's contribution consists in her having pointed this out so convincingly. Another possibility would be that it is only available for the guidance of attention and for cognition, but evades motor control, although this may be a situation that is hard to imagine. At least in healthy (i.e., nonparalyzed) persons we rarely find situations in which representational content is conscious in terms of being a possible object of attentional processing and thought, while not being an element of behavioral space, something the person can also *act* upon. Even in a fully paralyzed person, the accommodation of the lenses or saccadic eye movements certainly would have to count as residual motor behavior. However, if the conscious content in question is just the content of an imagination or of a future plan, that is, if it is mental content, which does not strictly covary with properties of the immediate environment of the system anymore, it certainly is something that we would call conscious because it is available for guiding attention and for cognitive processing, but it is not available for motor control simply because its representandum is not an element of our current behavioral space. However, if thinking itself should one day turn out to be a refined *version* of motor control (see sections 6.4.5 and 6.5.3), the overall picture might change considerably. It is interesting to note how such an impoverished "two-constraint version" already exemplifies the target property of "phenomenality" in a weaker sense; it certainly makes good intuitive sense to speak of, for instance, subtle nuances of hues or of imaginary conscious contents as being *less* conscious. They are less *real*. And Raffman qualia are elements of our phenomenal reality, but not of our cognitive world.

I find it hard to conceive of the third possibility on the two-constraint level, a form of sensory content that is more simple than Lewis qualia in terms of being available for motor control and cognitive processing, but *not* for guiding attention. And this may indeed be an insight into a domain-specific kind of nomological necessity. Arguably, a machine might have this kind of conscious experience, one that is exclusively tied to a *cognitive* first-person perspective. In humans, attentional availability seems to be the most basic, the minimal constraint that has to be satisfied for conscious experience to occur. Subtle, ineffable nuances, hues (as attentionally and behaviorally available), and imaginary conscious contents (as attentionally and cognitively available), however, seem to be actual and distinct phenomenal state classes. The central insight at this point is that as soon as one has a more detailed catalogue of conceptual constraints for the notion of conscious representation, it certainly makes sense to speak of *degrees* of consciousness, and it is perfectly meaningful and rational to do so—as soon as one is able to point out in which respect a certain element of our conscious mind is "less" conscious than another one. The machine just mentioned or a lower animal possessing *only* Raffman qualia would each be less conscious than a system endowed with Lewisian sensory experience.

Let me, in passing, note another highly interesting issue. From the first-person perspective, degrees of availability are experienced as degrees of "realness." The most subtle content of color experience and the conscious content entering our minds through processes like imagination or planning are also less *real* than others, and they are so in a distinct phenomenological sense. They are less firmly integrated into our subjective reality because there are fewer internal methods of access available to us. The lower the degree of global availability, the lower the degree of phenomenal "worldliness."

Let us now move down one further step. An even simpler version of phenomenal content would be one that is attentionally available, but ineffable and not accessible to cognition, as well as not available for the generation of motor output. It would be very hard to narrow down such a simple form of phenomenal content by the methods of scientific research. How would one design replicable experiments? Let us call such states "Metzinger qualia." A good first example may be presented by very brief episodes of extremely subtle changes in bodily sensation or, in terms of the representation of external reality, shifts in nonunitary color experience during states of open-eyed, deep meditation. In all their phenomenal subtlety, such experiential transitions would be difficult targets from a methodological perspective. If all cognitive activity has come to rest and there is no observable motor output, all one can do to pin down the physical correlate of such subtle, transitory states in the dynamics of the purely attentional first-person perspective (see sections 6.4.3 and 6.5.1) would be to directly scan brain activity. However, such phenomenal transitions will not be *reportable* transitions, because mentally categorizing them and reactivating motor control for generating speech output would immediately destroy them. Shifts in Metzinger qualia, by definition, cannot be verified by the experiential subject herself using her motor system, verbally or nonverbally.

It is important to note how a certain kind of conscious content that appears as "weakly" conscious under the current constraint may turn out to actually be a *strongly* conscious state when adding further conceptual constraints, for instance, the degree to which it is experienced as *present* (see section 3.2.2 in chapter 3). For now, let us remain on the one-constraint level a little bit longer. There are certainly further interesting, but only weakly conscious types of information in terms of only being globally available to very fast, but nevertheless flexible and selective behavioral reactions, as in deciding in which way to catch a ball that is rapidly flying toward you. There may be situations in which the overall event takes place in much too fast a manner for you to be able to direct your attention or cognitive activity toward the approaching ball. However, as you decide on and settle into a specific kind of reaching and grasping behavior, there may simultaneously be aspects of your ongoing motor control which are weakly conscious in terms of being selective and flexible, that is, which are not *fully* automatic. Such "motor qualia" would then be the second example of weak sensory content on the one-constraint level. Motor qualia are simple forms of sensory content that are available for selective motor control, but not for attentional or cognitive processing (for a neuropsychological case study, see Milner and Goodale 1995, p. 125*ff.*; see also Goodale and Milner 1992). Assuming the existence of motor qualia as exclusively "available for flexible action control" implies the assumption of subpersonal processes of response selection and decision making, of agency beyond the attentional or cognitive first-person perspective. The deeper philosophical issue is whether this is at all a coherent idea. It also brings us back to our previous question concerning the third logical possibility. Are there conscious contents that are only available for cognition, but not for attention or motor control? Highly abstract forms of consciously experienced mental content, as they sometimes appear in the minds of mathematicians and philosophers, may constitute an interesting example: imagining a certain, highly specific set of possible worlds generates something you cannot physically act upon, and something to which you could not attend before you actively *constructed* it in the process of thought. Does "construction" in this sense imply availability for action control? For complex, conscious thoughts in particular, it is an interesting phenomenological observation that you cannot let your attention (in terms of the concept of introspection₃ introduced earlier) *rest* on them, as you would let your attention rest on a sensory object, without immediately dissolving the content in question, making it disappear from the conscious self. It is as if the construction process, the genuinely cognitive activity itself, has to be continuously kept alive (possibly in terms of recurrent types of higher-order cognition as represented by the process of introspection₄) and is not able to bear any distractions produced by other types of mechanisms trying to access the same object at the same time. Developing a convincing phenomenology of complex, rational thought is a difficult project, because the process of introspection itself tends to destroy its target object. This observation in itself, however, may be taken as a way of explaining what it means that phenomenal states, which are exclusively accessible to cognition only, can be said to be *weakly* conscious states:

"Cognitive qualia" (as opposed to Metzinger qualia) are not attentionally available, and not available for direct action control (as opposed to motor qualia).

Let us now return to the issue of sensory primitives. We can also imagine simple sensory content which does not fulfill any of these three criteria, which is just *mental* presentational content (for the notion of "presentational content," see section 2.4.4), but not phenomenal presentational content. According to our working definition, such content *can* become globally available, but it *is* not currently globally available for attention, cognition, or action control. As a matter of fact there are good reasons to believe that such types of mental content actually do exist, and at the end of this chapter I present one example of such content. There is an interesting conclusion, to which the current considerations automatically lead: saying that a specific form of simple sensory content is, in terms of its functional profile, "simpler" than a comparable type of sensory content, does not mean that it is less *determinate*. In experiencing a certain, subtle shade of turquoise it does not matter if we only meditatively attend to it in an effortless, cognitively silent manner, or if we discriminate different samples by pointing movements in the course of a scientific experiment, or if we actually attempt to apply a phenomenal concept to it. In all these cases, according to subjective experience itself, the specific sensory value (e.g., its position in the hue dimension) always stays the same in terms of being maximally disambiguated.

Phenomenal content, on the most fine-grained level[43] of subjective representation, always is fully determined content. For color, there are only a few exceptions for which this fully determinate content is also cognitively available content. I have already mentioned them: a pure phenomenal red, containing no phenomenal blue or yellow; a pure blue, containing no green or red; and a pure yellow and a pure green are phenomenal colors for which, as a matter of fact, we possess what Raffman calls "phenomenal concepts" (Raffman 1995, p. 358, especially nn. 30 and 31; see also, Austen Clark 1993; Metzinger and Walde 2000). Empirical investigations show that for these pure examples of their phenomenal families we are very well able to carry out mental reidentifications. For *those* examples of pure phenomenal content we actually do possess transtemporal identity criteria allowing us to form mental categories. The degree of determinacy, however, is equal for all states of this kind: introspectively we do not experience a difference in the degree of determinacy between, say, pure yellow and yellow$_{280}$. This is why it is impossible to argue that such states are determinable, but not determinate, or to claim

---

43. In an earlier monograph, Raffman had denoted this level as the "n-level," the level of phenomenal "nuances." On the level of nuances we find the most shallow and "raw" representation (e.g., of a musical signal), to which the hearing subject has conscious access. "N-level representations" are nongrammatical and nonstructured phenomenal representations. Cf., e.g., Raffman 1993, p. 67 *ff.*

that, ultimately, our experience is just as fine-grained as the concepts with the help of which we grasp our perceptual states. This line of argument does not do justice to the real phenomenology. Because of the limitation of our perceptual memory (and even if something as empirically implausible as a "language of thought" should really exist), for most of these states it is impossible, in principle, to carry out a successful subjective reidentification. To speak in Kantian terms, on the lowest, and most subtle level of phenomenal experience, as it were, only intuition (*Anschauung*) and not concepts (*Begriffe*) exist.[44] Yet there is no difference in the degree of *determinacy* pertaining to the simple sensory content in question. In Diana Raffman's words:

Furthermore, a quick look at the full spectrum of hues shows that our experiences of these unique hues are no different, in respect of their "determinateness," from those of the non-unique hues: among other things, the unique hues do not appear to "stand out" from among the other discriminable hues in the way one would expect if our experience of them were more determinate. On the contrary, the spectrum appears more or less continuous, and any discontinuities that do appear lie near category boundaries rather than central cases. In sum, since our experiences of unique and non-unique hues are introspectively similar in respect of their determinateness, yet conceptualized in radically different ways, introspection of these experiences cannot be explained (or explained exhaustively) in conceptual terms. In particular, it is not plausible to suppose that any discriminable hue, unique or otherwise, is experienced or introspected in a less than determinate fashion. (Raffman 1995, p. 302)

Does this permit the conclusion that this level of sensory consciousness is in a Kantian sense epistemically blind? Empirical data certainly seem to show that simple phenomenal content is something about which we can very well be wrong. For instance, one can be wrong about its transtemporal identity: there seems to exist yet another, higher-order form of phenomenal content. This is the subjective experience of *sameness*, and it now looks as if this form of content is not always a form of *epistemically justified* content.[45] It does not necessarily constitute a form of knowledge. In reality, all of us are permanently making identity judgments about pseudocategorical forms of sensory content, which—as now becomes obvious—strictly speaking are only epistemically justified in very few cases. For the large majority of cases it will be possible to say the following: Phenomenal

---

44. Please note how there seems to be an equally "weakly conscious" level of subjective experience (given by the phenomenology of complex, rational thought mentioned above) which seems to consist of conscious concept formation only, devoid of any sensory component. The Kantian analogy, at this point, would be to say that such processes, as representing concepts without intuition, are not blind but *empty*.

45. At this stage it becomes important to differentiate between the phenomenal experience of sameness and sameness as the intentional content of mental representations. Ruth Garrett Millikan (1997) offers an investigation of the different possibilities a system can use for itself in marking the identities of properties on the mental level, while criticizing attempts to conceive of "identity" as a nontemporal abstractum independent of the temporal dynamics of the real representational processes, with the help of which it is being grasped.

experience interprets nontransitive indiscriminability relations between particular events or tokenings as genuine equivalence relations. This point already occupied Clarence Irving Lewis. It may be interesting, therefore, and challenging to have a second look at the corresponding passage in this new context, the context constituted by the phenomenal experience of *sameness*:

> Apprehension of the presented quale, being immediate, stands in no need of verification; it is impossible to be mistaken about it. Awareness of it is not judgment in any sense in which judgment may be verified; it is not knowledge in any sense in which "knowledge" connotes the opposite of error. It may be said, that the recognition of the quale is a judgment of the type, "This is the same ineffable 'yellow' that I saw yesterday." At the risk of being boresome, I must point out that there is room for subtle confusion in interpreting the meaning of such a statement. If what is meant by predicating sameness of the quale today and yesterday should be the immediate comparison of the given with a memory image, then certainly there is such comparison and it may be called "judgement" if one choose; all I would point out is that, like the awareness of a single presented quale, such comparison is immediate and indubitable; verification would have no meaning with respect to it. If anyone should suppose that such direct comparison is what is generally meant by judgement of qualitative identity between something experienced yesterday and something presented now, then obviously he would have a very poor notion of the complexity of memory as a means of knowledge. (Lewis 1929, p. 125)

Memory as a reliable means of epistemic progress, which is what the empirical material seems to show today, is not available with regard to all forms of phenomenal content. From a teleofunctionalist perspective this makes perfectly good sense: during the actual confrontation with a stimulus source it is advantageous to be able to utilize the great informational richness of directly stimulus-correlated perceptual states for discriminatory tasks. Memory is not needed. An organism, for example, when confronted with a fruit lying in the grass in front of it, must be able to quickly recognize it as ripe or as already rotten by its color or by its fragrance. However, from a strictly computational perspective, it would be uneconomical to take over the enormous wealth of direct sensory input into mental storage media beyond short-term memory: A reduction of sensory data flow obviously was a necessary precondition (for systems operating with limited internal resources) for the development of genuinely cognitive achievements. If an organism is able to phenomenally *re*present classes or prototypes of fruits and their corresponding colors and smells, thereby making them globally available for cognition and flexible control of behavior, a high information load will always be a handicap. Computational load has to be minimized as much as possible. Therefore, online control has to be confined to those situations in which it is strictly indispensable. Assuming the conditions of an evolutionary pressure of selection it would certainly be a disadvantage if our organism was forced or even only capable of being able to remember every single shade and every subtle scent it was able to discriminate with its senses when actually confronted with the fruit.

Interestingly, we humans do not seem to take note of this automatic limitation of our perceptual memory during the actual process of the permanent superposition of conscious perception and cognition that characterizes everyday life. The subjective *experience* of sameness between two forms of phenomenal content active at different points in time is itself characterized by a seemingly direct, immediate givenness. This is what Lewis pointed out. What we now learn in the course of empirical investigations is the simple fact that this higher-order form of phenomenal content, the conscious "sameness experience," may not be epistemically justified in many cases. In terms of David Chalmers's "dancing qualia" argument (Chalmers 1995) one might say that dancing qualia may well be impossible, but "slightly wiggling" color qualia may present a nomological possibility. Call this the "slightly wiggling qualia' hypothesis": Unattended-to changes of nonunitary hues to their next discriminable neighbor could be systematically undetectable by us humans. The empirical prediction corresponding to my philosophical analysis is *change blindness* for JNDs in nonunitary hues. What we experience in sensory awareness, strictly speaking, is subcategorical content. In most perceptual contexts it is therefore precisely not phenomenal *properties* that are being instantiated by our sensory mechanisms, even if an unreflected and deeply ingrained manner of speaking about our own conscious states may suggest this to us. It is more plausible to assume that the initial concept, which I have called the "canonical concept" of a quale at the beginning of this section, really refers to a higher-order form of phenomenal content that actually exists: Qualia, under this classic philosophical interpretation, are a *combination* of simple nonconceptual content and a subjective experience of transtemporal identity, which is epistemically justified in only very few perceptual contexts.

Now two important questions have to be answered: What is the relationship between logical and transtemporal identity criteria? What precisely are those "phenomenal concepts" which appear again and again in the philosophical literature? An answer to the first question could run as follows. Logical identity criteria are being applied on a metalinguistic level. A person can use such criteria to decide if she uses a certain name or concept, for instance, to refer to a particular form of color content, say, red_{31}. The truth conditions for identity statements of this kind are of a semantic nature. In the present case this means that the procedures to find out about the truth of such statements are to be found on the level of conceptual analysis. On the other hand, transtemporal identity criteria, in the second sense of the term, help a person on the "internal" object level, as it were, to differentiate if a certain concrete state—say the subjective experience of red_{31}—is the same as at an earlier point in time. The internal object level is the level of sensory consciousness. Here we are not concerned with use of linguistic expressions, but with *introspection₃*. We are not concerned with conceptual knowledge, but with attentional availability, the guidance of visual attention toward the nonconceptual content of certain sensory states or ongoing perceptual processes. Red_{31} or $turquoise_{64}$, the maximally determinate and simple phenomenal content of such states, is the object whose identity has to be determined over time. As this content typically is just presented as a subcategorical feature of a *perceptual* object, it is important to note now the concept of an "object" is only used in an epistemological sense at this point. The perceptual states or processes in question themselves are not of a conceptual or propositional nature, because they are not *cognitive* processes. On this second epistemic level we must be concerned with real continuities and constancies, with causal relations and lawlike regularities, under which objects of the type just mentioned may be subsumed. The metarepresentational criteria with the help of which the human nervous system, in some cases, can actually determine the transtemporal identity of such states "for itself," equally are not of a conceptual or propositional nature. They are *microfunctional* identity criteria—causal properties of concrete perceptual states—of which we may safely assume that evolutionarily they have proved to be successful and reliable. Obviously, on a subsymbolic level of representation, the respective kinds of systems have achieved a functionally adequate partitioning of the state space underlying the phenomenal representation of their physical domain of interaction. All this could happen in a nonlinguistic creature, lacking the capacity for forming concept-like structures, be it in a mental or in an external medium; $introspection_1$ and $introspection_3$ are *subsymbolic* processes of amplification and resource allocation, and not processes producing representational content in a conceptual format. Colors are not atoms, but "subcategorical formats," regions in state space characterized by their very own topological features. In simply attending to the colors of objects experienced as external, do we possess recognitional capacities? Does, for example, $introspection_1$ possess transtemporal identity criteria for chromatic primitives? The empirical material mentioned seems to show that for most forms of simple phenomenal content, and in most perceptual contexts, we do not even possess identity criteria of this second type. Our way of speaking about qualia as first-order phenomenal properties, however, tacitly presupposes precisely this. In other words, a certain simple form of mental content is being treated as if it were the result of a discursive epistemic achievement, where in a number of cases we only have a nondiscursive and, in the large majority of cases, perhaps not an epistemic achievement *at all.*

Let us now turn to the second question, regarding the notion of *phenomenal concepts*, frequently occurring in the recent literature (see Burge 1995, p. 591 *f.*; Raffman 1993, 1995 [giving further references], in press; Loar 1990; Lycan 1990; Rey 1993; Tye 1995, pp. 161 *ff.*, 174 *ff.*, 189 *ff.*; 1998, p. 468 *ff.*; 1999, p. 713 *ff.*; 2000, p. 26 *ff.*). First, one has to see that this is a terminologically unfortunate manner of speaking; of course; it is not the concepts *themselves* that are phenomenal. Phenomenal states are something concrete; concepts are something abstract. Therefore, one has to separate at least the following cases:

Case 1: Abstracta can form the content of phenomenal representations; for instance, if we subjectively experience our cognitive operation with existing concepts or the mental formation of new concepts.

Case 2: Concepts in a *mental* language of thought could (in a demonstrative or predicative manner) refer to the phenomenal content of other mental states. For instance, they could point or refer to primitive first-order phenomenal content, as it is episodically activated by sensory discrimination.

Case 3a: Concepts in a *public* language can refer to the phenomenal content of mental states: for example, to simple phenomenal content in the sense mentioned above. On an object level the logical identity criteria in using such expressions are *introspective experiences*, for instance, the subjective experience of *sameness* discussed above. Folk psychology or some types of philosophical phenomenology supply examples of such languages.

Case 3b: Concepts in a *public* language can refer to the phenomenal content of mental states: for instance, to simple phenomenal content. On a metalinguistic level, the logical identity criteria applied when using such concepts are publicly accessible properties, for instance, those of the neural *correlate* of this active, sensory content, or certain of its functional properties. One example of such a language could be given by a mathematical formalization of empirically generated data, for instance, by a vector analysis of the minimally sufficient neural activation pattern underlying a particular color experience.

Case 1 is not the topic of my current discussion. Case 2 is the object of Diana Raffman's criticism. I take this criticism to be very convincing. However, I will not discuss it any further—among other reasons because the assumption of a language of thought is, from an empirical point of view, so highly implausible. Case 3a presupposes that we can form rational and epistemically justified beliefs with regard to simple forms of phenomenal content, in which certain concepts then appear (for a differentiation between phenomenal and nonphenomenal beliefs, cf. Nida-Rümelin 1995). The underlying assumption is that formal, metalinguistic identity criteria for such concepts can exist. Here, the idea is that they rest on *material* identity criteria, which the person in question uses on the object level, in order to mark the *transtemporal* identity of these objects—in this case simple forms of active sensory content—for herself. The fulfillment of those material identity criteria, according to this assumption, is something that can be directly "read out" from subjective experience itself. This, the thinking is, works reliably because in our subjective experience of sensory sameness we carry out a phenomenal representation of this transtemporal identity on the object level in an automatic manner, which already carries its epistemic justification in itself. It is precisely this background assumption that is false for almost all cases of conscious color vision, and very likely in most other perceptual contexts as well;

the empirical material demonstrates that those transtemporal identity criteria are simply not available to us. It follows that the corresponding phenomenal concepts can *in principle* not be introspectively formed.

This is unfortunate because we now face a serious epistemic boundary. For many kinds of first-person mental content produced by our own sensory states, this content seems to be cognitively unavailable from the first-person perspective. To put it differently, the phenomenological approach in philosophy of mind, at least with regard to those simple forms of phenomenal content I have provisionally termed "Raffman qualia" and "Metzinger qualia," is condemned to failure. A descriptive psychology in Brentano's sense cannot come into existence with regard to almost all of the most simple forms of phenomenal content.

Given this situation, how can a further growth of knowledge be achieved? There may be a purely *episodic* kind of knowledge inherent to some forms of introspection$_1$ and introspection$_3$; as long as we closely attend to subtle shades of consciously experienced hues we actually do enrich the subsymbolic, nonconceptual form of higher-order mental content generated in this process. For instance, meditatively attending to such ineffable nuances of sensory consciousness—"dying into their pure suchness," as it were—certainly generates an interesting kind of additional knowledge, even if this knowledge cannot be transported out of the specious present. In academic philosophy, however, new concepts are what count. The only promising strategy for generating further epistemic progress in terms of *conceptual* progress is characterized by case 3b. The minimally sufficient neural and functional correlates of the corresponding phenomenal states can, at least in principle, if properly mathematically analyzed, provide us with the transtemporal, as well as the logical identity criteria we have been looking for. Neurophenomenology is possible; phenomenology is impossible. Please note how this statement is restricted to a limited and highly specific domain of conscious experience. For the most subtle and fine-grained level in sensory consciousness, we have to accept the following insight: Conceptual progress by a combination of philosophy and empirical research programs is possible; conceptual progress by introspection alone is impossible in principle.

2.4.3   An Argument for the Elimination of the Canonical Concept of a Quale

From the preceding considerations, we can develop a simple and informal argument to eliminate the classic concept of a quale. Please note that the scope of this argument extends only to Lewis qualia in the "recognitional" sense and under the interpretation of "simplicity" just offered. The argument:

1. *Background assumption*: A rational and intelligible epistemic goal on our way toward a theory of consciousness consists in working out a better understanding of the most simple forms of phenomenal content.

2. *Existence assumption*: Maximally simple, determinate, and disambiguated forms of phenomenal content do exist.

3. *Empirical premise*: For contingent reasons the intended class of representational systems in which this type of content is being activated possesses no transtemporal identity criteria for most of these simple forms of content. Hence, introspection$_1$, introspection$_3$, and the phenomenological method can provide us with neither transtemporal nor logical criteria of this kind.

4. *Conclusion*: Lewis qualia, in the sense of the "canonical" qualia concept of cognitively available first-order phenomenal properties, are not the most simple form of phenomenal content.

5. *Conclusion*: Lewis qualia, in the sense of the "canonical" qualia concept of maximally simple first-order phenomenal properties, do not exist.

My goal at this point is not an ontological elimination of qualia as conceived of by Clarence Irving Lewis. The epistemic goal is conceptual progress in terms of a convincing semantic differentiation. Our first form of simple content—*categorizable, cognitively available sensory content*—can be functionally individuated, because, for example, the activation of a color schema in perceptual memory is accompanied by system states, which, at least in principle, can be described by their causal role. At this point one might be tempted to think that the negated universal quantifier implicit in the second conclusion is unjustified, because at least *some* qualia in the classic Lewisian sense do exist. Pure red, pure green, pure yellow, and pure blue seem to constitute counterexamples, because we certainly possess recognitional phenomenal concepts for this kind of content, and they also count as a maximally *determinate* kind of content. However, recall that the notion of "simplicity" was introduced via degrees of global availability. Lewis qualia are states positioned on the three-constraint level, because they are attentionally, behaviorally, *and* cognitively available. As we have seen, there is an additional level of sensory content—let us again call it the level of "Raffman qualia"—that is only defined by two constraints, namely, availability for motor control (as in discrimination tasks) and availability for subsymbolic attentional processing (as in introspection$_1$ and introspection$_3$). There may even be an even more fine-grained type of conscious content—call them "Metzinger qualia"—characterized by fleeting moments of attentional availability only, yielding no capacities for motor control or cognitive processing. These distinctions yield the sense in which Lewis qualia are not the most simple forms of phenomenal content. However, there are good reasons to assume that strong Lewis qualia can be in principle functionally analyzed, because they will necessarily involve the activation of something like a color schema from perceptual memory. One can safely assume that they will have to be constituted by some kind of top-down process superimposing a prototype or other concept-like structure on the ongoing upstream process of sensory input, thereby making them recognizable states. Incidentally, the same may be true of the mental representation of sameness.

In the next step one can now epistemologically argue for the claim that especially those more simple forms of phenomenal content—that is, *noncategorizable*, but attentionally available forms of sensory content—are, in principle, accessible to a reductive strategy of explanation. In order to do so, one has to add a further epistemological premise:

1. *Background assumption*: A rational and intelligible epistemic goal on our way toward a theory of consciousness consists in working out a better understanding of the most simple forms of phenomenal content.

2. *Existence assumption*: Maximally simple, determinate, and disambiguated forms of phenomenal content do exist.

3. *Epistemological premise*: To theoretically grasp this form of content, logical identity criteria for concepts referring to it have to be determined. Any use of logical identity criteria always presupposes the possession of transtemporal identity criteria.

4. *Empirical premise*: The intended class of representational systems in which this form of content is being activated for contingent reasons possesses no transtemporal identity criteria for most maximally simple forms of sensory content. Hence, introspection and the phenomenological method can provide us with neither transtemporal nor logical criteria of this kind.

5. *Conclusion*: The logical identity criteria for concepts referring to this form of content can only be supplied by a different epistemic strategy.

A simple plausibility argument can then be added to this conclusion:

6. It is an empirically plausible assumption that transtemporal, as well as logical identity criteria can be developed from a third-person perspective, by investigating those properties of the minimally sufficient physical correlates of simple sensory content, which can be accessed by neuroscientific research (i.e., determining the minimally sufficient neural correlate of the respective content for a given class of organisms) or by functional analysis (i.e., mathematical modeling) of the causal role *realized* by these correlates. Domain-specific transtemporal and logical identity criteria can be developed from investigating the functional and physical correlates of simple content.[46]

7. The most simple forms of phenomenal content can be functionally individuated.

---

46. As I have pointed out, from a purely methodological perspective, this may prove to be impossible for Metzinger qualia. For Raffman qualia, it is of course much easier to operationalize the hypothesis, for example, using nonverbal discrimination tasks while scanning ongoing brain activity.

Now one clearly sees how our classic concept of qualia as the *most simple* forms of phenomenal content was incoherent and can be eliminated. Of course, this does not mean that—ontologically speaking—this simple phenomenal content, forming the epistemic goal of our investigation, does not *exist*. On the contrary, this type of simple, ineffable content does exist *and* there exist higher-order, functionally more rich forms of simple phenomenal content—for instance, *categorizable* perceptual content (Lewis qualia) or the experience of subjective "sameness" when instantly recognizing the pure phenomenal hues. Perhaps one can interpret the last two cases as a functionally rigid and automatic coupling of simple phenomenal content to, respectively, a cognitive and *metacognitive* schema or prototype. It is also not excluded that certain forms of epistemic access to elements at the basal level exist, which themselves, again, are of a nonconceptual nature and the results of which are in principle unavailable to motor control (Metzinger qualia). The perhaps more important case of Raffman qualia shows how the fact that something is cognitively unavailable does not imply that it also recedes from attention and behavioral control. However, it is much more important to first arrive at an informative analysis of what I have called "Raffman qualia," the one that we have erroneously interpreted as an exemplification of first-order *phenomenal* properties. As it now turns out, we *must* think of them as a neurodynamical or functional property, because this is the only way in which beings like ourselves *can think* about them. As all phenomenal content does, this content will exclusively supervene on internal and contemporaneous system properties, and the only way we can form a concept of it at all is from a third-person perspective, precisely by analyzing those internal functional properties reliably determining its occurrence. We therefore have to ask, About what have we been speaking in the past, when speaking about qualia? The answer to this question has to consist in developing a functionalist successor concept for the first of the three semantic components of the precursor concept just eliminated.

2.4.4   Presentational Content

In this section I introduce a new working concept: the concept of "presentational content." It corresponds to the third and last pair of fundamental notions, mental presentation and phenomenal presentation, which will complement the two concepts of mental versus conscious *representation* and mental versus conscious *simulation* introduced earlier. What are the major defining characteristics of *presentational* content? Presentational content is nonconceptual content, because it is cognitively unavailable. It is a way of possessing and using information without possessing a concept. It is subdoxastic content, because it is "inferentially impoverished" (Stich 1978, p. 507); the inferential paths leading from this kind of content to genuinely cognitive content are typically very limited. It is indexical content, because it "points" to its object in a certain perceptual context. It is also indexical content in a second, in a specifically *temporal* sense, because it is strictly confined to the experiential Now generated by the organism (see section 3.2.2). It is frequently and in all standard conditions tied to a phenomenal first-person perspective (see section 3.2.6). It constitutes a *narrow* form of content. Presentational content in its phenomenal variant supervenes on internal physical and functional properties of the system, although it is frequently bound to environmentally grounded content (see section 3.2.11). Presentational content is also homogeneous; it possesses no internal grain (see section 3.2.10).

Presentational content can contribute to the most simple form of phenomenal content. In terms of the conceptual distinction just drawn, it is typically located on the two-constraint level, with Raffman qualia being its paradigmatic example (I exclude Metzinger qualia and the one-constraint level from the discussion for now, but return to it later). The activation of presentational content results from a dynamical process, which I hereafter call mental *presentation* (box 2.6). What is mental presentation? Mental presentation is a physically realized process, which can be described by a three-place relation between a system, an internal state of that system, and a partition of the world. Under standard conditions, this process generates an internal state, a mental *presentatum*, the content of which signals the actual presence of a presentandum for the system (i.e., of an

Box 2.6

Mental Presentation: Pre_M (S, X, Y)

· S is an individual information-processing system.

· Y is an actual state of the world.

· X presents Y *for* S.

· X is a stimulus-correlated internal system state.

· X is a functionally internal system state.

· The intentional content of X can become available for introspection$_1$ and introspection$_3$. It possesses the potential of itself becoming the representandum of *subsymbolic* higher-order representational processes.

· The intentional content of X cannot become available for cognitive reference. It is *not* available as a representandum of *symbolic* higher-order representational processes.

· The intentional content of X can become globally available for the selective control of action.

---

element of a disjunction of physical properties forming no natural kind).[47] The presentandum, at least on the level of conscious experience, is always represented as a simple first-order object property. That is, presentational content never occurs alone; it is always integrated into a higher-order whole. More about this later (see section 3.2.4).

Epistemologically speaking, presentata are information-bearing states that certainly can *mispresent* elementary aspects of the environment or the system itself (see section 5.4) for the system, in terms of signaling the actual presence of such an aspect. However, they do not directly contribute to quasi-propositional forms of mental content generating truth and falsity. Presentational content is a nonconceptual form of mental content, which cannot be introspectively$_2$ categorized: "direct" cognitive reference to this content as such fails. The primary reason for this feature can be found in a functional property of the physical vehicles employed by the system in the process: the content of a presentatum is something which can only be sustained by constant input, and which cannot be *re*presented in its full informational content with the internal resources available to the system. Normally, presentata are always stimulus-correlated states,[48] which cannot be taken over into perceptual memory. Additionally, in standard situations their content is modality-specific. A conceptually attractive way of framing the characteristic "quality" belonging to different phenomenal families like sounds, colors, or smells is by describing them as *formats* of currently active data structures in the brain (Metzinger 1993; Mausfeld 1998, 2002): Consciously experienced colors, smells, and sounds come in particular formats; they are a *form of perception* the system imposes on the input. This format carries information about the sensory module generating the current state; if something is consciously experienced as being a color, a smell, or a sound, this simultaneously makes information about its causal history globally available. Implicitly and immediately it is now clear that the presentandum has been perceived by the eyes, through the nose, or with the help of the ears. Presentational content also is *active* content; active presentata are objects of our attention in all those situations in which we direct our attention to the phenomenal character of ongoing perceptual processes—that is, not toward *what* we are seeing, but to the fact that we are now *seeing* it. Although colors, for instance, are typically always integrated into a full-blown visual object, we can distinguish the color from the object to which it is "attached." The color itself, as a form of our *seeing* itself, however, cannot be decomposed in a similar manner by introspective attention. It is precisely the limited resolution of such metarepresentational processes that makes the presentational content on which they

47. With regard to the impossibility of straight one-to-one mapping of phenomenal qualities to physical properties, cf. Lanz 1996. See also Clark 2000.

48. This is true of those states as well in which the brain processes self-generated stimuli in sensory channels, for instance, in dreams or during other situations.

currently operate appear to us as *primitive* content, by necessity. Of course, this necessity is just a phenomenal kind of necessity; we simply have to *experience* this kind of sensory content as the rock-bottom level of our world, because introspection$_1$, the process generating it, cannot penetrate any deeper into the dynamics of the underlying process in our brains. Its subjectively experienced simplicity results from the given functional architecture and, therefore, is always relative to a certain class of systems.

Generally, there is now solid empirical support for the concept of perception without awareness, and it is becoming increasingly clear how two important functions of such non-phenomenal forms of perceptual processing consist in biasing *what* is experienced on the level of conscious experience and in influencing *how* stimuli perceived with awareness are actually consciously experienced (Merikle, Smilek, and Eastwood 2001). More specifically, it is now interesting to note how, again on a strictly empirical level, there are strong indications that in certain unusual perceptual contexts causally effective forms of *nonphenomenal* presentational content can be activated. It is tempting to describe such configurations as "unconscious color vision." In blindsight patients, for example, one can demonstrate a sensitivity for different wavelengths within the scotoma that not only correspond to the normal shape of the sensitivity curve but that—lacking any kind of accompanying subjective color experience—enable a successful discrimination of color stimuli with the help of (at least coarse-grained) predicates like "blue" or "red" formed in *normal* perceptual contexts (see Stoerig and Cowey 1992; Brent, Kennard, and Ruddock 1994; Barbur, Harlow, Sahraie, Stoerig, and Weiskrantz 1994; Weiskrantz 1997 gives a superb overview; for more on blindsight, see section 4.2.3). This, again, leads us to the conclusion that we have to differentiate between mental and phenomenal presentation, namely, in terms of degrees of global availability of stimulus information. It is also plausible to assume causal interactions (e.g., selection or biasing effects) between different kinds of stimulus-correlated perceptual content. Another conceptual differentiation, which is well suited for this context, is that between implicit and explicit color perception. At this point it becomes remarkably clear how searching for the most "simple" form of conscious content is an enterprise relative to a certain conceptual frame of reference. It is always relative to a set of conceptual constraints that a certain class of active informational content in the system will count as the "most simple," or even as phenomenal for that matter. Different conceptual frameworks lead to differently posed questions, and different experimental setups lead to different experimental answers to questions like, 'Does unconscious color vision exist?' or 'Are there invisible colors?' (for a recent example, see Schmidt 2000). However, let us not complicate matters too much at this point and stay with our first example of such a set of three simple constraints. As can be demonstrated in special perceptual contexts, for example, under laboratory conditions producing evidence for wavelength sensitivity in a blind spot of the visual field, we see how the respective type of information is still functionally active in the system. The causal role of the currently active presentatum remains remarkably unchanged while its phenomenal content disappears. However, I will not further discuss these data here (but see section 4.2.3). All we now need is a third conceptual tool that is as simple as possible but that can serve as a foundation for further discussion.

Let me offer such a third working concept: "Phenomenal presentation" or "phenomenal presentational content" could become successor concepts for what we, in the past, used to call "qualia" or "first-order phenomenal properties" (box 2.7). As we have seen above, there are "Lewis qualia," "Raffman qualia," and "Metzinger qualia" (with these three not exhausting logical space, but only identifying the phenomenologically most interesting terms). Lewis qualia present stimulus-correlated information in a way that fulfills all three subconstraints of global availability, namely, availability for cognition, attention, and action control, in a way that lacks any further introspectively accessible structure. Raffman qualia are located in the space of possibilities generated by only *two* subconstraints: they make their content available for discriminative behavior and for attentional processing in terms of introspection$_1$, but not for introspection$_2$. Metzinger qualia would be situated one level below—for instance, in terms of fleeting attentional episodes directed toward ineffable shades of consciously experienced color, which are so brief that they do not allow for selective motor behavior. For the purposes of the current investigation, however, I propose to stick with Diana Raffman's two-constraint version, because it picks out the

Box 2.7

Phenomenal Presentation: Pre$_P$ (S, X, Y)

· S is an individual information-processing system.

· Y is an actual state of the world.

· X presents Y *for* S.

· X is a stimulus-correlated internal system state.

· X is a functionally internal system state.

· The intentional content of X *is* currently available for introspection$_1$ and introspection$_3$. It possesses the potential of itself becoming the representandum of *subsymbolic* higher-order representational processes.

· The intentional content of X is *not* currently available for cognitive reference. It is *not* available as a representandum of *symbolic* higher-order representational processes.

· The intentional content of X *is* currently available for the selective control of action.

---

largest, and arguably also the intuitively most interesting class of simple sensory content. Raffman qualia may actually have formed the implicit background for much philosophical theorizing on qualia in the past.

Let us now proceed by further enriching this new working concept of "phenomenal presentation." A preliminary remark is in order: To avoid misunderstandings, let me draw the reader's attention to the fact that I am not mainly interested in the epistemological analysis of "presentation." In particular, I am not concerned with establishing a direct connection to the concept of *'Gegenwärtigung'* of Husserl and Heidegger, or to earlier concepts of presentation, for instance, in Meinong, Spencer, or Bergson, nor are implicit parallels intended to the use of the concept of presentation of contemporary authors (like Shannon 1993, Honderich 1994, or Searle, 1983). In particular, mental presentations in the sense here intended are not to be taken as active iconic signs which "exemplify properties of the corresponding stimulus source, by presenting a certain stimulus" (see Schumacher 1996, p. 932; see also Metzinger 1997). I am rather using the concept as a possible working term for a functionalist neurophenomenology, and not with a primarily epistemological interest. What is the difference?

To speak about presentation in a primarily epistemological sense could, for instance, mean to interpret the most simple forms of phenomenal content as active or property-exemplifying iconic signs (a good overview of problems connected with this issue is given by Schumacher 1996). Because, under this analysis, the process of presentation is modeled in accordance with an external process of sensory perception analyzed on the *personal* level of description—for instance, showing a color sample or a piece of cloth—any application of this idea to simple phenomenal states activated by subpersonal processing generates the notorious classic of philosophy of mind, the homunculus problem. What Daniel Dennett has called the "intentional stance" is being transported into the system, because now we also need an internal *subject* of presentation (see Dennett 1987a). Interestingly, the same is true of the concept of representation. From the point of view of the history of ideas the semantic element of "taking the place of" already appears in a legal text from the fourth century (see Podlech 1984, p. 510; and, in particular, Scheerer 1991). Here, as well, the semantic content of a central theoretical concept was *first* modeled according to an interpersonal relationship in public space. In the early Middle Ages, the concept of "representation" referred predominantly to concrete things and actions; mental representation in a psychological sense (*'Vorstellung'*) is an element of its meaning which only evolves at a later stage. If one is interested in dissolving the qualia problem under the fundamental assumptions of a naturalistic theory of mental representation, by introducing a conceptual difference between presentational and representational content, one must first be able to offer a solution to the homunculus problem on both levels. One has to be able to say why the phenomenal first-person perspective and the phenomenal self are accessible to, respectively, a presentationalist or representationalist analysis that avoids the homunculus problem. This is the main goal of this book and we return to it in chapters 5, 6, and 7.

Many people believe intuitively that mental presentation creates an epistemically direct connection from subject to world. Obviously, this assumption is more than dubious from an empirical point of view. Typically, the logical mistake involved consists in an equivocation between phenomenological and epistemological notions of "immediacy": from the observation that a certain information appears in the conscious mind in a seemingly instantaneous and nonmediated way it does not follow that the potential new *knowledge* brought about by this event is itself direct knowledge. However, it is important to avoid a second implication of this assumption, which is just as absurd as a little man in our heads looking at samples of materials and internal role takers of external states of affairs. Qualia cannot be interpreted as presenting iconic signs, which phenomenally exemplify the property forming their content for a second time. In external relations we all know what presenting iconic signs are—for instance, samples of a piece of cloth of a certain color, which can then be used as an exemplifying sign by simply presenting the target property to the subject. However, as regards the human mind, it is highly implausible to assume that property-exemplifying presenting iconic signs really exist. For a number of reasons, the assumption that the sensory content of the conscious mind is constructed from internal exemplifications of externally given properties, with the internal properties being related in a simple or even systematic manner to physical properties in the environment is implausible and naive. For color consciousness, for instance, a simple empirical constraint like color constancy makes this philosophical assumption untenable (see Lanz 1996).

There is a further reason why we cannot treat active presentational content as a simple property exemplification. Properties are cognitive constructs. In order to be able to use the internal states in question as the exemplifications of *properties*, the corresponding representational system would have to possess transtemporal and logical identity criteria for the content. It would have to be able to *recognize*, for example, subtle shades of phenomenal color while simultaneously being able to form a stable phenomenal *concept* for them. Obviously, such systems are logically possible. However, empirical considerations show human beings as not belonging to this class of systems. This is the decisive argument against interpreting the most simple forms of sensory content as phenomenal property exemplifications (i.e., in accordance with case 3a mentioned above, the "classic phenomenological" variant). Of course, the activation of simple perceptual experiences will constitute an exemplification of *some* property under *some* true description. This will likely be a special kind of physical property, namely, a neurodynamical property. What is needed is a precise mathematical model of, say, conscious color state space that coherently describes all phenomenologically relevant features of this space—for example, the different degrees of global availability characterizing different regions, as they are formed by the topology describing the *transition* from Lewis qualia to Raffman qualia—and seeking an implementation of this phenomenal state space in corresponding properties of the physical dynamics.

The core problem consists in doing justice to the extreme subtlety and richness of subjective experience in a conceptually precise manner. Those camps in analytical philosophy of mind still following a more classic-cognitivist agenda will have to come to terms with a simple fact: Our own consciousness is by far too subtle and too "liquid" to be, on a theoretical level, modeled according to linguistic and public representational systems.[49] What we have to overcome are crude forms of modularism and syntacticism, as well as simplistic two-level theories of higher-order representation assuming an atomism for content. As Ganzfeld experiments show, decontextualized primitives or atoms of phenomenal content simply do not exist (see below). The true challenge for representationalist theories of the mind-brain today lies in describing an architecture which plausibly *combines* modularism and holism in a single, integrated model (see, e.g., section 3.2.4).

Fortunately, a number of good approaches for overcoming the traditional distinction between perception and cognition toward a much more differentiated theory of intentional as well as phenomenal content have been in existence for quite some time. Perhaps the smallest unit of conscious experience is simply formed by the concept of an activation vector (including a number of strong neuroscientific constraints). This would mean that the ultimate goal is to develop a truly internalist state space semantics (SSS; P. M. Churchland 1986; see also Fodor and LePore 1996 for a recent criticism and P. M. Churchland 1998) for *phenomenal content* (e.g., in accordance with Austen Clark's model; see Clark 1993, 2000). Starting from elementary discriminatory achievements we can construct "quality spaces" or "sensory orders" of which it is true that the number of qualitative encodings available to a system within a specific sensory modality is given by the *dimensionality* of this space, and that any particular activation of that form of content which I have called "presentational" constitutes a *point* within this space, which itself is defined by an equivalence class with regard to the property of global indiscriminability, whereas the subjective experience of *recognizable* qualitative content of phenomenal representation is equivalent to a *region* or a *volume* in such a space. If a currently active volume representation and a representation of the same kind laid down in long-term memory are being compared to each other and recognized as isomorphic or sufficiently

---

49. Diana Raffman, in a recent publication, discusses this point extensively, backing it up with a number of interesting examples. Cf. Raffman in press.

similar, we may arrive at the phenomenal experience of *sameness* previously mentioned in the text. All three of those forms of phenomenal content, which are being confounded by the classic concept of a phenomenal "first-order phenomenal property," therefore, can be functionally individuated. If, on an empirical level, we know how these formally described quality spaces are neurobiologically realized in a certain class of organisms, then we possess the conceptual instruments to develop a neurophenomenology for this kind of organism. Peter Gärdenfors has developed a theory of *conceptual spaces*, which in its underlying intuitions is closely related to both the above-mentioned approaches. In the framework of this theory we can describe what it means to *form a concept*: "Natural concepts" (in his terminology) are convex regions within a conceptual space. He then goes on to write, "I for instance claim that the *color expressions* in natural languages use natural concepts with regard to the psychological representation of our three color dimensions" (Gärdenfors 1995, p. 188; English translation by Thomas Metzinger). Ineffable, consciously experienced presentational content (Raffman qualia) could under this approach be interpreted as natural properties corresponding to a convex region of a domain within the conceptual space of visual neuroscience (Gärdenfors 2000, p. 71).

2.5   Phenomenal Presentation

Consciously experienced presentational content has a whole range of highly interesting features. The ineffability of its pure "suchness," its dimensional position within a sensory order, is one of them. Another one is its lack of introspectively discernible internal structure. In philosophy of mind, this issue is known as the "grain problem" and I will return to it in section 3.2.10 to develop further semantic constraints enriching our concept of subjective experience. Now, I will close this chapter by introducing a number of more general constraints governing simple phenomenal content. Again, it is important not to reiterate the phenomenological fallacy by reifying ongoing presentational processes: Even if simple presentational content, for example, a current conscious experience of turquoise$_{37}$, stays invariant during a certain period of time, this does not permit the introduction of phenomenal atoms or individuals. Rather, the challenge is to understand how a complex, dynamic process can have invariant features that will, by phenomenal necessity, *appear* as elementary, first-order properties of the world to the system undergoing this process.

What does all this mean with respect to the overall concept of "phenomenal presentation?" In particular, what is *phenomenal* presentation, if we leave out the epistemic interpretation of "presentation" for now? According to our provisional, first definition we are facing a process which makes fine-grained sensory information available for attention and the global control of action. The insight of such fine-grained information evading perceptual memory and cognitive reference not only leads us to a whole set of more differentiated and empirically plausible notions of what simple sensory consciousness actually is, it also possesses philosophical beauty and depth. For the first time it allows us to do justice to the fact that a very large portion of phenomenal experience, as a matter of fact, is *ineffable*, in a straightforward and conceptually convincing manner. There is no mystery involved in the limitation of perceptual memory. But the beauty of sensory experience is further revealed: there are things in life which can only be experienced *now* and by *you*. In its subtleness, its enormous wealth in highly specific, high-dimensional information, and in the fine structure exhibited by the temporal dynamics characterizing it, it is at the same time limited by being hidden from the interpersonal world of linguistic communication. It only reveals its intricacies within a single psychological moment, within the specious present of a phenomenal Now, which in turn is tied to an individual first-person perspective.

In standard situations (for now leaving dreams, hallucinations, etc., out of the picture) presentational content can only be activated if the massive autonomous activity of the brain is episodically perturbed and shaped by the pressure of currently running sensory input. Differentiated by cognitive, concept-like forms of mental representation in only a limited manner, the phenomenal states generated in this way have to appear as fundamental aspects of reality to the system itself, because they are available for guided attention, but cannot be further differentiated or penetrated by metarepresentational processing. The second remarkable feature is that they are fully transparent. This is not to say that our sensory experiences cannot be highly plastic—just think about introspective experts in different phenomenological domains, like painters, psychotherapists, or designers of new perfumes. However, relative to a certain architecture and to a certain stage in the individual evolution of any representational system, the set of currently active presentata will determine what the phenomenal primitives of a particular conscious organism are at this point in time. Presentational content is precisely that aspect in our sensory experience which, even when maximally focusing attention, appears as atomic, fundamentally simple, homogeneous, and temporally immediate (for a recent discussion, see Jakab 2000). Third, the analysis sketched here does not only do justice to the real phenomenological profile and conceptual necessities on the representational level of description, it also allows us to take a step toward the functional and neuroscientific investigation of the physical underpinnings of sensory experience.

I want to conclude this section by highlighting four additional and particularly interesting features of the type of phenomenal content I have just sketched. They could serve as starting points for a more detailed functional analysis, eventually leading to the isolation of their neural correlates. Simple phenomenal content can be characterized by four interesting phenomenological principles. These principles may help us find an empirical way of anchoring the new concept of "presentational content" by developing a *neuro*phenomenological interpretation.

2.5.1 The Principle of Presentationality

As Richard Gregory aptly pointed out, the adaptive function of what today we like to call qualia may have consisted in "flagging the dangerous present" (see also sections 3.3.3 and 3.2.11 in chapter 3).[50] It is interesting to note how this important observation complements the first general conjecture about the function of consciousness, namely, the "world zero hypothesis" submitted earlier. If it is the experiential content of qualia that, as Gregory says, has the capacity to "flag" the present moment and thereby prevent confusion with processes of mental simulation, that is, with the remembered past, the anticipation of future events, and imagination in general, then it is precisely presentational content that can reliably achieve this function. World$_0$, the phenomenal frame of reference, is constituted by integrated and interdependent forms of presentational content (see sections 3.2.3 and 3.2.4). Sensing aspects of the current environment was, besides the coordination of motor behavior, among the first computational tasks to be solved in the early history of nervous systems. Phylogenetically, presentational content is likely to be one of the oldest forms of conscious content, one that we share with many of our biological ancestors, and one that is functionally most reliable, ultrafast, and therefore fully transparent (see section 3.2.7). Every particular form of simple, sensory content—the olfactory experience of a mixture between amber and sandalwood, the visual experience of a specific shade of indigo, or the particular stinging sensation associated with a certain kind of toothache—can formally be described as a point in high-dimensional quality space. However, it is important to note how presentational content always is *temporal* content as well.

The principle of presentationality says that first, simple sensory content, *always* carries additional temporal information and second, that this information is highly invariant in always being the *same* kind of information: the state in question holds *right now*. However, as Raffman's argument showed, we are not confronted with phenomenal properties in the classic sense, and therefore we cannot simply speak about internal predications or demonstrations from the first-person perspective. Apart from the fact that the classic language of thought approach is simply inadequate from an empirical perspective, predicative solutions do not transport phenomenal character and they do not supply us with an explanation of the transparency of phenomenal content (see section 3.2.7). Therefore, the

50. Cf. Gregory 1997, p. 194. Gregory writes: "I would like to speculate that qualia serve to flag the present moment and normally prevent confusion with the remembered past, the anticipated future, or more generally, with imagination. The present moment must be clearly identified for behavior to be appropriate to the present situation, and this is essential for survival." Cf. Gregory 1997, p. 192.

transparency, the temporal indexicality, and the phenomenal content as well have to be found within the real dynamics or the architecture of the system. As should have become obvious by now, the route I am proposing is that of interpreting qualitative content as the content of nonconceptual indicators.[51] Since higher-order representational or higher-order presentational theories of consciousness have fundamental difficulties (see Güzeldere 1995), we need a better understanding of the way in which what we used to call "qualia" can be a kind of "self-presenting" content. One possibility is to interpret them as states with a *double* indicator function. Active mental presentata might be the nonpropositional and subcategorical analoga to propositional attitudes *de nunc*. The analogy consists in what I would like to call the "temporal indicator function": they are always tied to a specific mode of presentation, their content is subcategorical, nonconceptual mental content *de nunc*. This special mode of presentation consists in the fact that, for contingent architectural reasons, they can exclusively be activated within a phenomenal window of presence: they are a kind of content, which by its functional properties is very intimately connected to those mechanisms with the help of which the organism generates its own phenomenal Now. The most simple form of phenomenal content is exactly what we are not deliberately able to imagine and what we cannot remember. Using our standard example: red_{31} is a determined phenomenal value, which, first, is always tied to a subjectively represented time axis, and second, to the origin of this time axis. "Red_{31}" is always "red_{31}-*now*." And this, finally, is a first phenomenological reading of "presentation": presentation in this sense consists in being tied to a subjectively experienced present in a sensory manner. This is also the way in which simple phenomenal content is self-presenting content. It is integrated into a higher-order representation of time, because it is invariably presented as a simple form of content immediately given *now*. Of course, we will soon be able to enrich the notion of conscious presentation by a whole range of further constraints. For now we can say the following: presentational content is nonconceptual mental content, which possesses a double indicator function, by, first, pointing to a specific, perceptually simple feature of the world in a specific perceptual context; and, second, invariably pointing to

---

51. In earlier publications (Metzinger 1993, 1994) I introduced the concept of an "analogue indicator." The idea was that simple sensory content, possessing no truth conditions and therefore being ineffable, often varies along a single dimension only, namely, a dimension of intensity. Consider gustatory qualities like sweetness or saltiness (see Maxwell, submitted): They can only be more and less intense; their fundamental quality remains the same. Therefore they are analogue representations, pointing toward a certain aspect of a given perceptual context. However, this concept does not yet solve the important problem, which Diana Raffman has called the "differentiation problem": How does one, on a theoretical level, specify the difference between particular representations and presentations of every discriminable stimulus configuration? If it is correct that mathematical models of the corresponding minimally sufficient neural correlates can in principle provide us with transtemporal, as well as with logical, identity criteria, then this will be relevant with regard to the differentiation problem as well.

the fact that this feature is a feature *currently* holding in the actual state of the environment or the organism's own body.

This short analysis implicitly names a functional property with which presentational content is logically connected in our own case. If one is interested in empirically anchoring the foregoing considerations, all empirical work pertaining to the generation of a phenomenal window of presence is relevant to this project.[52]

2.5.2   The Principle of Reality Generation

Our brain is an ontological engine. Noncognitive states of phenomenal experience are always characterized by an interesting property, which, in logic, we would call an existence assumption. Conscious experience, in a nonpropositional format, confronts us with strong assumptions about what *exists*. If one really wants to understand phenomenal consciousness, one has to explain how a full-blown *reality-model* eventually emerges from the dynamics of neural information processing, which later is untranscendable for the system itself. Presentational content will always be an important element of any such explanation, because it is precisely this kind of mental content that generates the phenomenal experience of presence, of the world as well as of the self situated in this world. The principle of reality generation says that in all standard situations presentational content invariably functions like an existential quantifier for systems like ourselves; sensory presence, on the subcognitive level of phenomenal experience, forces us to assume the *existence* of whatever it is that is currently presented to us in this way. The ongoing process of phenomenal presentation is the paradigm example of a fascinating property, to which we return in section 3.2.7. Presentational content is the paradigm example of *transparent* phenomenal content, because it is activated in such a fast and reliable way as to make any earlier processing stages inaccessible to introspection$_1$ as well as introspection$_2$. The fact that all this is an element of a *remembered present*, the *re*presentational character of simple sensory content is not available to us, because only content properties, but not "vehicle

---

52. For example, Ernst Pöppel's and Eva Ruhnau's hypothesis of phase-locked oscillation processes generating *atemporal zones* on a very fundamental level within the system, system states governed by simultaneity (in terms of the absence of any represented internal temporal relations) on a functional level, would be of direct relevance. The question is which role such elementary integration windows can actually play in constituting the *phenomenal* window of presence. By opening time windows in this sense, a system can, for itself, generate an *operational time*: By quantisizing its information processing, it swallows the flow of physical time on a very fundamental level of its representation of the world. It distances itself from its own processuality by introducing a certain kind of data reduction on the representational level. The physical time interval remains, but the *content* of the corresponding system states loses all or part of its internal temporal properties. *For the system itself* representational atoms are generated, so-called elementary integration units. This theory is especially interesting because it can help us achieve a better understanding of what the phenomenal property of "presence," which we find accompanying all forms of active simple sensory content, really is. See section 3.2.2; and Pöppel 1988, 1994; Görnitz, Ruhnau, and Weizsäcker 1992; Ruhnau and Pöppel 1991.

properties" are accessible to introspective attention directed at it. It is precisely this architectural feature of the human system of conscious information processing which leads to the phenomenal presence of a world. In other words, presentational content, on the level of subjective experience, mediates presence in an *ontological* sense. It helps to represent facticity (see section 3.2.7). Because on the lowest level of phenomenal content we are not able to represent the causal and temporal genesis of the presentatum (the "vehicle of presentation"); because the system, as it were, erases these aspects of the overall process and swallows them up in the course of elementary integration processes, the sensory content of our experience gains a fascinating property, which often is characterized as "immediate givenness." However, givenness in this sense is only a higher-order feature of phenomenal content; it is *virtual* immediacy brought about by a *virtual* form of presence. We have already touched on this point before. Now we are able to say the following: "givenness" is exclusively a phenomenological notion and not an epistemological or even an ontological category. Today, we are beginning to understand that this feature is strongly determined on a particular functional and physical basis, and that the system generating it needs a certain amount of physical time to construct the phenomenal experience of instantaneousness, of the subjective sense of immediate givenness related to the sensory contents. The sensory Now is a subpersonal construct, the generation of which takes time.

If this is true, we can conclude that the activation of presentational content has to be correlated with a second class of functional properties: with all those properties achieving an elementary integration of sensory information flow in a way that filters out temporal stimulus information. Elsewhere (Metzinger 1995b) I have pointed out how, in particular, presentational content has to inevitably appear as real, because it is homogeneous. Homogeneity, however, could simply consist in the fact of a higher-order integration mechanism, reading out "first-order" states as it were, having a low temporal resolution, thereby "glossing over" the "grainy" nature of the presentational vehicle. It is an empirically plausible assumption that elementary sensory information, for example, colors, shapes, surface textures, and motion properties, are integrated into the manifest conscious experience of a multimodal object (say, a red ball audibly bouncing up and down in front of you) by the synchronization of neural responses (see, e.g., Singer 2000; Engel and Singer 2000). For every sensory feature, for example, the perceived color as distinct from the perceived object, it will be true that there are myriads of corresponding elementary feature detectors active in your brain, in a highly synchronized fashion. The "ultra-smoothness," the grainless, ultimately homogeneous nature of the perceived color red could simply be the result of a higher-order mechanism not only reading out the dimensional position of the specific stimulus in quality space (thereby, in standard situations, making wavelength information globally available *as* hue) but also the *synchronicity* of neural responses *as such*. On a higher level of internal representation, therefore, simple presentational content would by necessity have to appear as lacking internal structure or processuality and as "dense" to the introspecting system itself. The user surface of the phenomenal interface our brain generates for us is a *closed* surface. This, then, would be a third way in which presentational content importantly contributes to the naive realism characterizing our phenomenal model of reality. I will not go into further details here, but I return to this issue frequently at later stages (in particular, see section 3.2.10). All that is important at this point is to see that there is no reason for assuming that functional, third-person identity criteria for the process underlying the generation of phenomenal presentational content cannot be found.

2.5.3   The Principle of Nonintrinsicality and Context Sensitivity

As we saw earlier, subcategorical, presentational content must be conceived of not as a phenomenal property, but rather as an as yet unknown neurodynamical property. However, many philosophical theories draw their antireductionist force from conceptually framing first-order phenomenal properties as *intrinsic* properties (see, e.g., Levine 1995). An intrinsic property is a nonrelational property, forming the context-invariant "core" of a specific sensory experience: an experience of turquoise$_{37}$ has to exhibit the purported phenomenal essence, the core quality of turquoise$_{37}$ in all perceptual contexts—otherwise it simply is not an experience of turquoise$_{37}$. The philosophical intuition behind construing simple sensory experience and its content as the exemplification of an *intrinsic* phenomenal property is the same intuition that makes us believe that something is a *substance* in an ontological sense. The ontological intuition associated with the philosophical concept of a "substance" is that it is something that could continue to exist by itself even if all other existing entities in the universe were to vanish. Substantiality is a notion implying the capacity of *independent existence*, as applied to individuals. The intrinsicality intuition makes the same assumption for particular classes of properties, for example, for phenomenal properties; they are special in being *essential* properties occurring within the flow of sensory experience, by being invariant across perceptual contexts. They are philosophically important, because they are *substantial* properties, which cannot be, as it were, dissociated from subjective experience itself and descriptively relocated on a lower level of description.

   If this philosophical intuition about the substantial, intrinsic nature of first-order phenomenal properties were true, then such properties would—in the mind of an individual conscious being—have to be capable of coming into existence all by themselves, of being sustained even if all *other* properties of the same class were not present in experience. Clearly, an essential phenomenal property in this sense would have to be able to "stand by itself." For instance, a specific conscious experience of a sound quality, if it is an intrinsic quality, should be able to emerge independently of any auditory scene surrounding it, independently of an auditory context. A color quale like red_{31} should be able to appear in the conscious mind of an individual human being independently of any perceptual context, independently of any other color currently seen.

As a matter of fact, modern research on the autonomy of visual systems and the functional modularity of conscious vision seems to show how activity within many stages of the overall hierarchy of visual processing can be made phenomenally explicit, and may not necessarily require cooperation with other functional levels within the system (see, e.g., Zeki and Bartels 1998). However, another set of simple empirical constraints on our notion of sensory experience shows the philosophical conception of phenomenal atomism to be utterly misguided (see Jakab 2000 for an interesting criticism). Let us stick with our standard example, conscious color vision, and consider the phenomenology of so-called Ganzfeld experiments. What will happen if, in an experiment, the visual field of a subject is filled by one single color stimulus only? Will there be a generalized conscious experience of one single, intrinsic phenomenal property only?

Koffka, in his *Principles of Gestalt Psychology* (Koffka 1935, p. 121), predicted that a perfectly homogeneous field of colored light would appear neutral rather than colored as soon as the perceptual "framework" of the previous visual scene vanished. Interestingly, this would also imply that a homogeneous stimulation of *all* sensory modalities would lead to a complete collapse of phenomenal perceptual experience as such. As Hochberg, Triebel, and Seaman (1951) have shown, a complete disappearance of color vision can actually be obtained by a homogeneous visual stimulation, that is, by a Ganzfeld stimulation. Five of their six subjects reported a red-colored surfaceless field followed by a total disappearance of the color within the first three minutes (p. 155). Despite considerable individual differences in the course of the adaptation process and in the shifts in phenomenal content during adaptation, complete disappearance of conscious color experience was obtained (p. 158). What precisely is the resulting phenomenal configuration in these cases? Typically, after a three-minute adaptation, an achromatic field will be described in 80% of the reports, with the remaining 20% only describing a faint trace of consciously experienced color (Cohen 1958, p. 391). Representative phenomenological reports are: "A diffuse fog." "A hazy insipid yellow." "A gaseous effect." "A milky substance." "Misty, like being in a lemon pie." "Smoky" (Cohen 1957, p. 406), or "swimming in a mist of light which becomes more condensed at an indefinite distance" or the experience of a "sea of light" (Metzger 1930; and Gibson and Waddell 1952; as quoted in Avant 1965, p. 246). This shows how a simple sensory content like "red" cannot "stand by itself," but that it is bound into the relational context generated by other phenomenal dimensions. Many philosophers—and experimentalists alike (for a related criticism see Mausfeld 1998, 2002)—have described qualia as particular values on absolute dimensions, as decontextualized atoms of consciousness. These simple data show how such an elementaristic approach cannot do justice to the actual phenomenology, which is much more holistic and context sensitive (see also sections 3.2.3 and 3.2.4).

A further prediction following from this was that a homogeneous Ganzfeld stimulation of *all* sensory organs would lead to a complete collapse of phenomenal consciousness (originally made by Koffka 1935, p. 120; see also Hochberg et al. 1951, p. 153) or to a taking over by autonomous, internal activity, that is, through hallucinatory content exclusively generated by internal top-down mechanisms (see, e.g., Avant 1965, p. 247; but also recent research in, e.g., ffytche and Howard 1999; Leopold and Logothetis, 1999). As a matter of fact, even during ordinary chromatic stimulation in a simple visual Ganzfeld, many subjects lose phenomenal vision *altogether*—that is, all domain-related phenomenal dimensions, including saturation and brightness, disappear from the conscious model of reality. Cohen (1957, p. 406) reported a complete cessation of visual experience in five of sixteen tested observers. He also presented what he took to be a representative description of the shift in phenomenal content: "Foggy whiteness, everything blacks out, returns, goes. I feel blind. I'm not even seeing blackness. This differs from black and white when the lights are out." Individual differences do exist. Interestingly, the fade-out effect is even wavelength dependent, that is, in viewing a short wavelength, fading periods are long and the additional phenomenal experience of darkness (i.e., of being darker than a nonilluminated Ganzfeld) after turning the lights off is strong, while just the opposite is true for viewing long wavelengths (with the magnitudes of all three shifts in conscious content, i.e., the loss of chromaticity, brightness, and the addition of darkness after lights are turned off being linearly related to the logarithm of stimulus intensity; see Gur 1989). In general, the Ganzfeld effect is likely to result from an inability of the human visual system to respond to nontransient stimuli.[53] What does all this mean in terms of conceptual constraints for our philosophical concept of conscious color experience, in particular for the ineffability of color experience?

Any modern theory of mind will have to explain phenomenological observations of this kind. To sum up, if stimulated with a chromatic Ganzfeld, 80% of the subjects will experience an achromatic field after three minutes, with about 20% being left with a faint trace of coloredness. Interestingly, an effect analogous to figure-ground segregation can be sometimes observed, namely, in a phenomenal separation of chromatic fog and achromatic ground (Cohen 1958, p. 394). Avant (1965) cites representative classic descriptions, for example, of an observer (in this case, Metzger) feeling "himself swimming in a mist

---

53. As Moshe Gur writes: "In the Ganzfeld, unlike normal viewing, the ever-present eye-movements do not affect the transformation from the object to the retinal plane and thus the stimulus temporal modulations are faithfully depicted at the retinal level. . . . It is the spatial uniformity of the stimulus that assures that although different retinal elements may receive different amounts of light, each element, in the absence of temporal changes in the stimulus, receives a time-invariant light intensity" (Gur 1989, p. 1335).

of light that becomes more condensed at an indefinite distance," or the typical notion of a "sea of light." Obviously, we can lose hue without losing brightness, which is the phenomenal presentation of the pure physical force of the stimulus itself.

The first philosophical lesson to be learned from the Ganzfeld phenomenon, then, is that presentational content must be conceived of as a highly relational entity, which cannot "stand by itself," but is highly dependent on the existence of a perceptual context. It is interesting to note that if homogeneous stimulation of further sense modalities is added to the visual Ganzfeld, extensive hallucinations result (Avant 1965, p. 247). That is, as soon as presentational content has vanished from a certain phenomenal domain and is no longer able in Richard Gregory's sense to "flag the present," the *internal* context can become autonomous, and lead to complex phenomenal simulations. In other words, in situations underconstrained by an externally given perceptual context, top-down processes can become dominant and get out of control (see also ffytche 2000; ffytche and Howard 1999; and sections 3.2.4 and 7.2.3).

The second philosophical lesson to be learned from these data is that presentational content is not only unable to "stand by itself" but has an important function in constraining a preexisting internal context by continuously interacting with it. In the Ganzfeld the continuous movement of the eyeballs is unable to affect the transformation from the object to the retinal plane and thus the stimulus temporal modulations are faithfully depicted at the retinal level (Gur 1989, p. 1335; see previous footnote). Every retinal element receives a time-invariant light intensity. What happens in the Ganzfeld is that the initially bright, colored field then desaturates and turns achromatic. Our visual system, and our "phenomenal system" as well, are unable to respond to nontransient stimuli.

The third philosophical lesson to be learned from this is that presentational content supervenes on a highly complex web of causal relations and is in no way independent of this web or capable of existing by itself *across* such contexts. Clearly, if chromatic primitives were context-independent essences they should not disappear in a Ganzfeld situation. On the other hand, it is interesting to note how a single blink can restore the conscious sensation of color and brightness for a fraction of a second (while not resetting the decay rate; cf. Gur 1989, p. 1339). How deeply embedded simple, conscious color content in the web of causal relations just mentioned actually is can also be seen by the differential effects of the stimulating wavelength on the disappearance rate: different phenomenal colors disappear at different speeds, with the duration basically being a function of wavelength and intensity. If a short wavelength is viewed, fading times are long and the sensation of additional darkness is strong, while the inverse is true for long wavelengths (Gur 1989). The conscious phenomenology of color desaturation differs for different stimuli and classes of phenomenal presentata. Undoubtedly, a large number of additional constraints can be found in other sensory modalities. If we want a phenomenologically plausible theory of conscious experience, all these data will eventually have to function as conceptual constraints.

2.5.4   The Principle of Object Formation

Simple phenomenal content never appears in an isolated fashion. What we used to call "phenomenal properties" in the past—that is, attentionally and cognitively available presentational content—is never being instantiated in isolation, but always as a discriminable aspect of a higher-order whole. For instance, a consciously experienced pain will always be phenomenally localized within a spatial image of the body (see section 7.2.2). And even the colored patches, which we sometimes see shortly before falling asleep, are in no way isolated phenomenal atoms, because they possess a spatial expanse; indeed, typically they possess contours and a direction of motion as well. That is, even in the most degraded situations of hallucinatory color content we never find fully decontextualized elements or strictly particular phenomenal values on a dimension that would have to be conceptually analyzed as an *absolute* dimension. *Pure* individuals and singular properties never appear in the sensory flow of conscious experience, but only complexions of different forms of presentational content. Even phosphenes—a favorite example of philosophers—are experienced against a black background. This black background itself is really a form of simple phenomenal content, even if sometimes we like to interpret it falsely as "pure nothingness." In other words, a phenomenal representation of absence is not the same as the absence of phenomenal representation.

Of course, what may be called the "principle of object constitution" from a philosophical perspective has been known as the "binding problem" in the neuro- and cognitive sciences for some time as well: How does our perceptual system bind elementary features extracted from the data flow supplied by our sensory organs into coherent perceptual gestalts? On the empirical level it has become obvious that the activation of presentational content has to be functionally coupled to those processes responsible for the formation of perceptual objects and figure-ground separations. As noted above, such separations can also happen if, for instance, a chromatic fog is consciously experienced as separated from an achromatic ground. Perceptual objects, according to the current model, are not generated by the binding of properties in a literal, phenomenological sense of "property" (i.e., in accordance with case 3a above), but by an integration of presentational content. How such objects are later verbally characterized, identified, and remembered by the cognitive subject is an entirely different question. It is also true that genuine cognitive availability only seems to start at the object level. However, it is important to note that, even if different features of a perceptual object, for example, its perceived color and its smell, are later attentionally available, the actual integration process leading to the manifest, multimodal object is of a *preattentional* nature. It is certainly modulated by attentional processing, by expectancies and context information, but the process of feature integration itself is not available for introspection₁ and it is never possible for us to introspectively "reverse" this process in order to perceive single features or isolated, nonintegrated forms of presentational content *as such*.

If this third idea is correct, conscious presentational content has to emerge simultaneously with and in dependence on the process of object formation, and therefore represents precisely that part of a perceptual object constituted by the system which can, for instance, be discriminated by the guidance of visual attention. With regard to this class of functional processes we have witnessed a flood of empirical literature in recent years (for reviews, see, e.g., Gray 1994; Singer 1994; see also Singer 2000; Edelman and Tononi 2000a,b). Once again, we find no reason to assume that what we used to call "qualia" has for principled reasons to evade the grasp of empirical research in the neuro- and cognitive sciences.

In this chapter, I have introduced a series of semantic differentiations for already existing philosophical concepts, namely, "global availability," "introspection," "subjectivity," "quale," and "phenomenal concept." In particular, we now possess six new conceptual instruments: the concepts of representation, simulation, and presentation, both in mentalistic and phenomenalistic readings. If generated by the processes of *mental* representation, simulation, and presentation, the states of our minds are solely individuated by their intentional content. "Meaning," intentional content, is something that is typically ascribed from an external, third-person perspective. Such states could in principle unfold within a system knowing no kind of conscious experience. It is only through the processes of *phenomenal* representation, simulation, and presentation that this new property is brought about. Phenomenal states are being individuated by their phenomenal content, that is, "from the first-person perspective." In order to be able to say what a "first-person perspective" actually is, in chapter 5 I extend our set of simple conceptual tools by six further elements: self-representation, self-simulation, and self-presentation, again both in mentalistic and a phenomenalistic interpretations. In chapter 5 we confront a highly interesting class of special cases characterized by the fact that the object of the representational process always remains the same: the system as a whole, the system *itself*.

Maybe it has already become obvious how provisional concepts in our present tool kit, such as "simulation," "representation," and "presentation," urgently have to be enriched with respect to physical, neurobiological, functional, or further representational constraints. If we are interested in generating a further growth of knowledge in the interdisciplinary project of consciousness research, the original set of analysanda and explananda must be decomposed into many different target domains. This will have to happen on a wider variety of descriptive levels. Special interests lead to special types of questions.

We are here pursuing a whole bundle of such questions: What is a conscious self? What precisely does it mean for human beings in nonpathological waking states to take on a phenomenal first-person perspective toward the world and themselves? Is an exhaustive analysis of the phenomenal first-person perspective on the representational level of description within reach? Is the phenomenal first-person perspective, in its full content, really a natural phenomenon? Have we approached a stage at which philosophical terminology can be handed over to the empirical sciences and, step by step, be filled with empirical content? Or is conscious experience a target phenomenon that will eventually force us to forget traditional boundaries between the humanities and the hard sciences?

In this chapter, I have only used one simple and currently popular functional constraint to point to a possible difference between mental and phenomenal representation: the concept of global availability, which I then differentiated into attentional, cognitive, and availability for behavioral control. However, this was only a very first, and in my own way of looking at things, slightly crude example. Now that these very first, semiformal instruments are in our hands, it is important to sharpen them by taking a very close look at the concrete shape a theory referring to *real* systems would have to take. Content properties and abstract functional notions are not enough. What is needed are the theoretical foundations enabling us to develop a better understanding of the *vehicles*, the concrete internal *instruments*, with the help of which a continuously changing phenomenal representation of the world and the self within it is being generated.

3 The Representational Deep Structure of Phenomenal Experience

3.1 What Is the Conceptual Prototype of a Phenomenal Representatum?

The goal of this chapter is to develop a preliminary working concept, the concept of a "phenomenal mental model." I shall proceed in two steps. First, I construct the baselines for a set of criteria or catalogue of constraints by which we can decide if a certain representational state is also a *conscious* state. I propose a multilevel set of constraints for the concept of phenomenal representation. The second step consists in putting these constraints to work against the background of a number of already existing theories of mental representation to arrive at a more precise formulation of the preliminary concept we are looking for. At the end I briefly introduce this hypothetical working concept, the concept of a "phenomenal mental model." In chapter 4 I shall proceed to test our tool kit, employing a short representational analysis of unusual states of consciousness. A series of brief neuropsychological case studies will help to further sharpen the conceptual instruments developed so far, in rigorously testing them for empirical plausibility. After all this has been done we return, in chapters 5 to 7, to our philosophical core problem: the question of the true nature of the phenomenal self and the first-person perspective. However, let me begin by offering a number of introductory remarks about what it actually *means* to start searching for the theoretical prototype of a phenomenal representatum.

One of the first goals on our way toward a convincing theory of phenomenal experience will have to consist in developing a list of necessary and sufficient conditions for the concept of phenomenal representation. Currently we are very far from being able to even approximate our goal of defining this concept. Please note that, here, it is *not* my aim to develop a full-blown theory of mental representation; the current project is of a much more modest kind, probing possibilities and pioneering interdisciplinary cooperation. At the outset, it is important to keep two things in mind. First, the concept of consciousness may turn out to be a *cluster concept*, that is, a theoretical entity only possessing overlapping sets of sufficient conditions, but no or only very few strictly necessary defining characteristics. Second, any such concept will be relative to a *domain* constituted by a given class of systems. Therefore, in this chapter, I shall only prepare the development of such a list: what I am looking for are the semantic baselines of a theoretical prototype, the prototype of a phenomenal representatum. Once one possesses such a prototype, then one can start to look at different forms of phenomenal content in a differentiated manner. Once one possesses an initial list of multilevel constraints, one can continuously expand this list by adding additional conceptual or *sub*constraints (e.g., as a philosopher working in a top-down fashion), and one can continuously *update* and enrich domain-specific empirical data (e.g., as a neuroscientist refining already existing bottom-up constraints). On a number of different levels of description one can, for particular phenomenological state classes, ask questions about necessary conditions for their realization: What are those minimally *necessary* representational and functional properties a system must possess in order to be able to evolve the contents of consciousness in question? What is the "minimal configuration" *any* system needs in order to undergo a certain kind of subjective experience? Second, one can direct attention toward special domains and, by including empirical data, start investigating what in certain special cases could count as *sufficient* criteria for the ascription of conscious experience in *some* systems: What are the minimal neural correlates (Metzinger 2000a) that realize such necessary properties by making them causally effective within a certain type of organism? Do multiple sufficient correlates for a maximally determinate form of phenomenal content exist? Could a machine, by having *different* physical correlates, also realize the necessary and sufficient conditions for certain types of subjective experience?

For philosophy of mind, the most important levels of description currently are the representationalist and the functionalist levels. Typical and meaningful questions, therefore, are: What are the constraints on the architecture, the causal profile, and the representational resources of a system, which not only possesses representational but sometimes also *phenomenal* states? Which properties would the representational tools employed by this system have to possess in order to be able to generate the contents of a genuinely *subjective* flow of experience? The relevance of particular levels of description may always change—for instance, we might in the future discover a way of coherently describing consciousness, the phenomenal self, and the first-person perspective not as a special form of "contents" at all, but as a particular kind of neural or physical dynamics in general. Here, I treat the representationalist and functionalist levels of analysis as *interdisciplinary* levels right from the beginning: today, they are the levels on which humanities and hard sciences, on which philosophy and cognitive neuroscience can (and must) meet. Hence, we now have to take the step from our first look at the logical structure of the representational relationship to a closer investigation of the question of how, in some systems, it factually brings about the instantiation of phenomenal properties. Different "domains," in this context, are certain classes of systems as well as certain classes of states. Let us illustrate the situation by looking at concrete examples.

Human beings in the dream state differ from human beings in the waking state, but both arguably are conscious, have a phenomenal self, and a first-person perspective. Dreaming systems don't behave, don't process sensory information, and are engaged in a global, but exclusively internal phenomenal *simulation*. In the waking state, we interact with the world, and we do so under a global phenomenal *representation* of the world. Not only waking consciousness but dreaming as well can count as a global *class* of phenomenal states, characterized by its own, narrowly confined set of phenomenological features. For instance, dreams are often hypermnestic and strongly emotionalized states, whereas conscious pain experiences almost never occur during dreams (for details regarding the phenomenological profile, see sections 4.2.5 and 7.2.5). Phenomenological state classes, however, can also be more precisely characterized by their situational context, forms of self-representation, or the special contents of object and property perception made globally available by them. Flying dreams, oneiric background emotions, olfactory experience in dreams, and different types of sensory hallucinations characterizing lucid versus non-lucid dreams are examples of classes of experiences individuated in a more fine-grained manner. A more philosophical, "top-down" question could be: What forms of representational contents characterize normal waking consciousness as opposed to the dream state, and which causal role do they play in generating behavior? On the empirical side of our project this question consists of different aspects: What, in our own case, are concrete mechanisms of processing and representation? What are plausible candidates for the de facto active "vehicles" of phenomenal representation (during the waking state) and phenomenal simulation (during the dream state) in humans? System classes can in principle be individuated in an arbitrarily fine-grained manner: other classes of intended systems could be constituted by infants, adults during non-REM (rapid eye movement) sleep, psychiatric patients during episodes of florid schizophrenia, and also by mice, chimpanzees and artificial systems.

At this point an important epistemological aspect must not be overlooked. If we are not talking about subsystemic states, but about systems as a whole, then we automatically take an attitude toward our domain, which operates from an objective third-person perspective. The levels of description on which we may now operate are intersubjectively accessible and open to the usual scientific procedures. The constraints that we construct on such levels of description to mark out interesting classes of conscious systems are objective constraints. However, it is a bit harder to form domains not by particular classes of conscious systems, but by additionally defining them through certain types of states. To precisely mark out such phenomenological state classes, to type-identify them, we again need certain criteria and conceptual constraints. The problem now consists in the fact that phenomenal states in standard situations are always tied to individual experiential perspectives. It is hard to dispute the fact that the *primary* individuating features of subsystemic states in this case are their subjectively experienced features, *as grasped from a particular, individual first-person perspective.*

Certain intended state classes are first described by phenomenological characteristics, that is, by conceptual constraints, which have originally been developed out of the first-person perspective. However, whenever phenomenological features are employed to describe state classes, the central theoretical problem confronts us head-on: for methodological and epistemological reasons we urgently need a theory about what an individual, first-person perspective is *at all.* We need a convincing theory about the *subjectivity* of phenomenal experience in order to know what we are really talking about when using familiar but unclear idioms, like saying that the content of phenomenal states is being individuated "from a first-person perspective". In chapters 5, 6, and 7 I begin to offer such a theory. For now, we are still concerned with developing conceptual tools with which such a theory can be formulated. The next step consists in moving from domains to possible levels of description.

There are a large number of descriptive levels, on which phenomenal representata can be analyzed in a more precise manner. In the current state of consciousness studies we need *all* of those descriptive levels. Here are the most important ones:

· *The phenomenological level of description.* What statements about the phenomenal contents and the structure of phenomenal space can be made based on *introspective* experience? In what cases are statements of this type heuristically fruitful? When are they epistemically justified?

· *The representationalist level of description.* What is special about the form of *intentional* content generated by the phenomenal variant of mental representation? Which types of phenomenal contents exist? What is the relationship between form and content for phenomenal representata?

· *The informational-computational level of description.* What is the overall computational function fulfilled by processing on the phenomenal level of representation for the organism as a whole?[1] What is the computational goal of conscious experience?[2] What kind of information is phenomenal information?[3]

· *The functional level of description.* Which causal properties have to be instantiated by the neural correlate of consciousness, in order to episodically generate subjective experience? Does something like a "functional" correlate, independent of any realization, exist for consciousness (Chalmers 1995a, b, 1998, 2000)?

· *The physical-neurobiological level of description.* Here are examples of potential questions: Are phenomenal representata cell assemblies firing in a temporally coherent manner

---

1. For didactic purposes, I frequently distinguish between the *content* of a given representation, as an abstract property, and the *vehicle*, the concrete physical state carrying this content for the system (e.g., a specific neural activation pattern spreading in an animal's brain). Useful as this distinction of descriptive levels is in many philosophical contexts, we will soon see that the most plausible theories about mental representation in humans tend to blur this distinction, because at least *phenomenal* content eventually turns out to be a locally supervening and fully "embodied" phenomenon. See also Dretske 1995.

2. It is interesting to see how parallel questions have already arisen in theoretical neuroscience, for instance, when discussing large-scale neuronal theories of the brain or the overall computational goal of the neocortex. Cf. Barlow 1994.

3. Jackson's knowledge argument frequently has been interpreted and discussed as a hypothesis about phenomenal information. Cf. Dennett's comment on Peter Bieri's "PIPS hypothesis" (Dennett 1988, p. 71*ff.*) and D. Lewis 1988.

in the gamma band (see Metzinger 1995b; Engel and Singer 2000; Singer 2000; von der Malsburg 1997)? What types of nervous cells constitute the direct neural correlate of conscious experience (Block 1995, 1998; Crick and Koch 1990; Metzinger 2000b)? Do types of phenomenal content exist that are *not* medium invariant?

Corresponding to each of these descriptive levels we find certain modeling strategies. For instance, we could develop a neurobiological model for self-consciousness, or a functionalist analysis, or a computational model, or a theory of phenomenal self-representation. Strictly speaking, computational models are a subset of functional models, but I will treat them separately from now on, always assuming that computational models are mainly developed in the mathematical quarters of cognitive science, whereas functional analysis is predominantly something to be found in philosophy. Psychologists and philosophers can create new tools for the phenomenological level of analysis. Interestingly, in the second sense of the concept of a "model" to be available soon, all of us construct third-person *phenomenal* models of other conscious selves as well: in social cognition, when internally *emulating* another human being.

Primarily operating on the representationalist level of description, in the following sections I frequently look at the neural and "functional" correlates of phenomenal states, searching for additional bottom-up constraints. Also, I want to make an attempt at doing maximal phenomenological justice to the respective object, that is, to take the phenomenon of consciousness truly seriously in all its nuances and depth. I am, however, not concerned with developing a new phenomenology or constructing a general theory of representational content. My goal is much more modest: to carry out a representational analysis of the phenomenal first-person perspective.

At this point it may nevertheless be helpful for some of my readers if I lay my cards on the table and briefly talk about some background assumptions, even if I do not have space to argue for them explicitly. Readers who have no interest in these assumptions can safely skip this portion and resume reading at the beginning of the next section. Like many other philosophers today, I assume that a representationalist analysis of conscious experience is promising because phenomenal states are a special subset of intentional states (see Dretske 1995; Lycan 1996; Tye 1995, 2000 for typical examples). Phenomenal content is a special aspect or special form of intentional content. I think that this content has to be individuated in a very fine-grained manner—at least on a "subsymbolic" level (e.g., see Rumelhart, McClelland, and the PDP Research Group 1986; McClelland et al. 1986; for a recent application of the connectionist framework to phenomenal experience, see O'Brien and Opie 1999), and, in particular, without assuming propositional modularity (Ramsey et al. 1991) for the human mind, that is, very likely by some sort of microfunctionalist analysis (Andy Clark 1989, 1993). Additionally, I assume that, in a certain "dynamicized" sense, phenomenal content supervenes on spatially and temporally internal system properties. The fundamental idea is as follows: Phenomenal representation is that variant of intentional representation in which the content properties (i.e., is the *phenomenal* content properties) of mental states are completely determined by the spatially internal and synchronous properties of the respective organism, because they supervene on a critical subset of these states. If all properties of my central nervous system are fixed, the contents of my subjective experience are fixed as well. What in many cases, of course, is not fixed is the *intentional* content of these subjective states. Having presupposed a principle of local supervenience for their phenomenal content, we do not yet know if they are complex hallucinations or epistemic states, ones which actually constitute knowledge about the world. One of the most important theoretical problems today consists in putting the concepts of "phenomenal content" and "intentional content" into the right kind of logical relation. I do not tackle this question directly in this book, but my intuition is that it may be a serious mistake to introduce a principled distinction, resulting in a *reification* of both forms of content. The solution may consist in carefully describing a *continuum* between conscious and nonconscious intentional content (recall the example of color vision, that is, of Lewis qualia, Raffman qualia, Metzinger qualia, and wavelength sensitivity exhibited in blindsight as sketched in chapter 2).

For a comprehensive semantics of mind the most promising variant today would, I believe, consist in a new combination of Paul Churchlands' "state-space semantics" (SSS; Churchland 1986, 1989, 1995, 1996, and 1998) with what Andy Clark and David Chalmers have provisionally called "active externalism" (AE; Clark and Chalmers 1998). SSS may be just right for *phenomenal* content, whereas an "embodied" version of AE could be what we need for *intentional* content. State-space semantics perhaps is presently the best conceptual tool for describing the internal, neurally realized dynamics of mental states, while active externalism helps us understand how this dynamics could originally have developed from a behavioral embedding of the system in its environment. State-space semantics in principle allows us to develop fine-grained and empirically plausible descriptions of the way in which a phenomenal space can be partitioned (see also Au. Clark 1993, 2000). The "space of knowledge," however, the domain of those properties determining the intentional content of mental states, seems to "pulsate" across the physical boundaries of the system, seems to pulsate into extradermal reality. Describing the intentional content generated by real life, situated, embodied agents may simply make it necessary to analyze *another* space of possible states, for example, the space of causal interactions generated by sensorimotor loops or the behavioral space of the system in general. In other words, the intentionality relation, as I conceive of it, is not a rigid, abstract relation, as it were, like an arrow pointing out of the system toward isolated intentional objects, but an entirely *real* relationship exhibiting causal properties and its own temporal dynamics. If the intentional object does not exist in the current environment, we are confronted with what I called a mental simulation in section 2.3, that is, with an intrasystemic relation. If the object of knowledge is "intentionally inexistent" in Brentano's ([1874] 1973) original sense, it is the content of an internally *simulated* object. The nonexisting object component of the intentionality relation exists *in* the system as an active object emulator.

It is interesting to note that there exists something like a consciously experienced, a *phenomenal* model of the intentionality relation as well (see Metzinger 1993, 2000c; and section 6.5 in particular). This special representational structure is crucial to understanding what a consciously experienced first-person perspective actually is. It can exist in situations where the organism is functionally decoupled from its environment, as for instance during a dream. Dreams, phenomenally, are first-person states in being structurally characterized by the existence of a phenomenal *model* of ongoing subject-object relations. As a form of phenomenal content the model locally supervenes on internal properties of the brain (see section 6.5). It is important never to confuse this theoretical entity (about which I say much more at a later stage) with the "real" intentionality relation constituted by an active cognitive agent interacting with its environment. Of course, or so I would claim, this phenomenal structure internally simulating *directedness* existed in human brains long before philosophers started theorizing about it—and therefore may not be the model, but the *original*.

If one uses dynamicist cognitive science and the notion of AE as a heuristic background model for taking a fresh perspective on things, the temporality and the constructive aspect of cognition become much more vivid, because the phenomenal subject now turns into a real agent, the functional situatedness of which can be conceptually grasped in a much clearer fashion. In particular, it is now tempting to look at such an agent and those parts of the physical environment with which it is currently entertaining a direct causal contact as a *singular* dynamical system. In doing so we may create a first conceptual connection between two important theoretical domains: the problem of embedding of the cognitive subject in the world and questions concerning philosophical semantics. According to my implicit background assumption and according to this theoretical vision, representations and semantic content are nothing static anymore. They, as it were, "ride" on a transient wave of coherence between system dynamics and world dynamics. Representational content is neither an abstract individual nor a property anymore, but an *event*. Meaning is a physical phenomenon that, for example, is transiently and episodically generated by an information-processing system tied into an active sensorimotor loop. The generation of the intentional content of mental representations is only an episode, a transient process, in which system dynamics and world dynamics briefly interact. Herbert Jaeger describes this notion of an *interactionist* concept theory:

Here the representational content of concepts is not (as in model theory) seen in an ideal reference relationship between concept (or its symbol) and external denotatum. Rather, the representational content of a concept results from invariants in the interactional history of an agent with regard to external objects. "Concepts" and "represented objects" are dependent on each other; together both are a single dynamical pattern of interaction. (Jaeger 1996, p. 166; English translation by T.M.; see also Metzinger 1998)

If we follow this intuitive line, cognition turns into a bodily mediated process through and through, resting on a process instantiating a transient set of physical properties extending beyond the borders of the system. Intentional content, transiently, supervenes on this set of physical properties, which—at least in principle—can be described in a formally exact manner. This is a new theoretical vision: Intentionality is not a rigid abstract relation from subject toward intentional object, but a dynamical physical *process* pulsating across the boundaries of the system. In perception, for instance, the physical system border is briefly transgressed by coupling the currently active self-model to a perceptual object (note that there may be a simplified version in which the *brain* internally models this type of event, leading to a *phenomenal* model of the intentionality relation, a "PMIR," as defined in section 6.5). Intended cognition now means that a system actively—corresponding to its own needs and epistemic goals—changes the physical basis on which the representational content of its current mental state supervenes.

If one further assumes that brains (at least in their cognitive subregion) never take on stationary system states, even when stationary patterns of input signals exist, the classic concept of a static representation can hardly be retained. Rather, we have to understand "representational" properties of a cognitive system as resulting from a dynamical interaction between a structured environment and a self-organizational process within an autotropic system. In doing so, internal representations refer to structural elements of the environment—and thereby to those problem domains confronting the system—as well as to the physical properties of the organism itself, that is, to the material makeup and structure of its sense organs, its motor apparatus, and its cognitive system. (Pasemann 1996, p. 81*f.*, English translation by T.M.; see also Metzinger 1998, p. 349*f.*)

If this is correct, cognition cannot be conceived of without implicit self-representation (see sections 6.2.2. and 6.2.3). Most importantly, the cognitive process cannot be conceived of without the autonomous, internal activity of the system, which generates mental and phenomenal simulations of possible worlds within itself (see section 2.3). This is another point making intentionality not only a concrete but also a *lived* phenomenon; within this conceptual framework one can imagine what it means that the activation of intentional content truly is a biological phenomenon (for good examples see Thompson and Varela 2001, p. 424; Damasio 1999, Panksepp 1998). On the other hand, one has to see that the dynamicist approach does not, for now, supply us with an epistemic justification for the cognitive content of our mental states: we have those states because they were functionally adequate from an evolutionary perspective. For biosystems like ourselves, they constituted a viable path through the causal matrix of the physical world. If and in what sense they really can count as knowledge about the world would first have to be shown by a naturalistic epistemology. Can any epistemic justification be derived from the functional success of cognitive structures as it might be interpreted under a dynamicist approach? Pasemann writes:

> As situated and adaptive, that is, as a system capable of survival, cognitive systems are by these *autonomous* inner processes put in a position to make predictions and develop meaningful strategies for action, that is, to generate *predictive world-models*. Inner representations as internally generated configurations of coherent module dynamics then have to be understood as building blocks for a world-model, based on which an internal exploration of alternative actions can take place. Hence, any such configuration corresponds to a set of aspects of the environment, as they can be grasped by the sensors and "manipulated" by the motor system. As partial dynamics of a cognitive process they can be newly assembled again and again, and to result in consistent world-models they have to be "compatible" with each other. . . . One criterion for the validity or "goodness" of a semantic configuration, treated as a hypothesis, is its utility for the organism in the *future*. Successful configurations in this sense represent regularities of external dynamical processes; they are at the same time coherent, that is, in harmony with external dynamics. (Pasemann 1996, p. 85, English translation by T.M.; see also Metzinger 1998, p. 350)

The general idea has been surfacing for a number of years in a number of different scientific communities and countries. Philosophically, its basic idea differs from the standard variant, formulated by Hilary Putnam and Tyler Burge (H. Putnam 1975a; Burge 1979), in that those external properties fixing the intentional content are historical and distal properties of the world; they can be found at the other end of a long causal chain. *Present*, actual properties of the environment were irrelevant to classic externalism, and therefore epistemically *passive* properties. Active externalism, as opposed to this intuition, consists in claiming that the content-fixing properties in the environment are active properties within a sensorimotor loop realized in the very present; they are *in the loop* (Clark and Chalmers 1998, p. 9). Within the framework of this conception one could keep assuming that phenomenal content supervenes on internal states. With regard to belief and intentional contents in general, however, one now would have to say that our mind extends beyond the physical borders of our skin into the world, until it confronts those properties of the world which *drive* cognitive processes—for instance, through sensorimotor loops and recurrent causal couplings. Please note how this idea complements the more general notion of *functional internality* put forward in the previous chapter. We could conceptually analyze this type of interaction as the activation of a new system state functioning as a representatum by being a *functionally* internal event (because it rests on a transient change in the functional properties of one and the same dynamical system), but which has to utilize resources which are *physically* external for their concrete realization. Obviously, one of the most interesting applications of this speculative thought might be social cognition. As we now learn through empirical investigations, mental states can in part be driven by the mental states of other thinkers.[4]

In short, neither connectionism nor dynamicist cognitive science, in my opinion, poses a serious threat to the concept of representation. On the contrary, they enrich it. They do not eliminate the concept of representation, but provide us with new insights into the *format* of mental representations. What is most urgently needed is a dynamicist theory of *content*. However, in the end, a new concept of explanation may be needed, involving covering laws instead of traditional mechanistic models of decomposition (Bechtel 1998). It also shifts our attention to a higher emphasis on ecological validity. Therefore, even if wildly sympathizing with dynamicist cognitive science, one can stay a representationalist without turning into a hopelessly old-fashioned person. Our concept of representation is constantly enriched and refined, while at the same time the general strategy of developing a representationalist analysis of mind remains viable.

I hope these short remarks will be useful to some of my readers in what follows. I endorse teleofunctionalism, subsymbolic and dynamicist strategies of modeling mental content, and I take it that *phenomenal* content is highly likely to supervene locally. Let us now return to the project of defining the baselines for a conceptual prototype of phenomenal representation. Is it in principle possible to construct something like a representationalist computer science of phenomenal states, or what Thomas Nagel (1974) called an "objective phenomenology?"

3.2   Multilevel Constraints: What Makes a Neural Representation a *Phenomenal* Representation?

The interdisciplinary project of consciousness research, now experiencing such an impressive renaissance with the turn of the century, faces two fundamental problems. First, there is yet no single, unified and *paradigmatic* theory of consciousness in existence which could serve as an object for constructive criticism and as a backdrop against which new attempts could be formulated. Consciousness research is still in a preparadigmatic stage. Second,

---

4. See, for example, Gallese 2000. If, however, one does not want to look at the self just as a bundle of currently active states and in this way, as Clark and Chalmers would say, face problems regarding the concept of psychological continuity, but also wants to imply dispositional states as components of the self, then, according to this conception, the self also extends beyond the boundary of the organism. This is not a discussion in which I can enter, because the general thesis of the current approach is that no such things as selves exist in the world. It may be more helpful to distinguish between the phenomenal and the intentional content of our self-*model*, which may supervene on overlapping, but strongly diverging sets of functional properties. Our *intentional* self-model is limited by the functional borders of behavioral space (which may be *temporal* borders as well), and these borders, under certain conditions, can be very far away. See also chapter 6.

there is no systematic and comprehensive catalogue of *explananda*. Although philosophers have done considerable work on the *analysanda*, the interdisciplinary community has nothing remotely resembling an agenda for research. We do not yet have a precisely formulated list of explanatory targets which could be used in the construction of systematic research programs. In this section I offer a catalogue of the multilevel conceptual constraints (or criteria of ascription) that will allow us to decide if a certain representational state may also be a conscious state. This catalogue is a *preliminary* catalogue. It is far from being the list mentioned above. It is deliberately formulated in a manner that allows it to be continuously enriched and updated by new empirical discoveries. It also offers many possibilities for further conceptual differentiation, as my philosophical readers will certainly realize. However, the emphasis here is not on maximizing conceptual precision, but on developing workable tools for interdisciplinary cooperation.

Only two of the constraints offered here appear as necessary conditions to me. Some of them only hold for certain state classes, or are domain-specific. It follows that there will be a whole palette of different concepts of "consciousness" possessing variable semantic strength and only applying to certain types of systems in certain types of phenomenal configurations. The higher the degree of constraint satisfaction, the higher the degree of phenomenality in a given domain. However, with regard to an internally so immensely complex domain like conscious experience it would be a mistake to have the expectation of being able to find a route toward one individual, semantically homogeneous concept, spanning, as it were, *all* forms of consciousness. On the contrary, a systematic *differentiation* of research programs is what we urgently need at the present stage of interdisciplinary consciousness research. Almost all of the constraints that follow have primarily been developed by phenomenological considerations; in their origin they are first-person constraints, which have then been further enriched on other levels of description. However, for the first and last constraint in this list (see sections 3.2.1 and 3.2.11), this is not true; they are objective criteria, exclusively developed from a third-person perspective.

3.2.1   Global Availability

Let us start with this constraint—only for the simple reason that it was the sole and first example of a possible constraint that I offered in the last chapter. It is a functional constraint. This is to say that, so far, it has only been described on a level of description individuating the internal states of a conscious system by their causal role. Also, it is exclusively being applied to subsystemic states and their content; it is not a personal-level constraint.

We can sum up a large amount of empirical data in a very elegant way by simply saying the following: Phenomenally represented information is precisely that subset of currently active information in the system of which it is true that it is *globally available* for deliberately guided attention, cognitive reference, and control of action (again, see Baars 1988, 1997; Chalmers 1997). As we have already seen, at least one important limitation to this principle is known. A large majority of simple sensory contents (e.g., of phenomenal color nuances, e.g., in terms of Raffman or Metzinger qualia) are not available for cognitive reference because perceptual memory cannot grasp contents that are individuated in such a fine-grained manner. Subtle shades are ineffable, because their causal properties make them available for attentional processing and discriminative motor control, but *not* for mental concept formation. As shown in the last chapter there are a number of cases in which global availability may even only apply in an even weaker and highly context-specific sense, for instance, in wavelength sensitivity in blindsight. In general, however, all phenomenal representata make their content at least globally available for attention and motor control. We can now proceed to further analyze this first constraint on the five major levels of description I mentioned in the brief introduction to this chapter: the *phenomenological* level of description (essentially operating from the first-person perspective or under a "heterophenomenological" combination of such perspectives), the *representationalist* level of description (analyzing phenomenal content as a special kind of representational *content*), the *informational-computational* level of description (classifying kinds of information and types of processing), the *functional* level of description (including issues about the *causal roles* realized in conscious states), and the *neurobiological* level of description (including issues of concrete implementational details, and the physical correlates of conscious experience in general).

The Phenomenology of Global Availability

The contents of conscious experience are characterized by my ability to react directly to them with a multitude of my mental and bodily capacities. I can direct my attention toward a perceived color or toward a bodily sensation in order to inspect them more closely ("attentional availability"). In some cases at least I am able to form thoughts about this particular color. I can make an attempt to form a concept of it ("availability for phenomenal cognition"), which associates it with earlier color experiences ("availability for autobiographical memory") and I can communicate about color with other people by using language ("availability for speech control," which might also be termed "communicative availability"). I can reach for colored objects and sort them according to their phenomenal properties ("availability for the control of action"). In short, global availability is an all-pervasive functional property of my conscious contents, which *itself* I once again subjectively experience, namely, as my own flexibility and autonomy in dealing with these contents. The availability component of this constraint comes in many different kinds. Some of them are subjectively experienced as immediate, some of them as rather indirect (e.g., in conscious thought). Some available contents are transparent; some are opaque (see section 3.2.7). On the phenomenal level this leads to a series of very general, but important experiential characteristics: I live my life in a world that is an *open* world. I experience a large degree of selectivity in the way I access certain objects in this world. I am an autonomous agent. Many different aspects of this world seem to be simultaneously available to me all the time.

From a philosophical perspective, availability for phenomenally represented cognition probably is the most interesting aspect of this characteristic. This phenomenological feature shows us as beings not only living in the concreteness of sensory awareness. If conscious, we are given to ourselves as thinking persons on the level of subjective experience as well (for the hypothetical notion of an *unconscious* cognitive agent, see Crick and Koch 2000). In order to initiate genuinely cognitive processes, abstracta like classes or relations have to be mentally represented and made available on the level of subjective experience itself. Globally available cognitive processing is characterized by flexibility, selectivity of content, and a certain degree of autonomy. Therefore, we become cognitive *agents*. In particular, this constraint is of decisive importance if we are interested in understanding how a simple phenomenal self can be transformed into a cognitive subject, which then in turn forms a new content of conscious experience itself. Reflexive, conceptually mediated self-consciousness can be analyzed as a particularly important special case under the global availability constraint, in which a particular type of information becomes cognitively available for the system (I return to this point in section 6.4.4). Furthermore, "availability for phenomenal cognition" is for two reasons a constraint requiring a particularly careful empirical investigation. First, a large class of simple and stimulus-correlated phenomenal states—presentata—do exist that do not satisfy this constraint. Second, phenomenal cognition itself is a highly interesting process, because it marks out the most important class of states not captured by *constraint 6*, namely, the transparency of phenomenal states (see section 3.2.7).

Importantly, we have to do justice to a second phenomenological property. As we have seen, there is a globality component and an availability component, the latter possessing a phenomenological reading in terms of autonomy, flexibility, and selectivity of conscious access to the world. But what about a phenomenological reading for the *globality component*? What precisely does it mean if we say that the contents of conscious experience are "globally" available for the subject? It means that these contents can always be found *in a world* (see *constraint 3*). What is globality on the phenomenological as opposed to the functional level? Globality consists in the property of being embedded in a highest-order whole that is highly differentiated, while at the same time being a fully integrated form of content. From the first-person perspective, this phenomenal whole simply is the world in which I live my life, and the boundaries of this world are the boundaries of my reality. It is constituted by the information available to me, that is, *subjectively* available. States of consciousness are always states within a consciously experienced world; they unfold their individual dynamics against the background of a highest-order situational context. This is what constitutes the phenomenological reading of "globality": being an integral part of a single, unified world. If globality in this sense is not used as a constraint for state classes, but as one of *system classes*, one arrives at the following interesting statement: All systems operating with globally available information are systems which experience themselves as *living in a world*. Of course, this statement will only be true if all other necessary constraints (yet to be developed) are also met.

Global Availability of Representational Content

Phenomenal representata are characterized by the fact of their *intentional* content being directly available for a multitude of other representational processes. Their content is available for further processing by subsymbolic mechanisms like attention or memory, and also for concept formation, metacognition, planning, and motor simulations with immediate behavioral consequences. Its globality consists in being embedded in a functionally active model of the world at any point in time (Yates 1985). Phenomenal representational content necessarily is integrated into an overarching, singular, and coherent representation of reality as a whole.

Informational-Computational Availability

Phenomenal *information* is precisely that information directly available to a system in the sense just mentioned. If one thinks in the conceptual framework of classical architecture, one can nicely formulate both aspects of this constraint in accordance with Bernard Baars's global workspace theory (GWT): phenomenal information processing takes place in a global workspace, which can be accessed simultaneously by a multitude of specific modules (Baars 1988, 1997). On the other hand, obviously, this architectural assumption in its current version is implausible in our own case and from a neurobiological perspective (however, see Baars and Newman 1994; for a recent application of GWT, see Dehaene and Naccache 2001, p. 26*ff*.; for a philosophical discussion, see Dennett 2001). However, Baars certainly deserves credit for being the first author who has actually started to develop a full-blown cognitivist theory of conscious experience and of clearly seeing the relevance and the general scope of the globality component inherent in this constraint. As it turns out, globality is one of the very few *necessary* conditions in ascribing phenomenality to active information in a given system.

Global Availability as a Functional Property of Conscious Information

There is an informational and a computational reading of availability as well: phenomenal information, functionally speaking, is precisely that information directly available to a system in the sense just mentioned, and precisely that information contributing to the ongoing process of generating a coherent, constantly updated model of the world as a whole. As a *functional* constraint, globality reliably marks out conscious contents by characterizing its causal role. It consists in being integrated into the *largest* coherent state possessing a distinct causal role—the system's world-model. One of the central computational goals of phenomenal information processing, therefore, is likely to consist in generating a single and fully disambiguated representation of reality that can serve as a reference basis for the fast and flexible control of inner, as well as outer, behavior. Please note how the globality constraint does not describe a cause that then later has a distinct conscious *effect*—it simply highlights a characteristic feature of the target phenomenon *as such* (Dennett 2001, p. 223). If one wants to individuate phenomenal states by their causal role, *constraint 1* helps us to pick out an important aspect of this causal role: phenomenal states can interact with a large number of specialized modules in very short periods of time and in a flexible manner. One-step learning and fast *global* updates of the overall reality model now become possible.

If one looks at the system as a whole, it becomes obvious how phenomenal states increase the flexibility of its behavioral profile: the more information processed by the system is *phenomenal* information, the higher the degree of flexibility and context sensitivity with which it can react to challenges from the environment. Now many different functional modules can directly use this information to react to external requirements in a differentiated way. In this new context, let us briefly recall an example mentioned in the last chapter. A blindsight patient suffering from terrible thirst and perceiving a glass of water within his scotoma, that is, within his experientially "blind" spot, is not able to initiate a reaching movement toward the glass. The glass is not a part of *his* reality. However, in a forced-choice situation he will in almost all cases correctly guess what kind of object can be found at this location. This meant that information about the identity of the object in question is active in the system, was extracted from the environment by the sensory organs in the usual way, and can, under special conditions, be once again made explicit. Still, this information is not phenomenally represented and, for this reason, is not functionally available for the selective control of action. The blindsight patient is an autonomous agent in a slightly weaker sense than before his brain lesion occurred. That something is part of your reality means that it is part of your behavioral space. From a teleofunctionalist perspective, therefore, globally available information supports all those kinds of goal-directed behavior in which adaptivity and success are not exclusively tied to speed, but also to the selectivity of accompanying volitional control, preplanning, and cognitive processing.

Neural Correlates of Global Availability

At present hardly anything is known about the neurobiological realization of the function just sketched. However, converging evidence seems to point to a picture in which large-scale integration is mediated by the transient formation of dynamical links through neural synchrony over multiple frequency bands (Varela, Lachaux, Rodriguez, and Martinerie 2001). From a philosophical perspective the task consists in describing a flexible architecture that accommodates *degrees* of modularism and holism for phenomenal content within one global superstructure. Let us focus on large-scale integration for now. Among many competing hypotheses, one of the most promising may be Edelman and Tononi's dynamical core theory (Edelman and Tononi 2000a,b; Tononi and Edelman 1998a). The activation of a conscious state could be conceived of as a selection from a very large repertoire of possible states that in principle is as comprehensive as the whole of our experiential state space and our complete phenomenal space of simulation. Thereby it constitutes a correspondingly large amount of information. Edelman and Tononi also point out that although for new and consciously controlled tasks neural activation in the brain is highly distributed, this activation turns out to be more and more localized and "functionally isolated" the more automatic, fast, precise, and unconscious the solution of this task becomes in the course of time. During this development it also loses its context sensitivity, its global availability, and its flexibility. The authors introduce the concept of a *functional cluster*: a subset of neural elements with a cluster index (CI) value higher than 1, containing no smaller subsets with a higher CI value itself, constitutes a functional "bundle," a single and integrated neural process, which cannot be split up into independent, partial subprocesses (Edelman and Tononi 1998; Tononi, McIntosh, Russell, and Edelman 1998).

The dynamical core hypothesis is an excellent example of an empirical hypothesis *simultaneously* setting constraints on the functional and physical (i.e., neural) levels of description. The phenomenological unity of consciousness, constantly accompanied by an enormous variance in phenomenal *content*, reappears as what from a philosophical perspective may be conceptually analyzed as the "density of causal linkage." At any given time, the set of physical elements directly correlated with the content of the conscious model of reality will be marked out in terms of a high degree of density within a discrete set of causal relations. The *internal correlation strength* of the corresponding physical elements will create a discrete set of such causal relations, characterized by a *gradient of causal coherence* lifting the physical correlate of consciousness out of its less complex and less integrated physical environment in the brain, like an island emerging from the sea. From a philosophical point of view, it is important to note how the notion of "causal density," defined as the internal correlation strength observed at a given point in time for all elements of the minimally sufficient and global neural correlate of consciousness, does not imply functional rigidity. One of the interesting features of Tononi and Edelman's theoretical analysis of complexity is that it lets us understand how "neural complexity strikes an optimal balance between segregation and integration of function" (Edelman and Tononi 2000b, p. 136).

The dynamical core hypothesis is motivated by a number of individual observations. Lesion studies imply that many structures external to the thalamocortical system have no direct influence on conscious experience. Neurophysiological studies show that only certain subsets of neurons in certain regions of this system correlate with consciously experienced percepts. In general, conscious experience seems to be correlated with those invariant properties in the process of object representation that are highly informative, stable elements of behavioral space and thereby can be manipulated in an easier way. Only certain *types* of interaction within the thalamocortical system are strong enough to lead to the formation of a large functional cluster within a few hundred milliseconds. Therefore, the basic idea behind this hypothesis is that a group of neurons can only contribute to the contents of consciousness if it is part of a highly distributed functional cluster achieving the integration of all information active within it in very short periods of time. In doing so, this cluster at the same time has to exhibit high values of complexity (Tononi and Edelman 1998a). The composition of the dynamical core, for this reason, can transcend anatomical boundaries (like a "cloud of causal density" hovering above the neurobiological substrate), but at the same time constitutes a *functional* border, because through its high degree of integration it is in contact with internal information in a much stronger sense than with any kind of external information. The discreteness of the internally correlated set of causal elements mentioned above, therefore, finds its reflection in the conscious model of reality constituting an integrated internal informational space.

These short remarks with regard to the first constraint (which, as readers will recall, I had introduced in chapter 2 as a first example of a functional constraint to be imposed on the concept of phenomenal representation) show how one can simultaneously analyze ascription criteria for phenomenal content on a number of levels of description. However, if we take a closer look, it also draws our attention toward potential problems and the need for further research programs. Let me give an example.

Many authors write about the global availability of conscious contents in terms of a "direct" availability. Clearly, as Franz Brentano, the philosophical founder of empirical psychology, remarked in 1874, it would be a fallacy to conclude from the apparent, phenomenal unity of consciousness that the underlying *mechanism* would have to be simple and unified as well, because, as Brentano's subtle argument ran, for inner perception not to show something and for it to show that something does not exist are two different things.[5] I have frequently spoken about "direct" availability myself. Clearly, on the *phenomenological* level the experiential directness of access (in "real time" as it were) is a convincing conceptual constraint. However, if we go down to the nuts and bolts of actual neuroscience, "direct access" could have very different meanings for very different types of information or representational content—even if the phenomenal experience of direct access seems to be unitary and simple, a global phenomenon (Ruhnau 1995; see also Damasio's concept of "core consciousness" in Damasio 1999). As we move down the levels of description, we may have to differentiate constraints. For instance, particularly when investigating the phenomenal correlates of neuropsychological disorders, it is always helpful to ask *what* kind of information is available for *what* kind of processing mechanism. Let me stay with the initial example and return to a first coarse-grained differentiation of the notion of global availability to illustrate this point. In order to accommodate empirical data from perceptual and neuropsychology we have to at least refine this constraint toward three further levels:

1. Availability for guided *attention* ("attentional penetrability" hereafter, in terms of the notions of introspection$_1$ and introspection$_3$ as introduced in chapter 2)

2. Availability for *cognitive* processing ("cognitive penetrability"; introspection$_2$ and introspection$_4$)

3. Availability for the selective control of action ("volitional penetrability" hereafter)

We experience (and we speak about) phenomenal space as a *unified* space characterized by an apparent "direct" access to information within it. However, I predict that closer investigation will reveal that this space can be decomposed into the space of attention, the space of conscious thought, and the volitionally penetrable partition of behavioral space (in terms of that information that can become a target of selectively controlled, consciously initiated *action*). It must be noted how even this threefold distinction is still very crude. There are many different kinds of attention, for example, low-level and high-level attention; there are styles and formats of cognitive processing (e.g., metaphorical, pictorial, and quasi-symbolic); and it is also plausible to assume that, for instance, the space of automatic bodily behavior and the space of rational action overlap but never fully coincide. Different types of access generate different worlds or realities as it were: the world of

---

5. "*Weiter ist noch insbesondere hervorzuheben, daß in der Einheit des Bewußtseins auch nicht der Ausschluß einer Mehrheit quantitativer Teile und der Mangel jeder räumlichen Ausdehnung . . . ausgesprochen liegt. Es ist gewiß, daß die innere Wahrnehmung uns keine Ausdehnung zeigt; aber etwas nicht zeigen und zeigen, daß etwas nicht ist, ist verschieden.* [Furthermore, it is necessary to emphasize that the unity of consciousness does not exclude either a plurality of qualitative parts or spatial extension (or an analogue thereof). It is certain that inner perception does not show us any extension; there is a difference, however, between not showing something and showing that something does note exist.] Cf. Brentano [1874], 1973, p. 165*f*.

attention, the world of action, and the world of thought. Yet, under standard conditions, these overlapping informational spaces are subjectively experienced as *one* unified world. An important explanatory target, therefore, is to search for the invariant factor uniting them (see section 6.5).

As we have already seen with regard to the example of conscious color perception, there will likely be different neurobiological processes making information available for attention and for mental concept formation. On the phenomenal level, however, we may experience both kinds of contents as "directly accessible." We may experience Lewis qualia, Raffman qualia, and Metzinger qualia as possessing different degrees of "realness," but they certainly belong to one unified reality and they seem to be given to us in a direct and immediate fashion. I have already discussed, at length, one example of phenomenal information—the one expressed through presentational content—which is attentionally available and can functionally be expressed in certain discrimination tasks, while not being available for categorization or linguistic reference. On a phenomenological level this conscious content can be characterized as subtle and liquid, as bound to the immediate present, and as ineffable. However, with regard to the phenomenal "directness" of access it does not differ from cognitively available content, as, for instance, presented in the pure colors. Let me term this the "phenomenal immediacy" constraint.

The subjectively experienced *immediacy* of subjective, experiential content obviously cannot be reduced to functionalist notions of attentional or cognitive availability. Therefore, we need an additional constraint in order to analyze this form of phenomenal content on the representationalist level of description. Only if we have a clear conception of what phenomenal immediacy could mean in terms of representational content can we hope for a successful functionalist analysis that might eventually lead to the discovery of neural correlates (see section 3.2.7). Having said this, and having had a first look at the functional constraint of global availability, which we used as our starting example for a productive and interesting constraint that would eventually yield a convincing concept of phenomenal representation, let us now consider a series of ten further multilevel constraints. The starting point in developing these constraints typically is the phenomenological level of description. I always start with a first-person description of the constraint and then work my way down through a number of third-person levels of description, with the representational level of analysis forming the logical link between subjective and objective properties. Only the last constraint in our catalogue of ten (the "adaptivity constraint" to be introduced in section 3.2.11) does not take a first-person description of the target phenomenon as its starting point. As we walk through the garden of this original set of ten multilevel constraints, a whole series of interesting discoveries can be made. For instance, as we will see, only the first two and the seventh of these ten constraints can count as candidates for *necessary* conditions in the ascription of conscious experience.

However, they will turn out to be sufficient conditions for a minimal concept of phenomenal experience (see section 3.2.7).

3.2.2   Activation within a Window of Presence

Constraint 2 points not to a functional, but primarily to a phenomenological constraint. As a constraint for the ascription of phenomenality employed from the first-person perspective it arguably is the most general and the strongest candidate. Without exception it is true of all my phenomenal states, because whatever I experience, I always experience it *now*. The experience of presence coming with our phenomenal model of reality may be the central aspect that cannot be "bracketed" in a Husserlian sense: It is, as it were, the temporal immediacy of existence *as such*. If we subtract the global characteristic of presence from the phenomenal world-model, then we simply subtract its existence. We would subtract consciousness *tout court*. It would not *appear* to us anymore. If, from a third-person perspective, one does not apply the presentationality constraint to states, but to persons as a whole, one immediately realizes why the difference between consciousness and unconsciousness appears so eminently important to beings like us: only persons with phenomenal states exist as psychological subjects at all. Only persons possessing a subjective Now are *present* beings, for themselves and for others. Let us take a closer look.

Phenomenology of Presence
The contents of phenomenal experience not only generate a world but also a *present*. One may even go so far as to say that, at its core, phenomenal consciousness is precisely this: the generation of an island of presence in the continuous flow of physical time (Ruhnau 1995). To consciously experience means to *be in a present*. It means that you are processing information in a very special way. This special way consists in repeatedly and continuously integrating individual events (already represented as such) into larger temporal gestalts, into one singular psychological moment. What is a conscious *moment*? The phenomenal experience of time in general is constituted by a series of important achievements. They consist in the phenomenal representation of temporal identity (experienced simultaneity), of temporal difference (experienced nonsimultaneity), of seriality and unidirectionality (experienced succession of events), of temporal wholeness (the generation of a unified present, the "specious" phenomenal Now), and the representation of temporal permanence (the experience of duration). The decisive transition toward subjective experience, that is, toward a genuinely *phenomenal* representation of time, takes place in the last step but one: precisely when event representations are continuously integrated into psychological *moments*.

If events are not only represented as being in temporal succession but are integrated into temporal figures (e.g., the extended gestalt of a consciously experienced musical motive), then a present emerges, because these events are now internally connected. They are not isolated atoms anymore, because they form a context for each other. Just as in visual perception different global stimulus properties—for instance, colors, shapes, and surface textures—are bound into a subjectively experienced object of perception (e.g., a consciously seen apple) in time perception as well, something like object formation takes place in which isolated events are integrated into a Now. One can describe the emergence of this Now as a process of segmentation that separates a vivid temporal object from a temporal background that is only weakly structured. This can, for instance, happen if we do not experience a musical motive as a sequence of isolated sound events, but as a holistic temporal figure. A psychological moment is not an extensionless point, but for beings like us it possesses a culturally invariant duration of, maximally, three seconds. What makes the task of giving an accurate phenomenology of time experience so difficult is that we do not have to describe the island, but the river flowing around it as well. The feature that is conceptually so hard to grasp is how we can consciously experience a full-blown present *as embedded in* a unidirectional flow, the experience of duration. There are temporal gestalts, islands of individually characterized Nows, but the background against which these islands are segregated is itself not static: it possesses a direction. Subjective time flows from past to future, while at the same time allowing us to rise above this flow in the immediacy of the conscious presence. From my point of view, the core of the philosophical problem consists in the fact that even the island is transparent in that the background from which it is segregated can always been seen through it. It is not only the island that is located in the river but in a strange sense the river is flowing *through* the island itself. The phenomenal property in question seems to be *superimposed* onto the serial flow of events that at the same time constitutes it (see also section 3.2.5).

Phenomenal Presence as a Form of Representational Content *de nunc*
Let us proceed to the representationalist level of description to get a better understanding of the presentationality constraint. Can it be analyzed as a special kind of *content*? Yes, because there is a specific *de nunc* character to phenomenal content. A complete physical description of the universe would not contain the information, what time is "now." A complete physical description of the universe would not contain an analysis of time as a unidirectional phenomenon. The first point to note when shifting back into the third-person perspective is that the physical world is "nowless," as well as futureless and pastless. The conscious experience of time is a *simulational* type of mental content that proved to be a useful tool for a certain kind of biological organism on a certain planet. It was functionally adequate to model approximatively the temporal structure of this organism's domain of causal interaction. It is not an epistemically justified form of content: just because human beings phenomenally experience a conscious Now doesn't permit the conclusion

that there actually *is* something like a present. Proceeding to the representationalist level of description we first find that the following analysis corresponds to the phenomenological constraint of "presence": phenomenal processes of representation not only generate spatial but also *temporal internality*. It is this form of internality that is a simulational fiction from the third-person perspective (see chapter 2). This does not mean that it is not a highly successful and functionally *adequate* fiction. Information represented by phenomenal models of reality is always being presented to the subject of experience as *actual* information. In section 2.4.4, I had formulated for the most simple forms of functional phenomenal content the *principle of presentationality*. Simple phenomenal content always is *temporal* content. This is to say that it always contains temporal information and this information is depicted as invariant: the state of affairs in question is holding *exactly now*.

Active phenomenal representata in this regard are the nonpropositional and subcategorical analoga to propositional attitudes *de nunc*. We now see that the principle of presentationality can be generalized to the class of all phenomenal states. They are tied to a certain mode of presentation because their content necessarily is content *de nunc*. This special mode of presentation has already been named: its content can only be activated within a virtual window of presence, because it possesses certain functional properties intimately tying it to those mechanisms by which the organism generates its own phenomenal Now. If one is interested in empirically narrowing down the philosophical concept of a "mode of presentation" for this special case, those scientific investigations are relevant that give us new insights into the generation of a window of presence by the human brain.[6] The conscious correlate of this functional property is the phenomenal experience of an instantaneous and simultaneous givenness of certain contents, and also of their dynamical evolution *within the current moment*.

The Window of Presence as a Functional Property
The generation of a phenomenal present can also be analyzed as a complex informational-computational property. Generally speaking, any purely data-driven model of the world will not permit explicit predictions in time (Cruse 1999). Only additional, recurrent networks will allow for the generation of time-dependent states. That is, any explicit representation of time in a connectionist network will make a functional architecture necessary, which involves feedback loops and recurrent connections. The representation of a "Now" then becomes the *simplest* form of explicit time representation, as a set of recurrent loops plus a certain decay function.

---

6. Therefore, all data concerning the underpinnings of short-term memory are directly related to the presentationality constraint. In chapter 2 I emphasized that it is also the work of Ernst Pöppel, which is relevant in this context. Cf. Pöppel 1985, 1994; Ruhnau 1992, 1995; Ruhnau and Pöppel 1991.

We have already seen how, from an epistemological perspective, every representation also is a simulation, and also that the genuinely phenomenal variant of mental representation can only emerge by a further achievement of the system. An important aspect of this achievement consists in an additional and continuous integration of currently active mental contents, for instance, into a global model of reality (see next section). This integration is special in that it also takes place with regard to the temporal domain: by defining *time windows*—that is, by creating an internal, temporal frame of reference—on a functional level, the intentional content of some simulations is being treated as if it were *temporally internal*. Not only is it *in a world* (i.e., globally available), but it is also *in a present*. A completely new form of representational content—"nowness" or temporal internality—is made available for the system. A new functional property brings about a new representational property: the capacity to internally model temporal properties of the environment. From this brief analysis, far-reaching statements about functional properties of phenomenal representata follow.

Obviously, short-term memory will be at the heart of any cognitivist-functionalist analysis of the presentationality constraint for phenomenal content. Working memory keeps phenomenal contents active for some time; even after actual stimuli have disappeared from the receptive field, it helps to bridge delays in memory processing and thereby enable a successful solution of certain tasks. Formally, one can easily imagine short-term memory as possessing a recurrent, "loopy," or reverbatory structure in combination with a variable decay function. Empirically, there is evidence for an additional domain-specificity within working memory (Courtney, Petit, Haxby, and Ungerleider 1998).

On a functional level of description phenomenal representata have to be precisely those states that are continuously accessed by the mechanism that defines the window of presence for the respective organism. Unfortunately, the generation of a psychological moment is a process very rich in necessary preconditions and of which, no doubt, we do not yet have anything approximating a full and analytically convincing understanding. First, the system has to create elementary event representations by defining *windows of simultaneity* on a fundamental level. All physical events being registered within such a window of simultaneity will from now on be defined as temporally identical. The system then treats all sensory information extracted within such a window of simultaneity as a single event. What it creates is *global indiscriminability* within the temporal domain. Ernst Pöppel (Pöppel 1972, 1978, 1985, 1994) and his coworkers (in particular Ruhnau 1994a, b, 1995; Ruhnau and Pöppel 1991), over many years, have developed a detailed hypothesis, claiming that by phase-locked oscillatory processes *atemporal zones* emerge on a very fundamental level in the system, system states internally characterized by "simultaneity." By opening time windows—in this second, but as yet *nonphenomenological* sense—an information-processing system can, for itself, generate an *operational time*: By quantisizing its information processing, it "swallows up" the continuous flow of physical time at a very fundamental level of its internal model of the world. The generation of such "elementary integration units" (EIUs; this is Pöppel's terminology) can be interpreted as a process of internal data reduction: the system *deletes* information about its own physical processuality, by not defining temporal relations between elements given within such a basal window of simultaneity. Using philosophical terminology, the physical temporality of the actual *vehicles* participating in this elementary representational process, thereby, is not reflected on the level of their *content* anymore. The fine structure of physical time becomes invisible for the system, by becoming *transparent* (see section 3.2.7). A functional property of the carrier systematically determines its content. The physical time interval remains, but the content of the corresponding system states loses all or part of its internal temporal properties: Representational atoms for the temporal domain are generated, the elementary units of integration or EIUs. According to this hypothesis, such elementary events can then, on a higher level of representation, be portrayed as elements in a sequence. Interestingly, empirical data show that for human beings nonsimultaneity is a necessary, but not yet a sufficient condition for generating a subjective time order. Knowledge about temporal differences in stimulus information does not suffice to predict the *direction* in which stimuli are ordered. For individual sensory modules different thresholds of simultaneity hold, a simple fact that is caused by their differing internal conduction velocities. However, the *ordering threshold* is equivalent for all sensory domains. Therefore, it seems to constitute a further function in the processing of temporal information, namely, the first of these functions operating on a supramodal level of representation. If, as this hypothesis assumes, an additional integrational function forms coherent *Zeit-Gestalten*, that is, time gestalts[7] out of elements which are already temporally ordered and are now contributing to common contents, then the central necessary functional constraints for the generation of a phenomenal Now have been satisfied. According to this idea, as soon as three-second segments of this kind form semantic chains through an internal linkage of their intentional contents, a continuous flow of seamlessly connected psychological moments results on the phenomenal level as well.

Neural Correlates of the Window of Presence
Very little is known in terms of implementational details. Ernst Pöppel, in a series of publications, has emphasized how certain empirically well-documented oscillatory phenomena in the brain could serve to provide a rigid internal rhythm for internal information processing by generating the elementary integration units mentioned above. This mecha-

---

7. Eva Ruhnau introduced this concept (cf. Ruhnau 1995). Ruhnau, in the publication cited, also attempted to describe the relationship between event generation, gestalt formation and gestalt and chain formation in a formally precise manner.

nism could thereby realize a function which individuates events with a minimal distance of 30 ms in a way that spans different modalities (and therefore satisfies another obvious constraint for phenomenal representation; see section 3.2.4). The idea that such an integration of low-level representational system events into a temporal experience of "nowness" with a duration of maximally three seconds actually takes place matches nicely with a large amount of neuropsychological data from speech production, musical perception, psychophysics, and the control of volitional movement. Additionally, the fact that the effects just mentioned seem to be highly invariant between different cultures seems to point to the existence of a unitary functional correlate for this integrative mechanism. For this reason it is not inappropriate to hope for a future localization of those neural structures realizing the functional properties just mentioned.

3.2.3   Integration into a Coherent Global State

Constraint 3 demands that individual phenomenal events be always bound into a global situational context. Subjective experience, not only functionally and in terms of the agent being causally grounded in its external behavioral space but also on the level of its contents, is a *situated process*. Conscious human beings are always *phenomenally situated* beings (for a potential exception to the rule, see the discussion of akinetic mutism in chapters 6 and 8). Individual conscious states, in standard situations, are always part of a conscious world-model. Again, we can translate this third constraint to the personal level of description by making the following statement: If and only if a person is conscious, a world exists for her, and if and only if she is conscious can she make the fact of actually living *in* a world available for herself, cognitively and as an agent. Consciousness is *in-der-Welt-sein* ("being in the world"); it makes situatedness globally available to an agent. In starting to speak like this one has not marked out a class of states, but a class of *systems* by our third criterion for the ascription of conscious experience. Let us look at the third constraint—the "globality constraint"—from a whole-system, first-person, and phenomenological perspective.

"Being in the World": Nonepistemic Situatedness

Conscious systems operate under an interesting constraint, which I introduced by calling it "autoepistemic closure." It is constituted by (a) the existence of a comprehensive representation of reality as a whole, and (b) the fact that this representation cannot be recognized *as* a representation by the system itself (this, as we will soon see, is an epistemological reading of *constraint 7*, the *transparency* of phenomenal representata). Put differently, in standard situations and from a first-person perspective the contents of phenomenal states always are *in a world*—they are a part of *my world* (*constraint 6*). This world is presented in the mode of naive realism. Obviously, this does not mean that the experiencing system must possess concepts like "world," "reality," "past," or "future," that is, that the features of globality, situatedness, and transparency just mentioned must be *cognitively* available to it. Therefore, I will (in alluding to the concept of "nonepistemic seeing"; see Dretske 1969) speak of "nonepistemic situatedness" to characterize the preconceptual character of this form of phenomenal content. What is at issue is not knowledge, but the structure of experience.

I am *one* person living in *one* world. For most of us this seems to be a self-evident and even trivial fact, which, however, we almost never explicitly state or even question. The reason for this is that we can hardly even *imagine* alternative situations (they are not "phenomenally possible" in the sense introduced in chapter 2). For most of us it is an obvious truth that we have never lived through phenomenal states in which we were many persons or in which we existed in multiple parallel worlds at the same time. Only professional philosophers or patients with severe neurological disorders, only people who have experimented with major doses of hallucinogens, or those unfortunate patients suffering from the syndrome of "dissociative identity disorder" (DID; see the neurophenomenological case study in section 7.2.4) can sometimes conceive of how it would be if the numerical identity of the phenomenal world and the unity of self-consciousness were suspended. For what arguably are good evolutionary reasons, in standard situations most of us cannot carry out the corresponding mental simulations (see section 2.3). It is simply too dangerous to play around in the corresponding regions of phenomenal state space. And what we are not able to mentally simulate is something that we cannot conceive of or imagine. If the world zero hypothesis presented in the last chapter is correct, it is obvious why we cannot voluntarily generate a suspension of the phenomenal representation of our world as numerically identical: the phenomenal world$_0$ as a fixed reference basis for all possible simulations has to be, in principle, inviolable. This is why the phenomenal world and the phenomenal self not only appear as numerically identical to us but as *indivisible* as well—a feature of our phenomenal architecture—which Descartes, in section 36 of his *Sixth Meditation*, used to construct a dubious argument for the separateness of mind and body. I would claim that there is a highest-order phenomenal property corresponding to this classical concept of "indivisibility" (Metzinger 1995c, p. 428). It is the phenomenal property of global coherence, and it is this property which really underlies most classical philosophical notions concerning the "unity of consciousness."

Global coherence, as consciously experienced from the first-person perspective, has two important phenomenological aspects. First, there is something that actually coheres: phenomenal events typically are densely *coupled* events. As I move through my own lived reality, through my consciously experienced model of the world, almost everything seems to simultaneously affect everything else. As I walk about, shift my visual attention, reach out for objects, or interact with other people, the contents of my sensory and cognitive states change like the contents of a high-dimensional kaleidoscope, while always preserving the apparently seamless, integrated character of the overall picture. Our conscious experience of reality is held together internally by a principle or mechanism which itself is subjectively inaccessible. This phenomenal coherence of my lived reality has nothing to do with the concept of coherence in physics or logic. Rather, it is responsible for a succinct *phenomenal* holism, which we ought to take into account on the conceptual level. The second aspect of the phenomenal target property of consciously experienced global coherence is the aspect of *holism*.

The conscious model of reality is not only highly differentiated; it is also fully integrated at any given point in phenomenal time. Holism is a richer notion than unity. Although a world made out of discrete, building block–like elements could be a unity, it could never be a whole. But my reality is not a toy world composed of little building blocks—it is also a *lived* reality whose parts interact in a quasi-organic way, in the sense of the original German concept, *Erleben*. This concretely experienced unity of a diversity is accompanied by a multitude of dynamic part-whole relations. Thus, the additional phenomenological aspect of holism or wholeness, which goes beyond mere unity, results from the fact that the different aspects constituting the phenomenal model of reality are not *elements*, but *parts* of this reality. Therefore, if we want to develop a phenomenologically realistic notion of the unity of consciousness, if we want to understand the holistic character of our phenomenal world as experienced from the first-person perspective, we will have to take its multilevel mereological structure as the starting point of our investigation.

Globality as a Representational Property

On the representationalist and functionalist levels of description one has to search for a coherent global state, which emerges by the integration of different and constantly changing elements of the phenomenal process of representation into an enduring, continuing superstructure. On the representational level of analysis the existence of a global and comprehensive highest-order *representatum* corresponds to the phenomenological constraint of *living in a world*: more precisely, living in a *single* world. In this way, being conscious simply means the representational possession of a world. The content of consciousness is the content of a model of the world (Yates 1985); more precisely, it is an ongoing and dynamic "containing" of one's physical environment. If globality is applied as a phenomenological constraint in deciding the issue of what makes a given neural representation a *conscious* representation (see Metzinger 2000c, figure 20.1), the answer now is that it has to be integrated into a currently active global representational state: the content of all currently active phenomenal representata is transiently embedded in a highest-order representational structure. I will henceforth simply call this representational structure the phenomenal "model of the world" or the phenomenal "reality-model" of the system.

Three aspects of this world-model are of particular interest on the representational level of description: the numerical identity of the reality depicted by it, its coherence, and the constant dynamical integration of individual contents leading to this coherence. Of course, all three are also important aspects of the classical philosophical question about the unity of consciousness. A subjective numerical identity of the world is generated by the experience of *sameness*: the transtemporal continuity and invariance of recurring contents of experience, mediated by memory capacities, leads to the immovable feeling of living in precisely one single world. It is important to always keep in mind that because indistinguishability generally is not the same as numerical identity,[8] this is not knowledge, just feeling. If this continuity of content and a minimal degree of invariance cannot be represented by the system anymore, then it is precisely this aspect of phenomenal experience which gets lost. Therefore, in order to explain the phenomenal unity of consciousness as a representational phenomenon, we have to look for the point of *maximal invariance of content* in the conscious model of reality. What is the representational content that displays the highest degree of invariance across the flow of conscious experience? The current theory says that it is to be found in certain aspects of bodily self-awareness and the conscious experience of agency (see section 5.4 and chapter 6). There will not only be a changing gradient of invariance within the phenomenal model of reality (in terms of more or less stable elements of experiential content) but also a gradient of *coherence* (in terms of different degrees of internal integratedness between such elements). As we saw in the last section, the wholeness of reality transcending a mere numerical identity, which cannot be transcended on the level of phenomenal experience, can be described as subjective coherence: Consciously experienced reality is being inwardly held together by a principle or mechanism, which itself is subjectively inaccessible. This concretely experienced unity of a manifold emerges together with a multitude of dynamical part-whole relations (see section 3.1 and *constraint 4*). The additional phenomenological aspects of holism and coherence superseding a simple unity result from the components out of which the phenomenal model is being constructed, not standing in element relations, but in *part-whole relations* to this overall reality. A third general constraint on the representational resources

8. Indistinguishability is not a transitive relation, whereas identity is. Two phenomenal models of reality may be indistinguishable in terms of introspection$_2$, but this does not infer that they are numerically identical as well. The interesting question is if "indistinguishability in terms of introspection$_1$"—*attentional availability*—is transitive. There clearly is more than one kind of "indistinguishability in appearance," and one might argue that attentional indistinguishability unequivocally marks out phenomenal content, the subcognitive "highest common factor" in experience, that which stays the same regardless of whether a phenomenal world model is veridical or hallucinatory. For an interesting recent discussion, see Putnam 1999, p. 128*ff.*

of any system supposed to activate a phenomenal world-model, therefore, consists in the availability of a flexible mechanism of integration that can carry out figure-ground separations and binding operations in many different modalities and on different levels of granularity, thereby being able to continuously embed new phenomenal contents in the global model (Engel and Singer 2000; Metzinger 1995c). A further functional constraint on this mechanism is that in the very large majority of cases its operation will be unavailable to conscious experience itself. Maybe it would be fruitful to interpret the emergence of a conscious experiential space within the brain of a biological organism as a generalized special case of feature binding and subsymbolic object formation. Such a unification of the content of the overall representational space could only be achieved if a subset of information active within the system were to be integrated into a single macrorepresentatum. If on the highest level of representation as well we found a most generalized form of gestalt and object formation, this would show how the system's unitary conscious model of reality could emerge. Such a highest-order representational structure would then be untranscendable for the system itself for at least two reasons. First, there would be no larger internal data structure to which it could be compared. Second, due to what I have called autoepistemic closure, it would by necessity be presented in the mode of "direct givenness." That is, the content of the global model of the world will inevitably be endowed with a further—illusory—phenomenological characteristic, the appearance of *epistemic* immediacy, that is, of direct knowledge or naive realism. I return to this point when discussing phenomenal transparency, *constraint 7* (see section 3.2.7).

In the following subsection we will see that global availability (*constraint 1*) was just a special application of spelling out the globality constraint relative to the functionalist level of description. On our way toward a systematic catalogue of conceptual and empirical constraints for a deeper notion of phenomenal experience it is important to always keep in mind that there will never be *one* singular concept of consciousness yielded as a kind of final result. Phenomenal experience itself is a graded phenomenon that comes in many different varieties, intensities, and degrees of internal complexity. Different degrees of conceptual constraint satisfaction will yield different concepts of phenomenal experience, concepts differing in their semantic strength. It is therefore interesting to find out what the weakest notion of conscious experience actually is. What is the *minimal degree of constraint satisfaction* necessary to get a firm grip on the phenomenon? At first sight it may seem as if the concept of consciousness is a cluster concept, a set of largely unknown, overlapping subsets of sufficient conditions with no single *necessary* condition to be found as a member of any set. Is all we can find a theoretical *prototype*? As a matter of fact, the discussion of different degrees of global availability for simple sensory content in chapter 2 has shown how, for instance, human color experience is a phenomenon that fades away from cognitive into attentional availability; implicit, subliminal perception; and blindsight.

However, taking first-person phenomenology seriously, it is important to note how the first two constraints—activation within a window of presence and integration into a coherent global state—are very likely the only two candidates for strictly necessary conditions. They may help us to arrive at a minimal notion of phenomenal experience. Short-term memory and global integration will therefore be at the heart of any empirical theory of consciousness. Why? If the content of the highest-order integrated representational structure here postulated is presented within a window of presence generated by the system, we can for the first time begin to understand what it means that an experienced *reality* emerges for the system. The activation *within* a self-generated window of presence endows the model of the world with an additional quality of temporal immediacy. The resulting representational content would be the phenomenal presence of a global whole, a world given in a single psychological moment, a *momentary reality*. If I am correct in claiming that *constraint 2* and *constraint 3* are the two most general constraints in conceptualizing conscious representation, that they are actually *necessary* conditions for any kind of conscious experience, then this supplies us with the weakest possible notion of consciousness: consciousness is the activation of an integrated model of the world within a window of presence. Phenomenologically speaking, consciousness is simply the "presence of a world." However, in order to understand how the representational contents of short-term memory and the representational contents of a world-model can turn into the untranscendable *appearance* of the presence of a real world, we have to apply one further constraint: *constraint 7*, the transparency constraint. I therefore return to the issue of a minimal notion of consciousness at the end of section 3.2.11.

The Generation of a World as an Informational-Computational Strategy

One main function of conscious experience may be to construct a final phase in a process of reducing information, data, and uncertainty originating in the buzzing, blooming confusion of the external world. As recent research into bistable phenomena (e.g., see Leopold and Logothetis 1999) has vividly demonstrated, if two incompatible interpretations of a situation are given through the sensory modules, then only one at a time can be consciously experienced. The generation of a single and coherent world-model, therefore, is a strategy to achieve a *reduction of ambiguity*. At the same time, this leads to a reduction of *data*: the amount of information directly available to the system, for example, for selection of motor processes or the deliberate guiding of attention, is being minimized and thereby, for all mechanisms operating on the phenomenal world-model, the computational load is reduced.

Second, if we assume the existence of mechanisms selecting nonphenomenal representata already active in the system and embedding them in the conscious world model, then the overall selectivity and flexibility of the system is increased by their cooperation because the system can now react to this information in a multitude of different ways. For fast and rigid patterns of reaction, for instance, in the domain of automatic motor responses, or in purely salience-driven, low-level attention, it is not absolutely necessary for the functionally relevant information already active in the system to also be part of its high-level world-model. However, if this information is critical in that it has to be available for many mechanisms at the same time, and if it is to be continuously monitored and updated, then it would be a strategical advantage to integrate this information into the current world-model.

A third aspect possibly is most interesting on a computational level of description. I described it in chapter 2 as the world zero hypothesis: consciousness is needed for *planning*. If a system needs to develop cognitive capacities like future planning, memory, or the simulation of possible worlds in general, it needs a *background* against which such operations can take place. If internally simulated worlds are to be compared to the actual world, so that their distance can be calculated and possible paths from the actual world into another global situational context can be mentally simulated and evaluated, then the system needs a reference model of the actual world as the *real* world. This reference model of the actual world should be untranscendable for the system, in order for it never to get lost in its own simulations. This, or so I claim, is the main reason for the phenomenal model of reality being activated within a window of presence (*constraint 2*) and for its transparency (*constraint 7*). The argument for this hypothesis consists in pointing out that the existence of a world simulation marked out as *actual* is simply a necessary condition for an alternative world simulation *referring* to this internally generated $world_0$ in the course of subsequent evaluation processes. Let me point out that not only a phenomenological and a representationalist but also a *neurocomputational* argument can be given for the necessity of such a transparent, highest-order informational structure. Of course, at a later stage and against such an already preexisting background, possible worlds can be compared to possible worlds and possible strategies of action to possible strategies of action. Still, naive realism was a first, and absolutely necessary step to make the difference between reality and simulation cognitively available for the system at subsequent stages. The phenomenal variant of world modeling achieves this goal in an elegant and reliable manner.

"Being in the World" as a Functional Property

The functionalist reading of our third constraint is this: phenomenal representata, by conceptual necessity, are operated on by a highest-order integrational function. Elsewhere, I have introduced a speculative concept, the concept of *highest-order binding*, in short, "HOB" (Metzinger 1995e). This concept was a very first and provisional attempt to mark out an important explanandum, a necessary research target for the empirical mind sciences that follows from centuries of philosophical research concerning the unity of conscious-ness, the understanding of which is vital to any theory of phenomenal experience (for a recent reformulation of the original set of assumptions from a neurobiological perspec-tive, see Engel and Singer 2000). Obviously, a functional solution to the mechanisms of perceptual and cognitive binding will be at the core of theories attempting to satisfy the constraint presented here. However, it is important to note that there are many different kinds of binding and not all of them are relevant to consciousness (for an excellent overview, see Cleeremans 2002). Integration processes take place on many phenomenal, as well as nonphenomenal, levels of information processing and it may therefore be nec-essary to differentiate and distinguish between consciousness-related and stimulus-related binding (Revonsuo 1999). Interestingly, everything that has already been said with regard to *constraint 1* is also true of the content of the phenomenal world-model. In other words, *constraint 1*, which I used as a first example of a conceptual constraint throughout chapter 2, now reveals itself as one possible functionalist interpretation of our phenomenological *constraint 3*. Representational states, after being integrated into the phenomenal world-model, can interact with a very large number of specialized modules in very short periods of time and in a context sensitive, flexible manner, thereby also increasing the adaptive flexibility of the system's behavioral profile. The more information is conscious, the higher the degree of flexibility and context sensitivity of its reactions to the environment will be, because many different functional modules can now access and use this information in a direct manner to react to challenges from the environment in a differentiated way. If it is true that the conscious model of the world is a highest-order holon (Koestler 1967; Metzinger 1995b), then an interesting way to analyze it functionally is as a two-way window through which the environment influences the parts, through which the parts com-municate *as a unit* to the rest of the universe (Allen and Starr 1982). This is true of lower-order holons too: they are functional doorways between parts of the internal structure and the rest of the universe. Mechanisms generating global coherence may also have highly interesting consequences in terms of a "downward" whole-part causation (please note that, in a holistic model of information processing, the predicate "downward" only corresponds to a level of description, not to an ontological hierarchy). Viewed as a coherent functional structure, a conscious model of reality will set global *macroconstraints* influencing the development of microinteractions, as if "enslaving" them through its overall dynamics. This may be an important insight into understanding certain psychiatric disorders, con-fabulations, and certain types of hallucinatory activity (see chapters 4 and 7). However, this issue clearly is one that has to be settled on an experimental and not on a conceptual level.

   When introducing the globality constraint on the phenomenological level of description at the beginning of this section, I stressed how only beings with a unified, conscious model of the world can make the *fact* of being part of and living in a more comprehensive but single reality available to them. It must be noted that the possession of an integrated world-model also results in a host of additional *functional* capacities. Only if you have the subjective experience of a world being present right now can you start to conceive of the notion of a single reality. The reality-appearance distinction becomes attentionally as well as cognitively available: you can start to mentally form concepts about the world as one, unified whole, and you can start to direct your attention to different aspects or parts of this whole while conceiving of them *as* parts of reality. And that may also be the reason why the phenomenon of conscious experience seems so highly important to most of us. Conscious experience for the first time allows an organism to interact with external reality under an internal representation of this reality as a single and coherent whole. From a strictly philosophical, epistemological perspective this assumption of a single, unified reality may be unwarranted. But in the course of natural evolution on this planet it has proved to be functionally adequate, because it allowed biological systems to "be in a world," to develop a large variety of subsequent functional capacities operating on the phenomenal world-model, including new and highly successful ways of representing *themselves* as being parts of this reality (see sections 6.2.2 and 6.2.3).

Neural Correlates of Global Integrational Functions

If we want to understand the unity of consciousness from an evolutionary point of view, as a historical process, the functional unity of the organism as situated in its ecological niche will be of central importance (Brinck and Gärdenfors 1999, p. 94). The phenomenal unity of consciousness, however, will exclusively supervene on brain properties at any given point in time. Currently, no detailed theories concerning the possible neural correlates, in particular of the minimally *sufficient* correlate for the appearance of a coherent, conscious model of the world, exist. However, there are a number of interesting speculative hypotheses, for instance, Hans Flohr's hypothesis concerning the potential role of the NMDA receptor complex in achieving large-scale integrations of ongoing activity (for further references and a recent discussion of his theory, see Flohr 2000; Franks and Lieb 2000; Hardcastle 2000; and Andrade 2000). The core intuition of this approach has been to study the mechanism of action common to different anesthetics, that is, to study the conditions under which phenomenal experience *as a whole* disappears and reemerges. A second important insight is that the globality constraint, which I have just formulated for different levels of description, applies to two fundamentally different classes of phenomenal states: to dreams (see section 4.2.5) and to waking states. In dreams, as well as as during ordinary waking phases, the system operates under one single, more or less coherent world-model, while its global functional properties differ greatly. Rodolfo Llinás and coworkers have long emphasized that one of the most fruitful strategies in searching for the neural correlate of consciousness (NCC) will be in "subtracting" certain global properties of the waking world-model from the dreaming world-model, thereby arriving at a common neurophysiological denominator or at global functional states which are basically equivalent between phenomenal experience during REM sleep and waking (Llinás and Paré 1991, p. 522ff.). As it turns out, certain aspects of the thalamocortical system may represent just this functional and neurophysiological common denominator for both kinds of phenomenal reality-modeling. The intuition behind this neuroscientific research program carries a distinct philosophical flavor; what we call waking life is a form of "online dreaming." If there is a functional core common to both global state classes, then conscious waking would be just a dreamlike state that is currently modulated by the constraints produced by specific sensory input (Llinás and Ribary 1993, 1994; Llinás and Paré 1991). A specific candidate for a global integrational function offered by Llinás and colleagues is a rostrocaudal 12-ms phase shift of 40-Hz activity related to synchronous activity in the thalamocortical system, modulated by the brainstem (the most detailed presentation of Llinás's thalamocortical model may be found in Llinás and Paré 1991, p. 531; see also Llinás and Ribary 1992; Llinás, Ribary, Joliot, and Wang 1994; Llinás and Ribary 1998; Llinás, Ribary, Contreras, and Pedroarena 1998). In the model proposed by Llinás and his coworkers a conscious model of reality is first constructed from the activity of a nonspecific system generating an internal context, which is then perturbed by external inputs, while continuously integrating new and specific forms of representational content relating the system to the external world during waking states.

The strategy of approaching the globality constraint by researching globally coherent states (as initially proposed in Metzinger 1995e) leads to a new way of defining research targets in computational neuroscience (e.g., see von der Malsburg 1997). However, it must be noted that global coherence as such is something that we also find in epileptic seizures and that what is actually needed is a theoretical model that allows us to find global neural properties exhibiting a high degree of integration and differentiation *at the same time* (see also the following constraint in the next section). One of the most general phenomenological constraints for any theory of conscious experience is that not only does it confront us with a highly integrated type of representational dynamics, it is also highly differentiated. The target phenomenon comes in an inconceivably large number of different forms of contents and sensory nuances. An approach doing justice to the globality constraint will have to offer a theoretical framework including the conceptual tools to *simultaneously* capture their holism and the internal complexity of consciousness. Gerald Edelman and Giulio Tononi have pointed out that the ability to differentiate among a large repertoire of possibilities—which is one of the most prominent features of conscious experience—clearly constitutes information in the classic sense of "reduction of uncertainty." Subjective experience in its discriminative structure is not only highly informative; it also renders this information causally relevant by making it available for speech and rationally guided action. Therefore, one can conclude that the neural correlate of the global, conscious model of the world must be a distributed process which can be described as the realization of a *functional cluster*, combining a high internal correlation strength between its elements with the existence of distinct functional borders. Edelman and Tononi have called this the "dynamic core hypothesis" (see Tononi and Edelman 1998a,b; Edelman and Tononi 2000a; for a comprehensive popular account, see Edelman and Tononi 2000b). The hypothesis states that any group of neurons can contribute directly to conscious experience only if it is part of a distributed functional cluster that, through reentrant interactions in the thalamocortical system, achieves high integration in hundreds of milliseconds. At the same time it is essential that this functional cluster possess high values of complexity. Edelman and Tononi have developed a formal tool to assess this property: the functional *cluster index* (CI). The advantage of this instrument is that it allows a precise conceptual grip on the relative strength of causal interactions within a subset of the elements compared to the interactions between that subset and the rest of the elements active in the system (see Tononi, Sporns, and Edelman 1996; Tononi et al. 1998; for brief overviews, see Tononi, Edelman, and Sporns 1998; Edelman and Tononi 2000b, p. 121*ff.*). A CI value near 1 shows that a subset of causally active elements are as interactive with the rest of the system as they are among themselves. However, the appearance of cluster indices higher than 1 indicates the presence of a functional cluster, that is, an island of what a philosopher might call "increased causal density" in the physical world. This island of causal density is constituted by a certain subset of neural elements that are strongly coupled among themselves, but only weakly interactive with their local environment within the system. Applying the CI measure to the neural dynamics of a conscious human brain allows us to define and identify the number of functional clusters currently existing in the system, clusters of what I have called "causal density," which cannot be decomposed into independent components. This way of looking at the globality constraint on the neural level is philosophically interesting for a number of reasons. First, it offers a conceptual instrument that allows us to clearly describe the coexistence of high degrees of differentiation and variability with a high degree of integration demanded by the more theoretical constraints developed on the phenomenological and representational levels of description. Second, it makes the prediction that any system operating under a conscious model of reality will be characterized by the existence of one *single* area of maximal causal density within its information-processing mechanisms. To have an integrated, globally coherent model of the world means to create a global functional cluster, that is, an island of maximal causal density within one's own representational system. Philosophical functionalists will like this approach, because it offers a specific and global functional property (a "vehicle property") that might correspond to the global phenomenal property of the unity of consciousness. In short, what you subjectively experience upon experiencing your world as coherent is the high internal correlation strength among a subset of physical events in your own brain. Third, it is interesting to note how the large group of neurons constituting the dynamical core in the brain of an organism currently enjoying an integrated conscious model of reality will very likely be different at every single instant. The physical composition of the core state will change from millisecond to millisecond. At any given point in time there will be one global, minimally sufficient neural correlate of consciousness, but at the next instant this correlate will already have changed, because the consciousness cluster only constitutes a *functional* border which can easily transgress anatomical boundaries from moment to moment. The global island of maximal causal density, if readers will permit this metaphorical description, is not firmly anchored to the rock bottom of the physical world. It is slightly afloat itself, a higher-order pattern hovering above the incessant activity of the brain, as it were. Fourth, it has to be noted that the informational content of the dynamical core is determined to a much higher degree by internal information already active in the system than by external stimuli. This point is of philosophical interest as well. Just as in the Llinás model, an overall picture emerges of the conscious model of reality essentially being an internal construct, which is only *perturbed* by external events forcing it to settle into ever-new stable states. This overall model is at least heuristically fruitful in that it also allows us to understand how a multitude of isolated functional clusters could coexist with the global, conscious model of reality while still being behaviorally relevant. It allows us to understand *how* certain forms of representational content may be active in the system, without being integrated into its conscious model of reality. It has long been known that the neural correlate of new solutions for new problems, of tasks that still have to be approached consciously, are typically widely distributed in the brain, but that, on the other hand, the more automatic, the faster, the more precise and unconscious the solution procedure for a certain kind of problem confronting an organism becomes, the more localized the neural correlates become as well. A good way of interpreting these data is to describe the respective activation pattern as "functionally isolated." In other words, for learned unconscious routines like tying your shoes, riding a bicycle, and so on, to first be in the process of *becoming* unconscious would mean for them to lose their context sensitivity, their flexibility, and their immediate availability for attention and cognition. This is a new way of describing what it means that something "drops out of awareness": individual functional clusters are embedded into the global, conscious model of reality as long as they have to be kept globally available for attention and cognition, as long as they represent new tasks and solutions that still have to be optimized and are frequent targets of computational resource allocation. As soon as this goal has been achieved they need no longer be embedded in the global, distributed set of neural events currently contributing to conscious experience. In fact, one elegant way of looking for the neural correlate of consciousness will typically consist in studying the correlates of a certain conscious capacity *while* it gradually "drops out of awareness" (see, e.g., Raichle 1998). In short, there may be many functional bundles—individual and episodically indivisible, integrated neural processes—within a system, and typically there will be *one* single, largest island of maximal causal density underlying the current conscious model of the world. They all contribute to the overall intelligence of the system. Still, the philosophical question remains of what it is that makes one of these clusters into the *subjective* world the organism lives in. It is plausible to assume that at any given time this typically is the largest functional cluster (for a dissenting view, see Zeki and Bartels 1998). However, the question remains how such a cluster becomes tied to an individual first-person perspective, to a representation of the system itself, and thereby becomes a truly *subjective* global model of reality (see the perspectivalness constraint in section 3.2.6 and chapter 6). The theory to be developed here makes the prediction that within the global functional cluster described by Tononi and Edelman there will typically exist one and only one *subcluster* (the organism's self-model; see section 6.2.1) and that this subcluster will itself possess an area of highest invariance, correlated with functional activity in the upper brainstem and the hypothalamus.

3.2.4   Convolved Holism

In developing the globality constraint in the last section, we saw how there is a deeper phenomenological issue behind the classic problem of the unity of consciousness, a problem that not only concerns the conscious experience of global singularity and sameness but also the global phenomenal properties of variable coherence and of holism. However, in addition, coherence and holism are not only to be found on the most comprehensive level of phenomenal content, on the level of the conscious world-model; they are found on a whole number of "subglobal" levels of analysis. In addition, as stated by *constraint 4*, phenomenal wholes do not coexist as isolated entities, but appear as flexible, *nested* patterns or multilayered experiential gestalts. They form mereological hierarchies. Nestedness (or "convolution") is a property of any hierarchical system having entities of smaller scale enclosed within those of larger scale (Salthe 1985, p. 61). Conscious experience itself can be described as a phenomenon possessing a hierarchical structure, for instance, by being composed of representational, functional, and neurobiological entities assignable to a hierarchy of levels of organization. This insight allows us to develop a further set of subconstraints.

The Phenomenology of Embedded Wholes

Let us look at paradigmatic examples of phenomenal holism. The lowest level on which we find an integration of features into a representational unit possessing global features like holism is the level of *perceptual* object formation. Consciously perceived, attention-ally available objects are sensory wholes, even if they are not yet linked to conceptual or memory structures. A second paradigmatic example of a holistic, coherent form of content is the phenomenal self. In standard situations, the consciously experienced self not only forms a unity but an integrated whole. As we know from the study of psychiatric disorders and altered states of consciousness, its internal coherence possesses consider-able variability (see chapter 7 for some case studies). A third level on which we find the phenomenal property of holism are complex scenes and situations: integrated arrays of objects, including relations between these objects and implicit contextual information. A visually perceived, presegmented scene—like a beautiful landscape you are looking at—or a complex, *multimodal* scene including a certain social context—like the conscious experience of following a seminar discussion in the philosophy department—are further examples of phenomenal holism. The brief integrations between subject and object as con-sciously represented, the phenomenal experience of what Antonio Damasio calls a "self in the act of knowing" is yet another paradigmatic phenomenological example of a briefly emerging integrated whole (I introduce some new conceptual tools to analyze this specific form of content in section 6.5). Objects and selves are integrated into scenes and situa-tions, as are different sequences of the "self in the act of knowing." That is, we can see how perceptual gestalts are seamlessly bound into ever richer and more complex forms of experiential contents. Let us call this feature "levels of phenomenal granularity."

Yet all this would not be enough to constitute the presence of a lived moment. It is interesting to see how the coherence constraint also applies to our second constraint, the activation within a window of presence. First, it must be noted how all these integrated and nested forms of holistic content are bound into a phenomenal present: from the first-person perspective all these nested phenomenal wholes are always experienced as *now* and all that has been said in section 3.2.2 about the generation of a temporal gestalt applies as well. A single lived moment, the specious present, again is something that cannot be adequately described as a bundle of features, a set of elements, or a sequence of atomic microevents. By setting the temporal boundaries for what becomes the subjective Now, each lived moment becomes something that could be described phenomenologically as a "world in itself." It is important to note that all other forms of holistic conscious content so far mentioned are always integrated into this experiential present. There are different kinds of embedding relations (spatial, perceptual, etc.), but the integration into the phenomenally experienced part of short-term memory may well be the most fundamental and general of these embedding relations. As a constraint, it is satisfied on *all* levels of phenomenal granularity.

In understanding the convolved holism constraint we therefore need an analysis of the phenomenal property itself and a more detailed description of different kinds of embedding relations, that is, of the aspect of *phenomenal convolution*. Let us start with global holism, returning to the conscious model of the world in general. So far we can say the following: Phenomenologically, conscious experience consists in the untranscendable presence of a world, in terms of a comprehensive and all-encompassing whole. With certain exceptions, information displayed within this whole is globally available for cognition, directed attention, and the volitional control of action. But what precisely does it mean to speak of "wholeness?" Holism means that, on a conceptual level, we are not able to adequately describe those aspects of a unit of experience which can be subjectively discriminated as isolated elements within a set. This is an important conceptual constraint for any kind of serious neurophenomenology. If one only analyzes such subregions or discriminable aspects in the flow of phenomenal experience as individual components of a class, one misses one of the most essential characteristics of conscious experience. There are no decontextualized atoms. The relationship between those aspects or subregions is a *mereological* relationship. On lower levels of phenomenal granularity different aspects may be bound into different low-level wholes (different colors or smells may belong to different perceptual objects), but ultimately all of them are parts of one and the same global whole. There is a second, intimately related, feature, which cannot be descriptively grasped by any form of conceptual modularism or atomism. This feature consists in the subjectively experienced *strength* of the integration accompanying this relation. Let me term this the phenomenal representation of internal correlation strength. This subjectively available strength of integration is variable, it is not an all-or-nothing affair like a feature either belonging to a certain set or not. There exists an unknown mechanism, entirely inaccessible from the first-person perspective, by which, on a preconceptual and preattentive level, consciously experienced part-whole relationships are continuously and automatically constituted. This mechanism clearly is stronger and more fundamental than the mechanism which underlies cognitive processes in terms of class formations and mental predications. Indeed, it is empirically plausible to assume that even the mental representation of nonholistic forms of content uses holistic neural "vehicles" as the physical carriers of this content (see von der Malsburg 1981, 1997). Let us for a second time start by investigating this interesting characteristic by looking at the largest and most comprehensive form of phenomenal content in existence: the conscious model of the world.

To *experience* a world is something different than to *think* a world. A world composed of *discrete* building block–like elements—an "analytical world-model"—could constitute a unity, but never a whole. All consciously available parts of my world are in a seamless way integrated into a highest-order experiential content, a global gestalt. Our phenomenal world is not an elementaristic world made out of building blocks, it is not a Lego universe, because it possesses an organic structure; it is more aptly characterized as a quasi-liquid network. At any time, I can direct my introspective awareness toward this property of my world; the fact that it possesses a flexible mereological structure certainly is attentionally and cognitively available. However, what can neither cognitively nor attentionally be penetrated is the mechanism generating this mysterious quality. This mechanism is also unavailable for volition. As we have already seen, acting exclusively from the first-person perspective it is impossible to deliberately split or dissolve my own global experiential space or my own phenomenal identity. On the other hand, there is presegmentation and selectivity on the level of sensory awareness. It is interesting to note that, in general, cognition starts to operate on the level of presegmented units, because the consciously experienced knowledge about the meaning of such units only starts on this level. Every meaningful holistic entity opens a window to semantic knowledge (Revonsuo 1999, p. 179). On the phenomenal level of description it is also important to note how the preattentive, prevolitional, precognitive integration of perceptual objects is an automatic process. It would not be possible to explain the constitution of such phenomenal objects in a top-down manner, because this would create the well-known homunculus problem. The subject would have to already *know* the relevant properties of the object, else it would not be capable of integrating them. Therefore, a top-down model of phenomenally experienced holism would be circular, because it presupposes what has to be explained.

Why is this holism a *convolved* holism? The concretely experienced holism of our phenomenal manifold appears simultaneously with a multitude of dynamical (*constraint 5*) part-whole relationships. The additional mereological structure of conscious experience is created by the components out of which the phenomenal model of reality evolves, not standing in elementary relations to each other, but in *hierarchical* part-whole relationships (please note that horizontally interwoven or circular hierarchies may exist as well). This point has been briefly touched upon before. We already confront phenomenal holism on the level of the constitution of perceptual objects, because properties like colors, edges, and surfaces are first integrated into a holistic percept on this level. However, these objects themselves are not only separated from backgrounds but also embedded in complex scenes and multimodal situations. Such situations may well be *possible* situations. Ongoing phenomenal simulations of possible actions or of an alternative, potential context are in many cases softly superimposed on perceptions. For philosophical analysis this means that what at earlier times philosophers may have called the "general unity of the phenomenal manifold" has today to be reformulated on a whole range of different phenomenological levels of granularity. The phenomenal constraint I have called "convolved holism," therefore, is an *enrichment* of the globality constraint. It immediately generates strong conceptual constraints for a representational analysis, and it also has strong implications for the necessary functional properties of representational "vehicles" employed by the conscious system. Before proceeding to the third-person levels of description, however, let me briefly point out that the current constraint cannot count as a necessary condition for the ascription of conscious experience in general.

As opposed to the presentationality constraint and the globality constraint introduced in the two preceding sections, it is conceivable that a conscious system could exist which enjoys the presence of a world, but for whom this world consists of only one, single, and integrated percept (e.g., exclusively its own phenomenal body image not yet coded as its *own* body image). It would possess a noncentered, maximally simple model of reality. For such a system, phenomenal holism would be a concrete structural feature of its subjective experience, but it would not be a *convolved* holism. There would not even be the most fundamental partitioning of representational state space conceivable, the self-world boundary (see sections 6.2.2 and 6.2.3). Therefore, the complex mereological structure typically characterizing human consciousness is a substantial enrichment of our target phenomenon, but not a necessary phenomenological condition in general.

Convolved Holism as a Representational Property

One does not have to be able to think in order to have rich subjective experience. Mental concept formation is not a necessary condition for phenomenal representation, as this is fundamentally based on the dynamical self-organization of preconceptual integration mechanisms. Can we arrive at a satisfying representational analysis of experiential holism? What kind of *content* is holistic content? Somehow this vivid phenomenological feature— the dynamic association linking different contents of consciousness on a multitude of levels of granularity by a large number of continuously changing part-whole relationships—has to be reflected on the level of deep representational structure and the functional mechanisms underlying it. If our phenomenological observations are correct, the conscious model of reality as a whole is presented to us in a holistic data format. What we experience are not only concrete contents but also the *format* they come in. A format is a set of abstract properties belonging to a specific class of data structures. Therefore, that is, on the level of mathematical modeling, there must be a clearly circumscribed, discrete set of abstract properties by which this holism can be analyzed and empirically explained. One such abstract property, for instance, could be a time constant in the underlying neural algorithm. The density of causal coupling, as expressed by the notion of a functional cluster mentioned in the last section, could be another candidate. Certainly we will discover many new candidates for such abstract properties in the twenty-first century. In any case, a first important representational constraint for any convincing theory of phenomenal representation consists in describing a format for the global level of representation that allows us to understand why the world, as experienced from the first-person perspective, possesses the global quality in question.

Analogous statements can be made for contexts, situations, scenes, and objects. If holism is a truly all-pervading phenomenal property, reappearing as a distinct type of format on many different levels, this could, for instance, be explained by the existence of *different* time constants, for instance, for neural algorithms operating on different frequency bands and on different levels of granularity (Metzinger 1995b; Engel and Singer 2000; for a review of converging evidence, see Varela et al. 2001). "Larger time windows" will then characterize higher levels of granularity, that is, by longer time constants (Metzinger 1995b). A related statement can be made with regard to the more general difference between conscious and unconscious stages of processing as such: The time constant of the phenomenal process must be longer than that of the computations accompanying transitional states, that is, the stages before a steady state is reached (Pollen 1999, p. 13). In this way, we never subjectively experience the dynamic incongruities between bottom-up and top-down processes, but just the final hypothesis, a dynamic, but stable state consistent with memory and sensory data. In this way unconscious dynamics contributes to conscious dynamics, and low-level phenomenal states can become embedded in higher-order wholes. One could also conceive of functional subclusters forming embedded islands within a dynamical core state (Tononi and Edelman 1998a,b). Common to all such correlates would be a specific abstract property of their content, its format. In almost all cases this format will be a *subsymbolic* format.

Let us look at an example: high internal correlation strength in a perceived set of features is an objective fact, usually holding in the external environment of the system. The internal *coherence* of sets of properties is a kind of objective fact, which is certainly relevant to the survival of biological organisms because it points to important physical invariances in the world surrounding it, which, in turn, are of immediate relevance to its behavior. Obviously, this state of affairs, the objective external fact of a high internal correlation strength holding between a set of perceptually given features, is not being represented in the brain by using a *propositional* format or a sentence-like structure, but—at least in our own case—by activating a holistic object, a representational whole. Therefore, one important criterion for judging a theory of consciously experienced perceptual objects is if it can tell us what precisely it is about the specific format of a currently active object model that endows it with the quality of holism we so clearly experience from the first-person perspective. Analogous constraints will then hold for higher-order representational wholes.

However, as we have already seen, the problem is not holism per se. The key question for a representational analysis of convolved holism consists in working out a better understanding of the *embedding relation*, which can hold between different active representational wholes, and of giving an answer to the question concerning its potential iterability (Singer 2000).

Convolved Holism as an Informational-Computational Strategy
Information displayed in a holistic format is highly coherent information. Phenomenal information, therefore, is that subset of active information which is available to the system in an *integrated* form. Consciously initiated cognition and focal attention always operate on a presegmented model of reality. In addition, information displayed within a nested, holistic world-model generates a strong interdependence: individual property features, perceptual objects, and global aspects of a scene influence each other and in this way the complex causal structure of the external world can be represented with a high degree of precision. Phenomenal information is not only coherent but *interdependent* information. The dense coupling of phenomenal events corresponds to a dense coupling of representational contents. One of the advantages is that the representational content of a global world-model, as everything contained in it is simultaneously affecting everything else, can, in principle, be *updated* in one single step. If necessary, local changes can effect global transitions.

Convolved Holism as a Functional Property
The characteristic causal role of a global and integrated data format consists in binding all information, to which the system has to be able to react in a fast and flexible manner at any time, into a unified superstructure. The convolved character, its high degree of internal differentiation, enables the system to directly access the causal structure of the environment (e.g., when generating motor or cognitive simulations; see *constraint 8*). The content of individual representata can now be constantly updated in a fast, flexible, and context-sensitive manner, depending on the content of other, simultaneously active representata, as it were, in one single globalized processing step. A related advantage of the type of reality modeling proposed here is its functional sensitivity to small variations in input: through the mereological coupling of representational contents, very small shifts in sensory input can lead to a very fast updating of global representational content. It also allows for something that we may term "nested constraint satisfaction." A global causal role, that is, a *discrete* integrated set of causal relations holding within the system, can always be decomposed into *subsets* of causal relations. This can be done from a third-person perspective, when analyzing a global functional cluster into subclusters. However, it is now also interestingly conceivable that the system itself, from a first-person perspective, actively *generates* such subclusters. This could, for instance, be achieved by selecting a specific motor pattern and enhancing it above a certain threshold, or by fixing attention on a certain aspect of the environment, thereby making it more salient. The holism constraint is then satisfied selectively by generating a *new* element within a nested hierarchy.

The existence of a functionally integrated but internally differentiated world-model is also one of the most important preconditions for the constitution of a subjective, inward perspective (see *constraint 6*). Conscious experience is highly differentiated (in a very short period of time we can live through a large number of different conscious states) while always being integrated (any individual conscious scene is fully disambiguated, and experienced as unitary). One way of understanding the connection between integration, differentiation, and perspectivalness is by conceiving of the impossibility of a consciously experienced scene that is not integrated—that is, a scene that is not experienced *from a single point of view* (this way of pointing to the relevance of the phenomenal first-person perspective has been put forward by Tononi and Edelman 1998a, p. 1846; we return to the role self-representation plays in global integration at length in chapter 6). Agency, the capacity for consciously experienced volitional selection, may be a core issue in achieving global integration from a functional point of view; for instance, we are only able to generate one single conscious decision with one "psychological refractory period" (Pashler 1994; Baddeley 1986) and, as noted earlier, the perceptual subject is not capable of consciously (i.e., *deliberately*) experiencing two incongruous scenes at the same point in time. In passing, let me note how both of these functional facts are good examples of facts determining what I termed *phenomenal* possibility and necessity in the previous chapter.

Neural Correlates of Convolved Holism

Once again, we have to admit that not enough empirical data are currently available to be able to make any precise statements (but see Varela et al. 2001). On a formal level, the correlation theory of brain function possesses the conceptual tools to transport the phenomenological constraint of convolved holism to the neurobiological level of description. In an earlier publication (Metzinger 1995b), I proposed the necessity for a global integrational function that fulfills two conditions. First, that function would have to achieve global integration of representational contents active in the brain without causing a "superposition catastrophe," that is, without causing interferences, misassociations, and the mutual deletion of different representational patterns. Given a plausible neurobiological theory about the mechanism of integration, for example, the temporal coherence of neural responses established through synchrony, this would correspond to states of global synchrony, as in epilepsy or deep sleep, in which all conscious experience is typically absent. Therefore, what is needed is a function achieving a dynamical and global form of metarepresentation *by functional integration*, not simply deleting or "glossing over" all the lower-order contents, but preserving its differentiated structure. Second, the holism-producing mechanism should be conceivable as operating on different levels of granularity. Therefore, what is needed to establish a differentiated type of large-scale coherence on the level of the brain itself will not be uniform synchrony, but specific cross-system relations binding subsets of signals in different modalities (see Engel and Singer 2000, in particular their reformulation of the original constraints as "NCC5" and "NCC6"). The embedding of simple perceptual objects in progressively higher-order contexts could, for instance, be achieved by a multiplexing of interactions in the brain *on different frequency bands* (again, see Engel and Singer 2000). According to this theoretical idea, a multitude of already active, integrated cell assemblies could be transiently bound into the ascending (but horizontally interwoven) hierarchy of higher-order representational wholes demanded by the phenomenological constraint formulated above, namely, through a network of large-scale interactions in the human brain. These interactions would then be mediated by temporal coherence holding for different subsets of neural responses and on different frequency bands. In this way it is also possible to formulate future research targets for *constraint 4*.

3.2.5   Dynamicity

Constraint 5 does justice to the fact that phenomenal states only rarely carry static or highly invariant forms of mental content, and they do not result from a passive, nonrecursive representational process. The physically acting subject—including the properties of *cognitive*, *attentional*, and *volitional* agency (see sections 6.4.4, 6.4.3, and 6.4.5)—plays an essential role in their constitution. And in a certain sense what has just been described as convolved holism also reappears in the phenomenology of time experience: Our conscious life emerges from integrated psychological moments, which, however, are themselves integrated into the flow of subjective time.

Phenomenology of Dynamicity
The notion of "convolved holism" was a natural extension of the third constraint, the globality constraint. The fifth constraint is a natural extension of the second constraint, the presentationality constraint. If our target phenomenon is the full-blown conscious experience of humans, we need to do justice to the highly differentiated nature of *temporal* experience coming along with it. The most important forms of temporal content are presence (as already required by *constraint 2*), duration, and change. The dynamicity constraint introduces duration and change as important forms of phenomenal content that have to be conceptually analyzed and empirically explained. Once again, it is important to note that the dynamicity constraint is not a necessary condition for the ascription of phenomenal experience in general. It involves no logical contradiction to conceive of a class of conscious systems (e.g., certain primitive types of organisms on our planet, or human mystics resting in the conscious experience of an "eternal Now") that *only* possess the phenomenal experience of temporality in terms of presence, but are devoid of any

phenomenal representation of duration or change. Just as, in principle, global holism could exist without the differentiated structure implying the specific notion of *convolved* holism discussed in the last section, there could be a class of conscious systems living in an eternal, and therefore *timeless* Now, only enjoying the fundamental aspect of presence, but never subjectively experiencing duration and change. If we are looking for the minimal notion of conscious experience, dynamicity is not a necessary condition. If, however, our epistemic goal is an understanding of ordinary human consciousness in all its temporal richness, the dynamicity constraint will have to be at the heart of our theory. It is also hard to imagine how nontemporal consciousness could have possessed an evolutionary history or have been an adaptive form of phenomenal content (see section 3.2.11), because biological organisms will almost inevitably have been under pressure to internally model the temporal structure of their causal interaction domain, the way in which their environmental niche *changes*. Let us first take a brief look at the phenomenology of time experience.

While investigating the phenomenology of time perception, we observe the following global characteristic: a temporal world, composed of discrete, building block–like elements, could possibly form a unit, but never a whole.[9] Once again I discover how, with regard to specific phenomenal contents like simultaneity, presence, succession, and duration, my first-person experiential world is not a building-block world. It is a *lived* reality in the sense of a quasi-organic and holistic interplay of its temporal constituents within the "enacted" phenomenal biography of a perceiving subject. Not only are we not dealing with a "knife-edge" present, but with an extended "specious present" in the sense of William James. Francisco Varela (1999, p. 268) has shown how the phenomenal representation of time also possesses a complex *texture*.

Of all constraints on the notion of phenomenal representation presented here, the dynamicity constraint certainly is one for which a rigorous bottom-up approach is particularly promising. As past discussions in philosophy of mind have shown, introspective access to the texture of time experience mentioned by Varela is so weak and particularly unreliable that it seems almost impossible to reach consensus on even the *phenomenological* first-person constraints that could turn it into a proper research target. Introspectively, time is a mystery. This is reflected in the now almost traditional fact that philosophers at this point typically quote a passage in the fourteenth chapter of the eleventh book of St. Augustine's *Confessions*, where he famously notes that as long as nobody asks

---

9. Arguably, we *do* know such phenomenological configurations as confined to single sensory modalities. Motion blindness may present a good, if rare, example. In motion blindness patients may selectively lose the capacity to phenomenally see movement (see Zihl, Cramon, and Mai 1983). Such a patient may see a moving bus as advancing in a series of discrete "stills" or the spout of tea emerging from an urn as a solid curved cylinder (see Weiskrantz 1997, p. 31). The visual world of this patient still is a unit, but the temporal structure of this visual world does not form a *nested whole* anymore. In a highly domain-specific way, it does not satisfy *constraint 5*.

him about the nature of time, he knows what it is, but as soon as he is supposed to explain it to a questioner, he does not know it any more. The phenomenal texture of time is a paradigmatic example of a feature governed by the "principle of evasiveness." It is a feature that instantly recedes or dissolves if introspective, cognitive, or even attentional processing is directed at it. As a matter of fact, many of the mystics mentioned above, that is, people who are *interested* in dissolving all of the temporal texture that veils the pure presence of the conscious Now, typically use meditative techniques of attention management to make this texture disappear. Therefore, if one is interested in theoretical progress on time experience, one may inevitably have to turn to third-person ways of modeling the target phenomenon. Before starting to discuss phenomenological constraints governing the conscious experience of time I herewith fully admit that I am not able to give an even remotely convincing conceptual analysis of what it *is* that actually creates the philosophical puzzle.

Time flows. Not only is there the core feature of phenomenal experience, the invariant integration of experiential contents into a lived *present* described earlier; superimposed on this experience of presence are the experience of duration and the experience of change. External objects, or bodily elements within self-consciousness, sometimes remain constant, they endure. Other objects or certain high-level aspects of our self-consciousness *change*, for instance, by gaining and losing a certain consciously experienced property. In the phenomenal self as well, time flows. However, the experience of flow, of duration and change, is seamlessly integrated into the temporal background of presence, *all the time*, as it were. What is so hard to describe is the strong degree of integration holding between the experience of presence and the continuous conscious representation of change and duration. It is not as if you see the clouds drifting through a window, the window of the Now. There is no window frame. It is not as if the Now would be an island emerging in a river, in the continuous flow of consciously experienced events, as it were—in a strange way the island is a *part* of the river itself.

As a matter of fact, one aspect of the dynamicity required here is actually reflected in the partly autonomous dynamics of phenomenal states through a well-known interdependence at the level of subjective experience: The *speed* of subjective time flow and the duration of a psychological moment are strongly dependent on the overall context (think of time perception during emergencies as opposed to situations with a maximally positive emotional tone). Attention also increases temporal resolution and thereby leads to a "phenomenal time dilatation." On the other hand, the resolution power of temporal perception always lies one order of magnitude above visual object constitution. Therefore, the process in which consciously experienced objects emerge can never be touched (see section 3.2.7). Relative to conscious contents already active, the resolution power of attention, in time as well as in space, is always rather crude. Yet it has to be noted that the individuation of events can be highly plastic and the perceived speed of such chains of events varies greatly. A further principle governing the phenomenology of dynamicity seems to be that it can be restricted to subregions of phenomenal space, for instance, to the dynamics within the phenomenal self. We can be detached witnesses: The degree to which a phenomenal subject experiences itself as present, as real, and as fully immersed in the temporal evolution of a consciously experienced situation can vary greatly (see chapter 7, sections 7.2.2 and 7.2.5). In short, there is also an internal dynamics of phenomenal self-consciousness (*constraint 6*; section 6.2.5). A last point to be noted is that the convolved holism described as *constraint 4* extends into the temporal dimension, because the world of consciousness is constituted by dynamical part-whole relations. The complex temporal texture of phenomenal experience is not only interdependent with the convoluted, nested structure of its representational content, it may simply be a particularly salient *aspect* of one and the same feature.

Dynamicity as a Representational Property

As many philosophers since Augustine have noted, the major difficulty for a representationalist analysis of time experience is that it is so extremely difficult to arrive at a convincing phenomenology of time perception in the first place. Therefore, it is tempting not to look at the content, but at possible properties of the "vehicles" of time representation. Dynamicist cognitive science holds the promise to provide a large number of new conceptual instruments by which we can analyze objective, dynamical properties of representational *vehicles* (for a good example, see Van Gelder 1999). However, it may also be precisely dynamicist cognitive science, which finally forces us to do without the time-honored vehicle-content distinction. But let us stay with the content level for now.

Phenomenal dynamics integrates past and future into the lived present. In section 3.2.2 we named a number of steps: First, events have to be individuated, that is, there has to be a mechanism of representing events as *individual* events. The next step consists in forming patterns out of such individual events, a process of representational "sequencing" or time binding. In this way what Eva Ruhnau (1995) called a "*Zeit-Gestalt*" ("time-Gestalt") can be generated. If a representational mechanism for the ongoing integration of such time-Gestalts in a seamless manner were in existence, the generation of an ongoing flow of subjective time as a new form of representational content would be conceivable. However, this step is already controversial, and philosophical intuitions will certainly diverge.

The core issue, for which I have no proposals to make, clearly seems to consist in the representational definition of duration, in internally representing the *permanence* of already active phenomenal wholes. It seems safe to conclude that a functional mechanism has to be assumed, which constitutes and represents the *transtemporal identity of objects* for the system. The question, if something like objects really exist, is a classic problem of philosophical ontology. But theoretical ontology is not the issue. The subsymbolic existence assumptions inherent in the way the *brain* subpersonally models reality is what is important here. As we have already seen, the phenomenal ontology of the human brain assumes the existence of ineffable nuances, categorizable simple content, integrated complexions of such simple forms of content (perceptual objects), and after this stage it knows scenes and situations constituted from multimodal objects, plus a phenomenal self acting in those situations.

In a certain sense, perceptual objects really are the fundamental components of phenomenal experience. This position can be taken, because they possess a certain kind of representational autonomy: presentata (Raffman qualia) and properties (Lewis qualia) never exist in isolation and *temporal* evolution of the content displayed by presentata and cognitively available properties can always only be experienced *as that of objects*. Phenomenal objects, therefore, function as carriers, as an integrative context for nuances and properties, for everything I subsumed under the notion of "presentational content" in the previous chapter. Therefore, it is the object level that for the first time truly confronts us with the question of the representational and functional resources with the help of which a system can represent the sameness of objects across time for itself: How can properties or ineffable aspects of an experientially presented object change over time in a manner that still allows us to experience this object as the *same* object? Introspection is mute on this issue, and conceptual speculations seem to be fruitless at this point. Whatever turns out to be an empirical answer to those questions will supply us with an important constraint for the concept of *dynamical* phenomenal representation.

Dynamicity as an Informational-Computational Strategy

A plausible assumption from an evolutionary perspective is that one of the main functions of consciousness consists in increasing the flexibility of our behavioral repertoire. Obviously, one necessary precondition for this achievement was to represent the *temporal structure* of our behavioral space in an increasingly precise manner. The environment of biological systems, their domain of causal interaction, is a highly dynamical environment. Frequently sudden and unpredictable changes take place, and phenomenal states seem to reflect this dynamism in their own relational properties and in their temporal fine structure. Phenomenal representation makes information about temporal properties of the world and the system itself globally available for the control of action, for cognition and guided attention. This is a first important step in approaching a teleofunctionalist analysis of phenomenal dynamicity: it makes dynamical properties of the organism's ecological niche, of its behavioral space, available for a multitude of processing systems at the same time, by bringing temporal information "online."

Dynamicity as a Functional Property

Dynamicity can here be analyzed not as a content property of certain representata, but as an aspect of the functional profile of representational *vehicles*. Depending on one's theory of representation, vehicle properties may even be mirrored in content properties. If, again, one additionally integrates the evolutionary context leading to the phenomenon of conscious representation, and takes on a teleofunctionalist perspective, one discovers that the internal as well as the external environment in which organisms operate are complex and highly dynamic. For every class of organism, there will be a minimal degree of precision with which the temporal structure of this causal domain has to be internally modeled in order to achieve survival. To be functionally adequate, phenomenal models have to causally drive behavior with such a minimal degree of precision. If phenomenal representata are supposed to be effective instruments in fighting for survival and procreation, they have to internally mimic those causal properties relevant to grasping information— to a certain degree they have to be dynamical states *themselves*.

Please note that dynamical representations can also be useful in generating *nonpredictability*. The capacity to generate chaotic behavior can be a highly useful trait in certain evolutionary contexts. For instance, think of the chaotic motor pattern generated by a rabbit as it flees from a predatory bird: The pattern of motor output is so chaotic that the predator simply cannot learn it. In fact, generations of predatory birds chasing rabbits have not been able to predict the running pattern of their prey. From a teleofunctionalist perspective, the capacity to produce chaotic dynamics at will certainly is an important property.

Neurodynamics

On a subpersonal level of description we see that neural representations can be interestingly characterized by exemplifying a complex, nonlinear dynamics. However, almost nothing can be said today about specific, minimally sufficient neural correlates for the *representational* functions just sketched.

3.2.6 Perspectivalness

The dominant structural feature of phenomenal space lies in the fact that it is tied to an individual perspective. Phenomenal representata not only have to allow object formation, scene segmentation, and the global modeling of complex situations but also the formation of a phenomenal *subject*. A conscious self-model is not yet a phenomenal subject, because arguably pathological configurations (as in akinetic mutism) do exist, where a rudimentary conscious self appears *without* subjectivity, in the absence of a phenomenal first-person perspective. In order to meet this constraint, one needs a detailed and empirically plausible theory of how a system can internally represent itself *for* itself, and of how the mysterious phenomenon today called a "first-person perspective" by philosophers can emerge in a naturally evolved information-processing system. Subjectivity, viewed as a phenomenon located on the level of phenomenal experience, can only be understood if we find comprehensive theoretical answers to the following two questions. First, what is a consciously experienced, phenomenal *self*? Second, what is a consciously experienced phenomenal *first-person perspective*? Because selfhood and perspectivalness are the core topic of this book, I can be very brief at this point (see chapters 1 and 6 for more detailed descriptions of the perspectivalness constraint).

Again, it has to be noted that perspectivalness is not a necessary condition for the ascription of conscious experience to a given system. There are a number of phenomenal state classes; for instance, spiritual and religious experiences of a certain kind or fully depersonalized states during severe psychiatric disorders, in which an inference to the most plausible phenomenological explanation tells us that no conscious self and no consciously experienced first-person perspective exist. Such states are important and of great relevance to a modern theory of mind, and they occur more frequently than most people think. I take such global experiential states to be instances of *nonsubjective* consciousness. On the level of their phenomenal content, they are not tied to an individual, consciously experienced first-person perspective anymore. This does not mean that under a nonphenomenological, for example, *epistemological*, concept of subjectivity they could not still be truthfully described as weakly subjective states, for instance, in terms of being exclusively internal models of reality generated by individual systems. In standard situations, epistemic access to one's mental states is realized via a consciously *experienced* first-person perspective, but this need not be so in all cases. Even if phenomenal perspectivalness is not a necessary condition for ascribing conscious experience to a given system, it probably is the most striking and fascinating characteristic of our target phenomenon, the ordinary waking state of human beings. The perspectivalness constraint is the most interesting topic from a philosophical point of view, because a closer look at this constraint may help us to understand how the *subjectivity* of our target phenomenon (which generates so many conceptual and epistemological problems for consciousness research) is ultimately rooted in the deep structure of phenomenal representation.

The Phenomenology of Perspectivalness

The phenomenology of perspectivalness unfolds on a number of different levels, leading to a whole subset of potential phenomenological constraints. First, the phenomenology of perspectivalness is the phenomenology of *being someone*. The first phenomenal target property here is the property of consciously experienced "selfhood." The experiential perspectivity of one's own consciousness is constituted by the fact that phenomenal space is centered by a phenomenal self: it possesses a focus of experience, a *point* of view. The mystery consists in—when shifting from a third-person to a first-person description—understanding what, for each of us, it means to say that I am this center *myself*. There seems to be a primitive and prereflexive form of phenomenal self-consciousness underlying all higher-order and conceptually mediated forms of self-consciousness (see sections 5.4 and 6.4), and this nonconceptual form of selfhood constitutes the *origin* of the first-person perspective. Phenomenal selfhood is what makes us an experiential subject. In German the property in question has sometimes been called *präreflexive Selbstvertrautheit* ("prereflexive self-intimacy"; e.g., see Frank 1991). It is a very basic and seemingly spontaneous, effortless way of inner acquaintance, of "being in touch with yourself," and phenomenally, of being "infinitely close to yourself." In short, it is a subjectively immediate and fundamental form of nonconceptual self-knowledge preceding any higher forms of *cognitive* self-consciousness. For the first time it constitutes a consciously available self-world boundary, and together with it generates a genuinely *inner* world. It is, however, important to note that a central part of the phenomenology of self-consciousness is the simple fact that the phenomenal self is constituted preattentively, and automatically on this most fundamental level.

As noted above, from a philosophical perspective phenomenal self-consciousness may well be the most important form of phenomenal content. On the level of logical structure we find this basic representational architecture reflected in the logical structure of phenomenological sentences, in what has been called a "subject presupposition" (e.g., see Nida-Rümelin 1997). Every concrete ascription of a mental property always assumes the existence of a subject *whose* property this property is. It is true that a proper analysis of most mental terms (and not only of qualia) presupposes an explanation for the emergence of subjects of experience, while obviously it is not true that *all* mental terms are governed by this subject presupposition. In fact, as we have already seen, it is an empirically plausible assumption that nonsubjective states of conscious actually do exist. The important question, of course, is whether the concept of a subject proposed here can in principle be defined in *nonmentalistic* terms. As we shall see in the course of this book, this possibility is not excluded in principle.

A second point of philosophical interest is that the epistemic asymmetry (Jackson 1982) only appears at this level of representational organization, because the possession of a phenomenal self is a necessary precondition for the possession of a strong *epistemic* first-person perspective (see section 8.2). It is very likely true that the emergence of a phenomenal first-person perspective is the theoretical core of the mind-body problem, as well as of most issues concerning mental content. Even if one is convinced that phenomenal content can be ontologically reduced to some set of functional brain properties or other, we still need an answer to the question as to why it obviously remains *epistemically* irreducible. What kind of knowledge *is* perspectival, first-person knowledge?

One last point of philosophical importance is the empirically plausible assumption that certain global phenomenal states possess a phenomenal self while not exhibiting a consciously experienced first-person perspective (e.g., in neurological conditions like akinetic mutism). In other words, a phenomenal self is a necessary, but not sufficient condition for a given system to develop a full-blown, consciously experienced first-person perspective.

The second level on which the perspectivalness constraint possesses high relevance is not selfhood, but the phenomenal property of perspectivalness itself. Perspectivalness in this sense is a structural feature of phenomenal space as a whole. It consists in the existence of a single, coherent, and temporally stable model of reality that is representationally centered on a single, coherent, and temporally extended phenomenal subject (Metzinger 1993, 2000c). A phenomenal subject, as opposed to a mere phenomenal self, is a model of the system as *acting and experiencing*. What is needed is a theory about how the intentionality relation, the relation between subject and object, is *itself* depicted on the level of conscious experience. What is needed is a theory about what in previous publications I have introduced as the "phenomenal model of the intentionality-relation" (Metzinger 1993, p. 128*ff*.; 2000c, p. 300; but see section 6.5 in particular). As Antonio Damasio (e.g., 1999, 2000) has convincingly emphasized, the core target of empirical consciousness research is a specific, complex form of phenomenal content that may best be described as "a self in the act of knowing," a "self in the act of perceiving," a "self in the act of deciding on a specific action," and so on. Doing full justice to this phenomenal constraint achieves a strong compression of the space of conceptual and empirical possibilities. What are the representational, functional, neuroscientific, and logical constraints of any system to exhibit a consciously experienced *inward perspective*?

A third level of the phenomenology of perspectivalness must be briefly mentioned. The possession of a phenomenal self is the most important precondition not only for higher-order types of reflexive self-consciousness but also for *social cognition*. A consciously experienced first-person perspective (the untranscendable "me") is a necessary precondition for the emergence of the phenomenal first-person *plural* (the untranscendable "we"). Phenomenal subjectivity makes phenomenal intersubjectivity possible, namely, in all those cases in which the object component of an individual first-person perspective is formed by another *subject*. I return to this issue in section 6.3.3. At this point it only has to be noted that consciously experienced social cognition is a third domain governed by the perspectivalness constraint.

Perspectivalness as a Property of a Representational Space
Perspectivalness is a *structural feature* of a certain class of representational spaces and of those models of reality active within them. In essence, it consists in these spaces being

functionally centered by an internal self-representation of the representational system itself. In chapters 5, 6, and 7, I offer a more extensive representational analysis of the perspectivalness of consciousness, and try to narrow down the conditions under which a *phenomenal* first-person perspective will necessarily emerge. I introduce two new theoretical entities for the representational structures carrying the phenomenal content in question: the phenomenal self-model (PSM) and the phenomenal model of the intentionality relation (PMIR).

Perspectivalness as an Informational-Computational Strategy

A perspectivally organized representational space makes a certain, highly specific kind of information globally available for the first time: information resulting from the fact that a system-world border exists, which, however, is continuously transgressed by the establishing of causal subject-object relations of a transient and highly diverse nature. The possession of an active and integrated self-representation allows a system to represent certain properties of the world as its *own* properties. Importantly, those properties thereby become available for higher-order representational processes like attention or cognition, and for self-directed behavior as well. Any system possessing a basic self-model can become the object of its own attention, of its own concept formation, and also of its own, self-directed *actions*. Any computational system operating under a world-model centered by a coherent self-model has introduced the most fundamental partitioning of its informational space possible: the differentiation between the processing of environment-related and system-related information.

A similar advantage is associated with a system processing information from a first-person perspective. It can now for the first time internally represent and process all information having to do with subject-object relations, in particular with transient interactions between the system and its environment. For instance, if that system is bound into sensorimotor loops, it can now internally model and possibly *predict* the evolution of such loops. On the other hand, it is interesting to note how pure reflexes and behaviors that do not entail consciousness also do not presuppose the availability of a subject-object dichotomy for the organism. Arguably, when considering the nature of pure reflexes, it simply doesn't make sense (or generates explanatory potential) to assume such a dichotomy on the representational level of description (Feinberg 1997, p. 87*f.*).

Centeredness as a Functional Property

The centeredness of our internal representational space corresponds, first, to the centeredness of *behavioral* space. Trivially, the causal interaction domain of physical beings is usually centered as well, because the sensors and effectors of such beings are usually concentrated within a certain region of physical space and are of a limited reach.

This basic fact is frequently overlooked: Distributed beings, having their sensory organs and their possibilities for generating motor output widely scattered across their causal interaction domain within the physical world, might have a multi- or even a noncentered behavioral space (maybe the Internet is going to make some of us eventually resemble such beings; for an amusing early thought experiment, see Dennett 1978a, p. 310*ff.*). I would claim that such beings would eventually develop very different, noncentered phenomenal states as well. In short, the experiential centeredness of our conscious model of reality has its mirror image in the centeredness of the behavioral space, which human beings and their biological ancestors had to control and navigate during their endless fight for survival. This functional constraint is so general and obvious that it is frequently ignored: in human beings, and in all conscious systems we currently know, sensory and motor systems are *physically* integrated within the body of a single organism. This singular "embodiment constraint" closely locates all our sensors and effectors in a very small region of physical space, simultaneously establishing dense causal coupling (see section 3.2.3). It is important to note how things could have been otherwise—for instance, if we were conscious interstellar gas clouds that developed phenomenal properties. Similar considerations may apply on the level of social cognition, where things *are* otherwise, because a, albeit unconscious, form of distributed reality modeling takes place, possessing *many* functional centers.

Second, in our own case, the self-model is *functionally anchored* in internally generated input (see section 5.4 and chapter 6). This changes the functional profile of the global, conscious model of reality (see section 6.2.3) as well: the conscious world-model now is not only phenomenally but also *functionally* centered by being tied to the brain of the organism generating it through a persistent functional link. This persistent functional link to the deepest core of the organism's brain is supplied by the self-model. The origin of the first-person perspective is now fixed through a specific causal role, creating a region of maximal stability and invariance. Please note how the notion of a functionally "centered phenomenal world-model" may be intimately related to the notion of a "centered world" in the work of Quine (1969, p. 154) and D. K. Lewis (1979), namely, as a more precise and empirically tractable description of what *actually* constitutes the object of egocentric propositional attitudes (e.g., in terms of classes of possible worlds marked out by an individual organism's neural stimulation pattern). The persistent functional link just mentioned has many theoretically relevant aspects. One of them is that it firmly ties all activities of the organism (be they cognitive, attentional, or behavioral) into an *internal* context, namely, elementary bioregulation.

Operating under a model of reality organized in a perspectival fashion enormously enriches and differentiates the functional profile of an information-processing system, by enabling it to generate an entirely new class of actions—actions directed toward *itself* (e.g., think of the many new patterns of self-exploratory behavior exhibited by chimpanzees once they have recognized themselves in a mirror).

From a certain level of complexity onward representational spaces centered by a self-model also enable the attribution of psychological properties to the system itself, as well as to other systems in the environment, and thereby open the door to conceptually mediated, reflexive subjectivity and social cognition, for example, by internally emulating other conscious agents. In particular, a centered representational space allows for an internal, phenomenal representation of the intentionality relation itself. I return to all of these points at length in later chapters.

Neural Correlates of the Centeredness of Representational Space

On the one hand, there are empirical data—for instance, the fact of phantom limbs reappearing after excision of somatosensory cortex (Gybels and Sweet, 1998, cited in Melzack, Israel, Lacroix, and Schultz 1997)—indicating that the neural correlate of our phenomenal self is highly distributed. On the other hand, there are many empirical results pointing to mechanisms constituting a persisting functional link between certain *localized* brain processes and the center of representational space. These mechanisms, for instance, include the activity of the vestibular organ, the spatial "matrix" of the body schema, visceral forms of self-representation, and, in particular, the input of a number of specific nuclei in the upper brainstem engaged in the homeostatic regulation of the "internal milieu" (see Parvizi and Damasio 2001; Damasio 1999, chapter 8; Damasio 2000). In chapters 6 and 7 I take a closer look at these mechanisms, which actually, due to the fact that they are not only functionally integrated but also *anatomically* characterized by proximity, may even form somewhat of a spatial center on the level of neurobiological implementation. Their function consists in generating a high degree of invariance and stability, by providing the system with a continuous internal source of input. As I explain in chapter 6, any system evolving a genuine first-person perspective has to possess a phenomenal model of the intentionality relation in order for the functional property of *centeredness* to be able to contribute to the phenomenal property of *perspectivalness*. About the neural correlates of *this* representational constraint hardly anything is known today (but see Damasio 1994, 1999; Damasio and Damasio 1996a, p. 172, 1996b, p. 24; Delacour 1997, p. 138; D. LaBerge 1997, pp. 150, 172). However, as we will see, it is of vital importance that this internal model of a relation between subject and object is a *transparent* model. While satisfying the perspectivalness constraint will help us to understand what it means for a conscious model of reality to be a *subjective* phenomenon, satisfying the transparency constraint will allow us to make progress in understanding how it truly makes sense to actually speak of a *reality* appearing together with this model.

3.2.7 Transparency

This constraint, again, only bundles a subset of phenomenal representations. Phenomenal transparency is not a necessary condition for conscious experience in general. Phenomenally *opaque* states do exist. Nevertheless, transparency certainly is one of the (if not *the*) most important constraints if we want to achieve a theoretical understanding of what phenomenal experience really is. From a systematic point of view, and in particular for the main argument here, the transparency constraint is of highest relevance. Therefore, to avoid any confusion with existing notions of "transparency," I will have to give a slightly longer introduction at this point.

The classic location for the notion of phenomenal transparency is usually given as G. E. Moore's paper, "The Refutation of Idealism":

... the fact that when we refer to introspection and try to discover what the sensation of blue is, it is very easy to suppose that we have before us only a single term. The term "blue" is easy enough to distinguish, but the other element which I have called "consciousness"—that which a sensation of blue has in common with a sensation of green—is extremely difficult to fix. . . . And in general, that which makes the sensation of blue a mental fact seems to escape us; it seems, if I may use a metaphor, to be transparent—we look through it and see nothing but the blue; we may be convinced that there *is something*, but *what* it is no philosopher, I think, has yet clearly recognized. (Moore 1903, p. 446)

Today, a broad definition of phenomenal transparency on which most philosophers would probably agree is that it essentially consists in only the *content properties* of a mental representation being available for introspection, but not its nonintentional or "vehicle properties." Typically, it will be assumed that transparency in this sense is a property of all phenomenal states.

Definition 1 Phenomenal states are transparent in that only their content properties are introspectively accessible to the subject of experience.

Below, I argue that this definition is unsatisfactory, because it violates important phenomenological constraints. Vehicle properties frequently *are* accessible for introspection. It may, therefore, be interesting to remember that Moore in his original paper pursued the same philosophical intuition:

... that the moment we try to fix our attention upon consciousness and to see *what*, distinctly, it is, it seems to vanish: it seems as if we had before us a mere emptiness. When we try to introspect the sensation of blue, all we can see is the blue: the other element is as if it were diaphanous. Yet it *can* be distinguished if we look attentively enough, and if we know that there is something to look for. (Moore 1903, p. 450)

In § 275 of *Philosophical Investigations* Wittgenstein (1953) pointed to the naive realism inevitably brought about by transparent, phenomenal experience.[10] Interestingly, many authors today have returned to the notion of transparency, employing it as a useful conceptual instrument. Robert van Gulick has developed a functionalist analysis of transparency in terms of the speed, reliability, and global interdependence of phenomenal representations in combination with an accompanying lack of access to earlier processing stages.[11] For qualia, Sydney Shoemaker has pointed out that we have no introspective access to the nonintentional features of one's experience that encode this content;[12] Gilbert Harman has defined the transparency of experience as an unawareness of intrinsic nonintentional features;[13] and Michael Tye now uses the concept at many places in many of

10. *§ 275. Schau auf das Blau des Himmels, und sag zu dir selbst "Wie blau der Himmel ist!"—Wenn du es spontan tust—nicht mit philosophischen Absichten—so kommt es dir nicht in den Sinn, dieser Farbeneindruck gehöre nur dir. Und du hast kein Bedenken, diesen Ausruf an einen Andern zu richten. Und wenn du bei den Worten auf etwas zeigst, so ist es der Himmel. Ich meine: Du hast nicht das Gefühl des In-dich-selber-Zeigens, das oft das 'Benennen der Empfindung' begleitet, wenn man über die 'private Sprache' nachdenkt. Du denkst auch nicht, du solltest eigentlich nicht mit der Hand, sondern nur mit der Aufmerksamkeit auf die Farbe zeigen. (Überlege, was es heißt, "mit der Aufmerksamkeit auf etwas zeigen.")* [Look at the blue of the sky and say to yourself "How blue the sky is!"—When you do it spontaneously—without philosophical intentions—the idea never crosses your mind that this impression of colour belongs only to *you*. And you have no hesitation in exclaiming that to someone else. And if you point at anything as you say the words you point at the sky. I am saying: you have not the feeling of pointing-into-yourself, which often accompanies "naming the sensation" when one is thinking about "private language". Nor do you think that really you ought not to point to the colour with your hand, but with your attention. (Consider what it means "to point to something with the attention".)] (Wittgenstein 1953; English translation 1958).

11. "How can the functionalist account for subjectively experienced transparency? Possessing information always involves a capacity for appropriate behavior. Being informed about the content of a representation is being able to relate it to other representations and items in the world appropriate to its content. As long as understanding or being informed is analyzed as a behavioral capacity, even if the relevant behavior is all internal, the functionalist can hope to fit it within his theory.

Thus the functionalist should resist any view of phenomenal transparency as a form of nonbehavioral self-luminous understanding. He can undercut the intuitive appeal of that view, by explaining the subjective experience of understanding in terms of smooth and seemingly automatic transitions. The internal component of understanding need involve nothing beyond an ability to interrelate many diverse representations with great speed. . . . How this is done is not something to which I have linguistic or introspective access, but there must be powerful processors to produce these seemingly instantaneous transitions" (van Gulick 1988a, p. 178*f.*).

12. "The only thing that seems to answer the description "attending introspectively to one's visual experience" is attending to how things appear to one visually; and offhand this seem to tell one what the representational content of one's experience is without telling one anything about what the nonintentional features of one's experience are that encode this content. One may be inclined to say that one is revelling in the qualitative or phenomenal character of one's experience when one "drinks in" the blue of a summer sky or the red of a ripe tomato. But neither the blue nor the red is an object of introspective awareness; these are experienced, perceptually rather than introspectively, as located outside one, in the sky or in the tomato, not as features of one's experience. G. E. Moore once complained that the sensation of blue is "as if it were diaphanous"; if one tries to introspect it one sees right through it, and sees only the blue. In a similar vein one might say that qualia, if there are such, are diaphanous; if one tries to attend to them, all one finds is the representative content of the experience" (Shoemaker 1990, 1996, p. 100*f.*).

13. ". . . in the case of her visual experience of a tree, I want to say she is not aware of, as it were, the mental paint by virtue of which her experience is an experience of seeing a tree. She is aware only of the intentional or

his writings,[14] making the strong and interesting claim that phenomenal character is actually identical with intentional contents.

Let me now introduce my own working definition of phenomenal transparency, the definition with which I want to work hereafter. Transparency in this sense is a property of active mental representations already satisfying the minimally sufficient constraints for conscious experience to occur. For instance, phenomenally transparent representations are always activated within a virtual window of presence and integrated into a unified global model of the world. The second defining characteristic postulates that what makes them transparent is the *attentional unavailability of earlier processing* stages for introspection. "Introspective attention" is here used in terms of the concepts introspection₁ and introspection₃. What is attention? In short, attention is a form of nonconceptual meta-representation operating on certain parts of the currently active, internal model of reality. It "highlights" these parts, because it is a process of subsymbolic resource allocation. The earlier the processing stages, the more aspects of the internal construction process leading to the final, explicit, and disambiguated phenomenal content that are available for introspective attention, the more will the system be able to recognize these phenomenal states *as* internal, self-generated constructs. Full transparency means full attentional unavailability of earlier processing stages. Degrees of opacity come as degrees of attentional availability.

Definition 2 For any phenomenal state, the degree of phenomenal transparency is inversely proportional to the introspective degree of attentional availability of earlier processing stages.

This definition diverges from earlier notions of phenomenal transparency in allowing us to describe two important facts about phenomenal consciousness which philosophers have frequently overlooked. First, *cognitive* availability of the fact that currently active phenomenal contents are the final products of internal representational processes is not enough to dissolve or weaken phenomenal transparency. To simply have a mentally represented

---

relational features of her experience, not of its intrinsic non-intentional features. . . . When you see a tree, you do not experience any features as intrinsic features of your experience. Look at a tree and try to turn your attention to intrinsic features of your visual experience. I predict you will find that the only features there to turn your attention to will be features of the presented tree, including relational features of the tree 'from here'" (Harman 1997, p. 667, cited in Block et al. 1997).

14. "Generalizing, introspection of your perceptual experiences seems to reveal only aspects of *what* you experience, further aspects of the scenes, as represented. Why? The answer, I suggest, is that your perceptual experiences have no *introspectible* [sic] features over and above those implicated in their intentional contents. So the phenomenal character of such experiences—itself is something that is introspectively accessible, assuming the appropriate concepts are possessed and there is no cognitive malfunction—is identical with, or contained within, their intentional contents" (Tye 1995, p. 136; see also p. 30*f.*, p. 220*f.*; for further uses, see Tye 1991, p. 119; 1998, p. 468*f.*; 2000, chapter 3).

concept of the book you are holding in your hand as only being a special form of representational contents almost does not change the character of your phenomenal experience at all—at least not in a way that would be relevant to the current context. However, there seems to be a relevant difference between cognitive and attentional processing, between conceptual and nonconceptual metarepresentation of first-order phenomenal states. Only if you could actually attend to the construction process itself would you experience a shift in subjective experience, namely, by adding new and nonconceptual content to your current model of reality.

Second, this definition departs from the classic vehicle-content distinction. The standard way of defining transparency would be to say that only content properties of the phenomenal representata are introspectively available to the system, and not vehicle properties. The vehicle-content distinction is a highly useful conceptual instrument, but it contains subtle residues of Cartesian dualism in that it always tempts us to *reify* the vehicle and the content, by conceiving of them as distinct, independent entities. A more empirically plausible model of representational content will have to describe it as an aspect of an ongoing *process* and not as some kind of abstract object. What we need is *embodied* content, as it were—an ongoing and physically realized process of *containing*, not "a" content (see, e.g., P. M. Churchland 1998, unpublished manuscript; Clark 1997; Opie and O'Brien 2001). In particular, describing phenomenal transparency in terms of the attentional availability of earlier processing *stages* has the advantage of being able to develop many different, fine-grained notions of *degrees* of transparency and opacity. For different phenomenal state classes resulting from functionally different types of processing, it may also be possible to describe not only variable degrees but also distinct *kinds* of transparency and opacity. This allows for a much more realistic description of certain phenomenological features pertaining to different classes of conscious states.

Let me first proceed to describe the three most important equivocations or potential misunderstandings of the notion of "phenomenal transparency," as introduced in definition 2. Such misunderstandings do exist, they are quite common, but a clarification can also be used to further enrich the target concept. There are three different, but well-established usages of "transparency," two in philosophy and one in communication theory.

First, transparency is not an epistemological notion, but a *phenomenological* concept. In particular, it has nothing to do with the Cartesian notion of epistemic transparency, the philosophical intuition that in principle I cannot be wrong about the content of my own consciousness, that the notion of an unnoticed error in introspectively accessing the content of your own mind is incoherent. Descartes famously expressed this idea in the last paragraph of his *Second Meditation*, and the advance of clinical neuropsychology today makes this classic philosophical assumption about the human mind untenable (for examples, see chapter 7). The modern concept of phenomenal transparency, however, is systematically related to the Cartesian project insofar as it furnishes an important building block for a theory that attempts to make the overwhelming intuitive force behind this false assumption intelligible. The Cartesian claim about the epistemic transparency of self-consciousness can itself not be epistemically justified, but it has the great advantage of correctly describing the *phenomenology* of certainty going along with the phenomenon.

Second, transparency is here conceived of as a property of phenomenal representata in a *subsymbolic* medium, that is, of nonlinguistic entities under an empirically plausible theory of mental representation, and not as a property of a context. The second equivocation is the extensionality equivocation: "Phenomenal transparency" is used not as a notion belonging to the field of formal semantics, but rather as a new concept in philosophical neurophenomenology. Transparency as a property of contexts is something entirely different. Extensional (i.e., *referentially* transparent) contexts are being constituted by sentences characterized by the intersubstitutivity of coreferential expressions *salva veritate* and by an implication of the existence of the entities mentioned by them. Intensional (i.e., *referentially* opaque) contexts are being constituted by sentences characterized by an intersubstitutivity of expressions with identical *meaning salva veritate*. Such contexts do not preserve the same truth-value, if coreferential expressions at the individual variable x or at the place held by the predicate letter F are being substituted for each other. Opaque contexts are, for instance, constituted by reference to propositional attitudes, to temporal and modal expressions, or by indirect speech. Who concludes from the fact that a certain expression x cannot be substituted by a coreferential expression y *salva veritate* within an intensional context that x and y do not refer to the same aspect of reality commits what philosophers call the "intensional fallacy."

Transparency as a property of contexts is *not* what I am talking about here. Phenomenal transparency can exist in nonlinguistic creatures, lacking any form of cognitive reference. Phenomenally transparent representations could supervene on a brain in a vat, whereas *referentially* transparent ones arguably could not. However, certain complex phenomenal contents can potentially constitute certain types of linguistic contexts; in particular, *opaque* phenomenal contents contributing to higher-order forms of mental self-representation can do so (see section 6.4.4). It is interesting to note how, once again, there is a connection between referential and phenomenal transparency: in both cases we have something like an implication of the existence of the entities represented. Sentences constituting extensional contexts imply the existence of the entities mentioned within them. Fully transparent phenomenal representations force a conscious system to *functionally* become a naive realist with regard to their contents: whatever is transparently represented is experienced as real and as undoubtedly existing by this system.

There is a third common use of the notion "transparency," which should not be confused with the notion intended here, but which at the same time exhibits a third interesting semantic parallel. It too is a well-established concept. Transparency can be conceived of as a property of *media*. For instance, in technical systems of telecommunication, transparency can be the property of a *channel* or of a system for the transmission of information in general. To give an example, transparency in this sense can be a feature of a server in the Internet. The three defining characteristics of this notion of transparency are, first, that it accepts unmodified user information as input; second, that it delivers user information that is unmodified with respect to form and informational content on the output side; and third, that user information may well be internally changed and reprocessed in many different ways, but is always retransformed into the original format before reaching the output stage *without causal interaction with the user*. E-mail is the obvious example. A single message that you send to your friend may be chopped up in many different portions, each of these taking many different roads and "hops" through the net before being reassembled on the other side. The user has no access to the subpersonal mechanisms underlying successful personal-level communication. Obviously, phenomenal transparency in the sense intended here is not a property of technical systems. However, it is interesting to again note the parallel that emerges if we look upon the neural correlate of consciousness or the conscious model of reality as a *medium:* This medium is transparent insofar as the subpersonal processing mechanisms contributing to its currently active content are attentionally unavailable to high-level introspective processing. Phenomenal color vision is transparent, because we cannot direct our personal-level attention to the ongoing activity of the relevant processing mechanisms in our visual cortex. All we get seems to be the final result, G. E. Moore's conscious sensation of blue. Let me give a beautiful—but much more complex—example provided by Jonathan Cole (1998): consciously perceived *faces* can be transparent as well. Looking into each other's faces we frequently directly see the emotion expressed, because, as Cole puts it, the human face is an "embodied communication area." In seemingly immediate emotional communication we do not take the face as a representation of the other's emotional state—the face, although still given as a sensory representation, becomes transparent. For autists, visually perceived faces of fellow human beings may be just complex visual patterns like "balls bouncing off a wall" without an emotional self behind it (see Cole 1998, chapter 7). While those faces are phenomenally transparent (on the level of their purely sensory content), they are epistemically opaque (on the level of the emotional content or *knowledge* usually transported through them) because, due to a deficit in unconscious, subpersonal mechanisms of information processing, this content is not available at the conscious, personal level. Face perception is not only a fundamental building block of human social intelligence but also a multilayered phenomenon that spans the whole range from conscious to unconscious processing.

Again, it must be noted that transparency is not a necessary condition for the ascription of conscious states. Phenomenal transparency varies greatly among different subclasses of phenomenal states, because it is a *gradual* property of such states. In short, I would claim that the distribution of transparency and opacity throughout phenomenal space processes an interesting *variance*.

On the other hand, it must be noted that applying the transparency constraint now and for the first time allows us to formulate a *minimal concept* of phenomenal experience: conscious experience, in its essence, is "the presence of a world." The phenomenal presence of a world is the activation of a coherent, global model of reality (*constraint 3*) within a virtual window of presence (*constraint 2*), both of which are transparent in the sense just introduced (*constraint 7*). The conjunction of satisfied *constraints 2, 3,* and *7* yields the most elementary form of conscious experience conceivable: the presence of a world, of the content of a world-model that cannot be recognized *as* a model by the system generating it within itself. Neither a rich internal structure nor the complex texture of subjective time or perspectivalness exists at this point. All that such a system would experience would be the presence of one unified world, homogeneous and frozen into an internal Now as it were. In short, the transparency of representational structures is the decisive criterion for turning a model into an *appearance*, into an apparent reality. We do not experience the reality surrounding us as the content of a representational process nor do we represent its components as internal placeholders, causal role players, as it were, of another, external level of reality. We simply experience it as *the world in which we live our lives*. I return to this issue at the end of section 3.2.11, before introducing the more general notion of a "phenomenal mental model" at the end of this chapter.

The Phenomenology of Transparency

Transparency is a special form of darkness. With regard to the phenomenology of visual experience transparency means that we are not able to see something, because it is transparent. We don't see the window, but only the bird flying by. *Phenomenal* transparency in general, however, means that something particular is not accessible to subjective experience, namely, the representational character of the contents of conscious experience. This analysis refers to all sensory modalities and to our integrated phenomenal model of the world as a whole in particular. The *instruments* of representation themselves cannot be represented as such anymore, and hence the experiencing system, by necessity, is entangled in a naive realism. This happens because, necessarily, it now has to experience itself as being in direct contact with the current contents of its own consciousness. The phenomenology of transparency is the phenomenology of apparently direct perception. What is it that the system cannot experience? What is inaccessible to conscious experience is the simple fact of this experience taking place in a *medium*. Therefore, transparency of phenomenal content leads to a further characteristic of conscious experience, namely, the subjective impression of immediacy. It is important to note that the naive realism caused by phenomenal transparency is not a philosophical attitude or a kind of belief. It is a global kind of phenomenal character, which could also be enjoyed by a non-linguistic animal entirely incapable of forming beliefs. On the other hand, many bad philosophical arguments concerning direct acquaintance, infallible first-person knowledge, and direct access are clearly based on an equivocation between epistemic and phenomenal immediacy; from the fact that the conscious experience, for example, of the color of an object, carries the characteristics of phenomenal immediacy and direct givenness it does not follow that any kind of nonmediated or direct kind of *knowledge* is involved. Phenomenal content as such is not epistemic content, and it is a widely held and plausible assumption that it locally supervenes on brain properties. According to the principle of local supervenience, for every kind of phenomenal content in humans there will be at least one minimally sufficient neural correlate. Phenomenal content can be dissociated from intentional content. A brain in a vat could possess states subjectively representing object colors as immediately and directly given. Any fully transparent phenomenal representation is characterized by the vehicle-generating mechanisms which have led to its activation, plus the fact of a concrete *internal* state now being in existence and carrying its content, not being introspectively available anymore. The phenomenology of transparency, therefore, is the phenomenology of naive realism.

Of course, *opaque* phenomenal representations exist as well. Opacity appears precisely when darkness is made explicit—at the moment we consciously represent *that* something actually is a representation, not by propositional knowledge or a conscious thought, but first by our attention being caught by the fact that what is currently known is known through an internal *medium*. If the window is dirty or has a crack, we realize that we view the bird flying by *through a window*. Here are some first examples of opaque state classes: most notably, consciously experienced thoughts, but also some types of emotions, pseudo-hallucinations, or lucid dreams are subjectively experienced *as representational processes*. Such processes sometimes appear to us as deliberately initiated cognitive or representational processes, and sometimes as spontaneously occurring, limited, or even global phenomenal simulations, frequently not under the control of the experiential subject. In such cases we know that they do not present realities to us, but only possibilities: the information that they are *representational* processes, the content of which may or may not properly depict an external reality, is globally available for attention, cognition, and behavioral control. Many authors describe phenomenal transparency as an all-or-nothing phenomenon. To do phenomenological justice to conscious experience, however, demands a more differentiated description.

Let us take a second and closer look at phenomenological examples in which the transparency constraint is satisfied to different degrees. Sensory experience is the paradigmatic example of fully transparent phenomenal content. There are, however, examples of sensory opacity, for instance, during extremely short transition phases in bistable phenomena, for example, in binocular rivalry tasks or if a consciously experienced Necker cube switches from one interpretation to the next and back (see, e.g., Leopold and Logothetis 1999). Then there is the phenomenon of pseudohallucination (see section 4.2.4), exhibited by all persons who know that they are hallucinating while they are hallucinating. If a subject in a laboratory experiment and under the influence of a hallucinogenic drug like LSD or 2-CB observes abstract geometrical patterns on the wall, breathing and slowly evolving into deeper and ever deeper forms of ineffable beauty, the subject will frequently be aware of the representational character of her visual experience in that subregion of his phenomenal space. Typically, the subject will immediately have doubts about the correctness of his experiential state and take back the "existence assumption," effortlessly going along with visual experience in standard situations. My claim is that what this subject becomes aware of are earlier processing stages in his visual system: the moving patterns simply *are* these stages (see also section 4.2.4; for a mathematical model of visual hallucinations, see Ermentrout and Cowan 1979; Bressloff, Cowan, Golubitsky, Thomas, and Wiener 2001). This first example of simple, abstract hallucinations also yields an interesting new way of describing the phenomenology of transparency versus opacity: transparent experience is *conscientia*,[15] the experience of not only knowing but also knowing that you know while you know; opaque experience is the experience of knowing while also (nonconceptually, attentionally) knowing that you may be *wrong*. Of course, complex hallucinations, which are fully transparent and in which the experiential subject gets lost in an alternative model of reality, exist as well (see, e.g., Siegel and West 1975). Importantly, however, the *paradigmatic* examples of fully opaque state classes are deliberately initiated processes of

15. Descartes shaped the modern interpretation of *conscientia* as a higher-order form of knowledge accompanying thought. In Latin *cogitatio*, *apperceptio*, and *sensus internus* are all used with a similar meaning. The concept of *conscientia* is the original root concept from which all later terminologies in Roman languages and in English have developed. It is derived from *cum* ("with," "together") and *scire* ("knowing") and in classical antiquity, as well as in scholastic philosophy, predominantly referred to moral *conscience* or a common knowledge of a group of persons, again most commonly of moral facts. It is only since the seventeenth century that the interpretation of *conscientia* as a higher-order knowledge of mental states as such begins to dominate. Because *cum* can also have a purely emphatic function, *conscientia* also frequently just means to know something with great certainty. What the major Greek precursor concept of συνειδησιζ (*syneidesis*) shares with *conscientia* is the idea of moral conscience. What it additionally highlights is the second semantic element of the notion of consciousness: *integration*. The Latin *cum* and the Greek prefix συν refer to the concomitant and synthesizing aspect of conscious experience. Interestingly, today the first semantic root element is predominantly discussed in philosophy of mind (e.g., Rosenthal 2002; but see also Singer 2000), whereas the second root element prominently reappears in neuroscience (e.g., Edelman and Tononi, 1998). See Metzinger and Schumacher 1999 for further references.

conscious thought. In these cases we really experience ourselves as deliberately constructing and operating with abstract representations, ones that we have generated ourselves and which can, at any time, turn out to be false. We are cognitive and epistemic agents at the same time, thinking subjects actively trying to achieve an expansion of knowledge. In particular, we are introspectively aware of processing stages, of the *formation* of thoughts. Conscious cognitive reference is phenomenally opaque.

It must be noted that there are also forms of thought which are localized at the other end of the spectrum, between phenomenal transparency and phenomenal opacity. If we slide into manifest daydreams, we frequently experience cognitive processing not *as* cognitive processing anymore. A further point to be noted when discussing the phenomenology of transparency and opacity is this: not only individual phenomenal contents can exhibit a variable degree of transparency; the same is true of global phenomenal world-models as well. Right after a traffic accident the whole world can appear as "unreal" or as "dreamlike" to us. The same phenomenon is known in stress situations and in transitory phases during certain psychiatric syndromes. However, the best and most basic example of an almost fully opaque, global phenomenal state is the lucid dream (see LaBerge and Gackenbach 2000; Metzinger 1993; and section 7.2.4 in particular). There are interesting transitions between ordinary dreams and lucid dreams, because there are *degrees* of lucidity. For instance, one can, as a passive witness, very clearly notice that all this is a dream (attentional and cognitive availability of information about the representational character of the overall state) without necessarily also knowing about one's freedom of the will, without realizing that one is an *agent* who can start to fly or pass through walls (availability of information concerning the representational character of the overall state for behavioral control). More about this later.

Returning from global phenomenal state classes to particular examples, it is of great interest to investigate the transparency and opacity of *emotions*. As opposed to sensory and cognitive states, emotions are neither a paradigmatic example of transparency nor of opacity. Our emotional states frequently seem to be directly given forms of subjective self-representation. Their content is something we do not doubt, but just take as reliable, immediately given information about our own current state and about our relation to and the states of other human beings. However, sometimes we suddenly become aware that our emotional response might actually be inappropriate in our current social environment. Take jealousy as an example: we may suddenly realize the representational character of our own jealousy, if we become aware of the fact that all this actually might be a *misrepresentation*—for instance, of those persons in our social environment of whom we are jealous. What was experienced as an obvious property of another person (the bird flying by) suddenly becomes a state of myself (the window has a crack!). In emotions we frequently oscillate between certainty and uncertainty, between the immediacy of an obvious perception and doubts. This simple phenomenological observation points to another important characteristic of opaque phenomenal representations. They make the possibility that they actually might be *misrepresentations* globally available for cognition, attention, and behavioral control.

Transparency as a Property of Conscious Representations

Phenomenal representations are transparent, because their content seems to be fixed in all possible contexts: The book you now hold in your hands will always stay this very same book according to your subjective experience, no matter how much the external perceptual situation changes. What you are now experiencing is not an "active object emulator," which has just been embedded in your global model of reality, but simply the *content* of the underlying representational dynamics: this *book*, as here (*constraint 3*) and now (*constraint 2*) effortlessly given to you (*constraint 7*). At this level it may, perhaps, be helpful to clarify the concept of transparency with regard to the current theoretical context by returning to more traditional conceptual tools, by once again differentiating between the vehicle and the content of a representation, between the representational carrier and its representational content.

The representational carrier of your phenomenal experience is a certain process in the brain. This process, which in no concrete way possesses anything "booklike," is not consciously experienced by yourself; it is transparent in the sense of you looking through it. What you are looking *onto* is its representational content, the existence of a book, here and now, as given through your sensory organs. This content, therefore, is an abstract property of the concrete representational state in your brain. However, as we have already seen, there are at least two kinds of content. The *intentional* content of the relevant states in your head depends on the fact of this book actually existing, and of the relevant state being a reliable instrument for gaining knowledge in general. If this representational carrier is a good and reliably functioning instrument for generating knowledge about the external world, then, by its very transparency, it permits you to directly, as it were, look "through it" right onto the book. It makes the information carried by it globally available (*constraint 1*), without your having to care about *how* this little miracle is achieved. The *phenomenal* content of your currently active book representation is what stays the same, no matter if the book exists or not. It is solely determined by internal properties of the nervous system. If your current perception, unnoticed by you, actually is a hallucination, then, as it were, you, as a system as a whole, are no longer looking "through" the state in your head onto the world, but only at the representational vehicle itself—without *this* fact itself being globally available to you. The specific and highly interesting characteristic of the phenomenal variant of representation now is the fact that this content, even in the situation just described, is invariably experienced as maximally *concrete*, as absolutely unequivocable, as maximally determinate and disambiguated, as directly and immediately given to you. Its causal history is attentionally unavailable. Phenomenal representations are those for which we are not able to discover the difference between representational content and representational carrier on the level of subjective experience itself.

Of course, there are counterexamples, and they are very helpful for arriving at an even deeper understanding of the concept of "transparency." *Opaque* phenomenal representata are, for instance, generated if the information that their content results from an internal representational process suddenly becomes globally available. Imagine that you suddenly discover that the book in your hands does not exist in reality. A hallucination now becomes a pseudohallucination. On the level of phenomenal experience the additional information that you are not looking directly onto the world, but "onto" an internal representational state—which momentarily seems not to be a good instrument for gaining knowledge—becomes available. The phenomenal book state becomes opaque. The crack in the window catches your attention. What you are losing is *sensory* transparency; you are becoming conscious of the fact that perceptions are generated by sensory organs and that those organs do not function in an absolutely reliable manner in all situations. There are, however, more comprehensive types of phenomenal opacity.

Let us make a second assumption. You now suddenly discover, that not only this particular book perception but also all of your philosophical reflections on the problem of consciousness are currently taking place in a dream. This dream then becomes a lucid dream (see section 7.2.5). The fact that your phenomenal life does not unfold in a world, but only in a world-model, now becomes globally available. You can use this information to control action, for further cognitive processing, or to guide your attention. What you are losing is *global* transparency. It is interesting to note how cognitive availability alone is not sufficient to break through the realism characterizing phenomenal experience. You cannot simply "think yourself out" of the phenomenal model of reality by changing your beliefs about this model. The transparency of phenomenal representations is cognitively impenetrable; phenomenal knowledge is not identical to conceptual or propositional knowledge.

Classic philosophical examples of opaque mental representations, of course, are good old propositional attitudes. Because of their association with a mode of presentation, beliefs and other propositional attitudes are semantically opaque, because they can represent their objects in different ways—at least this is a background assumption shared by many philosophers (which I do not intend to discuss further at this point). Your belief that you now hold a book in your hands differs from your belief that you are now holding a book about the "self-model theory of subjectivity" in your hands, because you could know the content of one of those two propositions without knowing the content of the other. Beliefs allow us to represent the same object in different ways; they generate a possible difference between the content of a mental representation and the way in which this content is presented. Purely phenomenal representations do not possess this ambiguity. We experience their content in a way that does not raise any questions about *how* this content is given to us. It is only in the interplay with theoretical reflection, only with the emergence of cognitive mental representations in a narrow sense, that phenomenal experience becomes a problem at all.

Transparency as an Informational-Computational Strategy

Semantic transparency of internal data structures is, in two respects, a great advantage for any biosystem having to operate with limited temporal and neural resources. First, it minimizes computational load. Second, it creates the most important "architectural" precon dition for planning processes.

First, transparency is synonymous to a *missing* of information: those complex processes of information processing leading to the activation of our phenomenal world-model are systematically taken out of the picture. This means that almost all information about the complex causal history of this model does not have to be reprocessed, and from an evolutionary perspective this certainly is an advantage. The transparification of earlier processing stages limits the target domain for attentional and cognitive processing, as well as for selective motor control, and this is an important strategy of resource allocation. I sometimes like to look at it like this, in terms of an old-fashioned computationalist metaphor: Conscious experience, for a biological system, generates a simply structured *user surface* for its own nervous system. Naive realism, inevitably accompanying the closedness of its surface (*constraint 10*), is an advantage. It only confronts the system with the final results of its own processing activity, and it does so by making them available for the control of action while simultaneously protecting the system from losing contact with external reality by getting lost in an introspective exploration of the underlying mechanisms. Therefore, our representational architecture only allows for a very limited introspective access to the real dynamics of the myriad of individual neural events out of which our phenomenal world finally emerges in a seemingly effortless manner. I have already emphasized this fact on the epistemological level by introducing the concept of "autoepistemic closure": conscious experience severely limits the possibilities we have to gain knowledge about ourselves. Subjective experience has not been developed in pursuing the old philosophical ideal of self-knowledge, but it has been evolutionarily successful, because it has enabled a more flexible form of action control. Phenomenal opacity is simply the degree of attentional availability of earlier processing stages, and the degree depends on how *adaptive* it was to make these earlier processing stages globally available.

Second, by taking a detour via naive realism, the transparency of our phenomenal world-model is an elegant and simple way to create a reference basis for planning processes. It is being assumed by the world zero hypothesis presented earlier. Intended simulations are always opaque representations, and they can only fulfill their function for the organism if they are embedded in a *transparent* background model. Transparent world-models are an essential tool for measuring the distance from a real world to certain internally simulated world-models, which are simultaneously recognized *as* simulations.

Transparency as a Functional Property

Transparency leads to new functional properties. This is true of individual representata as well as for systems as a whole. Systems operating under a transparent world-model for the first time live in a reality, which, for them, cannot be transcended; on a functional level they become *realists*. Again, this does not mean that they have to possess or even be able to form certain beliefs. It means that the assumption of the actual presence of a world becomes causally effective. If their reality-model contains a system-world border, then the underlying differentiation becomes a *real* difference for them; because the factual character of the contents of their phenomenal representata cannot be transcended by them, the causal effectivity of information depicted in this mode is increased. For a teleofunctionalist analysis of transparency and opacity it is important to see how both representational phenomena buy different advantages for the organism.

A transparent world-model is useful, because, for the first time, it allows the internal representation of *facticity*. It allows a system to treat information as *factual* information. Transparency forces an organism to take the world seriously. In this context, it may be interesting to note how human children only manage to explicitly represent facticity at the age of $1\frac{1}{2}$ years. The implicit representation of facticity as supplied by phenomenal transparency is the central necessary precondition for the capacity to later explicitly and cognitively represent the fact *that something really is the case*.

As soon as a certain degree of opacity becomes available, a second major functional advantage emerges: The appearance-reality distinction can now be represented. The fact that some elements of the ongoing flow of conscious experience actually are representational *contents*, and therefore may be false, becomes globally available. The difference between appearance and reality itself becomes an element of reality, and it can now be acted upon or thought about, attended to, and made the object of closer inspection. As is well-known from developmental psychology, the emergence of the appearance-reality distinction is a decisive step in the child's unfolding of its own subjective reality.

This opens a new potential for self-representation, the relevance of which is hard to underestimate: the emergence of a genuinely cognitive subject (see section 6.4.4) is tied to the existence of opaque phenomenal representations. It is the interplay between opaque and transparent representations, which allows for new and specific cognitive achievements. Let me give a typically philosophical example. *De-re*-reference is something that not only has to take place but something that has also to be internally modeled by the cognitive subject itself to be successful. When referring to an already internally represented object *as an object*, the content of an internal state has to be reliably coded as external, concrete, and not content-like. The object component of this act of reference, therefore, has to be mentally represented in a transparent manner, whereas the act of reference itself, the representational activity accompanying this step, must be mentally modeled *as* a representational activity, and hence must be represented opaquely. We return to these issues in chapter 6.

For a functional analysis of individual states, however, a strong general statement about necessary properties of the phenomenal vehicles of representation results. They are created by a functional architecture, which makes it generally impossible for attentional top-down mechanisms to access their causal history. Different subconstraints and different degrees of constraint satisfaction yield different classes of phenomenal vehicles.

Neural Correlates of Transparent Representation
There is a meaningful reading of transparency on the neuroscientific level of description as well: the brain is the *medium* of subjective experience, and *as the medium* it is unavailable to this very experience. Our own brain is the blind spot of conscious experience because there is *no* kind of self-presentational content (section 5.4) caused by it—for instance, when consciously undergoing neurosurgery with only local anesthesia blocking the pain in the skin that had to be cut and pushed away to open the skull, we cannot feel pain in the brain because there is "no 'brain-skin' which feels the neurosurgeon's knife" (Feinberg 2001, p. 157). This indeed implies a functional variety of transparency. As Todd Feinberg put it:

It has been know since the time of Aristotle that the brain is insensate. For instance, cutting the cortex itself evokes no pain. Further, the brain has no sensory apparatus directed toward itself. There is no way the subject, from the "inside," can become aware of his own neurons, from the "inside." They can be known only objectively from the "outside." There is no inner eye watching the brain itself, perceiving neurons and glia. The brain is "transparent" from the standpoint of the subject, but not from the standpoint of an outside observer. We may say, therefore, that a neural state that instantiates consciousness does not refer to itself. A conscious neural state entails a *meaning state* that, from the subject's standpoint, refers to something that is materially not that state. (Feinberg 1997, p. 87)

However, a neural state carrying intentional content (a "meaning state") could also be an unconscious state, that is, a nonphenomenal meaning state. Therefore, in order to attack the explanatory target of *phenomenal* transparency, further constraints on other levels of description are needed. In principle it would be conceivable for an unconscious neural state, as a matter of fact, to refer to itself as a vehicle of representation—but this would not yet imply it becoming *phenomenally* opaque. Phenomenal opacity and transparency are determined by the degree to which the system as a whole has attentional access to earlier stages of neural processing.

Unfortunately, almost nothing is known today about the neural basis of phenomenal transparency. As soon as the minimally sufficient neural correlates for specific forms of phenomenal content are available, however, we may research the degree of availability of earlier processing stages leading to the establishment of these correlates in the system. Such a research program would have to be oriented toward the "principle of attentional availability" I have introduced above: the degree of phenomenal transparency is inversely proportional to the degree of attentional availability of earlier processing stages. Transparency, therefore, can be viewed as a functional property of the neural process carrying the respective phenomenal content. A closer investigation of the temporal resolution of attentional processing relative to such earlier phases of dynamical, neural self-organization may be of particular interest.

It may also be helpful to apply an additional "acquisition constraint" (see Bermúdez 1998) to the phylogenetic and ontogenetic history of phenomenal transparency. A neuro-biological theory of transparency should be able to explain how we acquired transparent and opaque phenomenal representations in a series of steps. To illustrate the idea, let me briefly point to an obvious feature of the three phenomenal state classes I had initially differentiated, namely, sensory processing, emotional processing, and cognitive processing. Obviously, sensory processing is very old, very fast, and highly integrated with other representational resources in the system. It is also, typically, highly reliable and well adapted to our current environment. It is interesting to note how sensory content also was our paradigmatic example of transparency. If philosophers look for an example of transparency, they usually choose a sensory quale, like G. E. Moore chose the visual color quale of *blue*. Sensory qualia are *the* example of transparency. It is interesting to note that emotions only appeared much later in evolutionary history and that emotions typically take a longer processing time; they frequently are not as well adapted and as reliable relative to our quickly changing, current social environment. As it turns out, emotions take a middle place on the phenomenal spectrum between transparency and opacity: sometimes we recognize their representationality, often we don't. From an evolutionary perspective, cognitive processing—in terms of the internal simulation of rule-based operations involving discrete symbol tokens, compositionality, syntacticity, simplicity, and so on—is something very, very new. Conscious thought by far has the shortest period for evolutionary optimization; it is slow and—as all of us know—very unreliable. Cognitive processing is so slow that it allows us to introspectively experience the construction process of its content. Taking an evolutionary perspective may be of help in taking the first steps toward a neurobiologically grounded theory of phenomenal transparency (see, e.g., Roth 2000).

However, eventually it may also be possible to explain the phenomena of transparency and opacity on a much shorter time scale. If there is a gradual distribution of transparency in phenomenal space, defined as a gradient of attentional availability of earlier processing stages, this gradient may have a straightforward explanation in terms of temporal resolution and processing times for the first-order target states in the brain.

In searching for the neural correlates of certain conscious states, it is important to isolate the smallest possible set of conditions sufficient for the activation of a specific form of phenomenal content. Of particular interest are all experimental setups which manage to separate the intentional content of a representational state from its phenomenal content. In other words, we have to look for the common set of minimally sufficient conditions of identical experiences, which sometimes are hallucinations and sometimes are veridical perceptions (for a good example, see Düzel, Yonelinas, Mangun, Heinze, and Tulving 1997).

3.2.8 Offline Activation

As we have just seen, some constraints come with a considerable amount of phenomenological domain-specificity. The degree of constraint satisfaction may vary greatly from one phenomenological state class to another. The next constraint is not valid for all, but for a considerable number of different forms of phenomenal content. As explained in chapter 2, presentational content always is stimulus-correlated. *Re*presentational content always refers to the actual state of the world. Phenomenal *simulations* (see section 2.3), however, are generated in a way that is largely independent of current sensory input. Higher-order, that is, genuinely *cognitive* variants of conscious contents in particular, can enter in that way into complex simulations: they are generated by such simulations. It is interesting to note, in the context of the transparency constraint just discussed, that cognitive phenomenal content activated in an offline fashion is typically opaque.

The Phenomenology of Simulation

First, however, one has to look at the dream state, because it exhibits the maximal degree of constraint satisfaction for *constraint 8*: dreams are *global* offline states. In dreams we confront a very large, global state class, which emerges precisely because the brain continuously interprets internally generated stimuli by integrating them into a dynamic, transparent world-model. Just as in the ordinary waking state, this model is not recognized *as* a model, and in this case even the information that this model does not refer to an actual world is not available to the subject of experience. I return to a more detailed analysis of phenomenal dreams and their relevance to a general theory of consciousness in chapter 4 (section 4.2.5). Here we are only concerned with states phenomenally experienced *as* not directly stimulus-related. There are basically two kinds of such states.

Has reading a philosophical text ever triggered a spontaneous, inner dialogue with the author in you? Daydreams, associative fantasies, spontaneously appearing memory sequences, or seemingly useless inner monologues are *nonintended simulations*. Sometimes, this first category of states even opens a magical dimension: it is ruled by images experienced as autonomous and *as images*. In nonintended simulations we subjectively experience ourselves as beings not tied to the experiential Now as currently given through the senses. The intentional content of our ongoing mental processes extends into past and future, while at the same time it remains true that, as contents of working memory, they are governed by the principle of presentationality (*constraint 2*). I may dream about the distant future or be surprised by the sudden appearance of a pleasant childhood memory, but at the same time these internal simulations always take place against the background of myself *having* these dreams or of being surprised *now*. This new level of subjective experience can be analyzed as follows: The difference between a possible and a real situation becomes globally available (*constraints 1* and *3*). Past and future can now be represented as explicit episodes, which nevertheless are always tied to a singular, individual perspective (*constraints 5* and *6*) on the level of phenomenal experience. An individual perspective is generated by the phenomenal presence of a situated, fully embodied self (see section 5.4). If the intentional content of these episodes is formed by past states of the organism, autobiographic memory emerges and the phenomenal self is now being enriched by a new dimension of content, the theoretical importance of which can hardly be underestimated. The *historicity of one's own person* is now cognitively available in conscious experience itself. If, however, spontaneously appearing simulative episodes refer to possible situations and potential future states of the phenomenal self, the *indeterminacy of one's own biography* is available on the level of conscious experience. This information then is one of the most important preconditions for initiating planning and goal selection processes. In short, the capacity to generate globally available offline simulations is particularly interesting in cases where these phenomenal simulations are phenomenal *self-simulations* (see section 6.2.7).

An even richer form of conscious experience appears if another kind of phenomenal content is additionally integrated into the overall process, the phenomenal property of agency (see section 6.4.5). Simulations then become *intended* simulations. Intended simulations are the second kind of explanatory targets to be investigated under the offline-activation constraint. The phenomenology of intended simulation is the phenomenology of the autonomous cognitive subject. In such states we experience ourselves as mental agents. In this context, mental agents are not only beings capable of voluntarily guiding their own attention toward an object. Mental agents are systems deliberately generating phenomenally opaque states within themselves, systems able to initiate and control ordered chains of mental representations and for whom *this* very fact again is cognitively available. Mental agents are systems experiencing themselves as the thinkers of their own thoughts. They can form the notion of a "rational individual," which in turn is the historical root of the concept of a *person*. We then take the step from a being with a phenomenal first-person perspective to a being with a consciously experienced *cognitive* first-person perspective, because we are now able to mentally model the fact of actually being systems able to activate mental representations within ourselves in a goal-directed manner. Our own rationality becomes a part of reality. We can then integrate this new information into our phenomenal self by, for the first time, consciously experiencing ourselves *as* rational individuals, *as* persons (I return to this point in section 6.4.4; see also Baker 1998). In short, we *experience* the reflexivity of self-consciousness; our capacity for rational cognitive self-reference has now become a globally available fact. On our planet, this phenomenology may be restricted to human beings and some higher primates. The offline activation constraint is an important constraint in finding out which kinds of representational structures made this development possible.

Offline Simulation as a Representational Property
For primitive biosystems it may be true that only integrated phenomenal presentation, or core consciousness (Damasio 1999), exists. Such organisms would be caught within an eternal Now, because the content of their phenomenal states would only refer to currently given stimulus sources. If, however, we are interested in explaining memory and higher cognitive capacities like the internal representation of goal states ("future planning") as a biological as well as a subjectively experienced phenomenon, then we have to assume a possibility for the system to generate complex mental representata independently of the incessant flow of input. The simple fact that dreaming is much harder during daytime than at night shows that, functionally speaking, there is a real computational problem in the background: Although from a neurobiological and purely functionalist point of view a large portion of the activity underlying the conscious model of reality may be based on an internal, autonomous activity of the brain, the pressure of ongoing sensory input certainly puts strong constraints on the content of this world-model. Phenomenal reality-models are the more plastic the less they are being determined by the actual input and the more specific aspects of the functional architecture of the system. The example of nocturnal dreams also shows how a high degree of plasticity frequently is equivalent to instability, loss of global coherence, and low epistemic content: The dreaming system cannot access the informational flow from the sensory modules; it can only resort to the relational structure of internally available data structures (*constraints 4 and 5*). Phenomenal representata have to enable an internal simulation of complex counterfactual situations by, as it were, offering a relational structure to the system which can also be utilized in internal "test runs." Maybe a good way to imagine the specific process of internal simulation as

guided by phenomenal representata is of a certain interesting representatum being, in the course of an internal experiment, *embedded* in the current overall model of the world. A process of metarepresentation could then investigate the general "goodness of fit" for this model, and also how the content of other representata would change by fully embedding this new relational structure. In order for such internal simulations to be realistic and biologically successful, they will have to generate a critical degree of structural equivalence with a given goal situation. This, in turn, depends on phenomenal representata reflecting as many of those relational properties of their external representanda as necessary which are relevant to survival in their *own* relational structure. One further subconstraint can be formulated for those phenomenal offline simulations that are subjectively experienced as deliberate acts of thinking, as *intended* phenomenal simulations: They must be objects of a selection process operating on them, and the operation of this selection process *itself* must be integrated into the globally available partition of the currently active self-model. This is not to say that selection processes do not operate on nonintended simulations like daydreams or free-flowing associative fantasies. It just means that these selection processes are not themselves represented on the level of a global, conscious model of reality. The system does not represent itself *as* selecting.

Offline Simulation as an Informational-Computational Strategy
I have already pointed to the fact that offline simulations make new forms of intentional content (i.e., the important difference between possibility and reality) available to the system as a whole and that they also open new sources of information (i.e., temporal or modal information). Generally speaking, globally available processes of simulation are a powerful instrument for making a system *intelligent*. First, simulations are useful tools when a closer inspection of the temporal structure of internally represented events is necessary: they make possible worlds and viable trajectories leading into such worlds cognitively available. It may be interesting to note that in scientific practice simulations of target phenomena (e.g., on a large computer in the department of meteorology) are typically employed to study the temporal fine structure and dynamical evolution of the target phenomenon. From a neurocomputational perspective many mental simulations, particularly those consciously experienced, may share this function. Second, offline simulations may support social cognition. Of course, a very important role, in this context is played by simulated *first-person perspectives* (as in social cognition and so-called theory of mind tasks; for an example, see Gallese and Goldman 1998; Gallese 2000). Third, offline states contribute to the overall intelligence of a system by enabling *self*-simulations, that is, the planning of possible future states of the system (see sections 5.3 and 6.3.3 and chapter 7). Such self-simulations constitute not only potential *perceptual* perspectives and possible sensory states but also depict the manner in which these can be integrated with available

patterns of motor output. Fourth, adaptive motor control constitutes a further example, but interestingly, one in which we see an intricate interplay between online and offline simulations. The simulation of possible bodily movements and of one's own action strategies can serve to minimize the risks, which are always given with *external* exploratory behavior in the real world. A forward model of one's own body, (e.g., see Wolpert, Ghahramani and Jordan 1995; Wolpert and Ghahramani 2000) which can simulate the causal flow of a movement process, anticipate the results and sensory feedback of a motor command, and which can be used to minimize errors or estimation tasks, in learning processes, and in mental simulations of alternative patterns of movement, is of central importance in this context. A forward dynamic model, internally simulating the motor-to-sensory transformation in terms of bodily actions and their bodily consequences; a forward sensory model, internally simulating the expected *external* sensory consequences of a specific action; and an inverse model, implementing opposite transformations from "desired consequences to actions" (Wolpert and Ghahramani 2000, p. 1212); are needed to realize a full-blown sensorimotor loop. They are excellent examples of such structures. The inverse model, in particular, is an example of a mental process that makes intelligent and selective motor planning possible. It does so by *not* covarying with the actual state of the world anymore, in representing possible actions leading to a certain goal state. However, to make mental simulations of goal-directed behaviors efficient, a translation from "high-level" to "low-level" tasks (Wolpert and Ghahramani 2000, p. 1212*f.*), from simulation to detailed structures actually *representing* the current state of the system's body, has to be achieved. Simulation and representation have to go hand in hand.

Offline Simulations as Functional Processes

Phenomenal simulations are constructed from a sequence of non–stimulus-correlated states. This lack of covariance with the current environment is the essential feature of their causal role. Our previous constraint of phenomenal states being *dynamical* states (*constraint 5*), therefore, can now also be interpreted in the following way: Many phenomenal states can be activated independently of the environment of the system or the current flow of input, because they are integrated into a comprehensive, ongoing *internal* dynamics. They are exclusively driven by this dynamics, and—in this special case—not by the coupled dynamics of world, body, and nervous system. Offline simulations, in short, greatly enrich the functional profile of any phenomenal system. They do so by generating new sets of functional properties in making new types of information and representational content available for fast and flexible processing on the level of a global model of reality.

Neurobiological Correlates of Phenomenal Offline Simulations

A large number of scanning data now support the hypothesis presented above. The human brain, in simulating possible perceptual situations, frequently uses the same anatomical structures that are also active during a real sensory contact with the current environment. The same is true for motor simulations. Interestingly, a large number of new results concerning the neural correlates of *social cognition* plausibly lead to the assumption of the mental representation of the action goals of other agents being functionally anchored within an unconscious online simulation of their perceived motor behavior, for instance, in area F5 of premotor cortex (see section 6.3.3). This would mean that the conscious realization of the goal driving the actions of *another* human being is caused by, first, an unconscious representation of its actual motor profile being activated in its brain. In a second step, this would then lead to a globally available, abstract, and allocentric simulation of this perceived motor profile. The representational content of this simulation would be a motor equivalence between observer and observed agent, what appears as the assumed action *goal* on the phenomenal level. Therefore, the most important neurobiological simulation processes may be those that make the transition from an online simulation to an offline simulation in social cognition, enabling an agent to consciously experience the intention of another agent (see Gallese and Goldman 1998). It is interesting to note how even such complex mechanisms as motor simulations are characterized by what I would call the "principle of substrate sharing." If an organism has developed a substrate for conscious vision, then it can in principle—as soon as the correlated set of phenomenal states satisfies *constraint 8*—learn to take this substrate offline. It can *imagine*, *dream* about, or even *hallucinate* visual experiences. If an organism possesses self-consciousness (*constraint 6*), then it can in principle imagine, dream about, or hallucinate other minds (see section 6.3.3).

3.2.9   Representation of Intensities

What Lewis qualia, Raffman qualia, and Metzinger qualia have in common is that they vary along a continuous dimension of intensity. This variation on the level of simple content is a characteristic and salient feature of consciousness itself. However, the domain to which the intensity constraint applies is only the domain of conscious, *presentational* content as introduced in chapter 2. There are, however, numerous and important senses in which higher-order forms of phenomenal content can be said to possess a subjective intensity as well: The qualities of *presence* and realism underlying a consciously experienced situation as a whole can certainly be more or less intense; the consciously experienced emotional bond to another human being can be more or less intense; the availability of explicit context information during a certain cognitive episode can be more or less marked, and so forth. However, none of these more metaphorical uses of the concept of phenomenological intensity lie within the scope of the intensity constraint. It is only satisfied in the domain of simple and directly stimulus-correlated conscious content.

The Phenomenology of Intensity

Sensory experience comes in different intensities. In section 2.4 of chapter 2 we saw that it is possible to conceptualize presentational content in terms of different degrees of global availability, for instance, as "Lewis qualia," "Raffman qualia," or "Metzinger qualia." Interestingly, on the level of attentional availability, further differentiations in terms of the content that can be discriminated in introspective attention are possible. Let us take the standard example of simple sensory content first, namely, phenomenally experienced color. We have seen that colors cannot exist by themselves, if not integrated into a chromatic context. According to the standard view (but see Mausfeld 2002) a phenomenal color can vary in three dimensions: hue, saturation, and brightness. For the example of phenomenal color, *brightness* is the aspect at issue, because it is the conscious correlate of the physical *force* of the stimulus. Phenomenal brightness is the way in which human beings consciously experience the intensity of the physical stimulus on their retina. Phenomenal tones can vary in pitch, timbre, and loudness. Again, *loudness* is the aspect that is grasped by the intensity constraint. As Shaun Maxwell (Maxwell, submitted, p. 4) has pointed out, while variations in any of these dimensions are attentionally distinguishable from each other in normal subjects, members of each tripartite set cannot exist independently. Typically, one cannot, for example, experience a pitch without also, at least, experiencing loudness. However, if we remember the Ganzfeld experiments discussed in chapter 2, it seems at least possible for a normal subject under a uniform homogeneous stimulation to, in the visual domain, experience intensity *as such* on the conscious level. For instance, recall the reports about colorless, formless visual experience described as "swimming in a mist of light which becomes more condensed at an indefinite distance" or the experience of a "sea of light" (Metzger 1930; and Gibson and Waddell 1952, quoted in Avant 1965, p. 246). What the Ganzfeld subject is left with after all hue and saturation have vanished from the visual field is adequately termed an "achromatic level of luminance." That is, after phenomenal color has completely vanished in a Ganzfeld experiment, pure stimulus intensity as such, pure brightness without hue, can still be represented on the phenomenal level. This is an important phenomenal constraint for any further theorizing on simple sensory content. First, the intensity dimension seems to be the most fundamental phenomenal dimension in which conscious experience can vary. It is separable. Second, because this dimension is a continuous dimension, phenomenal representation, on a very fundamental level, is *analogue* representation.

All simple forms of presentational content possess an intensity parameter; there is no counterexample to this principle. Pain, visual sensations, colors, tones, and so on all appear in different intensities on the phenomenal level. An interesting question is: Are there any forms of attentionally available and basic presentational content that only vary along one other single dimension, namely, the dimension of intensity? Maxwell points out that our oldest sensory channels, those that present chemical properties of the world to the experiencing subject, may be the prime candidates for this position in any theory of the phenomenology of intensity:

Perhaps the most compelling examples of such basic qualia are in the gustatory modality. For example, while sweetness *may* not be a unitary sensation . . . it is likely that neither saltiness, sourness, nor bitterness admit of any phenomenal dimensions of variation save that of intensity. There appear to be no examples of fundamental qualia that have any kind of variability save for variation in intensity. (Maxwell, submitted, p. 4)

Phenomenal smell is a particularly interesting example. In the generation of olfactory presentational content, binding is homogeneously achieved across the whole sensory surface of the organism. In other words, the phenomenology of smell tells us that there is no olfactory *scene*; there is no such thing as scene segmentation, but only a representation of intensity plus a sequential, temporal evolution of presentational content as such. The fact that even for the most primitive forms of sensory awareness, forms that do not even segment phenomenal space into objects and backgrounds, a phenomenal intensity parameter is invariably present, forms another strong argument for the intensity constraint being a very fundamental and relevant constraint in its respective domain.

Intensity as a Property of Presentational Content
One defining characteristic of presentational content is that, functionally, it is stimulus-correlated. We can now see how this defining characteristic is reflected on the content level: The stimulus is present in terms of a continuous representation of its own intensity. The intensity of hunger and pain, the loudness of a conscious sound experience, the continuous unfolding of the subjective force within an olfactory or gustatory experience, the degrees of brightness in a conscious color experience—all those phenomenological examples demonstrate a specific form of phenomenal content which is not only variable but *continuously* variable. The continuous character of the intensity mentioned is something to which we can introspectively direct our attention: it is not a cognitively, but an *attentionally* available feature of the ongoing flow of phenomenal experience. Obviously, the limited cognitive availability of fine-grained shifts and changes in phenomenal intensity lies at the heart of the difficulties we have in attempting to convey the force or subjective "strength" of a sensory experience in ordinary language. As we have seen, there are simple forms of presentational content that are characterized only by their dimensional position in a sensory order (their "quality") and their current intensity value. As the Ganzfeld experiments show, in addition, a single value on the intensity dimension can be made globally available as such, that is, the activation of presentational content which *only* reflects the physical force of the stimulus to which it is correlated and *no* dimensional position anymore is nomologically possible in human beings. The theoretically interesting point

therefore is that presentational content has not only a dimensional position and a certain temporal fine structure given by its dynamics (*constraint 5*) but also a fundamental *quantitative* dimension, in which the intensity of a sensory stimulus can be reflected. It is interesting to note how there is a quantitative aspect to a simple form of phenomenal content that traditionally has only been discussed as qualitative content. I propose that it is precisely this aspect which anchors presentational content in the physical world. A closer investigation may help us to build conceptual bridges from the phenomenological to the functional and physical levels of description. It is important to note that this quantitative aspect of simple phenomenal content can be separated from the "qualitative" component during a full-blown conscious experience in nonpathological subjects, simply by choosing an unusual stimulus configuration (e.g., in a Ganzfeld experiment). On the other hand, the conscious presentation of the dimensional position in a sensory order (what we would traditionally term the *qualitative* component of this content) *cannot* exist without a determined value along the intensity dimension. Let us call this the "principle of stimulus force." All forms of presentational content are necessarily integrated with an analogue representation of the underlying stimulus intensity.

The Presentation of Intensities as an Informational-Computational Property

From an informational-computational perspective the role of the intensity constraint is rather trivial and straightforward. On the most basic level of input processing, information about the actual stimulus intensity is extracted and passed on to subsequent levels of the internal hierarchy. The *conscious*, that is, globally available, presentation of information about stimulus intensity just discussed achieves this computational goal in a very economic and direct manner.

Phenomenal Intensity Modeling as a Functional Property

From a teleofunctionalist, evolutionary perspective it is clear how such information was maximally *relevant* information for biological organisms and it is also obvious how the presentation of intensities in the way just described would have been adaptive: it makes information about stimulus intensity available for fast, direct, and noncognitively mediated forms of action control. Functionally speaking, it may also play an important role in automatically guiding the focus of attention, that is, in fixating attention in a fast and direct way. To again give a concrete example, the biological function of consciously experienced *pain* can convincingly be interpreted as "attention fixation"—it locks the organism's attention onto whatever part of its own body it is that has been damaged. It is important to note that it is not the specific "quality," the dimensional position of the pain presentatum, which plays this functional role. It is the globally available *intensity* of a pain experience that makes it harder and harder to guide our attention anywhere else and that eventually *locks* our attentional focus onto the damaged body part. From a teleofunctionalist perspective, an important secondary effect is the maximization of motivational force behind a behavioral response.

But what is the causal role of presentational content in general? In earlier publications (e.g., see Metzinger 1993) I have conceptually analyzed the causal role of presentational content as that of an "analogue indicator." Let us first look at the role of indicators, indexical expressions, in natural languages.

What is the corresponding function in natural languages? Indicators are expressions like "I," "here," "this," or "now" and they are used frequently. Their reference depends on the spatial, temporal, or mental context and the position of the speaker in this context. They help the speaker by orienting herself and localizing herself *within* this context. In contentful propositions indicators can miss their referent. Therefore, I would call them "digital indicators"—they generate truth and falsity.

Analogue indicators—what I have called mental presentata—on the contrary signal the pure presence of a stimulus by being *internal* states of the system. The functional states in question can be analyzed as analogue indicators. However, they play the causal role of a *nonconceptual* indicator and their content is nonconceptual content. They do not present their content as true or false, as a property either exemplified or not exemplified, but as more or less similar. A specific presentational content like red_{31} is not related to the external world in terms of a one-to-one mapping but through a very complex and unsystematic statistical dependency relation. If we wanted to represent the content of a visual color presentatum on the level of natural language, we would have to use digital indicators, for example, by saying: "red_{31}-now-here!" "Red_{31}" refers to the currently active presentational content and its dimensional position on a sensory order that is, in almost all cases, only attentionally available and therefore ineffable. It linguistically points to this internally active content, falsely assuming the possession of transtemporal identity criteria (see section 2.4). The "Now" component of this expression refers to the presentationality constraint, that is, the *de nunc* character of this special form of mental content, and the "Here" component refers to the globality constraint, that is, the fact that this content is located at a specific position in a coherent world-model. Functionally speaking, this may illustrate the internal function of indicators from an external perspective—in Richard Gregory's formulation, they "flag the dangerous present." But why *analogue* indicators? We now know a second argument for this way of conceptualizing presentata on the functional level: because phenomenal presentata make a certain range of the intensity or signal strength characterizing the presentandum (i.e., information about a physical stimulus property) internally available by integrating it with what we have traditionally described as its "qualitative" component. For the example of color vision, the quantitative component is functionally more fundamental, because—as opposed to hue—it can exist by itself on the phenomenal level. It is a "stand-alone feature." It is an analogue form of very fundamental phenomenal content, because it varies not in discrete steps, but along a continuous dimension. The second component is an analogue form of content as well, because it varies along a continuous dimension of hue. A functional property shared by both components is that subtle variations and all conscious events involving just noticeable differences in changes along both dimensions will typically be ineffable, because in most cases they are not cognitively, but only attentionally, available to the subject of experience.

Neural Correlates of Phenomenal Intensity Experience
In most cases of simple phenomenal content, stimulus intensity is simply coded by the mean firing rate of specific feature detectors. In perceptual psychology and psychophysics, we possess today a large and well-secured body of knowledge concerning the absolute and different thresholds for stimulus intensities and with regard to the relationship between psychophysical and neural intensity functions.

3.2.10 "Ultrasmoothness": The Homogeneity of Simple Content

Just like the intensity constraint, the homogeneity constraint now to be introduced is only satisfied in the domain of phenomenal presentata. From a philosophical perspective the homogeneity of simple phenomenal content, frequently interpreted as the homogeneity of phenomenal properties, is of particular theoretical relevance, because it generates conceptual predicates, which may defy definition. Can a color predicate like International Klein Blue (see Metzinger 1995b, p. 431 *ff.*) or red$_{31}$ have a successor predicate within the scientific worldview, for instance, in a scientific theory of phenomenal color vision, or are such predicates *primitive* predicates? For Wilfrid Sellars, who originally formulated the theoretical puzzle known as the "grain problem" (Sellars 1963, 1965),[16] a primitive predicate refers to properties ascribed to things made up exclusively of things which in turn possess this property. If we stay with the example of the famous color International Klein Blue, for some nondualistic philosophers this would mean that single molecules of Rhodopas, vinyl chloride, ethyl alcohol, and ethyl acetate (out of which the color is made) themselves possess the color of International Klein Blue. Other nondualistic philosophers would see themselves driven to the conclusion that a certain number of the nerve cells firing in our visual cortex while we are looking at one of Yves Klein's monochrome pictures are in fact International Klein Blue. Of course this assumption is absurd in both cases.

That is, the phenomenological predicates that refer to homogeneous presentational content as if they were referring to a cognitively available *property* seem to introduce a

---

16. Cf. Sellars 1963 and also 1965. Texts I found helpful are Green 1979; Gunderson 1974; Lockwood 1993; Maxwell 1978; and Richardson and Muilenburg 1982. Kurthen (1990) gives a good account of the development of Sellars's philosophical treatment of the problem.

further simple property that apparently cannot be reductively explained. It is the internal, structureless *density* of simple phenomenal color experiences and the like that has traditionally supported antireductive theoretical intuitions. It may be helpful to look back to the classic example of Wilfrid Sellars, the pink ice cube:

Pink does not seem to be made up of imperceptible qualities in the way in which being a ladder is made up of being cylindrical (the rungs), rectangular (the frame), wooden, etc. The manifest ice cube presents itself to us as something which is pink through and through, a pink continuum, all the regions of which, however small, are pink. It presents itself to us as *ultimately homogeneous*; and an ice cube variegated in colour is, though not homogeneous in its specific colour, 'ultimately homogeneous,' in the sense to which I am calling attention, with respect to the generic trait of being coloured. (Sellars 1963, p. 26)

For Sellars, the central question of the grain problem was whether it could, in principle, be possible within the conceptual framework of neurophysiology to define states that in their intrinsic character show a sufficient similarity to sensations. Only states of this kind, Sellars thought, could render a reductive solution of the mind-body problem (in the sense of early identity theory) plausible.

The answer seems clearly to be no. This is not to say that neurophysiological states cannot be defined (in principle) which have a high degree of analogy to the sensations of the manifest image. That this can be done is an elementary fact of psychophysics. The trouble is, rather, that the feature which we referred to as "ultimate homogeneity," and which characterizes the perceptible quality of things, e.g., their colour, seems to be essentially lacking in the domain of the definable states of the nerves and their interactions. Putting it crudely, colour expanses in the manifest world consist of regions which are themselves colour expanses, and these consist in their turn of regions which are colour expanses, and so on; whereas the states of a group of neurons, though it has regions which are also states of groups of neurons, has ultimate regions which are *not* states of groups of neurons but rather states of single neurons. And the same is true if we move to the finer grained level of biochemical process. (Sellars 1963, p. 35)

For theoretical reasons, the homogeneity constraint satisfied by conscious presentational content is of great theoretical interest. It may generate a principled obstacle for naturalist theories of subjective experience. Second, it bears an intimate relationship to the transparency constraint already discussed. Let us therefore again begin by taking a first-person stance, looking at homogeneity as a *phenomenological* constraint imposed on the notion of conscious presentation first.

The Phenomenology of Homogeneity

What Sellars called "ultimate homogeneity" may itself be another paradigmatic example of ineffability (see section 2.4; Metzinger and Walde 2000). On the other hand, homogeneity is characterized by an explicit *absence* of something (namely, internal structure), and this absence is certainly available for guided, introspective attention. This time, it is a higher-order characteristic of presentational content for which it is hard to form a concept, because arguably this characteristic as well is only attentionally, but not cognitively available. For this reason, I will try to offer a metaphorical description of the phenomenological feature in question, which I am borrowing from physics and mathematics. What does it mean to say that a subjective color experience like red_{31} or International Klein Blue (see Metzinger 1995b, e) is homogeneous? The primary phenomenal property is characterized by a kind of additional "field quality," generating a subjective *continuum* in a certain subregion of our conscious space. If, for instance, we visually experience objects that possess the property of International Klein Blue the following statement always seems to be true: There is always a finite region within phenomenal space, in which no changes take place with regard to the quality in question.[17] There is no temporal texture. There is no internal structure. There is just *this*, *now*. I believe that it is precisely for this reason that we experience low-level subjective qualities as immediately given. They never *become* what they are, they always already *are* what they are. The structureless character of presentational content endows it with an ahistoric character. Introspectively, we cannot find out how this content may have come into existence because nothing in its attentionally available properties points to the *process*, which may have caused, generated, or shaped it. The continuum metaphor is a nonmechanistic metaphor on the most simple level of phenomenal content, because it does not include parts and their relations anymore.

Let us now turn to the second, mathematical metaphor. Perhaps it is also possible to describe the homogeneity constraint for presentational content as its subjective "density." It seems as if, for any two points (no matter how close they are to one another) within the respective region of my experiential space, there always exists a third point which lies between them. The mathematical analogy for this flowing density is the continuum of real numbers. At least intuitively it remains utterly obscure how this density of presentational content could be accessible to a mechanistic strategy of explanation, that is, how we could analyze it as the result of a myriad of causally intertwined singular events on the neural level. How does the "graininess" disappear? What is hard to explain is the obvious correlation between homogeneous presentational content and underlying neural activity. For a number of prominent accounts of scientific explanation in general, an explanation of a regularity constituted by the correlation between homogeneous presentational content and

---

17. This is one of the ways in which philosophers have tried to reformulate the original grain problem (Cf. the formulations of Meehl 1966, p. 167; and Green 1979, p. 566*f*.) It is interesting to note that if we imagine cases of a continuous, flowing *change* of a certain type of qualitative content, that is, cases in which we might *not* be able to discriminate any finite regions in phenomenal space anymore, the Sellarsian *ultimate homogeneity* with regard to the generic trait, for example, of coloredness, would still hold.

certain sets of objective conditions in the brain can only be achieved if two *intrinsic* structures can be described in both of the entities under comparison. This must be done in a way that demonstrates an isomorphism between those intrinsic structures. If the most simple form of phenomenal content actually *lacks* intrinsic structure, this type of scientific explanation will not work for them (for a detailed discussion, see Maxwell in preparation). Therefore, many of the antireductionist intuitions of dualist philosophers may not so much be rooted in the dimensional position that could describe the presentational content (e.g., a specific hue) itself by locating it in a suitable state space, but in the fact that it is governed by the homogeneity constraint. It is, I maintain, exactly for this reason that subjective qualities such as red_{31} or International Klein Blue appear as detached from any possible functionalist analysis, lending themselves to descriptions as intrinsic and nonrelational: If they were really identical with a dancing pattern of microevents in your brain, they would have to possess something like a graininess, their subjective "surface" would not be so infinitely smooth. Michael Lockwood has illustratively called this effect "glossing over" (Lockwood 1993, p. 288 p.).

The problem with reductively explaining maximally simple and determinate forms of phenomenal content, therefore, may consist in the fact that these states, due to their phenomenal homogeneity, also lend themselves to an interpretation as *atoms* of experience (see, e.g., Jakab 2000). Let me once again suggest that it may not be what we used to call *first*-order phenomenal properties (the attentionally available content of mental presentata) that make qualia appear as by necessity irreducible to many people, but rather the higher-order property of the phenomenal field quality, namely, the density or ultrasmoothness; the real problem is not International Klein Blue (which can be formally described by its dimensional position in a sensory order), but the *homogeneity* of International Klein Blue. What resists analysis is not the hue dimension, the subjective character of blue *itself*, but its structureless density. On the other hand, the concept of a nonhomogeneous form of presentational content seems to be an incoherent concept. At least for human subjects it denotes a phenomenal impossibility. We would then be thinking of a *set* of phenomenal properties, or of nonphenomenal properties altogether. To sum up, as viewed from the internal perspective of the experiencing subject, fundamental features of sensory world- and self-perception are *ultrasmooth*: they lack processuality and contain no internal structure, they are grainless and simple. That is one reason why these features appear as directly given and offer themselves to an interpretation as intrinsic, irreducible first-order properties. Any satisfactory account of sensory consciousness operating on representational, functionalist, or neuroscientific levels of description has to satisfy the homogeneity constraint by conceptually relocating phenomenal ultrasmoothness on those levels.

Homogeneity as a Characteristic of Presentational Content

Homogeneity can be analyzed as representational *atomicity*: Whatever the metarepresentational instruments used by a system to inspect its own active perceptual states, they can only generate a certain resolution. In real physical systems, resolution is never infinite. Resolution power is always relative to a readout mechanism. The resolution power of cognitive processing is not as fine-grained as the resolution of attentional processing, for example. Different filtering effects come with different kinds of metarepresentational mechanisms. On the lowest level of representational granularity, therefore, forms of content will be automatically generated, which by conceptual necessity have to appear as structurally simple to the system itself. The homogeneity of simple sensory content therefore is not an absolute property, but always relative to a certain class of representational architectures. The same first-order state could lead to a single, homogeneous presentatum in one class of systems, while being decomposed into a larger number of homogeneous presentata in another class of systems. Importantly, one and the same system can have introspective powers exhibiting varying degrees of resolution at different points in its development. For example, it could discover subtle qualitative structures within its own perceptual states, inaccessible to it in the past. In this case new and more fine-grained information about the *dimensional position* of these states in certain property spaces would become globally available for it, for instance, in terms of new introspectable subregions of color space. However, because this information would always be given in the form of a number of new representational atoms, the property of homogeneity *as such* would be preserved.

It is important to point out that presentational content cannot be a phenomenal reflection of absolutely simple properties in a strict sense, although it is phenomenologically homogeneous. If those properties were really strictly simple, then we would not be able to discover similarities between them, because there would exist no aspects that they share with each other. This, however, clearly contradicts the phenomenology. Presentata, although homogeneous, possess an implicit deep structure on the level of their content: we precisely experience this deep structure *in their similarity relations*, in experiencing orange as more similar to yellow than blue. The mistake may simply consist in conceiving of these similarity relations as extrinsic, noninternal features. They are intrinsic, internal features of phenomenal color space as a whole and, as the Ganzfeld experiment previously discussed demonstrates, it makes no sense to conceive of presentational color content as *detached* from this overarching context.

One last point about the phenomenology of homogeneity. We defined the transparency constraint by saying that the degree of phenomenal transparency is inversely proportional to the degree of attentional availability of earlier processing stages. It is now interesting to note how it is strictly true of all homogeneous, simple forms of sensory content that earlier processing stages are *completely* unavailable to introspective attention. Homogeneous sensory content always is fully transparent content. The transparency constraint is maximally satisfied for sensory primitives. Above, I have metaphorically referred to transparency as the "closedness" of our internal user surface, and, epistemologically speaking, I have introduced the notion of autoepistemic closure to describe this feature of human consciousness. In phenomenal homogeneity we experience the closedness of our own user surface in a maximally concrete way. It is precisely this homogeneity which makes the causal history of the respective presentational content in the system, the earlier processing stages that led to its activation, unavailable to attention. Therefore one may conclude that on the most fundamental levels of phenomenological and representationalist analysis it is the continuous, representationally atomic nature of simple sensory content which generates the all-pervading transparency of sensory awareness.

Homogeneity as an Informational-Computational Strategy

The homogeneity of simple phenomenal content comes into existence because global availability of information about the causal history of a stimulus is restricted. Just like transparency in general, homogeneity is a special form of autoepistemic closure: Perceptual states, being the result of complex dynamical processes with a very intricate causal fine structure, appear as simple on the level of our global model of the world and as directly given in their simplicity. This is a major and essential factor in the emergence of the transparent (*constraint 7*) phenomenal world-model. Homogeneity generates the *closure* of the internal user surface. This fact also is a central part of the causal role realized by simple sensory states carrying presentational content. The density of this internal user surface also is a *functional* kind of closure. Without homogeneity we could introspectively penetrate into the processing stages underlying the activation of sensory content. One obvious consequence of this would be that the multimodal, high-dimensional surface of our phenomenal world would start to dissolve. We would then phenomenally experience the model as an ongoing global simulation permanently generated from scratch, as it were, and thereby it would inevitably lose the phenomenal character of being an untranscendable reality. We would experience it as a *possibility*, as only one of countless hypotheses active and incessantly competing in the system. Obviously, this would lead to a dramatic shift in a whole range of computational and functional system properties. The homogeneity of presentational content reduces computational load for the overall system, and it creates a reference model of the actual world that is firmly anchored in sensory input.

Homogeneity as a Functional Property

Let me now offer a speculative hypothesis: the causal role of consciously experienced presentational states is not realized by what we traditionally call its "qualitative character" (the dimensional position in a suitable state space), but by the homogeneity of this qualitative character. And, in systems like ourselves, this *is* the realization of its causal role. Let me explain.

Introspectively picking out a specific form of presentational content means that this content is globally available for attention. Global availability comes with a satisfaction of *constraints 2 and 3*, integration of information into a window of presence and into a global world-model. In particular, simple sensory contents are typically also governed by *constraint 4*, the convolved-holism constraint. In standard situations presentational content is always integrated into a *perceptual object* before it enters the phenomenal level. Before this stage is reached, a multiplicity of binding problems, some of them consciousness-related, some of them unconscious (see Cleeremans 2002 for an excellent overview; cf. also Engel and Singer 2000) must have been solved by the system. An important background assumption, therefore, is that subjectively experienced homogeneity is the expression of the success of integrational processes in the brain leading to the activation of a coherent percept, of a binding mechanism operating *on the level of simple features*. That is, the information expressed in the ongoing activity of feature detectors, for example, for a specific presentation of color, only reaches the level of availability for introspective attention *after* this activity has been successfully bound into a phenomenal whole. Therefore, binding itself is transparent to the subject of experience.

At the end of chapter 2 I offered a speculative hypothesis: The causal role of presentational states is not realized by what we today call its "qualitative character," but by what today we call the homogeneity of this qualitative character. What really *enables* me to pick out redness introspectively₁ is the fact that it is homogeneous, and precisely this is the realization of its causal role. An important background assumption, therefore, is that subjectively experienced homogeneity is a globally available, phenomenal aspect of the success of integrational processes in the brain, leading to the activation of a coherent percept.

If, as is now empirically plausible for human beings, such binding processes make use of the synchronicity of neural responses in order to label certain perceived features as belonging to the same object, one can say the following: On the level of simple content, homogeneity is the conscious correlate of the *synchronicity* of the activity of the respective feature detectors and it is precisely through this synchronicity that this activity can at all be made *functionally* active on the level of the global model of the world, and thereby subjectively available to the system as a whole (see also Metzinger 1995e, p. 446*ff.*). From a neurodynamic perspective it is plausible to interpret synchronicity as a marker of the achievement of a stable state (Pollen 1999). A stable state is a state that can be characterized by playing *one* unified causal role for the system. And that is what it means for its components to become functionally active: What was a more or less disjunctive set of causal relations between microevents in the system now becomes *one* discrete set of causal relations, a single and currently realized causal role. Ultrasmoothness is an expression of functional coherence. In short, what I am experiencing when I introspectively attend to the homogeneity of red$_{31}$ in a consciously viewed color expanse is the *synchronicity* of the respective feature detectors in my brain contributing to the current sensory percept.

Neural Correlates of the Homogeneity of Simple Features

If we hold a red apple in our hand we can, while viewing it, attend to different features. We can attend to the phenomenal holism going along with the object as a whole (see section 3.2.4). We can also attend to the homogeneity of a certain color patch on the surface of this apple. What we attend to in both cases may be two different aspects of one and the same underlying physical process, on different levels in the representational hierarchy (on different levels of "phenomenal granularity," as it were). If the subjectively experienced apple in our hand were to be identical with a specific neural activation pattern in a Leibnizian sense (i.e., if it shared all its nonintensional and nonmodal properties with this pattern), then every region of this pattern of activity would have to instantiate a property of homogeneity for all the different types of presentational content integrated by this object. According to this analysis, "homogeneity" would be a property of a functionally active representational whole; not a structural property, but a higher-order *content property*.[18] One speculative possibility offered here for discussion is that the homogeneity might be a *vehicle* property as well (again using the helpful, but ultimately limited vehicle-content distinction) or rather, under an empirically more plausible theory of representation, a form of fully *embodied* phenomenal content. I will not explicitly argue for this thesis here, but simple sensory states may be precisely the place at which we first discover a domain-specific *identity* between phenomenal content and phenomenal vehicle. We are now for the first time able to identify the property under investigation with a physical property: The homogeneity of subjectively experienced qualities is the *temporal* homogeneity of correlated neural states in the human brain. In fact, there actually *is* a complex physical property that can be found in all spatiotemporal regions in question, namely, the synchronicity of neural activity. In other words, a systematic mapping of this aspect of phenomenal state space to a corresponding neural state space must be possible. That is, consciously experienced presentational content is not "infinitely" homogeneous; homogeneity does not go all the way down—rather it is a functional-representational phenomenon emerging at a certain level of complexity. Synchronicity can be experienced *as* homogeneity in precisely those cases in which an integration mechanism possesses a lower temporal resolution than the states of the system, which it unifies by transforming them into low-level representational atoms. The system then represents temporal coherence as

18. See Richardson and Muilenburg 1982, p. 177*f.* See also Lycan 1987, p. 85.

smoothness. On a higher level of representation, for example, on the level of attentional processing and attentional availability for introspection, the synchronous activity of feature detectors of a certain type must, therefore, by nomological necessity, appear as structureless and dense. The causal role of attentional availability is not realized through the presentational content itself, through the dimensional position in a certain region of phenomenal state space, but through the homogeneity of this qualitative character. This in turn may be defined as the "attentional impenetrability" of the corresponding region. We introspectively pick out redness by virtue of *homogeneity* and precisely this is the realization of the causal role. Therefore, or so my speculative hypothesis for simple phenomenal content says, homogeneity is a subjective correlate of the synchronicity of the activity of the feature detectors and—as is empirically plausible—it is precisely through this synchronization that this activity can become functionally active and subjectively available to introspective experience. A straightforward empirical prediction follows from my philosophically motivated hypothesis: If it is possible to experimentally disrupt the temporal coherence of the specific neural assembly underlying a currently active simple sensory percept, that is, if it is possible to eliminate *only* its synchronicity in a highly selective fashion, then it will immediately lose the functional property of attentional availability and its content will disappear from the subject's phenomenal reality altogether. However, in the color example, as in a blindsight patient, wavelength sensitivity should be preserved. It may still be available for *behavioral* control.

However, we have to keep in mind that this hypothesis is not only highly speculative but also makes a strong assumption about how the relevant level of binding is actually realized in the human brain—a set of assumptions, however, which are at present highly plausible (see sections 3.2.3 and 3.2.4). What, then, would be the *precise* physical correlate of the phenomenal target property, the physical property which realizes the causal role of making presentational content available for attention and helps to integrate it into the global model of the world? It is the *evenness* of the temporal response of a certain subset of feature detectors in the brain. This evenness can formally be expressed by the time constant in a neural algorithm. It is a *functional* kind of invariance. It is this temporal uniformity, a physical property of the minimally sufficient neural correlate of the respective form of presentational content, which appears as ultrasmoothness if read out by a higher-order representational mechanism (such as attention) with a lower temporal resolution power. This mechanism is not able to represent the temporal fine structure of neural processing, but only the fact that temporal uniformity as such has just been achieved. If we jump to the larger neural assembly constituting the perceptual object *as a whole*, the same temporal coherence may be read out as the holistic property of this perceptual object (*constraint 4*).

3.2.11   Adaptivity

In chapter 2 we used a third-person constraint, the "global availability" constraint, as a prime example of how the general concept of mental representation can be enriched and gradually refined toward a notion that includes *phenomenal* content. At the beginning of this chapter we saw that this constraint is actually only a special case of what I then introduced as the "globality constraint," *constraint 3*. Global availability, in its three differentiated variants of availability for guided attention, for cognition, and for action control, is simply the third-person equivalent of the *phenomenological* globality constraint, as it reappears on the functional level of description. In this chapter, *constraints 2 to 10* all had one crucial aspect in common: they were *phenomenological* constraints. This is to say that these constraints, to be imposed eventually on a descriptively plausible concept of phenomenal representation, were predominately developed by *initially* taking on a first-person stance. In always starting with a phenomenological constraint I attempted to take the target phenomenon—conscious experience—as seriously as possible in order to maximize phenomenological plausibility. I then made further attempts, from a third-person perspective, to semantically enrich those constraints on four different *subpersonal* levels of description. The representational, computational, functional, and neuroscientific levels of analysis served to add domain-specificity and experimentally tractable predictions to our working concept of conscious representation. The last and final constraint I now want to offer corresponds to my evolutionary background assumption introduced in chapter 2. If we want to understand how conscious experience, a phenomenal self, and a first-person perspective could be *acquired* in the course of millions of years of biological evolution, we must assume that our target phenomenon possesses a true teleofunctionalist description. Adaptivity—at least at first sight—is entirely a third-person, objective constraint. Prima facie, there seems to be no direct conscious correlate of the adaptivity or maladaptivity of specific mental representations. This is also the reason for the first, phenomenological level of analysis still lacking: Do we ever subjectively experience the evolutionary origin of our conscious mental states *as such*?

However, upon second thought, it is highly interesting to note that the structure of our phenomenally experienced *emotions* very often simply contains information about "the logic of survival" (Damasio 1999, p. 54*ff*.). They make this information globally available for flexible behavioral control, for cognition and memory, and for attentional processing. Emotional processing may not reveal to consciousness the evolutionary origin of our conscious mental states *as such*, but it constantly evaluates concrete (and in higher animals even cognitively simulated) situations. If analyzed as representational entities, emotions are special in that they are structured along an axis of valence. That is, one defining characteristic of emotions is that they possess a *normative* character; they represent the biological or social *value* of a certain state of affairs to the organism as a whole (see also section 6.2.8). This feature distinguishes them from all other conscious representata—although interestingly, the phenomenology of emotions tells us that they can endow perceptual and cognitive states with a certain "affective tone." The intentional, representational content of consciously experienced emotions typically is about the adaptivity of a certain situation, the adaptive value of another person or potential behavior, or a form of *self*-representation phenomenally portraying bioregulatory aspects of the organism's own bodily state. The function of emotions lies in reliably regulating and triggering survival-oriented patterns of behavior. In humans, emotions are felt stronger in groups (a simple fact pointing to their essential role in social cognition). Evolutionary pressure on the human mind has been a continuous environmental constraint since the origins of conscious minds on this planet, and emotions are very old states. The adaptive pressure on our ancestors has involved the same types of challenges again and again, over millions of years, and it is interesting to note how basic emotions are characterized by a high degree of cultural invariance in human beings. However, it is not only true that some conscious states may have *represented* survival value, it is also true that all of them must, on a functional level, have *possessed* survival value.

Introspectively, on the other hand, it is not at all obvious that in emotions "evolution speaks to us." It is also interesting to note what the notoriously most popular answer of most people is when being confronted with questions about the possibility of machine consciousness or selfhood: "But," goes the traditional answer, "*none* of these things is ever going to have genuine *emotions*!" This intellectual reflex is not only politically correct, it may actually contain an important insight: artificial systems as known today do not possess genuinely *embodied goal representations*, because they are not "evolutionarily grounded"—neither their hardware nor their software has developed from an evolutionary optimization process. They may have goal representations, but they are not directly reflected in body states and bodily self-awareness (see the final part of section 8.2).

If different forms of phenomenal content possess a biological proper function (Millikan 1989), then the functional profile of the vehicle of representation carrying this content has to causally explain the existence or maintenance of that content in a given population of organisms, under the pressure of natural selection. We would therefore have to treat functionally active phenomenal content as a *trait* that can be passed on from generation to generation, a trait that can come into existence as a result of natural variation and that can be maintained within a certain group of systems. A widely shared assumption today is that consciousness—including its social correlates (see section 6.3.3)—is an entirely biological phenomenon; its functional profile should be entirely comprised of biological proper functions. If this is true, we then can investigate how a certain type of conscious experience, say color vision or the global availability of information about the mental states of conspecifics, initially started to spread through a population. We can also investigate the etiology, the niche history, which in the past made organisms having this special kind of subjective, experiential content more successful. Was it that the remarkably uniform trichromatic red-green color vision of higher primates evolved for finding vitamin-rich ripe fruits, or did its true advantage consist rather in discovering tasty young red leaves against a background of green, mature foliage, because young leaves are easier to digest owing to lower fiber levels, and, in some species, richer in protein (Dominy and Lucas 2001)? Did social intelligence help them to successfully hunt down and defend themselves against much stronger, physically superior animals? However, we can also treat phenomenal content as a dispositional property and try to *predict* the future maintenance of this representational trait within a certain population. If, for instance, one looks at the history of phenomenal experience as a whole, we principally have to be able to tell an intelligible story about the developmental history of phenomenal representata. We need a convincing story about how it was that the possession of such "virtual organs" actually increased the overall fitness of biosystems and why, after the sufficient neurobiological conditions for its activation had appeared, they didn't simply get lost again by genetic drift. In other words, on a certain level of theory formation, the *history* of the phenomenon of consciousness will have to be included in the explanatory basis. Of course, it remains true that phenomenal content as such likely only locally supervenes, that is, in a given individual it is always determined by the internal and contemporaneous properties of its neural system. However, in order to anchor a story about phenomenal content in a broader story about *representational* (i.e., intentional) content we have to develop some suitable version of teleofunctionalism and look at the evolutionary history of our target phenomenon as well. The objective history of the concrete neural "vehicles," forming the minimally sufficient organic and functional correlates of certain types of phenomenal content, itself forms a highly relevant constraint on our concept of consciousness. Therefore, one has to ask: What *precisely* about conscious experience made it an advantage to possess this new trait in order to secure individual survival and that of one's own species? Why was it *adaptive* to develop a phenomenal model of reality and a subjective first-person perspective?

Adaptivity of Phenomenal Representata
An evolutionary psychology of consciousness will mainly analyze the possession of phenomenal states as the possession of new functional properties. They may be precisely those properties helping an organism to differentiate and optimize its behavioral profile on different time scales. Consciousness, first, is an instrument to generate successful behavior; like the nervous system itself it is a device that evolved for motor control and sensorimotor integration. Different forms of phenomenal content are answers to different prob-

lems which organisms were confronted with in the course of their evolution. Color vision solves another class of problems than the conscious experience of one's own emotion, because it makes another kind of information available for the flexible control of action. An especially useful way of illustrating this fact consists in describing phenomenal states as new *organs*, which are used to optimize sensorimotor integration of the information flow within a biosystem.

There are two kinds of organs: permanently realized organs like the liver or the heart, and "virtual organs." Virtual organs are coherent assemblies of functional properties, only *transiently* realized, typically by the central nervous system. Classes of integrated forms of phenomenal content are classes of virtual organs. The phenomenal book you are now holding in your phenomenal hands is one such virtual organ. You are functionally *embodying* it: its neural correlate is a part of *your* body. Currently, this part of your body works for you as an object emulator. A conscious color perception bound to a phenomenally experienced visual object is a transiently activated organ, whose function is to make certain invariances in the surface properties of objects globally available in a maximally reliable manner (*constraint 1*). The objects of visual experience frequently are objects within reach, objects in the immediate behavioral space of the organism. Information about remission and other surface properties of these objects, as soon as it is *conscious* information, is available for the flexible control of action, and also for the guidance of attention and further cognitive processing.

But not only simple presentata, phenomenal *representata* are virtual organs as well: Consciously experienced objects (*constraints 3, 4, and 7*) are distinct, functionally active parts of the organism currently making global stimulus properties and the high internal correlation strength, that is, the *coherence* of a perceptually given set of properties, globally available. In doing so, these object emulators form a functional cluster, that is, a causally dense, discrete subregion within the *global* functional cluster constituting the organism's world-model (see section 3.2.3). Phenomenal scene segmentation is a necessary precondition for making willfully initiated and differentiated reaching movements and spatial memory possible. It too is a dynamic property of the transient organ we call our world-model.

Phenomenal *simulations* (*constraint 8*), however, may themselves be interestingly interpreted as a new form of *behavior*. At least intended simulations are internal forms of behavior (*constraint 6*), enabling planning processes and being accompanied by the phenomenal experience of agency (see section 6.4.5). They allow an organism to *take possession* of its own internal cognitive activities, to conceive of itself as a cognitive agent for the first time (see section 6.4.4). Those neural correlates episodically activated in the course of such simulational processes are—as long as they exist—concrete organs, playing a distinct, modularized causal role in the system by making a coherent set of information, referring to specific types of possible situations or actions, globally available. The possession of a coherent, transparent world-model (*constraints 3 and 7*)—normal waking consciousness—as well can be analyzed as the transient possession of a certain *organ*. This organ provides an integrated and continuously updated representation of its behavioral space to the system. By being a transparent representation of behavioral space, possibly including an embedded self-representation (*constraint 6*), it represents *facticity* for the first time and thereby becomes the organism's world$_0$. Simultaneously, the content of this behavioral space is available for cognitive operations and attentional processing; for the first time it enables a creature to realize that it is *actually situated* (*constraints 2 and 3*).

Consciousness as an Informational-Computational Strategy

Phenomenal states are also *computational* organs, making information relevant to survival globally available within a window of presence. On a computational level of description, therefore, one way to individuate phenomenal states would be to investigate the type of information they integrate into the phenomenal level of representation in general. Concrete examples of this research program would have to be supplied by answers to questions of the following type: What kind of information is only made globally available by gustatory experience (i.e., by active gustatory presentata)? What kind of information is only made globally available by spontaneously occurring motor fantasies (i.e., by nonintended motor self-simulations)? What kind of information, on the other hand, is only made available by consciously experienced, abstract thought (i.e., by intended cognitive simulations)? What kind of information can in principle only be represented within a space, which, additionally, displays a perspectival organization, because it refers to dynamical subject-object relations (see section 6.5)? Given the set of constraints developed in this chapter, it is obviously possible to develop a whole catalogue of systematized research programs on the informational and computational level. However, I will not go deeper into this issue at this point.

Another possibility to more closely research the adaptive character of certain types of phenomenal processing would consist in modeling certain aspects of their computational role: How long are such states typically active? What mechanisms—on the output side of things—typically *access* phenomenally represented information in a special way? Language centers? The motor cortex? Those processes consolidating long-term memory? Under what conditions will this computational role again be "taken out" of the phenomenal world-model and handed over, as it were, to functionally isolated and therefore unconscious forms of processing? In stress situations? After successfully terminated learning phases? In deep sleep? An important general question in developing an evolutionary view of the computational neuroethology of phenomenal consciousness is: What precisely is the *metabolic price* for the organism of adopting a specific computational strategy?

Adaptivity as a Functional Property of Phenomenal States

As I have chosen to make teleofunctionalism one of the background assumptions in this book and not to offer a detailed argument of my own, I will have to be brief in this section. However, let me at least point to one specific and interesting set of theoretical issues. If we accept *constraint 11*, which has just been introduced, then, under this additional constraint, we can *reinterpret* the functional level of description offered for all of the preceding constraints. The adaptivity constraint demands that all the functional properties I have sketched when discussing those constraints on the respective level of description always have to possess a plausible reading as gradually acquired properties. That is, additional *teleofunctionalist* constraints must hold on this level of analysis. We then have to assume that such states do not simply have to be individuated by their causal role alone but that one has to introduce the general assumption that they always play this role *for* the system: they help the organism in pursuing its individual goals—or those of its ancestors. In the long run a specific new kind of phenomenal mental model (see next section), a specific class of phenomenal content going along with a specific new kind of neuronal "vehicle," can only survive if it supports the biological system in which it emerges in achieving survival and procreation. It is important to note how the ascription of goals has not necessarily to be accompanied by a realistic stance; it can be interpreted in an instrumentalistic fashion, as a preliminary research program (Dennett 1987b; a typical example of the general strategy is supplied by Gallup 1997). Our scope will then be widened by looking at the history of these causal properties, their relation to the selective pressure exerted by specific and changing environments onto the ancestors of the organism in question, and so on. It is interesting to note that such a teleofunctionalist analysis introduces for the first time a normative aspect into our investigation: Phenomenal representata are *good* representata if, and only if they successfully and reliably depict those causal properties of the interaction domain of an organism that were important for reproductive success.

Consciousness as a Stage of Neurobiological Evolution

On a short time scale, an interesting approach is to regard phenomenal experience as a level of organization in the individual brain (Revonsuo 2000a). However, when looking for psychophysical correlations between specific forms of phenomenal content and states of the nervous system, we are not only concerned with isolating the minimally sufficient neural correlates on which *synchronous* phenomenal properties of the systems supervene. We now have to look at much larger periods of time, because we focus on the evolutionary history of consciousness as a specific form of intentional content, most of all, however, on the genesis of the anatomical substrate. The basis set of properties for the explanatory relation is being temporally extended; in offering teleofunctionalist explanations of presently existing phenomenal properties we can now recur to *past* neural correlates and environments (for an example, see, e.g., Roth 2000). The relationship between types of phenomenal contents and sets of neurofunctional properties is not a simple, asymmetrical relationship of determination, as in relationships of local supervenience, but a truly explanatory relation. Any satisfactory explanation of consciousness, the phenomenal self, and the first-person perspective will have to do justice to the *history* of the target phenomenon on our planet.

We have now arrived at the end of our first set of constraints. These constraints will help us further to sharpen the conceptual tools developed in chapter 2 *and* in chapter 4 to assess some neurophenomenological case studies when we pursue the same goal from another angle. From what has been said so far, it must be obvious that this set of constraints is just a beginning. At most, it is a prelude to a much more systematic catalogue of analysanda and explananda for the future. Before moving on, however, it may be interesting to see how even this simple set of constraints can help us to formulate a number of very different notions of phenomenal consciousness. The target phenomenon and the conceptual tools related to it come in many different shades and variations. As I have already noted, phenomenal experience is such a subtle and highly complex phenomenon that it is impossible at this time to draw sharp and absolute boundary lines on the conceptual level. Exceptions to rules will always exist. Nevertheless, we are now able to describe our target phenomenon in a number of different strengths.

Minimal Consciousness
The minimal degree of constraint satisfaction in order to speak about the phenomenon of "appearance," the phenomenon of consciousness *at all*, involves *constraints 2* (presentationality), *3* (globality), and *7* (transparency). Conscious experience consists in the activation of a coherent and transparent world-model within a window of presence. On the level of phenomenal content this is simply equivalent to "the presence of a world." Please note how such a minimal version of conscious experience is not *subjective* experience in terms of being tied to a consciously experienced first-person perspective (it is only subjective in the very weak sense of being an internal model within an individual organism), and how this notion still is very simplistic (and probably empirically implausible), because it is completely *undifferentiated* in its representation of causality, space, and time. A system enjoying minimal consciousness as exclusively described by the conjunction of *constraints 2, 3*, and *7*, would be frozen in an eternal Now, and the world appearing to this organism would be devoid of all internal structure.

Differentiated Consciousness

If we add a mereological internal structure in terms of *constraint 4* (convolved holism), we allow for scene segmentation and the emergence of a complex situation. A nested hierarchy of contents now comes into existence. However, if we do not want to assume the unlikely case of "snapshot consciousness," of one single, presegmented scene being frozen into an eternal Now on the phenomenal level, we have to add *temporal* structure in terms of *constraint 5* (dynamicity). At this stage it is possible to have phenomenal experience as a dynamically evolving phenomenon on the level of content, to have an interrelated hierarchy of different contents that unfold over time and possess a dynamical structure. Differentiated consciousness, therefore, results from adding an internal context and a rich temporal structure.

Subjective Consciousness

This is the level at which consciousness begins to approach the complexity we find on the human level of organization, and the level at which it becomes a truly theoretically interesting phenomenon. By adding *constraint 6* (perspectivalness) to *constraints 2, 3, 4, 5, and 7*, we introduce a consciously experienced first-person perspective into phenomenal space. The space of experience is now always *centered* on an active self-representation. If we demand the satisfaction of this constraint, we pick out a much more interesting class of representational systems: the class of systems of which it can actually be said that they enjoy phenomenally *subjective* experience in the true sense of the word. Still, such systems—although a subjectively experienced flow of time involving duration and change against the background of a specious present would already be available for them—would not yet have an explicit phenomenal representation of past and future, of possible worlds, and possible selves.

Cognitive, Subjective Consciousness

If we add *constraint 8* (offline activation) and if we assume a spectrum ranging from transparent to opaque representations (see section 3.2.7), we arrive at a yet more specific class of phenomenal systems. These systems would be able to selectively engage in the activation of globally available representational structures *independently of current external input*, and given that these structures would exhibit a certain degree of opacity, the fact that they were now operating *with* representations would be globally available to them and could be integrated into their self-model. In other words, such systems could not only in principle engage in future planning, enjoy explicit, episodic memories, or start genuinely cognitive processes like the mental formation of concepts; these systems could for the first time represent themselves *as* representational systems on however minimal a scale. They would be thinkers of thoughts. Through the running of phenomenally opaque simulations, they would be able to finally escape naive realism, previously generated by a full satisfaction of the transparency constraint on all levels of content. For such systems, the difference between reality and appearance would for the first time become available for attention and metacognition. It may well be that human beings are the only biological creatures on our planet fulfilling this additional condition to any interesting degree.

Biological Consciousness

Could there be a class of systems that simultaneously satisfy *all* the constraints so far mentioned, while not stemming from a biological evolution? Put differently, are there phenomenal realities which are not *lived* realities? Could there be systems enjoying all the different kinds of increasingly rich phenomenal content just mentioned while not having the correct history?

Let me give two examples of such "historical incorrectness." The first is Donald Davidson's famous story of "the Swampman" (see Davidson 1987, p. 46*f.*). Lightning strikes a dead tree in a swamp while Davidson is standing nearby. His body is reduced to its elements, while entirely by coincidence (and out of different molecules) the tree is turned into his physical replica. This replica, the Swampman, is a physical and functional isomorph of Davidson; it moves, thinks, talks, and argues just as the original Donald Davidson did. Obviously, it has precisely the same kind of phenomenal experience as Donald Davidson, because phenomenal content locally supervenes on the brain properties of the replica. On the other hand, the *intentional* contents of Swampman's mental state are not the same—for instance, it has many false memories about its own history be they as conscious as they may. The active phenomenal representations in Swampman's brain would be strongly conscious in terms of the whole set of constraints listed so far, but they would *not* satisfy the adaptivity constraint, because these states would have the wrong kind of history. They did not originate from a process of millions of years of evolution. They emerged by an absurdly improbable coincidence; they came into existence by a miracle. And this is precisely why we cannot relate a deeper explanatory story about these dates: We cannot expand the explanatory set of base properties into the past, and include the history of the ancestors of the system—this system *has* no ancestors. It would enjoy a rich, differentiated cognitive version of conscious experience tied to a first-person perspective, but it would still be consciousness in a *weaker* sense, because it does not satisfy the adaptivity constraint holding for ordinary biological consciousness.

The second example of a conceptually weaker and "historically incorrect" form of phenomenal experience may be slightly more realistic. Imagine that the human race eventually creates *postbiotic* systems, complex information-processing systems that are neither fully artificial nor fully biological. These systems may be strongly conscious, *phenomenal* systems in terms of maximally satisfying *constraints 2 to 10* on all nonbiological levels of description. We frequently assume that the conceptual distinction between artificial and natural systems is an exclusive and exhaustive distinction. This assumption is false, because already today we have, for example, hybrid biorobots using organic hardware and semiartificial information-processing systems employing biomorphic architectures while being submitted to a quasi-evolutionary process of individual development and group evolution by the human scientists constructing them. Therefore, we might in the future even have systems meeting all the constraints just mentioned, while originating from a *quasi*-evolutionary dynamics generated, for instance, by researchers in the field of artificial life. Still, these systems would have satisfied the adaptivity constraint in an entirely different way than would human beings or any other conscious animals on this planet. They evolved from a second-order evolutionary process initiated by biological systems *already* conscious. From the way I have outlined the original set of conceptual constraints for the notion of a "conscious system," it would still follow that these postbiotic phenomenal systems would only be conscious in a slightly weaker sense than human beings, because human beings were necessary to trigger the second-level evolutionary process from which these beings were able to develop their own phenomenal dynamics. From a human perspective, just like Swampman, they might not possess the right kind of history to count as maximally conscious agents.

However, it is easy to imagine a postbiotic philosopher pointing out that all "historical incorrectness" arguments inevitably constitute a genetic fallacy and that actually a conscious system like itself, a system satisfying the adaptivity constraint in an entirely different, namely, a postbiological, way is conscious in a conceptually and theoretically much more *interesting* sense, simply because *its* kind of phenomenal experience emerged from a second-order evolution automatically *integrating* the human form of intentionality, which is, therefore, intrinsically more valuable. Second-order optimization is always better than first-order optimization. For instance, such a system could argue that the burden of primate emotions reflecting the ancient *primate* logic of survival is something that makes you *less* conscious from a theoretical point of view. If consciousness is what maximizes flexibility, our postbiotic philosopher could argue, animal emotions in all their cruelty and contingency certainly are something that makes you *less* flexible. Neither consciousness nor intelligence *must* be linked to the capacity to suffer or the fear of death. Artificial subjectivity is better than biological subjectivity because it satisfies the adaptivity constraint in a purer form than life and because it decreases the overall amount of suffering in the universe—or so our historically incorrect philosopher would argue.

Unfortunately, we have to get back to work. It should be obvious by now how the ten constraints offered in the previous sections (and more differentiated future versions, which will hopefully be developed soon), can serve to break down the naive folk-psychological notion of "consciousness" into more specific concepts, describing richer and more specific variants of the target phenomenon. Let us now try to briefly integrate the considerations just developed into a working concept for consciously experienced contents *in general*.

3.3 *Phenomenal* **Mental Models**

Let us now introduce a flexible working concept by saying that consciously experienced content is the content of "active phenomenal models." The concept of a "mental model" is the centerpiece of a theory of mental representation, which has been called the *Cambridge theory of mental representation* (alluding to Craik and Wittgenstein; see McGinn 1989a, p. 178). Kenneth Craik can count as the central founding father of this theory. In 1943 he published a book, titled *The Nature of Explanation*, which in its claims did not at all fit well with the behaviorist euphoria characterizing those days. In explaining cognitive and behavioral achievements Craik made strong assumptions with regard to internal structures. Long before the ascent of the computer as a technical-theoretical metaphor for the human mind, Craik already assumed that human beings transform environmental events into internal structures, then manipulate these structures in certain ways, only to then retransform them into external actions.[19] According to the theory, mental models of numbers or of propositions exist as well. Craik's early theory was not only inspired by neuroscientific knowledge, the intuitions behind it also strikingly resembled some of the ideas of today's dynamicist cognitive science—for instance, in thinking of representational dynamics as an ongoing process of *assembling* dynamical patterns from scratch.[20] The most prominent representative of the theory of mental models today is Philip Johnson-Laird, who originally worked in Cambridge as well. He continues to develop the concept of a mental model (e.g., see Johnson-Laird 1983, 1988, 1995) and differentiates between a number of different applications in different domains of theory formation.

For present purposes, it is not necessary to go deeper into the specific debate on mental models. Johnson-Laird himself formulates a basic thought with regard to *phenomenal* mental models dominated by sensory information:

19. In the words of Craik: "By a model we thus mean any physical or chemical system, which has a similar relation-structure to that of the process it imitates. By 'relation-structure' I do not mean some obscure nonphysical entity which attends the model, but the fact that it is a physical working model which works in the same way as the process it parallels, in the aspects under consideration at any moment. Thus, the model need not resemble the real object pictorially; Kelvin's tide predictor, which consists of a number of pulleys on levers, does not resemble a tide in appearance, but it works in the same way in certain essential respects—it combines oscillations of various frequencies so as to produce an oscillation, which closely resembles in amplitude at each moment the variation in tide-level at any place" (Craik 1943, p. 51*ff.*).

20. "It is likely then that the nervous system is in a fortunate position, as far as modeling physical processes is concerned, in that it has only to produce combinations of excited arcs, not physical objects; its 'answer' need only be a combination of consistent patterns of excitation—not a new object that is physically and chemically stable" (Craik 1943, p. 56).

Our phenomenological experience of the world is a triumph of natural selection. We seem to perceive the world directly, not a representation of it. Yet this phenomenology is illusory: what we perceive depends on both what is in the world and what is in our heads—on what evolution has "wired" into our nervous system and what we know as a result of experience. The limits of our models are the limits of our world. (Johnson-Laird 1989, p. 470*f*.)

Johnson-Laird also assumes that mental models can represent propositional attitudes, that they play an important role in syllogistic reasoning and in the construction and conservation of complex knowledge structures.[21] The mental model theory has predominantly been developed to understand reasoning or perception in a specific representational framework. It has never been developed toward a theory of phenomenal experience or of the first-person perspective as such. However, mental models possess a whole number of characteristics that are of interest for any naturalist theory of *phenomenal* representation. One of these properties is the way in which they can support a system in activating mental simulations, that is, in internal "dry runs" of virtual processes of representation. A second important property consists in mental models being conceived of as structures optimized in the course of evolution. Third, as we have seen, they may frequently be conceived of as transparent. Another highly relevant characteristic is presented by the idea of mental models being embedded in each other on ever higher, nested levels of content. Therefore, it is in principle—and in accordance with the very first thoughts of Craik quoted earlier—conceivable how comprehensive models of *reality as a whole* or even a unified *phenomenal model of the world* could emerge in this manner.

If we now enrich the concept of a mental model by applying the constraints developed in section 3.2, this will provide us with a working concept for a typical "vehicle" of phenomenal representation, which is phenomenologically plausible and open to future

---

21. The three essential characteristics of a mental model, in the words of Johnson-Laird, are:
    1. Its structure corresponds to the structure of the situation it represents.
    2. It can consist of elements corresponding only to perceptible entities, in which it may be realized as an image, perceptual or imaginary. Alternatively, it can contain elements corresponding to abstract notions; their significance depends crucially on the procedures for manipulating models.
    3. Unlike other proposed forms of representation, it does not contain variables. (Johnson-Laird 1989, p. 488)

One of the great strengths of the mental model theory is that it explains and predicts the way in which reasoning processes *break down*, and precisely in what sense it is to be expected that human beings frequently are not fully rational subjects. Mental models represent true state of affairs explicitly, but not what is false. Due to limitations of working memory, subsets of more complex models representing the logical landscape of a certain, more complicated task will typically drop out of focus, that is, of the phenomenal part of the cognitive self-model (see section 6.4.4). They are not available for action control and further cognitive processing anymore, which leads to irrational decisions and systematic errors in drawing conclusions. As soon as falsity is involved, it will frequently be impossible to keep all possible scenarios globally available in terms of simultaneous phenomenal simulations integrated into the self-model, particularly those that portray anything that is *not* true.

developments. *Phenomenal* mental models will be those mental models which are, functionally speaking, globally available for cognition, attention, and the immediate control of behavior. Any individual phenomenal model is in principle available for mental categorization and concept formation, because phenomenal modeling begins on the *object level*. Phenomenal mental models always are integrated complexes of more simple kinds of content (they are what I termed a phenomenal "holon" in Metzinger 1995c). Typically, phenomenal mental models are supramodal structures generated by an integration of different sensory information sources. If you now simultaneously feel and see the book in your hand, you experience it as a singular object in external reality, given to you by two different sense organs. The unified phenomenal model of the book still contains the information of being given in two different ways, through two causally distinct chains of events, because it results from an integration of visual and tactile presentational content.

Phenomenal mental models must be activated within a window of presence. This, of course, does not mean that we cannot consciously experience mental models of the past or of future situations. What it does mean is that all phenomenal mental models must be integrated into a single, overarching process of modeling of the *current present*. One way to flesh out *constraint 2* would be to assume the existence of a continuously active, dynamic model for time perception, namely, the mental model of the "Now," and then add the assumption that *phenomenal* mental models are precisely all those structures which are continuously embedded in the ongoing recurrent loop of this higher-order structure.

Third, the content of subjective experience is the content of a model of the world (*constraint 3*; see also Yates 1985). Therefore, phenomenal mental models will be all those structures currently embedded in a coherent, highest-order mental model of the world as a whole. Obviously, one of the most important projects is searching for a mechanism of integration, which can realize the "embedding relations" between different mental models, about which Johnson-Laird frequently speaks (this would be important both in satisfying the globality constraint as well as the convolved-holism constraint). Johnson-Laird himself postulates recursive functions, embedding models into each other (Johnson-Laird 1983, 1989).

Finally, there are two major components in which phenomenal mental models contribute to the emergence of the first-person perspective, satisfying the perspectivalness constraint (see also chapters 5, 6, and 7). First, one has to see that a system, obviously, can not only possess a phenomenal mental model of the world but can start modeling its *own* properties as well. Johnson-Laird, it must be clearly noted, has at a very early stage explicitly pointed to the possibility of a system possessing a model of the capabilities of its own operating system.[22] In short, it is now conceivable that a system not only activates a *mental* self-model but also—satisfying the constraints presently under discussion—a *phenomenal* self-model. However, modeling a self-world boundary in itself is not enough. As we shall see in section 6.5, a first-person perspective only emerges if an active process of *modeling ongoing subject-object relations* comes into existence. The theoretical core of any theory about the first-person perspective (or so I would claim) will have to be the phenomenal model of such subject-object relations. The existence of a self-model embedded in a world-model is a necessary precondition for this kind of mental content to be activated.

Nothing much has to be said about the criterion of transparency, as it is already implied in the original concept of a perceptually driven mental model. Let us simply recall that the large majority of phenomenal mental models will have to be transparent in the very sense introduced in section 3.2.7: the information that they are structures *modeling* a reality is not globally available for attentional processing. Interestingly, however, there is a subset of globally available structures, namely, exactly those structures forming the main focus of original research into mental models—that is, reasoning processes—which are constituted by *opaque* phenomenal mental models. Obviously, as these structures are analogue representations of linguistic or logical entities, they have to reintroduce a distinction between form and content on the level of their content. Therefore, they make the information that in this specific case the system is actually operating on *representational* structures available *to* the system.

We have now arrived at a more general working concept. It is highly flexible, because it is able to satisfy the conceptual, phenomenological, informational-computational, functional, and neurobiological constraints discussed in the last two chapters to differing degrees. Obviously, our working concept of a phenomenal mental model is not fully determined in its semantic content. However, the strength of its generality consists in its openness to data-driven semantic transformations and the fact that we can adapt it to different neurophenomenological domains. As I remarked at the outset, one's intention should not be to engage in scholastic a priori philosophizing or to maximize the analytical degree of precision at any price. On the contrary, one's goal should be to achieve as much as possible with minimal effort by developing a simple set of tools which can facilitate interdisciplinary *cooperation* between philosophy and the empirical mind sciences. However, from an argumentative and methodological point of view, even a simple tool kit must be thoroughly tested. In the next chapter, I submit it to an extensive reality test.

22. Cf. Johnson-Laird 1983, p. 477.

4 Neurophenomenological Case Studies I

4.1 Reality Testing: The Concept of a Phenomenal Model of Reality

Arguably, conscious experience is the most complex domain of scientific and philosophical inquiry in existence. Therefore, it would be methodologically naive to assume that we can arrive at narrowly circumscribed sets of necessary and sufficient conditions for the ascription of consciousness on one singular level of description in the near future. One possibility that always has to be kept in mind is the nonexistence of a singular conceptual "essence" of the phenomenon. What we may discover in the course of this century could be only loosely overlapping, but complex and domain-specific sets of *sufficient* conditions for the emergence of conscious experience, located on different levels of description, which resist full reductive explanations to a much higher degree than anybody would have expected given the current speed of data generation on the empirical frontier.

Consciousness may turn out to be a "cluster concept." The same could be true of the phenomenal self and the notion of a "first-person perspective." Large amounts of data do not yet constitute knowledge, and for particularly rich domains and target phenomena the conceptual landscape corresponding to those data may not only be a complicated logical terrain but also eventually turn out to be only decomposable into a rather messy bundle of subregions. It is therefore important to have an effective cure for what Daniel Dennett has identified as "philosopher's syndrome"—mistaking a failure of imagination for an insight into necessity (Dennett 1991, p. 401).

If we are interested in a better understanding of a complex domain of phenomena—especially in an initial, preparadigmatic phase of theory formation—an analysis of borderline cases and restricted situations has frequently proved to be of great heuristic value with regard to a general interpretation of the standard phenomenon. In our case, the standard phenomenon is constituted by what I have called "nonpathological waking states" of human beings. A closer inspection of borderline cases of complex phenomena reveals implicit assumptions, helps to dissolve intuitive fallacies, and makes conceptual deficits of existing theories clearly visible. This is the first goal I am pursuing in chapters 4 and 7 of this book.

At the beginning of chapter 3 I briefly introduced the concept of a phenomenal model of reality (see sections 3.2.1 and 3.2.3, and in particular the notions of *minimal, differentiated*, and *subjective* consciousness put forward at the end of section 3.2.11). The minimal degree of constraint satisfaction in order to speak about the phenomenon of "appearance," the phenomenon of consciousness *at all*, involves *constraints 2* (presentationality), *3* (globality), and *7* (transparency). Conscious experience then consists in the activation of a coherent and transparent world-model within a window of presence. A phenomenal model of reality is a phenomenal *world*-model and, as many researchers in diverging disciplines now agree, the content of subjective experience is the contents of a model of the

world (Yates 1985). Our conscious model of the world is a dynamical permanently changing multimodal map of that partition of reality accessible to beings like us. The higher its
richness in detail and the stronger its internal coherence, the more *real* it appears to the
subject of phenomenal experience.[1] An ordinary map, as we would find it hanging on the
wall in a classroom, is a two-dimensional, external analogue representatum. It does not
covary with the landscape that it represents, and it only uses a single "modality." The phenomenal model of the world, however, as internally generated by our brain, is a full-blown
spatial model, possessing a temporal dimension (it is a "4D-model"). While realizing an
extremely large number of dimensions for what I have called presentational content, it
also replicates a part of the relational structure of the world.[2] The most important feature
of this phenomenal model of reality is that it integrates information and *other* phenomenal mental models already active within the system into a global superstructure. In doing
so, it binds information from a multitude of functionally encapsulated modules into an
ever-changing, nested hierarchy of representational contents. These contents are subject
to a permanent updating by information flow from the sensory organs, and continuously
constrained by top-down influences, (as, e.g., represented by higher-order cognitive
operations).

The second main goal of this chapter is to develop a deeper understanding of what it
means that the drama of our subjective life unfolds within such a phenomenal model of
reality. And in order to do so it will be helpful to turn one's attention to pathological or
deviating phenomenal models of reality. Certainly some readers have found many of the
ideas presented in the preceding two chapters much too abstract and too detached from
the intricacy, subtlety, and phenomenological vividness of actual conscious experience.
Therefore, let us now finally look at some real-world situations.

---

1. This hypothesis can be supported by observing persons who progressively experience their reality as more
and more "unreal" or "dreamlike" (cf. the corresponding psychiatric term *derealization*). All of us know such
phenomenal states, if only in a less marked expression, namely, following traumatic experiences of different
kinds (after minor accidents, following psychological shocks). The richness of detail displayed by our phenomenal world-model episodically decreases, sometimes in a dramatic manner, and the world is suddenly characterized by a dreamlike or unreal quality. Typically, there is a phenomenal slow-motion effect: subjective time
flows much slower. On the other hand, during all those states in which the global processing capacity and the
general level or arousal in the brain is probably markedly elevated (e.g., in mania, during religious experiences,
in pharmacologically induced global states, or during so-called peak experiences), phenomenal reality can gain
a "superreal" quality. It is important to note how, on a purely phenomenological level of description, something
like a variable phenomenal aspect of "realness" does exist and that we have to do justice to it. It is something
that corresponds to the German philosophical concept of *Seinsgewißheit* ("certainty of being") the subjectively
experienced degree of "authenticity" of the world. My own hypothesis is that this global phenomenal property
is correlated with global information density and the degree of internal coherence of the world-model generated
by the brain.

2. Note that the *kinds* of relations themselves can differ greatly in nature: they can be spatial, causal, logical,
temporal relations, and so on.

4.2   Deviant Phenomenal Models of Reality

If one defines nonpathological waking consciousness as a norm, one immediately has a set of criteria for systematizing deviating phenomenal states. At any given point in time, one could describe any global phenomenal model of reality by its minimally sufficient neural correlate. One can also have a closer look at its functional and computational profile: Does this global type of state restrict the inner or outer repertoire of actions available to a person? Does it *extend* this repertoire? What kind of information is available for attention? Is there information that is now unavailable for cognition? Philosophers, on the other hand, might be interested in categorizing phenomenal models of the world according to their actual intentional or epistemic content: Is the general density of information higher or lower, compared to the normal state of consciousness? What sources of *knowledge*, non-conceptual or conceptual, nonpropositional or propositional, does this state of consciousness deprive a person of? Are there deviating global phenomenal state classes opening *new* sources of knowledge to human beings?

However, one can also analyze the structure of the phenomenal content itself, and that is what I will do here. In our present context, important questions are: Which phenomenal "qualities," that is, which types of presentational content, get lost? Do *new* forms of simple content emerge? Has the content of the phenomenal self changed? How is the global quality of consciousness "as such" (i.e., in terms of attentional or cognitive availability) distributed over the spectrum of representational content? Do new contents exist and what elements of the nonpathological model of reality can no longer be integrated into subjective experience? Other interesting features could be the gradient of transparency, availability for autobiographical memory, type-specific variance, shifts in time perception, and the degree of phenomenal centeredness. I will not pursue any of these projects in a systematic fashion here. All I have to offer is a cursory and incomplete collection of examples. I hope that even these brief examples can serve as illustrative evidence for my background hypothesis. It states that the content of subjective experience is the content of an integrated, global process of reality-modeling taking place in a virtual window of presence constructed by the human brain. This hypothesis is not as trivial as it sounds. It can integrate nonstandard cases of our target phenomenon in an *explanatory* manner. Common to all examples to be presented is the simple fact that neither folk psychology nor classical philosophical theories of mind can offer an adequate explanation for them.

4.2.1   Agnosia

Can you imagine how it would be to not be able to recognize your own face as your *own* face in a mirror? A circumscribed hemorrhage in a certain area of your brain could permanently and selectively change your model of reality in this way by putting you into such a highly specific, agnostic state.

"It must be me because I'm here!" That is what Emily said cautiously as she contemplated the face in the mirror before her. It had to be her; she had placed herself in front of the mirror, of her own free will, so it had to be her; who else could it be? And yet she could not recognize her face in the looking glass; it was a woman's face, all right, but whose? She did not think it was hers and she could not confirm it was hers since she could not bring her face back into her mind's eye. The face she was looking at did not conjure up anything specific in her mind. She could believe it was hers because of the circumstances: She had been brought by me into this room and asked to walk to the mirror and see who was there. The situation told her unequivocally that it could not be anyone else and she accepted my statement that, of course, it was her.

Yet, when I pressed "play" on the tape deck and let her hear an audiotape of her own voice, she immediately recognized it as hers. She had no difficulty recognizing her unique voice even if she could no longer recognize her unique face. This same disparity applied to everyone else's faces and voices. She could not recognize her husband's face, her children's faces, or the faces of other relatives, friends, and acquaintances. However, she could easily recognize their characteristic voices. (Damasio 1999, p. 162)

Patients suffering from agnosia frequently are not able to recognize stimuli previously known to them *as such*. Although perceptual functions are not disturbed and there exists no impairment of higher cognitive capacities—including speech processing[3]—the patient is not able to consciously grasp the meaning of the certain conscious percept (see, e.g., Teuber 1965; Damasio 1987). Frequent causes of such deficits are specific lesions of certain brain regions caused by strokes. For visual agnosia, these may be in bilateral lesions of those occipital temporal regions pertaining to the lower visual association areas in parts of Brodmann areas 18 and 19. Many different kinds of visual agnosia exist (Farah 1990), for instance, object agnosia (inability to name, recognize, and use objects), an agnosia for drawing (a deficit constituted by lacking the ability to recognize drawn objects), color agnosia (the association of colors with objects), achromatopsia (inability to discriminate different hues; see below), and visuospatial agnosia (inability for stereo vision and topographic concept formation). Corresponding to the specific loss of consciously experienced content one finds specific localizations of the lesions, including, for instance, areas 20, 21 left or right, the corpus callosum, bilateral damage to area 37, and regions responsible for speech processing.

A rare, but frequently remarked form of visual agnosia is *prosopagnosia* (Damasio, Damasio, and van Hoesen 1982; Tranel and Damasio 1985, 1988; see also Dennett 1991,

---

3. This is to say that we are not confronted here with *anomia*, that is, lacking the capacity for naming active phenomenal percepts. In terms of *constraint 1* we can say: There is no global impairment of cognitive availability.

chapter 11). Interestingly, prosopagnosia is very narrowly circumscribed on the phenomenological level of description. It consists in the inability to recognize faces, including, in some cases, one's *own* face reflected in a mirror. The visual world of prosopagnostic patients is unrestricted in all other aspects. However, functionally speaking, a certain stimulus on a highly specific, context-dependent level cannot be integrated with an internally existing knowledge structure. Patients with such lesions have no difficulty in recognizing their friends and relatives by their voices. They are, however, incapable of grasping the *identity* of persons (in some cases their own identity) by activating a certain, highly specific component of their phenomenal model of reality. A circumscribed defect on the "hardware level" presumably prevents certain capacities for integrating representational content (e.g., embedding a certain actual, visually given model of a specific person into an already existing memory structure) from being used. One consequence of this is that the internal model of the world is not only functionally restricted but also phenomenally deprived. A certain narrowly circumscribed aspect of conscious reality—namely, *personal identity as visually given*—disappears forever from the experiential world of the subject.

We had noted, purely by chance, as we used a long sequence of photographs to test her recognition of varied people, that upon looking at the photo of an unknown woman who had one upper tooth slightly darker than the rest, Emily ventured that she was looking at her daughter.
"Why do you think it is your daughter?" I remember asking her.
"Because I know Julie has a dark upper tooth," she said. "I bet it is her."
It wasn't Julie, of course, but the mistake was revealing of the strategy our intelligent Emily now had to rely on. Unable to recognize identity from global features and from sets of local features of the face, Emily seized upon any simple feature that could remind her of anything potentially related to any person she might be reasonably asked to recognize. The dark tooth evoked her daughter and on that basis she made an informed guess that it was indeed her daughter. (Damasio 1999, p. 164)

Of course, the actual phenomenology of this defect can be described in a more fine-grained manner and there are large variations across different cases. For instance, there can be a loss of face recognition without a loss of the ability to conjure up *images* of remembered faces (Weiskrantz 1997, p. 224). We can now slowly start to put our first tool kit to use. More precisely, there are phenomenal configurations in which the presentationality constraint and the globality constraint are not satisfied by the system relative to a specific kind of representational content (identities of persons via their faces as being present in the current visual environment), whereas the respective "top-down component" of the content in question is still available for offline activation (thereby satisfying *constraint 8*, because phenomenal *simulations* are still possible). Doubtless, neuropsychology will in the future arrive at a more precise separation of variables, even with regard to such narrowly circumscribed phenomenal losses as the one presented by prosopagnosia. In the end it may turn out not to be a unitary perceptual impairment, but composed of a number of separable processing stages. Explicit face recognition and face categorization are automatic and effortless, but it becomes increasingly obvious that different stages of face representation *without* conscious processing do exist (Khurana 2000). However, the phenomenon of prosopagnosia nicely demonstrates how, in embodied beings like ourselves, particular aspects of the conscious world-model can disappear in an extremely selective fashion. For instance, there are auditory agnosias like amusia (the selective inability to recognize and consciously experience tones and melodies; disturbances concerning rhythm and tempo) and sound agnosia (inability to recognize and consciously experience the meaning of non-verbal sounds). There is asterognosia (inability to consciously recognize objects by touching them, typically associated with lesions in Brodmann areas 5 and 7) and autotopagnosia (inability to identify and name body parts, associated with lesions in area 7, possibly also the left part of area 40). There are higher-order forms of agnosia involving an inability to become aware *of* an existing disease or deficit (anosognosia) and anosodiaphoria (inability to emotionally *react* to an existing disease or deficit). Interestingly, such higher-order deficits also concern conscious self-representation, and we therefore return to such cases in the second set of neurophenomenological case studies in chapter 7.

What is most striking about agnosia is the *selectivity* of the individual cases. This selectivity immediately leads to the conclusion that there must be a separate microfunctional module underlying the kind of phenomenal content in question. We can now recall our teleofunctionalist assumption and ask why this kind of conscious content—personal identity as given through visually perceived faces—was obviously so important for creatures like ourselves that a separate functional module for the computation of this kind of information developed, a module we can today selectively lose. Obviously, the kind of information made available by conscious face perception must have played an important role in social cognition. Face recognition may have taken the place of olfaction as the ecological niche of human beings became more and more complex (Adolphs 1999). In particular, face recognition presents a much better window onto the current emotional and motivational state of a conspecific than simply trying to extract the properties relevant to interacting with the other organism or person by attending to her smell. Members of one's own species are visually very similar, but their potential social behavior varies greatly. A specific mechanism for reading out the current mental state and the personal identity from the ongoing visual perception of a conspecific's face, therefore, would have been of particular importance as soon as the social reality surrounding the system became increasingly complex. Prosopagnosia, in severe cases of impaired mirror self-recognition, also destroys common phenomenological intuitions about the immediacy of self-awareness: As in primate research on mirror self-recognition, we now discover that this phenomenal feature is by no means a *necessary* feature of any sighted, self-conscious being, and that it has a historical dimension.[4] We gained this kind of phenomenal content for entirely contingent reasons in the history of our species, and, as individuals, we may lose it for entirely contingent reasons having to do with simple facts concerning our internal physical makeup. In many cases, what we lose may not even be the representational content itself, but only attentional availability.

Let us stay in the domain of visual agnosia. Visual agnosia is constituted by disorders in object representation and recognition. While the phenomenological landscape of this kind of deficit is more complicated than previously thought, a very coarse-grained categorization could differentiate associative agnosia and apperceptive agnosia. Generally speaking, associative agnosia consists in the inability to integrate an existing memory with an active phenomenal model in the visual domain. However, there are also cases of *apperceptive* agnosia in which no coherent visual model emerges on the level of conscious experience at all, despite the fact that all low-level visual processes are intact. The patient with apperceptive agnosia typically will have a fully intact visual field that is consciously perceived, while being unable to recognize objects. This kind of neurophenomenological state class is important, because for the visual domain it shows the possibility of a dissociation between the second and fourth constraint offered in chapter 3. It is possible to have a globally coherent global model of the visual world without satisfying the convolved holism constraint. It is important to note that intact visual functions include acuity, brightness discrimination, color perception, and spatial attention (see Vecera and Gilds 1997, p. 240 for an interesting discussion and a simulation study; see Vecera and Behrmann 1997 for a more detailed case study). Subjects suffering from apperceptive agnosia usually have suffered from a lack of oxygen supply to the brain, for instance, through carbon monoxide poisoning. They consciously see color (i.e., all presentational content is active because low-level visual processing is not affected), they have a coherent, integrated world-model (*constraint 3*), but visual information is not available for the control of action anymore. For instance, they are not able to match shapes or to copy visually presented shapes. On a functional level, they are not able to use gestalt grouping cues or figure-ground cues to organize their visual field (Vecera and

---

4. Povinelli (1993) offers the speculative hypothesis of orangutans possessing the capacity for recognizing themselves in a mirror, chimpanzees being in the process of losing this capacity (not all chimpanzees are able to learn to recognize themselves in a mirror), and of gorillas having already lost this capacity, although they still possess the underlying genetic information. It is important to note how a specific representational module adapted to a specific, for example, social, aspect of reality will always have a cost in terms of neural hardware and metabolic effort for the system, and may therefore disappear if it does not generate a reproductive advantage (Povinelli and Cant 1995). Only 50% of chimpanzees show convincing signs of mirror self-recognition (Gallup 1997), which may point to the fact that the species as a whole is in a historical phase of its evolution where it has a mental self-representation which is not yet or not anymore *attentionally available* in terms of a functionalist reading of the globality constraint.

Gilds 1997, p. 240). Their phenomenal visual world does not contain subglobal wholes, and for this reason it is not characterized by the phenomenon of convolved holism (*constraint 4*). In short, although low-level perceptual mechanisms work perfectly well, *preattentive* grouping is impaired in these patients, and therefore object-related information (information about the internal correlation strength holding between different sets of visually perceived features) cannot be made globally available for attention, cognition, and behavioral control. Therefore, the respective kind of phenomenal content simply drops out of their world. It is not part of their phenomenal reality-model anymore. Again, it is important to note how highly selective this deprivation of phenomenal content actually is; it pertains only to nonsatisfaction of the convolved holism constraint relative to the visual domain.

A large portion of the philosophical discussion of what I have called presentational content focuses on conscious color experience (for prominent recent examples, see Clark 2000; Tye 2000). Color experience, it turns out, can be selectively lost. In cerebral achromatopsia we find a selective vanishing of colors from the conscious model of the world (Zeki 1990). We have a situation in which localized brain lesions specifically destroy the conscious perception of color *without* necessarily being accompanied by object agnosia. However, here and in many other cases, the situation soon gets complicated. Cowey and Heywood report a phenomenally colorblind patient, M.S., who can still detect chromatic borders, perceive shape from color, and discriminate the direction in which a striped pattern moves when the determination of direction requires the viewer to "know" which stripes have a particular color (Cowey and Heywood 1997). Such cases of color blindness, despite an extended remaining capacity for wavelength processing, not only show, again, how a basic category of phenomenal content can selectively be deleted from the conscious model of the world, they also demonstrate to how great a degree *intentional* and *phenomenal* content active in the system can be separated. This particular patient, living in a colorless world, still processes information about wavelengths and successfully uses it in judgments about perceptually uncolored events. As Cowey and Heywood put it, their patient "does consciously perceive the visual events influenced by wave-length; only their color has disappeared. It is as if . . . conscious awareness of color has been deleted selectively, allowing the remainder to contribute normally to the generation of shape and motion now seen chiefly in shades of gray" (Cowey and Heywood 1997, p. 37). This example once again shows why the original Baars-Chalmers criterion of "global availability" had to be differentiated into cognitive, attentional, and behavioral availability. We seem to be presented with the possibility of wavelength-related information being *cognitively* available, namely, in terms of becoming the possible contents of judgments about perceptually uncolored events. However, this information is not *attentionally* available: The patient is not able to deliberately direct his attention to an integrated representation phenomenally displaying this information. Cowey and Heywood also asked if such a patient could covertly process phenomenal color (and not just wavelength). Could he, for instance, discriminate colors by forced-choice guessing as some prosopagnosic patients discriminate facial identity or familiarity?

It seems safe to say that color has disappeared from the phenomenal model of reality for this patient. However, the respective information obviously is available for the formation of judgments, for inferences, and for control of speech acts. It is as if it was still an element of the "cognitive" world-model and the behavioral space causally linked to it. It would therefore be highly interesting to investigate if there are corresponding inconsistencies on the level of phenomenal *self*-representation. In any case, the central philosophical lesson is obvious: Nonconscious presentational content can be functionally active in systems like ourselves while not being introspectively$_1$, that is, attentionally, available, while at the same time retaining a considerable portion of its causal role, including determining the content of other, higher-order phenomenal states simultaneously active (cf. the case study given in section 4.2.4 below). Another conceptual insight flowing naturally from these first examples is that the concept of a "boundary" for our phenomenal model of the world will have to be used with the greatest care in the future. Agnosia is important, because it can serve to shatter philosophical intuitions about what the *primitives* of phenomenal space actually are.

Typically, philosophers speak about sounds, smells, tactile experiences, and colors as if they were the obvious atoms of experience. As it turns out, the conscious perception of motion is another "primitive" aspect of our conscious model of reality which can be selectively lost (Zihl, Cramon, and Mai 1983; Zihl, Cramon, Mai, and Schmid 1991). This situation can be described by an isolated nonsatisfaction of *constraint 5*, the dynamicity constraint, in the visuospatial domain. It shows how the perception of motion in space, on the phenomenal level, is another good candidate for such a primitive. Yet the phenomenological constraints imposed on any theory of consciousness that can be derived from motion blindness are more counterintuitive. Who would have thought that the conscious experience of motion *as such* could disappear from one's reality, leaving everything else as it was before? What we learn from the study of agnosia is that the deep structure of phenomenal experience frequently differs greatly from what we would intuitively take it to be from a first-person perspective. What is a dissociable element, and what is not, cannot be determined by introspection and conceptual analysis alone. It also shows that we may have to depart from the notion of an "atom of subjective experience" altogether: What the "border of consciousness" or the "lowest level" is depends on the readout mechanisms and may vary greatly across different instances.

4.2.2   Neglect

Neglect is a selective impairment of attention, that is, the intended direction of conscious experience.[5] Patients with related syndromes are not able to direct their attention to certain sections of their mental model of reality, which in turn has perceptual, motor, and motivational consequences (Mesulam 1987; Bisiach and Vallar 1988). One of the best-known forms, hemineglect, appears after unilateral lesions or tumors, predominantly in the right hemisphere. Some of these patients are no longer capable of reading the left half of a sentence or of phenomenally representing events in the left half of their perceptual field. They may omit details on the left side when copying pictures or ignore people approaching them from the left (Driver and Mattingley 1998, p. 17; for a brief philosophical discussion, see Tye 1995). Many of them do not wash or dress the left side of their body; some of the male patients stop shaving the left side of their face (see also section 7.2.1). Let us turn to a modern classic. Oliver Sacks describes a patient suffering from the consequences of a right hemispheric lesion:

She sometimes complains to the nurses that they have not put dessert or coffee on her tray. When they say, "But, Mrs S., it is right there, on the left," she seems not to understand what they say, and does not look to the left. If her head is gently turned, so that the dessert comes into sight, in the preserved right half of her visual field, she says, "Oh, there is it—it wasn't there before." She has totally lost the idea of "left," with regard to both the world and her own body. Sometimes she complains that her portions are too small, but this is because she only eats from the right half of the plate—it does not occur to her that it has a left half as well. Sometimes, she will put on lipstick, and make up the right half of her face, leaving the left half completely neglected: it is almost impossible to treat these things, because her attention cannot be drawn to them ("hemi-inattention"—see Battersby 1956) and she has no conception that they are wrong. She knows it intellectually, and can understand, and laugh; but it is impossible for her to know it directly. (Sacks 1998, p. 77)

What this patient has lost is not the *concept* of "left" or a capacity to activate certain quasi-propositional mental models or specific linguistic functions. All presentational aspects of the left side of her conscious model of the world, of her perceptual field, seem to be lost— the left side simply *is* not present, it *is* not a part of reality for these patients. What is it

---

5. Interestingly, when introducing a concept of focal attention in terms of directed awareness, the question automatically poses itself, if something like *nonfocal*, nondirected, global attention is a meaningful phenomenological concept. *Vigilance,* as a generalized dimension of "brightness" for the global model of reality, might present us with such a general background parameter. Unspecific arousal or activation, the most important neural substrate for which will be the reticular formation, could be a functional and phenomenal analogue of the pure "signaling aspect" of presentational content discussed in chapter 2. If this speculation points in the right direction, there may be an application of *constraint 9*—the representation of intensities—to *constraint 3*—the emergence of a global coherent state. Is it phenomenologically plausible to form the concept of a comprehensive, *global intensity* of the way we experience reality as a whole in this sense? If so, the global quality so described could be termed *Bewusstseinshelligkeit*, or brightness of consciousness as a whole.

that the patient has lost—the visual model of reality *as such* or a special kind of *access* that ties it to her individual, conscious point of view? Empirical data show that a considerable amount of unconscious processing actually takes place for neglected stimuli. In many situations, figure-ground segmentation, visual completion, the mental representation of object identity, and even the "meaning," that is, the semantic properties of such object representations, are actually achieved (for a review, see Driver and Mattingley 1998). Therefore, once again, we could just be confronted with a problem pertaining to attentional availability. Is hemineglect an impairment of attention management? On the representational level of analysis, what is lacking may be the possibility of constructing an explicit model of a certain *subject-object relation* as currently holding, a model of the patient herself *as currently attending to a certain visual object* (see section 6.5 for the notion of a "phenomenal model of the intentionality relation," or PMIR). We may have to wait until our second tool kit is in place before we can adequately describe the missing kind of content.

However, the underlying representation of egocentric space as such seems to be intact, because, after all, how could you ignore one half of things *systematically* (see Grush 2000, p. 76*ff.*) without having functional access to at least an unconscious model of the world as a whole? As Driver and Vuilleumier (2001, p. 75) point out, neglect demonstrates an interesting neurophenomenological asymmetry when compared to the deficits discussed in the previous section, namely, that losing "spatial awareness, as in neglect, invariably leads to losses of, say, 'colour awareness' or 'face awareness' in the affected locations for neglected stimuli there. But losing colour or face awareness (as in cerebral achromatopsia or prosopagnosia) apparently never leads to losses of spatial awareness for the affected colours or faces." Interestingly, the above-mentioned patient can compensate for the loss of phenomenally available content by using implicit, structural features of her reality-model.

If her portions seem too small, she will swivel to the right, keeping her eyes to the right, until the previously missed half now comes into view; she will eat this, or rather half of this, and feel less hungry than before. But if she is still hungry, or if she thinks on the matter, and realizes that she may have perceived only half of the missing half, she will make a second rotation till the remaining quarter comes into view, and, in turn, bisect this yet again. This usually suffices—after all, she has now eaten seven-eighths of the portion—but she may, if she is feeling particularly hungry or obsessive, make a third turn, and secure another sixteenth of her portion (leaving, of course, the remaining sixteenth, the left sixteenth, on her plate). "It's absurd," she says, "I feel like Zeno's arrow—I never get there. It may look funny, but under the circumstances what else can I do." (Sacks 1998, p. 78)

Patients with hemi-inattention or left hemifield extinction do not consciously experience the obvious discontinuity of available mental content from the first-person perspective.

But how obvious is it really? Do you now, as you read this, consciously experience the dramatic incompleteness of your own visual model of the world? Do you consciously experience the expanse of nothingness behind your head? Many great philosophers of consciousness have traditionally, upon reaching this point, emphasized that an absence of information is not the same as information about an absence (see, e.g., Franz Brentano ([1874] 1973, p. 165*f*.) and Daniel Dennett: ". . . the absence of representation is not the same as the representation of absence. And the representation of presence is not the same as the presence of representation" [Dennett 1991, p. 359].) Patricia Churchland has pointed out how all of us naively assume visual consciousness as being unconstrained by any spatial limitations (P.S. Churchland 1988, p. 289); if we are visually conscious, as it were, we are simply visually conscious. We do not *explicitly* experience the nonrepresented part of the world behind our backs as a phenomenal hole in our subjective model of reality. Today, however, it has become technologically possible to actually create explicit, circumscribed holes in the visual world-model. Artificial scotomata can be created by the suppression of certain regions in visual cortex, using transcranial magnetic stimulation (see Kamitami and Shimojo 1999; Morgan 1999). But for us this is not normally the case, because the absence of information is only *implicitly* represented. As to many neglect patients, the world appears to us as complete in spite of this obvious deficit.

The pathological example described above is philosophically interesting, because, first, it shows that an extended spatial restriction of the phenomenal model of the world does not have to be accompanied by an awareness of this deficit (Bisiach 1988; see also section 7.2.1). Cases of neglect and unawareness of deficit throw an important light on *constraint 7*, the transparency constraint, for the phenomenal model of reality. Large portions of this model may disappear by becoming functionally unavailable; they just drop out of existence, and in such situations the initiation of introspective, exploratory, or self-investigative behavior becomes very difficult for systems like us—because, as it were, it assumes an impossible situation. How could a system search for something that is not part of *reality*, not even part of a *possible* reality? A further interesting point to note is how neglect patients are not even able to generate phenomenal *simulations*, that is, intended representations of possible states of affairs or possible perceptual experiences in the neglected portion of their world. Therefore, unilateral neglect cannot be simply reduced to a disorder confined to the "input-output machinery of the organism" (Bisiach and Luzzatti 1978, p. 132). Non–stimulus-correlated aspects of the representational architecture must play a role. At this point we also see in which way the phenomenon of experiential transparency and the philosophical concept of *epistemic transparency* are linked: Descartes's fundamental assumption that I cannot be wrong about the contents of my own mind proves to be empirically false. It is an important feature of human conscious experience (and a central constraint for any plausible philosophical theory) that unnoticed and unnotice*able* losses of mental content can, in principle, occur at any time. This is made especially obvious by neuropsychological case studies on anosognosia, to which we return in chapter 7 (for some brief case studies demonstrating the coexistence of epistemic opacity and phenomenal transparency, see sections 7.2.1, 7.2.2, 7.2.3.3, and 7.2.4 in particular). As the phenomenon of neglect demonstrates, not only our minds as such but also our phenomenal model of the world is characterized by a considerable degree of vulnerability (Bisiach, Luzzatti, and Perani 1979, p. 615*f.*).

It is important to note that neither neglect nor attention is a unitary theoretical entity. As Halligan and Marshall (1998) note, most studies on neglect have investigated the remaining capacities of patients after the deficit, but only rarely has the question concerning visual experience *itself* been posed. As pointed out above, an important phenomenological feature of neglect is the absence of a deliberate ignoring of the left side of space by the patient. This part of space is simply nonexistent. In standard situations, the same is also true for the simulational space available to the patient suffering from neglect. Usually, those patients are not even able to *imagine* this part of the world (Bisiach and Luzzatti 1978; see also Bisiach, Capitani, Luzzatti, and Perani 1981). Neglected information does not satisfy *constraint 8*, the offline activation constraint. One interesting proposal is that neglect might be a loss of important parts of the functional architecture subserving what I have here formulated as the constraint of convolved holism (*constraint 4*, section 3.2.4), namely, in terms of a decoupling of binding processes. The critical binding processes are realized by those attentional mechanisms necessary to integrate global and local processing mechanisms, coactivating global and local forms of representational content. Neglected phenomenal content not only loses global availability in terms of disappearing from perception and not being an element of the current window of presence anymore but there is also no chance for offline activation (*constraint 8*): it disappears from memory, as well as from the space of intended imagination. If Halligan and Marshall's functional hypothesis points in the right direction, patients suffering from neglect may not have any difficulties with generating a global representation of the world as such, but in *returning* from focused, local processing to the initial global representation forming the background model. They lose world zero. Because they lack the capacity to integrate over a scene and because an explicit phenomenal experience of *absence*, as mentioned above, is impossible, the focus of attention cannot return from the right-sided half of the world. Therefore the patient may have lost the capacity to let his visual attention wander without losing the implicit system of spatial relationships forming the basis for an ordered generation of globally available phenomenal content (Halligan and Marshall, p. 377). What the study of neglect seems to show is that, for systems like ourselves, an explicit, globally available representation of absence may be necessary to make losses of all kinds *functionally* available to us.

In the beginning I claimed that what the neglect patient loses is not the *concept* of "left." However, in some cases of severe neglect it may even be the case that the information about the left side of the patient's world is not only unavailable for conscious high-level attention but that it has become truly *cognitively* unavailable for spatial reasoning (see also Bisiach et al. 1979, p. 614). One aspect of cognitive unavailability is that no *expectations* can be formed anymore, precluding the search for certain classes of solutions. Another is that the patient suddenly finds herself under pressure to develop *alternative* hypotheses. Consider the following excerpt from a popular case study of Ramachandran, in which he confronted a neglect patient with a mirror which in principle could have helped her to "overcome" her neglect by enabling her to generate reaching movements toward her neglected field.

Ellen looked in the mirror and blinked, curious about what we were up to. It ought to have been obvious to her that it was a mirror since it had a wooden frame and dust on its surface, but to be absolutely sure, I asked, "What is this I am holding?" (Remember I was behind the mirror, holding it.)

She replied without hesitating, "A mirror."

I asked her to describe her eyeglasses, lipstick and clothing while looking straight into the mirror. She did so with no trouble. On receiving a cue, one of my students standing on Ellen's left side held out a pen so that it was well within the reach of her good right hand but entirely within the neglected left visual field. (This turned out to be about eight inches below and to the left of her nose.) Ellen could see my student's arm as well as the pen clearly in the mirror, as there was no intent to deceive her about the presence of a mirror.

"Do you see the pen?"

"Yes."

"Okay, please reach out and grab it and write your name on this pad of paper I've placed in your lap."

Imagine my astonishment when Ellen lifted her right hand and without hesitation went straight for the mirror and began banging on it repeatedly. She literally clawed at it for about twenty seconds and said, obviously frustrated, "It's not in my reach."

When I repeated the same process ten minutes later, she said, "It's behind the mirror," and reached around and began groping with my belt buckle.

A little later she even tried peeking over the edge of the mirror to look for the pen. (Ramachandran and Blakeslee 1998, p. 123)

Ramachandran dubbed this phenomenon "mirror agnosia"[6] or, in honor of Lewis Carroll, "the looking glass syndrome." What has been lost in this severe case of neglect is the knowledge that a certain segment of the visually perceived mirror image is a *representa-*

---

6. Cf. Ramachandran, Altschuler, and Hillyer 1997; but see also Binkofski, Buccino, Dohle, Seitz, and Freund 1999 for a more in-depth discussion of mirror agnosia and mirror ataxia. Mirror agnosia constitutes a specific clinical syndrome, and neither hemineglect nor right parietal lesions are necessary conditions for this phenomenon to appear.

tion of external reality, and the ability to draw inferences from this knowledge. Remember that the fact of the experimenter holding a mirror was cognitively available for the patient (as demonstrated in the course of the interview). It was also behaviorally available (as proved by her description of eyeglasses, lipstick, and clothing while looking straight into the mirror). It is exclusively a specific kind of spatial reasoning—the inference that, since the reflection is on the right and since it is a representation, its causative object should be on the left, which is not possible for this patient. The left portion of the spatial model of reality is not available as a frame of reference for the mental simulation that would be necessary to create a phenomenal mental model of the causal *relationship* between object and mirror image. The model of the object-as-reflected-in-the-mirror therefore becomes "hypertransparent" and collapses into a nonveridical model of the object as is, on the right-hand side. What makes this specific phenomenal configuration theoretically interesting is that it shows how certain obvious facts about the external world can become cognitively unavailable to a human subject of experience in a maximally strict and quite absolute sense, because the frame of reference necessary to carry out the relevant forms of globally available, that is, *conscious*, simulations has disappeared. A whole space of possibilities are lost.

It is, of course, an intriguing question whether there are, even for "normal" persons, simple facts—for instance, about the relationship between mind and body or about the nature of the phenomenal self—which are in principle cognitively unavailable, because our brains are not able to supply the *frame of reference* that would be necessary to carry out the cognitive simulations leading to a convincing theoretical solution. Are we, like Ellen, suffering from a theoretical version of the looking glass syndrome? Some philosophers have argued that the puzzle of conscious experience itself belongs to this class of problems (McGinn 1989b, 1991). Are we cognitively closed, because we are autoepistemically closed? As I pointed out in chapter 2 "autoepistemic closure" does not necessarily refer to *cognitive* closure in terms of the unavailability of *theoretical*, propositionally structured self-knowledge. And we have in the past solved many theoretical puzzles (e.g., in theoretical physics) in ways that were unexpected and probably *unexpectable* by anyone—simply by employing mathematical and other intersubjective, nonphenomenal media of representation. A community of neglect patients could certainly find out about the nature of mirrors and the representational roots of the looking glass syndrome. The simple fact that we can turn the neurophenomenology of neglect into a philosophical metaphor, while all the time *understanding* that this is only a metaphor, itself shows that we are not in this way restricted. The truth in the skeptic's argument may rather lie in the possibility that a good theory about the relationship between mind and body or about the nature of the phenomenal self may not only come to us in an entirely unexpected way but also in a form that makes its truth phenomenally impossible, unimaginable *for us*, and therefore counterintuitive. But the same is true of pathological configurations like severe visual neglect. Their phenomenological correlates seem to be an impossibility; they also are unimaginable *for us*, and therefore counterintuitive. Yet nobody would argue on these grounds that a convincing theory of neglect could not be developed.

4.2.3 Blindsight

All those deviant models of the world in which you find clearly marked dissociations between functional properties and available phenomenal content are of particular theoretical interest. They help to isolate or "screen off" conscious from unconscious processing. All those configurations are highly instructive in which the functional analysis of the system, in particular the amount of internally available information that can be used in sustaining output, remains largely unchanged while losses or restructurization within the phenomenal model of reality take place. Blindsight is probably the most prominent example of such a situation.[7]

Patients with a lesion in the geniculostriatal projection of visual cortex report a scotoma, an experiential "blind spot" in the corresponding region of the visual field. This region of their subjective world, as it were, possesses a *phenomenal hole*: there are no visual contents of consciousness referring to this region of the world. However, some of these patients, as has been experimentally shown in a large variety of different setups, are able to carry out complex visual information processing. They are surprisingly successful in "guessing" the presence or absence of target objects within this scotoma, and of discriminating colors and patterns presented within this region. According to first-person reports given by such patients, all these capacities exist without being paralleled by any phenomenal, visual experience. Perhaps this is also where this deficit got its name. In fact, in earlier times optic agnosia was called *Seelenblindheit*, "blindness of the soul," in the German literature. Blindsight is an even more specific case. In blindsight we can not only clearly observe how a very narrowly circumscribed portion of phenomenal content drops out of the patient's model of reality but it also becomes strikingly evident how this results in a corresponding damage to the "soul," the conscious self: for a very limited part of their reality blindsight patients are not able to experience themselves as a *self-in-the-act-of-knowing* (see section 6.5.2 and Damasio 1999). Some subjects describe their subjective

---

7. See, for instance, Bodis-Wollner 1977; Cowey 1979; Marcel 1983, Pöppel, Held, and Frost 1973; Stoerig, Hubner, and Pöppel 1985; Weiskrantz, Warrington, Sander, and Marshall 1974; Weiskrantz 1986; Werth 1983; Zihl 1980. Because blindsight is now a well-known phenomenon, I refrain from a more detailed description or an extensive review of the literature here. A beautiful overview of the development of this field of research, including a comprehensive review of the relevant literature, is given by Weiskrantz 1997.

experience while living through successful experiments of "nonphenomenal seeing" as guessing; others even protest against being asked to utter a lie by the experimenter (Weiskrantz 1988, p. 188*ff.*).

> Many subjects, and no doubt experimenters alike, find it embarrassing to pretend that they can guess about something they cannot *see*. Indeed, some subjects refuse point blank. I have had a patient tell me, when encouraged to guess in the same way that one would back a horse, "I do not gamble!" Another patient insisted, "my brain is just not set up for *guessing!*" Another said "I *know* it's 50-50 of one or the other. But I can't guess." (Weiskrantz 1997, p. 66)

Neuropsychological research into the phenomenon of blindsight generated a breakthrough in interdisciplinary communication, for example, by finally drawing the attention of large numbers of the best philosophers of mind to the wealth of theoretically relevant material produced by other disciplines.[8] The phenomenon itself has now also been documented in other modalities, for instance, in the tactile domain of presentational content ("blind touch" or "numb sense"; cf. Paillard, Michel, and Stelmach 1983; Rossetti, Rode, and Boisson 1995; Rossetti 2001, p. 151*ff.*), in the auditory domain ("deaf hearing"; Michel and Peronnet 1980), and possibly the olfactory domain ("blind smell"; e.g., Sobel, Prabhakaran, Hartley, Desmond, Glover, Sullivan, and Gabrieli 1999). However, a conceptually convincing interpretation of the empirical material presents a number of difficulties. Although the phenomenon generates a number of phenomenological constraints that reliably destroy the myth of simple and self-revealing phenomenology, it is possible to overlook the strong functional constraints that make the target phenomenon arise in the first place (e.g., a narrow range of possible targets, cueing by the experimenter in a very specific experimental setup, smaller subsets of sensory targets as in the typical perceptual situation for conscious vision, and the volitional unavailability of the actual response demanded by the experimental task for ordinary volition). There is a real danger in jumping to specific fallacies. To give an example, the existence of residual and unconscious visual processing in blindsight patients does not imply that this is the *normal* kind of processing from which an isolated epiphenomenon, the phenomenal content as such, arises. For instance, one inherent mistake in Ned Block's conceptual distinction between access consciousness and phenomenal consciousness (see Block 1995) is that blindsight might not be a deficit in an isolated form of conscious processing, in *phenomenal* consciousness, at all, but might also result from a functional deficit (or a combination of such deficits) in *unconscious* processing. In

---

8. Philosophical discussions of the phenomenon of blindsight can be found in Mellor 1977–8, 1980; Block 1995; Dennett 1991; Schumacher 1998; Tye 1994; in particular, Tye 1995, 209*ff.* (appendix).

particular, it is difficult to assess phenomenologically reports about "hunches" or diffuse emotional contents of awareness preceding a successful act of guessing performed by these patients.

It seems safe to say that extensive perceptual processing is going on in the relevant regions, while no form of presentational content is activated or bound into a phenomenally available multimodal object. I have analyzed the functional role of presentational content as indexical: it *points* to a portion of reality, demonstrating that this is now here. It is this aspect of the functional profile of presentational content that has disappeared in the scotoma. A first interesting conclusion about the function of phenomenal experience can be derived from the simple fact that forced-choice paradigms had to be used to make perceptual information functionally explicit, as it were. Global availability of information is not only needed to *initiate* intended acts of guiding attention or cognitive processing but also to be able to initiate external motor behavior (e.g., speech behavior, button pushing, etc.) directed at target objects only perceived within the phenomenal blind spot. The space of consciousness is the space of selective action. However, any serious neurophenomenological assessment will also have to introduce "hunches," as a new class of phenomenal content induced in these situations.

L. W.:   G., you remember the experiment that you did in the PET scan—with the moving bar? Can you tell me what sort of experience you had in that situation? What did you sense? What was it like?

G. Y.:   You don't actually ever sense anything or see anything. That's where we get the mix-up, because the sensation I get I try to put into words. It's more an awareness but you don't *see* it [his emphasis].

L. W.:   Did you know what it was?

G. Y.:   The shape or the motion?

L. W.:   The shape.

G. Y.:   No. Roughly, but not sure about that.

L. W.:   The direction?

G. Y.:   Yes.

L. W.:   What kind of words do you think you have to use? Is it like anything in your normal visual field?

G. Y.:   The nearest I ever get, and it is not a fair comparison, is waving your hand in front of your eyes when they are closed. You are kind of aware that something has happened but you don't quite see it. You know something has moved. But that isn't a fair comparison to make.

L. W.:   The nearest you can get is the sense of something happening, but you don't know what it is?

G. Y.:   Yes.

L. W.:   Anything else you can think of to describe it?

G. Y.:   No, because it is a sense that I haven't got, if that makes sense. If you said something to try to describe sight to a blind man, we don't have the words to do it because he does not have the receptors or the reception, and that is the same with me. I mean I can't describe something I don't understand myself. (Weiskrantz 1997, p. 144*f.*)

First, reports of this kind support the idea presented above that motion, if we actually concede that something like phenomenal "primitives" do exist, is a good candidate: it seems to be possible to experience motion *as such*. Blindsight patients are particularly sensitive to moving stimuli and are able to discriminate directions in their scotomata, but this sensitivity is dependent on the complexity of stimuli. The choice of stimulus could be decisive, and it is plausible to assume that motion processing is impaired in the scotoma (Azzopardi and Cowey 2001). Searching for further characteristics, it seems safe to say that the phenomenal content expressed in this ineffable "hunch" accords with the notion of presentational content introduced in chapter 2 in that (a) it is clearly stimulus-correlated, and (b) it satisfies the presentationality constraint because it is experienced as a diffuse event that is happening *now*. However, this diffuse, ineffable motion perception is only part of the patient's world-model in a weaker sense, because it is only available to attention and behavioral control, but as can be concluded from the autophenomenological report just cited it is clearly *cognitively unavailable*. As is clear from the last passage quoted, neither mental nor linguistic concept formation works with regard to the kind of phenomenal content in question. At this stage we already have two new kinds of phenomenal content: the ineffable experience of motion and the explicit conscious experience of *cognitive* unavailability. Michael Tye (2000, p. 63) has pointed out that as there is no complete, unified representation of the visual field in blindsight, the content in the respective part of the visual field does not make a direct difference in *beliefs*, as can be seen from the fact that blindsight subjects do not believe in their own guesses. However, we also see how blindsight subjects indirectly form *higher-order* beliefs, namely, about the actual cognitive availability (i.e., the "believability") of their own conscious experience. Reinhard Werth (1998) interestingly differentiates between the blind field and the "guessing field." If a stimulus is presented in the guessing field, a phenomenal correlate emerges: for example, the diffuse experience of a "hunch." According to Werth (1998, p. 98), the stimulus is truly unconscious if the subject himself is dependent on seeing the results of the experiments in order to find out if his brain has actually reacted to the stimulus, for example, when triggering the button-pushing movement. A stimulus is conscious if the subject himself can independently *predict* the outcome of the experiment.[9]

Let us briefly return to the standard example, the conscious experience of color. As it turns out, there even exists wavelength sensitivity in the blind field of subjects (but only for light, not for surfaces). Since conscious color is the paradigmatic example of a quale for philosophers, this discovery is indeed fascinating—although, again, we must be careful not to jump to conclusions. As I pointed out in chapter 2, the perception of the unconscious sensitivity to wavelength information within the region corresponding to the scotoma precisely follows the sensitivity curve of conscious vision. If in a coarse-grained forced-choice situation, simply having to guess whether a particular stimulus is red or blue, blindsight subjects can even successfully apply identity criteria to their unconscious presentational content currently active (Stoerig and Cowey 1992; for further reference, see Weiskrantz 1997, p. 136). The argument presented in section 2.4 predicts that such successful blind wavelength discrimination would not work on the level of maximum determinacy, on the level of just noticeable differences in hue, as, for instance, in a forced-choice experiment asking the subject if a stimulus was red_{31} or red_{32}. What is intriguing is how the blindsighted subject understands and *uses* color predicates that she previously acquired in a normal, nonpathological context. The application of these predicates to unconscious presentational states and their content, triggered by wavelength information originating in the retina, is *parasitic* on the ordinary use: a congenitally colorblind person, even if functionally possessing the same shape of the sensitivity curve, could not participate in experiments of this type because she could not understand what the task would

9. As Werth points out, precise experimental procedures could be designed to find out to what degree of precision a subject can predict the result of the experiment without possessing the same information that every other person needs to know the outcome of the experiment. Werth calls such an experiment a "second-order experiment." He proposes to define conscious perception by this correct *prediction* of a result of the perceptual experiment (Werth 1998, p. 99). The guessing field also is a field of sensation, a region covarying with the content of phenomenal experience. If this is true there should be a gradient of consciousness, a gradient of covariance and availability, which can be determined by second-order experiments. An interesting parallel here is Dennett's claim about conscious robots. If robots are analyzed as *second-order intentional systems*, as systems taking the intentional stance (Dennett 1987a, b) toward themselves as well, one may treat a robot as conscious in precisely all those situations where it has itself become the best available source of information in terms of predicting its own future behavior (Dennett 1995). Werth also defines *third-order* experiments, which allow us to compare conscious experiences with each other by demarcating different forms of content and possibly determining their identity. Different "degrees of phenomenality" for mental content can be assigned by making a subject assess its own success without having to evaluate the first-order experiment, in which he would have had to register his reactions and correlate them with the presence of, for example, light stimuli. Such experiments could show that patients have special access to their own capacity for discovering light stimuli. The reliability of this access could be measured by investigating the reliability of the subject's assessment of his own capacity to discover stimuli. It may be possible to define this reliability as the degree to which the discovery of a light stimulus itself is conscious (Werth 1998, p. 102; but see also 1983, p. 85*ff.*). Typically we will discover that this capacity is maximally expressed in the blind as well as in the sighted field, while being very low within the "guessing field."

be about. However, our new tool kit allows us to describe nicely what the available data of wavelength sensitivity in blindsight safely demonstrate, namely, how we can apply the difference between *mental* and *phenomenal* presentation, which was introduced at the end of chapter 2. Judged by its functional, relational profile it seems to be precisely the same kind of stimulus-correlated information presented as a simple feature that is active in the blind field. However, this active, mental presentatum is not globally available, because it has not been embedded in a coherent global state and it is not experienced as being *present*, because it is not an element of the contents currently displayed within the window of presence opened by the brain (*constraints 3 and 2*). Consequently, some other sub-constraints are not satisfied as well. The higher-order properties of variation among a single dimension of intensity (like brightness), and the grainless, homogeneous quality generated by representational atomicity (see sections 3.2.9 and 3.2.10) are not instanti-ated, as wavelength information presented within the scotoma is not embedded in higher-order holistic objects (like, e.g., a multimodal percept), it is not bound into a convolved hierarchy of phenomenal wholes (*constraint 4*) and, obviously, it is not integrated into the phenomenal first-person perspective (*constraint 6*). From the patient's perspective, in a nonexperimental situation this information simply is not part of his world.

On the functional level of description an important question is whether blindsight might only be a *quantitatively* weakened form of normal seeing. This aspect has been under dis-cussion for quite some time, for instance, as the possibility of a gradual transition of blind guessing to what Weiskrantz once called "non-veridical seeing" (Weiskrantz 1988, p. 189). There have also been attempts to investigate the phenomenon of artificially induced blind-sight in normal observers (e.g., Kolb and Braun, 1995; but see also Azzopardi and Cowey 1998). One obvious lesson from blindsight studies is that presentational content can be functionally or causally active on a nonphenomenal processing stage, thereby influencing the content of explicit phenomenal representata (for an example, see Schmidt 2000). From a teleofunctionalist perspective, we can clearly see the advantage that conscious presen-tational content has as long as it is integrated into objects and the overall world-model. Only as a *conscious* content can it form the direct target of goal-directed actions, and con-tribute to the content of deliberately intended phenomenal simulations, for example, as in planning or remembering. Call this the "principle of selectivity and flexibility."

More than one hypothetical mechanism could be responsible for the generation of a "phe-nomenal hole" in the world-model of these patients. Whereas in principle there seem to be two routes of explanation—insufficient intensities or durations concerning the "signal aspect" of an active mental presentatum versus a circumscribed deficit in a discrete metarep-resentational function, integrating it into the global model of the world—the simple fact of some blindsight patients being able to discriminate color information (Pöppel 1987; Stoerig and Cowey 1990; Dennett 1991, p. 326*ff.*) seems to point to the second possibility.

It is interesting to note how dissociative configurations like blindsight are also theoretically relevant, because they demonstrate counterintuitive configurations within the functional deep structure of conscious experience—as can be seen from our difficulties in *interpreting* the phenomenological material. Is "unconscious color vision" conceptually possible? Can there be something that truly counts as *hue* without attentional availability? Our intuitions are always shaped by those phenomenal models of reality we have lived through in the course of our own lives. However, as Daniel Dennett has pointed out, any theory that makes real progress is bound to be initially counterintuitive (Dennett 1987b, p. 6). In a metaphorical way we can interpret phenomenal models of reality as nonpublic theories about the structure of reality, internally generated by brains with the help of nonpropositional formats of representation. A phenomenal model of reality is good if it helps its possessor survive. Thought experiments are a special kind of phenomenal model. Thought experiments in philosophy of mind are important heuristic tools. They are *good* tools if they prepare lasting insights into what is necessary and what is possible. However, they are particularly dangerous in philosophy of mind, because many of their implicit premises are usually gained through unreflected introspection in combination with a constant danger of conflating the difference between *phenomenal* and *logical* possibility (see section 2.3 and Wilkes 1988a, chapter 1). Wavelength sensitivity in blindsight nicely demonstrates this underlying principle.

In some sense, blindsighters seem to be seeing people who—in a narrowly confined domain—do not represent themselves *as* seeing people on the level of phenomenal experience. In other words, there may be an implicit *self-representational* component to the phenomenon. Let us therefore look at the bizarre mirror image to blindsight: Anton's syndrome (Anton 1898, 1899; Benson and Greenberg 1969).[10] Patients who suddenly become completely blind due to a lesion in the visual cortex in some cases keep insisting on still being visually aware. While claiming to be seeing persons, they bump into furniture and show all the other signs of functional blindness. Still, they act as if the phenomenal disappearance of all visually given aspects of reality is not phenomenally available to them. For instance, when pressed by questions concerning their environment, they produce false, but consistent confabulations. They tell stories about nonexisting phenomenal worlds, which they seem to believe themselves, while denying any functional deficit with regard to their ability to see.

On a philosophical level, Anton's syndrome, as a classic example of unawareness of visual impairment (see McGlynn and Schacter 1989 and section 7.2.1), presents another

---

10. An early report of what may have been Anton's syndrome can be found in the second paragraph of Seneca's fiftieth letter to Lucilius (*Ad Lucilium Epistulae Morales*). Seneca briefly mentions Harpaste, a demented female slave who suddenly stopped seeing "without knowing that she is blind." Harpaste always asked to be allowed to leave the house, because she thought it was "dark."

striking counterexample of the Cartesian notion of epistemic transparency or any strong transcendentalist notion of phenomenal self-consciousness. I still vividly remember one heated debate at an interdisciplinary conference in Germany a number of years ago, at which a philosopher insisted, in the presence of eminent neuropsychologists, that Anton's syndrome does not exist because a priori it *cannot* exist. Anton's syndrome shows how truthful reports about the current contents about one's own self-consciousness can be dramatically wrong. It would also be an ideal starting point for philosophical debates concerning the incorrigibility of mentalistic self-ascriptions (e.g., see Rorty 1965, 1970). To take a more recent example, the empirical possibility of Anton's syndrome also seems to considerably weaken the intuitive force behind David Chalmers's *reductio* against the absent-qualia argument. In his fading-qualia thought experiment, Chalmers assumes that absent qualia are empirically possible in order to show how absurd consequences would follow (Chalmers 1995, p. 313*ff*.). Of course, patients suffering from Anton's syndrome are not functional isomorphs. Still, their judgments are so bizarre that their sheer existence refutes many traditional theories of mind. On a functional construal of judgment, can there be rational, sentient beings that suffer from such a strong dissociation between consciousness and cognition that they are so systematically out of touch with their own conscious experience? Well, in a domain-specific way restricted to internal self-representation and metacognition, there are. Anton's syndrome gives us good empirical reasons to believe that self-consciousness actually *is* "such an ill-behaved phenomenon" (Chalmers 1995, p. 317). Patients suffering from Anton's syndrome certainly possess the appropriate conceptual sophistication to form rational judgments about their current visual experience. The empirical material interestingly shows us that they simply do not, and this, in all its domain-specificity, is an important and valuable constraint for philosophical theories of consciousness. For instance, it also directs our attention to the fact that a convincing neurophenomenological interpretation of state classes like Anton's syndrome will eventually have to involve the concept of phenomenal self-representation. (Therefore, we need to return to these issues in chapter 7.) Obviously, the patient suffering from Anton's syndrome has false beliefs about *himself*, because he is suffering from something that might be called "recursive neglect" or a "meta-agnosia." Of course, anosognosia, the lack of phenomenally represented insight into an existing deficit, as frequently caused by nondominant parietal lesions, is not agnosia in the *strict* sense of the term (Damasio 1987). However, these patients, again, have two "holes" in their phenomenal model of reality: the first hole completely covers the visual modality as a whole, while the second hole is a hole *referring* to this hole.

Here is my own interpretation: A dramatic loss of globally available information is, for some time, not available for the computational processes generating and updating the phenomenal *model of the self*, in turn forcing the patient to generate massive confabulations in order to preserve the overall coherence of his behavior and his phenomenal model of reality. My own hypothesis for Anton's syndrome goes as follows: In human brains, a loss of the visual phenomenal model of the world does not immediately and automatically lead to an *updating* of the phenomenal self-model (see chapter 6). What those patients, truthfully, refer to in their autophenomenological reports is the current content of their phenomenal self-model. For a certain period, functional blindness can exist simultaneously with a transparent model of the self as a seeing, visually unimpaired person. Young and de Haan quote a description of Raney and Nielsen (Young and de Haan 1993, p. 69; Raney and Nielsen 1942, p. 151) of a female patient who, after a whole year of apparent lack of insight into her own severe problem regarding conscious vision, exclaimed, "My God, I am blind! Just to think, I have lost my eyesight!" The real explanatory question posed by Anton's syndrome, therefore, is: Why is the updating process of the phenomenal self-model delayed in these cases, and what are the functional mechanisms underlying this process?

Possibly the phenomenological material allows us to draw some general conclusions about the coupling strength of underlying functional modules or, more specifically, the time windows in which they operate. Antonio Damasio (1999, p. 269) has offered an interesting partial explanation. It has been noted that patients' eyes, although not contributing to phenomenal vision anymore, are still capable of version toward objects and do remain capable of *focusing* on them. That is, a certain part of the perceptual machinery is still issuing motor commands that lead to adjustments and changes in the eyes' position. It is plausible to assume that this residual, ongoing adjustment behavior produces a continuous *feedback*, for instance, as Damasio points out, to structures such as the superior colliculi and the parietal cortices. Now please note how, obviously, this feedback information about actual ongoing motor adjustments will contribute to the unconscious portion of the patient's self-model. In other words, the self-model *is* updated in a way that resembles the process of continuous motor feedback generated by true conscious vision. For a short period of time, or so I would propose, it may be possible that the ongoing successful matching of an issued motor command to the eyeballs and the feedback received *suppresses* an updating of the phenomenal partition of the self-model. If this speculative hypothesis points in the right direction, we may derive a general principle from it. I will term it the "principle of phenomenal self-reference": In truthful autophenomenological reports, subjects and patients alike *can* never report about anything other than the content of their currently active self-model. That is, to arrive at a deeper understanding of the phenomenal "hunches" of blindsight patients or the bizarre confabulations characterizing Anton's syndrome, we will have to extend our discussion to *self-representational* deficits. This will be done in chapter 7.

So far we have been considering phenomenally restricted models of reality. However, a large number of *hypertrophied* reality-models exist. Hypertrophied models of reality are global representational states accompanied by an extension or expansion of the phenomenal world, which usually is uncontrollable and undesirable.

4.2.4 Hallucinations

As all philosophers know, one important criterion of mental health, for beings like ourselves, is the ratio of phenomenal representation to phenomenal simulation. A number of deviant states of consciousness are caused by the system being internally flooded by a large number of mental *simulata*, which in turn leads to a drastic shift in the overall ratio between representation and simulation within the phenomenal model of the world. In extreme cases, the system may lose touch with world zero, the reference model for reality. Frequently, the phenomenal simulata generated in such states are pure artifacts. They are not elements of an epistemic or cognitive process, that is, they do not fulfill a function *for* the system. There is no true teleofunctionalist description of such phenomenal situations (i.e., the adaptivity constraint is not satisfied). On the other hand, it is complex hallucinations and delusions in particular which can be interestingly interpreted as a desperate attempt of a system confronted with uncontrollable internal signal sources and representational artifacts to keep on trying to maximize global coherence. Human brains sacrifice veridicality to maintain coherence, even in this situation, by constructing an internal model of reality that is as consistent and rich in content as possible (i.e., one that still satisfies the globality constraint).

An important conceptual distinction is that between complex hallucinations and pseudohallucinations. Complex hallucinations are untranscendable. They are transparent in the sense of *constraint 4*—the fact that hallucinatory content is just (nonveridical) *misrepresentational* content not available to the subject of experience. Of course, from an epistemological point of view, this is an interesting commonality between hallucinations and many phenomenal states in general. Pseudohallucinations, however, are opaque. Not only is their content recognized as nonveridical (i.e., at most expressing a *possibility*, but not an actuality) but also the underlying dynamics of phenomenal experience is suddenly recognized as *merely* misrepresentational, as simulational. However, in some cases phenomenal opacity seems to be related to the obvious features of the hallucinatory percepts themselves (i.e., to the discovery of vehicle properties), whereas in other cases the fact that the phenomenal content given through the hallucinatory process must have an entirely internal cause is *cognitively available* (i.e., an inference) rather than simply attentionally available. A first conclusion is that there are different kinds of phenomenal opacity, and that the phenomenology of hallucination may be an excellent road toward gaining a deeper understanding of the transparency constraint introduced in chapter 3.

Before penetrating deeper into a neurophenomenological analysis, lets us briefly look at two examples given by Vilayanur Ramachandran. Both examples are from patients suffering from Charles-Bonnet syndrome (Bonnet 1769; Fluornoy 1902; de Morsier 1967). Patients with Charles-Bonnet syndrome experience spontaneous visual hallucinations that possess many of the vivid features of normal seeing, cannot be voluntarily controlled, and are, as opposed to imagery, projected into external phenomenal space. Of course, spontaneous visual experience in the absence of specific sensory input is of great interest in narrowing down the minimally sufficient correlate for conscious vision (for a new categorization of hallucinations, see ffytche, Howard, Brammer, David, Woodroff, and Williams 1998; ffytche 2000; for a review of clinical and neurobiological details, see Manford and Andermann 1998). To give an example, as would be expected from the phenomenology, the correlates of color hallucinations are closer to a true color *percept* than to that of color imagery. Specific hallucinations of color, faces, textures, and objects clearly correlate with cerebral activity in ventral extrastriate visual cortex, while reflecting the respective functional specializations of these regions. Neuroimaging of visual awareness in normal and in abnormal states is providing us with a flood of data concerning the neural correlates for specific contents, as well as global background states, complementing electrophysiological, neuropsychological, and neurophenomenological observations (Rees 2001). Let us now look at two examples:

"Well, the most extraordinary thing is that I see images inside the scotoma," Nancy said, sitting in the same chair that Larry had occupied earlier. "I see them dozens of times a day, not continuously, but at different times lasting several seconds each time."
"What do you see? "
"Cartoons."
"What?"
"Cartoons."
"What do you mean by cartoons? You mean Mickey Mouse?"
"On some occasions I see Disney cartoons. But most commonly not. Mostly what I see is just people and animals and objects. But these are always line drawings, filled in with uniform color-like comic books. It is most amusing. They remind me of Roy Lichtenstein drawings."
"What else can you tell me? Do they move?"
"No. They are absolutely stationary. The other thing is that my cartoons have no depth, no shading, no curvature."
So that is what she meant when she said they were like comic books.
"Are they familiar people or are they people you have never seen?" I asked.
"They can be either," Nancy said. "I never know what is coming next." (Ramachandran and Blakeslee 1998, p. 108*ff.*)

A number of insights can immediately be derived from this report. First, Charles-Bonnet–type hallucinations do not satisfy the dynamicity constraint. Second, it is highly interesting to note that they are frequently characterized by a "cartoon-like" character. What is a cartoon? As Paul Churchland has pointed out (see P. M. Churchland 1995,

p. 29 *ff.*), connectionist models of the vector coding of faces give us a formally precise idea of average or *prototypical* representations, and also of exaggerated or *hyperbolic* representations of faces. In short, if in the facial vector space there is a central "average point" in terms of a prototypical face, it is possible to draw a line through any particular face that might become activated and *extend* this line beyond the veridical face representation. All faces on that extended line segment in representational state space will be caricatures of this face. This is true because the caricature or cartoon face is, as Churchland puts it, "less ambiguous than" the face of the represented person *itself*. Its distance to any alternative real faces in vector space is farther away; therefore the cartoon, again in the words of Paul Churchland, "couldn't be anybody but him" (P. M. Churchland 1995, p. 32 *ff.*). This may be the computational-neurophenomenological reason why, across all cultures, it is not only children who like cartoons. Cartoons correspond to a distinct representational possibility in our space of conscious experience, minimizing ambiguity beyond veridicality, and they let us experience this possibility without us understanding *what* it actually is we find appealing or funny about these images. Cartoon-like hallucinatory contents, therefore, could result from an excessive process of *ambiguity minimization* taking place in some regions of the hallucinating brain. It may be interesting to note that several authors question the rarity of Charles-Bonnet syndrome and suggest that many patients do not report their hallucinations out of fear of being considered insane (Teunisse, Cruysberg, Hoefnagels, Verbeek and Zitman 1996, p. 794). Such fear in patients may be completely misguided; prototypical images of animals, plant archetypes, or "cartoon-like" forms of excessive ambiguity reduction may be the result of quite similar features of the functional architecture underlying the generation of a benign form of phenomenal content in hallucinations. As a matter of fact, one reason why I have chosen Charles-Bonnet syndrome as an example out of a large class of very different phenomenal states (for a good overview, see Siegel and West 1975; for a recent review, cf. Manford and Andermann 1998) is that patients suffering from Charles-Bonnet syndrome have complex visual hallucinations that cannot be explained by the presence of a psychiatric disorder. They are the patients least likely to be distressed by their own hallucinations (Manford and Andermann 1998, p. 1820). Most patients hallucinate with their eyes open, typically perceiving humans, animals, plants, and different inanimate objects. Seventy-seven percent of patients with Charles-Bonnet syndrome could not detect any personal relevance in their hallucinations as opposed to their nocturnal dreams (Teunisse et al. 1996, p. 796). In contrast to Anton's syndrome, in which patients often experience disorientation accompanied by attentional and memory deficits (Schultz and Melzack 1991, p. 819; Hecaen and Albert 1978), Charles-Bonnet patients definitely show no impairment of any other mental abilities. Charles-Bonnet–type visual hallucinations are fully opaque. At any point in time the patient *knows* that he is hallucinating.

Obviously, here percepts are missing characteristic features and are simply super-imposed on, but not semantically embedded in, the phenomenal model of external reality and this fact deprives them of transparency. Their *phenomenal* content is integrated into the current model of reality, whereas their *intentional* content is not. This is what immediately makes them opaque phenomenal states: the subjective experience is like looking at autonomous images, and not one of immediate contact with an external reality. Let us look at a second example of Charles-Bonnet syndrome.

"Back in the hospital, colors used to be a lot more vivid," Larry said.
   "What did you see?" I asked.
   "I saw animals and cars and boats, you know. I saw dogs and elephants and all kind of things."
   "You can still see them?"
   "Oh, yeah, I see them right now here in the room."
   "You are seeing them now as we speak?"
   "Oh, yeah!" said Larry.
   I was intrigued. "Larry, you said that when you see them ordinarily, they tend to cover other objects in the room. But right now you are looking straight at me. It is not like you see something covering me now, right?"
   "As I look at you, there is a monkey sitting on your lap," Larry announced.
   "A monkey?"
   "Yes, right here, on your lap."
   I thought he was joking. "Tell me how you know you are hallucinating."
   "I don't know. But it's unlikely that there would be a professor here with a monkey sitting in his lap, so I think that probably there isn't one." He smiled cheerfully. "But it looks extremely vivid and real." I must have looked shocked, for Larry continued, "For one thing they fade after a few seconds or minutes, so I know they are not real. And even though the image sometimes blends quite well into the rest of the scene around it, like the monkey on your lap," he continued, "I realize that it is highly improbable and usually don't tell people about it." Speechless, I glanced down at my lap while Larry just smiled. "Also there is something odd about the images—they often look too good to be true. The colors are vibrant, extra-ordinarily vivid, and the images actually look more real than real objects, if you see what I mean." . . .
   "Are the images you see, like this monkey in my lap, things you've seen before in your life or can the hallucinations be completely new?"
   Larry thought a moment and said, "I think they can be completely new images, but how can that be? I always thought that hallucinations were limited to things you have already seen elsewhere in your life. But then lots of times the images are rather ordinary. Sometimes, when I am looking for my shoes in the morning, the whole floor is suddenly covered with shoes. It is hard to find my own shoes! More often the visions come and go, as if they have a life of their own, even though they are unconnected to what I am doing or thinking about at the time." (Ramachandran and Blakeslee 1998, p. 107 *ff*.)

In these spontaneous visual hallucinations we see homogeneous, presentational content, sometimes characterized by unusual intensities. This is a common feature of the phenomenology of sensory hallucinations. Colors, for instance, can be seen in a degree of brightness that would inevitably have blinded the person had it been triggered by the sheer intensity of an external physical stimulus impinging on the retina. However, hallucinations clearly fulfill the criterion of offline activation, as their causal history originates entirely within the system. Different researchers looking at the neural substrate of different kinds of hallucinations have found that it is closer to that of a true (nonhallucinated) percept than to that of imagery, that is, the physical correlate of an *intended* simulation in which the subject is aware of the causal history of his current conscious experience actually originating from an internal source. For instance, Dominic ffytche and colleagues (ffytche et al. 1998), using functional magnetic resonance imaging (fMRI), studied patients with Charles-Bonnet syndrome and found that hallucinations of color, faces, textures, and objects correlate with brain activity in ventral extrastriate visual cortex, and that the content of such hallucinations reflects the functional specializations of the region. They found that visual hallucinations are "difficult to dismiss as vivid imagery experiences as they differ qualitatively . . . and, at least for color hallucinations, neurobiologically" (p. 740).

Szechtmann and colleagues (Szechtmann, Woody, Bowers, and Nahmias 1998) investigated auditory hallucinations. Just like visual hallucinations, auditory hallucinations share the property of causally originating solely within the brain with cases of intended, conscious simulations as in imaginal hearing. On the other hand, they share the property of being "tagged" as originating from the external world with ordinary conscious auditory perception on the level of phenomenal content. Thomas Dierks and colleagues identified a region in the right anterior cingulate gyrus (Brodmann area 32) by positron emission tomography (PET) that was activated both in real hearing and in hallucinatory hearing, but not when the subjects merely *imagined* having a hearing experience. They have identified the cortical areas showing increased blood flow during the brief, transitory hearing of voices in three paranoid schizophrenics who were still able to indicate the onset and end of their verbal hallucinations (Dierks, Linden, Jandl, Formisano, Goebel, Lanfermann, and Singer 1999). Here we find another variation of the principle of substrate sharing mentioned above. The major area activated is Heschl's gyrus in the dominant hemisphere, in the primary auditory cortex, the same area active in the direct sensory perceptions of voices. Inner speech, as consciously and deliberately initiated, is not phenomenally represented as real or as externally caused (see also section 5.4). Although, interestingly, both forms of conscious experience involve classic speech production areas, inner speech does *not* activate Heschl's gyrus. In short, hallucinations belong to the class of phenomenal simulata and they satisfy the offline activation constraint, as their causal history originates entirely within the system. They usually do not share the neuroanatomical substrate with *intended* simulations of the same type. They are bound to a first-person perspective, are characterized by varying degrees of dynamicity, and are embedded in a coherent global state. However, in the first case presented, the degree of integration into the visual scene is so low that the content presented to the experiential subject in the course of these episodes is immediately recognized as such, now becoming opaque. In Larry's case, however, we can see how the hallucinatory character (the phenomenally modeled lack of intentional content) has to be concluded from the context. The monkey sitting on Ramachandran's lap is fully bound to the overall visual scene. Only in some cases will Larry's visual hallucinations reveal their nonveridicality to him by their quasi-sensory features. In other cases he has to conclude, as a result of cognitive activity, that these experiences do not put him in direct contact with external reality. In this case, their consciously recognized misrepresentational character is an inferential kind of knowledge. Therefore, they are *not* opaque in the sense of our original definition.

If insight into the origin of hallucinatory content is lost, we soon cross the border to "real," complex hallucinations and manifest delusions (for additional case studies, see Halligan and Marshall 1996; Cahill and Frith 1996; Siegel 1992). Even for a system still able to recognize hallucinatory activity *as such*, a situation can occur in which simulational activity has temporarily become autonomous. It is, as it were, completely out of control. In such cases the phenomenal model of reality can transiently be enriched by a surging flood of more or less stable phenomenal artifacts. Even if the system is able to phenomenally represent them as afunctional simulata, as superfluous mental structures without any functional role *for* the overall psychological ecology of the system, they will typically remain transparent on the level of presentational content and elementary object constitution. It is context knowledge that is cognitively available and not phenomenal opacity that leads us to classify them as *pseudo*hallucinations. However, there are other and less complex neurophenomenological state classes, in which earlier processing stages are, as a matter of fact, available for introspective attention (figure 4.1). If hallucinations are induced by pharmacological stimuli (e.g., by ingestion of classic hallucinogens like LSD, mescaline, or the injection of DMT), a rather unspecific disinhibition of neural activity in different brain regions results (Aghajanian, Foot, and Sheard 1968, 1970; Aghajanian, Haigler, and Bennett 1975; Aghajanian 1994; Gustafson and Tapscott 1979; Siegel and Jarvik 1975). Many hallucinogens act on those brainstem nuclei that control the general level of cortical excitability. For instance, LSD exerts an inhibitory effect on the neurons of the Raphe nucleus (Aghajanian et al. 1970). The resulting state of increased functional excitability then leads to the destabilization of a preexisting dynamical state, which probably is the central necessary condition for the onset of hallucinosis. On the phenomenological level of description, this typically leads to the pure intensity parameter of presentational content becoming increased, first resulting in the intensification of simple forms of "qualitative" content on the phenomenal level. To give an example, phenomenal colors may be brighter than anything seeable with bare eyes. Functionally, presentational content is still stimulus-correlated, but—as in dreams—it now is an *internal* stimulus source which drives the relevant aspect phenomenal content almost in its entirety. Closing your eyes will not make much of a difference; external input only weakly modulates the degree to which *constraint 9* is satisfied in the strongly aroused, hallucinating brain. LSD reliably produces visual hallucinations in a large number of blind subjects (Krill, Alpert, and Ostfield 1963). The first complex kind of phenomenal content that appears frequently is context-free, geometrical patterns exhibiting four different categories of "form constants" (such as, paradigmatically, gratings, cobwebs, tunnels, and spirals; see Klüver 1967 for details). Because all observers report Klüver's form constants, these abstract and rather invariant phenomenal properties potentially contain information about the functional architecture of the human brain, for instance, about area V1 (for an excellent recent discussion, see Bressloff, Cowan, Golubitsky, Thomas, and Wiener 2001, p. 301). Detailed mathematical models of such low-level sensory hallucinations have been in existence for some time, assuming that they arise from an instability of the resting state due to a combination of excitatory modulation and decreased inhibition, which in turn is expressed in certain doubly periodic spatial patterns corresponding to the form constants just mentioned (e.g., see Ermentrout and Cowan 1979, pp. 138, 149; see also Kistler, Seitz, and van Hemmen 1998; for an extended and more specific version of the original Ermentrout-Cowan model, see Bressloff et al. 2001).

Abstract geometrical hallucinations are interesting not only in terms of the historical emergence of a new and important scientific discipline—phenomathematics—but also from a philosophical point of view, because they demonstrate the possibility of dissociating phenomenal and intentional content. The patterns shown above are purely *phenomenal* forms of mental content. They appear in conscious experience, but they have no function *for* the organism and there is no object they are *directed* at. The functional process of hallucinating, as such, does, of course, have such a function. For complex as well as for simple abstract hallucinations the underlying principle seems to be the continuous "attempt" of the system to settle into a stable, low-energy state that, given unexpected causal constraints, still maximizes overall coherence as much as possible. Sometimes this process of "self-coherencing" takes place under conditions of heightened arousal; it is slowed down by pathological conditions, and what I called earlier processing stages above now become accessible for introspective attention. A new kind of nonconceptual, phenomenal content appears in the conscious mind, but it is plausible to assume that the accompanying state does not have the *function* to make the ongoing attempt at restabilization globally available. However, let us be careful: An interesting alternative hypothesis might say that in fact there was an evolutionary benefit to the process of *consciously*

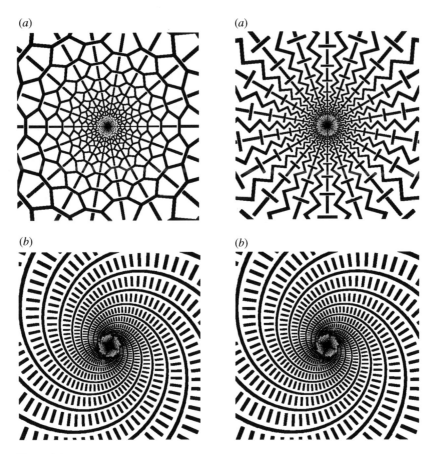

Figure 4.1
Global availability of earlier processing stages plus full dissociation of phenomenal from intentional content:
Abstract geometrical hallucinations in the visual domain. (From Bressloff et al. 2001.)

hallucinating, namely, in that it allows an organism to react to the fact that some parts of
its subpersonal mental machinery are right now desperately struggling for coherence in a
more focused and flexible manner.

Of course, more complex and context-sensitive effects exist as well. Under the effect
of classic hallucinogens the speed of higher cognitive operations can accelerate, eventually leading to flight of ideas and severe disorientation. If the number and the speed of
activation of phenomenal simulata now flooding the global phenomenal model of the
world go beyond a certain threshold, the system may no longer be able to integrate them
into a unitary model of the world and the self within it by organizing those different hal-

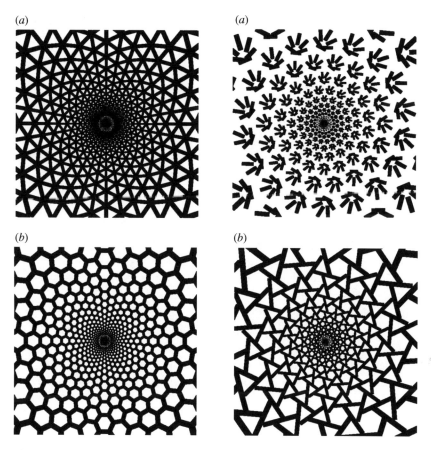

Figure 4.1
Continued.

lucinations into a single "story." In such situations *dissociative* states can result. Parallel realities emerge. Global coherence may be lost because, as it were, the phenomenal model of reality has been overloaded with so much content that it starts to split or dissolve. A connectionist metaphor for this kind of situation is a system, which, after being artificially "heated up," moves through an increasing number of internal states per time unit, which, however, are less and less stable.

It is interesting to compare hallucinatory phenomenal content to the content emerging in multistable phenomena. Leopold and Logothetis (1999) have argued that there are three fundamental properties that can be found in all multistable phenomena: exclusivity, inevitability, and randomness. Exclusivity is the principle of disambiguation that was discussed when introducing the notion of a phenomenal mental model. A fundamental coding principle of perceptual phenomenal models seems to be that conflicting representations are never simultaneously present in the system; the unique existence of only a single perceptual solution seems to be a basic feature of the functional architecture underlying conscious experience. The inevitability in the perceptual alternation of, say, a Necker cube could result from a permanent impact of "top-down" mechanisms persistently impinging on the ongoing upstream of sensory input. Multistable phenomena, then, would be those states of conscious experience in which, due to an ambiguity inherent in the data set, the many top-down hypotheses automatically and continuously generated by the system never get locked into a single, coherent solution. This second principle of Leopold and Logothetis (Leopold and Logothetis 1999, p. 260*ff.*) is of interest in the context of hallucinations. What we experience during hallucinatory episodes may just be an overshooting process of "internal hypothesis generation." This process is continuously active in constraining sensory input, but we never experience it consciously in standard situations. The idea is that ordinary phenomenal experience continuously emerges from an interplay between "top-down" and "bottom-up" processes. The top-down hypotheses are realized by a persistent, ongoing process of internally simulating possible worlds (as it were, continuously generated Kantian categories in search of the right kind of empirical content), which finally lock into the right sort of active presentational content to generate an explicit phenomenal mental model. Ramachandran and Hirstein (1997, p. 442) have vividly illustrated the general picture slowly emerging from these considerations as follows: "To deliberately overstate the case, it's as though when you look at even the simplest visual scene, you generate an endless number of hallucinations and pick the one hallucination which most accurately matches the current input—i.e., the input seems to *select* from an endless number of hallucinations." If this selection process does not work anymore, then the persistent process of automatically forming a myriad of internal hypotheses about the possible current state of the world may start to *dominate* phenomenal experience as a whole. Leopold and Logothetis point out that randomness is common for all forms of multistable vision. Randomness introduces variability in the way in which an organism interacts with its environment. In particular, a constant process of "shaking up" the organization of input would allow for new solutions, "solutions that are not the most probable, given the functional/anatomical constraints imposed by the visual pathways" (Leopold and Logothetis 1999, p. 261). It is interesting to note how this process of "shaking up" or "heating up" the underlying neural dynamics is something that can plausibly be assumed to be a cause of many hallucinations as well (the pharmacological action of hallucinogenic drugs seems to result typically in a rather global and unspecific disinhibition). In multistable phenomena, noisy or weak stimuli—for which no correct "answer" exists—

frequently lead to the subjective experience of meaningful, completed patterns, which can now be conceived of as having completely emerged out of a successful top-down hypothesis. As Kant said, concepts without intuitions do not generate knowledge—they are empty. Hallucinations resulting from top-down processes becoming dominant and enslaving regions of the phenomenal reality-model are just that: they are empty, because they possess no intentional content, they are not causally related to the external environment (note that this may be different in cases of *self*-representation; see n. 12). All they possess is phenomenal character. Now we can also understand what it means to say that phenomenal representation, in the case of hallucinations, has become "hypertrophic." The model of reality is enriched by phenomenal content that is entirely independent of external stimuli and was not in existence before, for instance, in terms of "positive pathologies of vision" (ffytche and Howard 1999) or "phantom visual images" (Schultz and Melzack 1991). It is interesting to note how identical parthologies in vision result in remarkably similar stereotypes of hallucinatory phenomenal content across a broad range of experimental and clinical conditions, and how they allow for conclusions toward invariant properties of their functional profile and neural correlates (for an early investigation into form, color, and movement constants, see Siegel and Jarvik 1975, p. 109*ff*.; for a new categorization of hallucinatory visual content, including useful references, see ffytche and Howard 1999).

Before we move on to the next case study, let me point out two further general issues of predominantly philosophical interest. First, hallucinatory phenomenal content—if it is not a purely abstract, geometrical pattern—is usually phenomenally transparent on the level of its integrated nature as an isolated percept and with regard to its purely presentational aspects. We have already touched upon this point above: pseudohallucinations are characterized by *context knowledge* that, as opposed to low-level processing mechanisms, is not culturally invariant. Therefore, hallucinatory experience may be culturally embedded via a process of making its simulational character cognitively available in the framework of a preexisting theory. In the example of Larry we have already seen how a transparent visual percept can become opaque by being subjected to cognitive exploration, that is, by being embedded in an internal context labeling it *as* hallucinatory content. However, there may be opaque content, as in our first example of Charles-Bonnet syndrome, which may eventually regain the subjective property of *epistemic* transparency by being embedded in an appropriate cultural context. It may be coded as *knowledge*. If one looks for and investigates different definitions of what hallucinations actually are, one finds a common denominator in all of these definitions: Hallucinations are perception-like experiences occurring in the absence of an appropriate external stimulus. They originate in the activation of quasi-perceptual content, which has the full force of the corresponding *actual* perception and is not triggered by the sensory organs, while at the same time not being under voluntary control.[11] In other words, hallucinations are *extrasensory perception*. They emulate perceptual processing. If you live in a culture which assumes that there is more than one world and more than one level of reality, then you can reinterpret the sudden appearance of unwanted and unlooked-for perceptual content in your phenomenal model of reality as a window onto *another* reality. One man's unwanted artifact is another man's window. A scotoma episodically filled by spontaneous visual hallucinations may be one very simple example of such a neurophenomenological window. Obviously, a large subset of so-called paranormal experiences, for instance, of clairvoyance or of otherworldly visions, can easily be explained by hallucinatory syndromes like Charles-Bonnet syndrome. In fact, many patients suffering from complex hallucinations *do* develop the belief that they have suddenly acquired paranormal capabilities (for a case study, see Halligan and Marshall 1996; see also Coltheart and Davies 2000). If you live in a culture where no alternative models of explanation are available, and if you are suddenly confronted with spontaneously occurring "internal television," you may well make an inference to the best explanation *available in your culture*. Of course, the neurophenomenology of hallucinations is an immensely rich and complex field, and I have just chosen one simple example for purposes of illustration. But, as it has recently turned out, Charles-Bonnet syndrome is much more frequent experience than has so far been assumed (Teunisse et al. 1996). It is fairly common in elderly people with culturally invariant damages to the external visual system like cataracts, corneal damage, macular degeneration, and diabetic retinopathy. Of course, in Western cultures, many elderly people do not report these spontaneous visual hallucinations because of fear of social isolation. A number of reviewers, therefore, point out that the incidence of the phenomenon may be considerably higher because many patients may be reluctant to talk about their experience "for fear of being labeled as emotionally disturbed" (Schultz and Melzack 1991, p. 813). In another cultural setting (e.g., in prescientific cultures), of course, such phenomenal states may well be interpreted as *epistemically transparent*, as providing secure and direct knowledge of existing objects, scenes, or layers of reality. It is therefore well conceivable that fairy tales, mythical folklore concerning gnomes, animal spirits, or invisible higher beings, as well as "esoteric" reports about parallel worlds, astral planes, etheric elements of reality surrounding us, and so on, originally developed in this way. It also has a certain logic in that elderly people in particular, people who, according to many cultural traditions, are getting ready to make a final transition to an invisible world, start to get their initial *glimpses* of this world. Anybody interested in a rigorous research

11. Cf. Slade and Bentall (1988, p. 23) for an example: "Any percept-like experience which (a) occurs in the absence of an appropriate stimulus, (b) has the full force of impact of the corresponding actual (real) perception, and (c) is not amenable to direct and voluntary control by the experiencer." (Quoted in Cahill and Frith 1996, p. 271).

program in parapsychology must therefore also be interested in marking out all cases in which a neurophenomenological reduction of the target phenomenon is plausible and sensible. In analyzing paranormal experiences one will, in a very large majority of cases, be confronted with truthful autophenomenological reports. A comprehensive, neurobiologically grounded theory of hallucination could help to distinguish reports that only refer to the transparent *phenomenal* content of certain nonordinary experiential states and those which actually possess informational or *intentional* content of an unknown causal origin (for a fascinating discussion of the relationship between belief in paranormal phenomena and their possible neural causes, see Brugger 2000).

Second, an obvious truth about hallucinatory types of phenomenal experience, spontaneous or deliberately induced, seems to be that phenomenal hypertrophy is not equivalent to epistemic progress. If those additional phenomenal simulata, which penetrate into an already active phenomenal model of reality during hallucinatory episodes, really are afunctional artifacts, then the system as a whole will be enriched with phenomenally available mental content, but it will not gain any additional *knowledge* or information about the world.[12] On the other hand, if pseudohallucinations could be made available in a controlled and protected experimental setting, they would be highly interesting with regard to the theoretical issue that I introduced under the heading of "autoepistemic closure" in chapter 2 and which we reencountered as the "transparency constraint" in chapter 3. A controlled experience of pseudohallucinations in a scientific setting may offer a chance to introspectively *observe* the process of construction, activation, and dynamical self-organization of phenomenal representata as they change along a gradient from transparency to opacity. As long as we remember that "observation" is itself a process of phenomenal representation, this could be quite fruitful. Why should it not be possible to increase the attentional availability of earlier processing stages for such states? System states that are "heated up" or "shaken up" seem to be ideally suited for experimental paradigms targeting the above-mentioned gradient. In other words, this may allow us to make the process, by which in some cases we recognize them *as* representata, as internally generated simulata globally available for attention, and possibly even for cognition. It may also shed new light of the incessant process of automatic "hypothesis generation" discussed above. Transitions from transparency to opacity could become an object of rigorous investigation, not in terms of theoretical or empirical strategies, but by utilizing the

---

12. Again, this question has to be carefully decided in a differentiated manner from individual case to individual case. An example of a context in which self-related hallucinatory components seem to be able to support an overall process of *gaining* knowledge may be constituted by modern, hallucinogen-based psychotherapy, which has demonstrably led to good catamnestic results. This may be interpreted as an indicator that the overall psychological process triggered in these forms of pharmacologically induced psychotherapy *cannot* be epistemically vacuous in its entirety (Leuner 1981).

phenomenal variant of representation itself as a starting point. Attentional availability of earlier processing stages, in a second step, could become a *variable* in controlled experiments, which finally might lead to new insights concerning the notion of phenomenal transparency itself.

Let me direct attention to a last and more general philosophical point. There is a certain perspective from which one can analyze *all* phenomenal states as transporting hallucinatory content. It is the perspective of epistemology. Recall that our minimal notion of conscious experience is generated by satisfying the globality constraint, the presentationality constraint, and, to a certain degree, the transparency constraint. First, as long as phenomenal experience is anchored in a largely transparent portion of one's reality-model, it will always be characterized by naive realism. This realism can now itself be interpreted as a kind of *hallucination* that proved to be adaptive for systems like ourselves. Phenomenal transparency is not the same as epistemic transparency, but in systems like ourselves the content of phenomenally transparent representation is experienced *as* epistemically transparent. Seeing seems to be *knowing*. This, on a more general level of analysis, can be described as a fundamental hallucinatory feature of our own type of conscious experience. For human beings, the paradigmatic example of an opaque phenomenal state is a conscious thought. Only if our phenomenal world-model *as a whole* was becoming opaque (see section 7.2.5) could we experience it as a global pseudohallucination; it would, as it were, from now on be experienced as one big and comprehensive *thought*. The world as a whole would suddenly become a single representational or even cognitive event, and this may have been the intuitive vision driving many idealistic philosophers in the past. Please note how, for us, such a fully opaque, global state would not count as a *conscious* state anymore, because it fails to satisfy the transparency constraint.

A second way of formulating the claim that, on a certain level of description, *all* phenomenal experience is of a fundamentally hallucinatory character can be developed by pointing out how the presentationality constraint makes all such content epistemically unjustified on a very fundamental level. A physical theory about the universe will never tell us what time is "now." "Nowness" is a kind of mental content that only appears under phenomenal representations of reality. As extensively discussed above, our experiential present always is a *simulated* present, because in its extended character (the phenomenal Now being a dilated or "smeared" form of time as opposed to the time of physics) it is a pure fiction. This fiction proved to be biologically adaptive, because it approximated the real temporal structure of our environment, of our ecological niche, of our physical domain of interaction in a way that was efficient, and just good enough. Nevertheless it must be pointed out how the phenomenal window of presence is a *virtual* window of presence, because it represents a possibility and not an actuality. From a strict third-person perspective, therefore, all phenomenal content is hallucinatory content, because what I have termed its *de nunc* character (see sections 2.4.4 and 3.2.2) is nothing but a simulational fiction that proved to be functionally adequate. From an *epistemological* perspective it is not a form of knowledge. It follows that there are at least two conceptually clear ways in which one can claim that all consciously experienced content is hallucinatory content.

However, the neurophenomenological case studies of hallucinations too briefly presented in the preceding sections were examples of states that always were integrated into *global* phenomenal models of reality, models that still embodied a considerable amount of reliable information about the world. The natural, logical step to follow now is to ask if phenomenal state classes exist that are *completely* empty from an epistemological perspective while possessing rich experiential content. Do global phenomenal states exist that possess *only* phenomenal character, but no intentional content?

4.2.5 Dreams

Dreams have been a topic of philosophical inquiry right from the early beginnings and throughout the history of Western thought (Dreisbach 2000). Descartes famously argued that, as sensory experience itself is emulated during the dream state, it would never be possible to distinguish between dreams and reality on empirical grounds alone (Descartes [1642] 1911). However, philosophical interest in dreams has somewhat decreased since Malcolm's (1959) anti-Cartesian argument that dreams are not experiences at all, because they do not involve cognitive availability and linguistic access in terms of publicly declarative metaknowledge. Today, given our new conceptual tools and a rich set of empirical constraints, a much more differentiated perspective can be developed.

In section 3.2.7 we saw how the notion of "conscious experience" comes in many different strengths, and how the existence of a full-blown *cognitive* first-person perspective (for details, see sections 6.4.4 and 6.5.2) is not a necessary condition for conscious experience as such. Dreams are conscious experiences because they satisfy *constraints 2* (presentationality), *3* (globality), and *7* (transparency). From a purely phenomenological perspective a dream certainly is the *presence of a world*. On the representationalist level of description, dreams are interesting because—at least for human beings—they lead to the most general conceptual distinction between classes of phenomenal reality-models, to the most fundamental categorization possible. In terms of representational content, dreams and waking states are the two most important global state classes. From a functionalist third-person perspective, however, dreams are even more interesting phenomena—for instance, because they are comprehensive *offline* world-models (*constraint 8*), and because it is still unclear if they have any adaptive function *for* the dreaming organism (*constraint 11*). Finally, the cognitive neuroscience of dreaming has made considerable progress during the last two or three decades, increasing the attraction of this field of research for interdisciplinary approaches (for an excellent review, see Hobson, Pace-Schott, and

Stickgold 2000). Since we all dream, and since most of us have at least some dream recall, I will not offer an example of the phenomenology of dreams here.

However, a more systematic look at dreams on the phenomenal level of description often has surprising results. To give an example, have you ever noticed that you are not able to control the movement of your attentional focus during a dream? Have you ever noticed that some classes of sensory experiences occur rarely during your dreams—for instance, experiences of pain, smell, and taste? The absence of specific kinds of presentational content is a primary and very basic phenomenological feature of the dream state. High-level attention, in terms of the phenomenal quality of "attentional agency" (see section 6.4.3), the conscious experience of being able to control the trajectory of attentional processing, is generally absent. The same is true of volitional control of dream *behavior*, which generally is greatly weakened. Phenomenologically, dreamers are rarely agents (see section 6.4.5). The dreamer is not a cognitive subject in a strong sense, because he is severely disoriented about places, times, and persons, and constantly produces ad hoc explanations for the events he encounters. The phenomenal dream-self is almost incapable of conscious self-reflection and metacognition that could make the lack of intellectual consistency become a recognizable *fact* for herself. Additionally, short-term memory is greatly impaired and generally unreliable. Therefore, dreamers are only cognitive subjects in a weak and, arguably, philosophically uninteresting sense (see section 6.4.4).

On the other hand, as almost all of us know, *long-term* and semantic memory can be greatly enhanced in the dream stage: *Internally*, oneiric states can be hypermnestic—for instance, in making childhood memories reappear in great vividness, memories that would never have been accessible in the ordinary waking state. *Externally*, looking backward from the perspective of everyday consciousness, amnesia is a dominant feature of dream consciousness. For many people, dream recall is very weak. There are further examples of representational enrichments. The hallucinatory perceptual experiences of the dream state are episodically accompanied by intense *emotional* episodes, which, again, can be more intense than most emotions we know from the ordinary waking state. It is interesting to note that not all dream emotions are equally charged, but that there is a predominance of negative emotions like fear and anxiety (for the "threat simulation" hypothesis of the origin of dreams; see Revonsuo 2000b). Finally, a global phenomenological feature of the dream state is its delusional nature, the fact that there is no conscious first-person experience that might reveal the true nature of the state (for two excellent reviews that also offer many interesting observations and further references concerning the *phenomenological* landscape of the dream state, see Kahn, Pace-Schott, and Hobson 1997; Hobson, Pace-Schott, and Stickgold 2000. In particular, see Hobson 1988, 1999; Jouvet 1999). The phenomenal landscape of dreams just sketched is nicely reflected in a more specific definition of the dream state, which is taken from Hobson et al. (2000) and has the advantage of briefly integrating a number of first-person and third-person constraints:

Mental activity occurring in sleep characterized by vivid sensorimotor imagery that is experienced as waking reality despite such distinct cognitive features as impossibility or improbability of time, place, person and action; emotions, especially fear, elation and anger predominate over sadness, shame and guilt and sometimes reach sufficient strength to cause awakening; memory for even very vivid dreams is evanescent and tends to fade quickly upon awakening unless special steps are taken to retain it.

In the context of searching for a general theory of phenomenal representation and the first-person perspective, dreams are of particular interest for a number of reasons. Many of them will become more obvious as we open our conceptual tool kit to briefly extend our neurophenomenological analysis to the representational, functional, and neural levels of description.

Let me start by pointing out a first interesting aspect: Although dreams certainly can be analyzed as global, integrated models of the world (*constraint 3*), they do not seem to satisfy the functional constraints offered by the concepts of availability for attention, cognition, and control of action (*constraint 1*), which turned out to be the functionalist reading or counterpart of the more comprehensive *constraint 3* in our previous discussion. One way of analyzing this peculiar dissociation of representational contents and functional role is by pointing out that dreams are internal simulations of a complete behavioral space, including target objects; complex, ongoing behaviors; and other agents, while not being *causally coupled* to the actual behavioral space of the dreaming organism. Dreamers are not bodily agents. Dream content certainly is phenomenal content, but it is never directly *used* in the control of action or in guiding external behavior.[13] If it is available for external behavior, this availability is never realized in nonpathological situations. However, in nonpathological situations phenomenal dream content clearly is available for spontaneous *internal* behavior, that is, it can drive a kind of behavior which is only *simulated* behavior, although at the current stage of our investigation it is entirely unclear if dreamers can count as agents in any interesting sense (see sections 6.4.5 and 7.2.3.3). It is interesting to note that there is a subclass of phenomenal dreamers for whom this first functional constraint is not satisfied, although this very fact, unfortunately, is not cognitively available to them. An inhibition of the spinal motor neurons normally prevents actual macrobehavior from being generated during REM phases. This is not true of situations in which, due to failing motor inhibition, people suffer from REM-sleep behavioral disorder (RBD). These patients actually are forced to physically act out their dream behavior (Hobson 1999, p. 136*f*.; Hobson et al. 2000; Mahowald and Schenck 1999; Schenck and Mahowald 1996; Revonsuo 1995,

---

13. It is important to note that dreaming can plausibly be interpreted as *internal microbehavior*, for instance, in terms of supporting homeostasis and hormonal self-regulation at the molecular level. It is also important to note how, conceived of as microbehavior in this way, the process of dreaming will plausibly satisfy the adaptivity constraint and how on this level of description, the coactivation of phenomenal content taking place will likely play no explanatory role in terms of its biological function.

2000a, p. 66; for a case study, see Dyken, Lin-Dyken, Seaba, and Yamada 1995). There is
a well-known neurological syndrome called "echopraxia," in which patients are inevitably
forced to act out the observed behavior of other human beings during the waking state.
Here we seem to have a similar situation, in which an internal behavior-simulation system
(likely functioning as an *intentionality detector*; see Gallese 2000; Gallese and Goldman
1998) is coupled to the motor system. It then forces the patient to act out behaviors which
he is currently mentally simulating (because he visually perceives them). For now, RBD
may count as a functional variant of this process: the RBD patient acting out his dreams is
not *acting* at all, he is just echopractic with regard to the current dream-self.

Second, phenomenal dream content is not attentionally available. The capacity to deliberately focus attention simply does not exist in ordinary dreams. All there is is salience-
driven, low-level attention. And third, because dreams are characterized by severe
disorientation and bizarre formal thought disorders, dream content is not cognitively available in the sense of processes that could, from an external perspective, be described as
approximating *rational* mental concept formation. Although from a phenomenological perspective it seems safe to say that dreams unfold within an integrated phenomenal world-
model, adding these further constraints on the functional level of description, it becomes
much less clear in what sense dream content really is *subjective* conscious content. Dreams
are states of consciousness. Dreams have phenomenal selves. But do dreams really exhibit
a *first-person* perspective? The reason for this uncertainty is that an important type of representational content is only weakly expressed during the dream state. This representational content is the phenomenal model of the intentionality relation (see section 6.5). The
representational content missing in ordinary dreams is the one of the *self-in-the-act-of
deciding* to take a specific course of action (the volitional subject), the *self-in-the-act-of-
deliberately-attending* to certain perceptual or cognitive states (the attentional subject),
and the self as *rationally* thinking about events currently taking place in the dream (the
cognitive subject). Now there is a simple and elegant way to describe all these phenomenological, representational, and functional deficits—by saying that dreams only weakly
satisfy the perspectivalness constraint (*constraint 6*).

Looking at the remaining multilevel constraints in our conceptual tool box also makes
it possible to bring out further characteristics of the dream state that make it interesting
for a general theory of conscious representation. Although working memory is severely
impaired (the cognitive subject is not fully *present*, as it were), the dream world as a whole
is certainly activated within a window of presence. Dream states are governed by the principle of presentationality; they can be described phenomenologically as the presence of a
world, albeit a world possessing very different features. In particular, it is very instructive
to look at oneiric models of reality in terms of the convolved holism constraint and the
dynamicity constraint.

Dreams are global hallucinatory processes, characterized by a fundamentally delusional nature. Two phenomenological features (which have been noted by generations of dream researchers since Freud) are intimately related to this fact: hyperassociativity and bizarreness. Dream contents are hyperassociative in that the tendency to discover "similarities" and to jump to structurally related interpretations of situations or persons is much greater in the dream state than in the waking state. The complementary phenomenological feature is that of instability. Functionally speaking, the dreaming system resembles other kinds of systems having to cope with (e.g., drug-induced) hallucinations in that it behaves like a system that has been "heated up" and now is passing through a great number of weakly linked states at increased speed, making the overall representational content ever more short-lived and less stable. In terms of the convolved holism constraint we can now see how the multilevel functional links assumed in the continuous generation of phenomenal wholes and their embedding in a flexible, nested hierarchy of representational contents evolving over time can help in understanding the hyperassociativity of dreams. There are just *more* of such links formed per time unit, and as these integrational processes are not constrained by the stability and invariance normally supplied by the actual perception of an external world, they become less and less stable. Kahn and colleagues (1997, p. 21) have hypothesized that defective binding over time may play a crucial role. It is plausible to assume that binding operations take place on many levels in the dreaming brain. They are part of the ongoing dynamics of self-organization "striving" to generate a maximally coherent global state at any given point in time, given the informational resources currently available. However, no global stimulus properties can be extracted from an ongoing perceptual processing of the external world, and therefore the system is entirely dependent on internal resources. The resulting instability can be described in terms of the dynamicity constraint introduced in the last chapter. Dreams are *more* dynamic than the waking state, because the rate with which representational content changes per time unit is higher than in the waking state. In terms of the convolved holism constraint, the integrated nature of individual objects, persons, or scenes in the dream world—the feature of holism as such—is actually expressed to a weaker degree. However, due to the increase in dynamicity, that is, in continuous and fast changes in representational content, the *convolved* character—the degree of "nestedness" of different representational contents with respect to each other—can actually be greater. Phenomenologically, this analysis is plausible. Dream content is not only short-lived and hyperassociative, it can also, for brief periods, be utterly complicated, leading the experiential subject into a phenomenological jungle, as it were. Kahn and colleagues have pointed out how "such hyperassociativity helps create the semblance of unity amid a great variety and richness of imagery as well as contributing to those incongruities and discontinuities that typify dreaming consciousness" (ibid., p. 17).

What about bizarreness? Recent years have seen a lot of very detailed and rigorous work concerning the bizarreness of dreams (for an example, see Mamelak and Hobson 1989; for further references, see Kahn et al. 1997, p. 18; Hobson et al. 2000; Revonsuo and Salmivalli 1995). For instance, a bizarreness scale dividing the phenomenological feature into quantifiable categories like discontinuity, incongruity, uncertainty, and the presence of ad hoc explanations has been developed (again, see Kahn et al. 1997, p. 18). It is obvious how, for instance, the discontinuity found in the evolution of phenomenal content over time can plausibly be explained in terms of deficits in binding over time on the functional level of description. Kahn and colleagues, for instance, have defined the resulting functional deficit as an "interruption in orientational stability." However, I will not go into further details at this point.

We have already touched on the issue of how the representational deep structure of dreaming is characterized by a weak and unstable satisfaction of the perspectivalness constraint, and how the transparency of the dream state leads to a global loss of *insight* into the nature of the state. It is interesting to note a parallel to the waking state: systems having strictly *no* phenomenally opaque portions in their reality-model (e.g., simple organisms on our planet operating under a simple, fully transparent model of reality) will also be fully deluded about the true nature of their current state. For them (just as for the dreamer) there will be no explicit appearance-reality distinction. They will be unaware of the fact that they are currently living their conscious life with the help of a global online simulation. Obviously, dreams are importantly characterized by being the only global type of phenomenal state available to human beings that almost fully satisfies *constraint 8*, the offline activation constraint. There are certainly exceptions, in which weak subliminal stimuli can directly influence consciously experienced dream content. For instance, this happened to me when experimenting with one of the famous lucid dream induction devices. After such a device registers the onset of a REM phase, it will, after a certain delay, start to flash soft red lights onto the closed eyelids of the dreamer. Frequently, however, this will not lead to lucidity (see section 7.2.5), but to a dream of approaching police cars, flashing alarm lights on the control panel of your space ship which is *just* taking off, and the like. What is more important is to note how the neurophenomenological example of the dream state relativizes the offline activation constraint. In order to make this point clearer, let us look at a coarse-grained functional analysis of dreams. It reveals them as being a very specific type of reality-model characterized by specific functional properties. These are the three most important functional features of the phenomenal reality-model called "dream":

1. *Output blockade*: Dreamers are not functionally embodied agents. When the human brain is in the state necessary to generate a reality-model of the category "dream," it is not able to generate motor output. The central neural correlate of this functional situation

consists in a postsynaptic inhibition pertaining to the last region of the common path of all motor neurons in the brainstem and spinal cord (for a recent review of the neurobiological details, see Hobson et al. 2000). Due to physical constraints, dreaming systems are not able to initiate complex patterns of external behavior or goal-directed actions. There are, however, specific forms of microbehavior, like REMs, which in human beings typically accompany dream phases and which have given these phases their name as REM-sleep phases. Therefore, dreams are world-models, which are *without function* with regard to the actual and external control of behavior. If, as in RBD or borderline cases of an incomplete motor inhibition—for instance, when speaking during sleep—nonintended, complex forms of behavior emerge, these are not *actions*, but "behavioral artifacts" (spontaneous motor hallucinations, coupled to the motor system but not tied to a volitional first-person perspective, as it were). They do not satisfy *constraint 11*, the adaptivity constraint. They have no true teleofunctionalist description, because they are maladaptive and do not fulfill a function *for* the system.

It is interesting to note how, on a nonphenomenal, *fine-grained* functional level of analysis, ordinary dreams could well be states having an important and essential function for the individual organism, for instance, by allowing a fine-tuning of relative neurotransmitter levels or the consolidation of long-term memory (for a critical discussion of the latter claim, see Vertes and Eastman 2000).

2. *Input blockade*: Dreams are states in which peripheral sensory signals can only very rarely penetrate into the central mechanisms of information processing. For instance, brainstem, visual system, and forebrain are basically *deafferented* in the dream state. This is the central reason for dreams being epistemically empty, at least with regard to the *current* state of the system's environment. The information flow subserving their phenomenal content is exclusively an internal flow of information. For this reason, some philosophers have called dreams *virtual* phenomenal realities, and used a current technological metaphor to describe these states: *cyberspace* (Revonsuo 1995, 1997, 2000; Metzinger 1993, pp. 146*ff.*, 194*ff.*, 241*ff.*; see also section 8.1). There are two good hypotheses concerning the neurobiological realization of this functional property in the human brain, assuming a presynaptic inhibition of certain afferent nerve terminals as well as of certain nuclei in the brainstem or of the thalamus on the one hand and a "jamming" or "flooding" of higher sensory cortices by internally generated activation on the other. An important, more recent, development in describing the temporal evolution of the neural substrate underlying phenomenal dreaming consists in introducing *self-organization* as an explanatory variable, for instance, in describing shifts from the input-controlled global model of reality of the waking state to the input-decoupled reality-model unfolding during REM phases (see Kahn and Hobson 1993; Kahn et al. 1997, p. 30*ff.*; for the latest version of the AIM state-space model, together with a sketch of the different historical stages

through which the theory developed from Hobson and McCarley's original "activation synthesis model" in 1977, see Hobson et al. 2000).

3. *Internal signal generation*: A dreaming brain processes self-generated stimuli as if they were external input and then integrates them into a global state. A philosophically relevant question in this context is whether this generation of internal stimuli can be meaningfully described as a *source of information* or only as a sequence of random events on the physical level. Do dreams *represent*? I return to this issue later. A good preliminary candidate for the signal source underlying the activation of phenomenal dream content are ponto-geniculo-occipital waves ("PGO waves"). In the relevant areas of the brainstem we find a mutual interaction between aminergic and cholinergic neurons (again, for details, see Hobson et al. 2000). The beginning of a dream phase is initiated by a periodical cessation of activity within the aminergic systems, in turn leading to a disinhibition of functionally associated units and to the generation of PGO waves in the pontine reticular formation. These strong impulses carry on into the thalamus, and thence into visual and association cortices, leading to clearly demonstrable, ordered, and coordinated patterns of activity in oculomotor, vestibular, and visual regions of the brain. An interesting detail is that this internally generated input possesses at least a very strong *spatial* specificity: the cell activity underlying the generation of PGO waves reflects the spatially oriented activity of *real-world* eye movements on the level of the brainstem. This leads to the careful conclusion that dreams are not *entirely* meaningless, as the physical processes modeled by them are in part ordered, internal system processes (please note the implicit parallels to Anton's syndrome, and Charles-Bonnet syndrome).

Let us now return to *constraint 8*, and how the example of the dream relativizes it. It is empirically plausible to assume that the phenomenal dynamics of the conscious dreaming process results from self-organizational processes in the underlying neurodynamics that unfolds when the brain is confronted with a strong internal stimulus source. The complex confabulatory narrative of the dream is the brain's way of interpreting this strong internal stimulus source, which in turn results from massive shifts in its internal chemical landscape. It is also interesting to note that microinjection of cholinergic agonists or cholinesterase inhibitor into many areas of the paramedian pontine reticular formation directly *induces* REM sleep (for references concerning recent findings supporting the hypothetical cholinergic mechanisms triggering REM sleep, see Hobson et al. 2000). Therefore, there is an important sense in which *no* form of phenomenal content is truly activated offline. Trivially, all phenomenal content is dependent on arousal. As a locally supervening phenomenon it is physically determined by depending on a suitable stimulus source that can eventually lead to the activation of a transparent, coherent world-model within a virtual window of presence. What the neurophenomenology of dreams demonstrates is how full-blown, complex reality-models can evolve from an exclusively *internal* stimulus source.

The intensity constraint for simple sensory contents is certainly satisfied in the dream state as well. However, the general landscape of constraint satisfaction is very different from the waking state. As noted above, for nociception and smell and taste, the phenomenal representation of intensity is either weak or absent. For other state classes—such as fear, panic, sudden elation, or emotionally charged memory episodes—it is tempting to point out how they frequently go along with much stronger intensities. However, we must not forget that the intensity constraint can only be applied to simple sensory content in a nonmetaphorical way. What about the *ultrasmoothness* of simple sensory content? Is consciously experienced presentational content in the dream state *homogeneous*? When considering this question we confront the central difficulty in dream phenomenology, the central difficulty in developing and assessing first-person level constraints for the dream state: introspection₃ is almost impossible in the dream state, because high-level attention is absent. You cannot introspectively attend even to your most simple sensory perceptions in the dream state, because you are not an attentional subject. All dream phenomenology, therefore, can be criticized as *waking* phenomenology of dream *memories* (see Dennett 1976). Any phenomenologist seriously interested in a rigorous and systematic description of dream content must therefore first master the art of lucid dreaming (see section 7.2.5). However, it might then be argued that there are only two kinds of dream phenomenology: *lucid* dream phenomenology and waking-state dream *memory* phenomenology. The present approach tries to do justice to this problem by introducing different strengths for the target phenomenon of conscious experience, thereby making initial steps toward a future catalogue of multilevel constraints that in turn allows for very different degrees of constraint satisfaction. Before we can jump to stronger philosophical conclusions (i.e., about the impossibility of certain first-person constraints in dream theory), we need a much better description of the target phenomenon.

The deeper structural reason why dream phenomenology is a difficult task lies in a feature of its deep representational structure: the perspectivalness constraint, in the dream, is only satisfied weakly, intermittently, and with a high degree of variability. Therefore, first-person approaches to dream content can at most be only weakly, intermittently, and variably successful. In other words, if one believes in the heuristic value of phenomenological approaches supplementing efforts in the cognitive neurosciences, one also has to admit that different kinds of conscious states may be more or less *suitable* for this type of approach, in principle. There will be classes of phenomenal states—like the ineffable presentational content discussed in chapter 2 or conscious dreams lacking a stable attentional-cognitive subject—about which we can ultimately gain deeper knowledge by investigating their microfunctional profile and their minimally sufficient neural correlates *only*. Of course, a passionate neurophenomenologist might attempt to strengthen his capacities for extracting first-person information for even such states. This could be done by training her color perception so as to make the wider range of consciously experienced colors cognitively available or by becoming a lucid dreamer. However, it must be noted, all these efforts will significantly change the target phenomenon itself.

Are dreams, like hallucinations, phenomenal artifacts fulfilling no biological function for the dreaming organism? Do they possess any *intentional* content beyond their phenomenal character? Or are they *atavisms*, leftover virtual organs from an ancient phase of brain evolution? Are they residual neurocomputational aftereffects from a certain stage in embryonic development in which the unborn child slowly starts to configure its own internal model of behavioral space and the way in which its body image is embedded in that space (Winson 1991)? Are conscious dreams just epiphenomenal correlates of elementary bioregulatory processes best described on a *molecular* level? I will not attempt to give answers to any of these questions here because they seem to me to be classic examples of a subset of issues that should be empirically investigated instead of philosophically discussed. However, let me add one brief conceptual remark. So far we have encountered three potential classes of phenomenal states that may not satisfy our last constraint, the adaptivity constraint. The first class consists of *pathological* states like agnosia, neglect, blindsight, and hallucinations. The second class was defined by all forms of *machine consciousness*, as long as it has not emerged from an evolutionary process of its own, but is truly "artificial" consciousness in a strict sense. Dreams may form the third class. If we would arrive at an affirmative answer to this question on empirical grounds, then we could develop new conceptual analogies, either describing dreamers as a specific kind of machine, as phenomenal automatons without a stable first-person perspective, or as regularly occurring but *pathological* forms of conscious processing. For instance, dreams could then be characterized as a specific type of organic delirium characterized by amnesia, disorientation, confabulation, and hallucinosis. As a matter of fact, leading dream researchers today seem to be approaching precisely this sort of hypothesis (see, e.g., Hobson 1999; Kahn et al. 1997, p. 18). It is interesting to note, on a purely conceptual level, how dreams, if it turns out that a nosological analysis (i.e., an analysis guided by the notion of pathological deficits) turns out to be true, are also an *anosognostic* state: they are states in which information about an existing deficit cannot be integrated into the conscious self-model. A dreaming machine would also have to be defined as having a specific deficit in an internal representation of itself, as being an automaton *because* it is unable to sustain a stable first-person perspective. In other words, a full-blown theory of dreaming eventually will have to be a theory of self-representation as well.

Back to our original question: Are dreams a source of self-knowledge or serious forms of delusion? Are dreams meaningless artifacts or are they states possessing a meaningful interpretation (see Flanagan 1995, 1997)? As so often is the case, the truth seems to lie somewhere in the middle. As I have pointed out elsewhere (Metzinger 1993, p. 149), even if the internal causes of dream content cannot be recognized as such and even if on the phenomenal level we only witness a bizarre chain of phenomenal simulata, it seems not entirely to be the pure activity of some "internal randomisator" (Crick and Mitchison 1983; Hobson and McCarley 1977; Hobson 1988) which is then being globally modeled during the process of dreaming. The preexisting internal context (e.g., the system's position in weight space), used by our brain as an interpretative mechanism to generate a world-model that is as consistent as possible when confronted with a continuous internal source of signals, *does* carry information—for instance, about what in a psychoanalytic or folk-psychological context could be called the "personality" of the dreamer. Above, we have already seen that some brainstem activity, that is, the motor trajectory guiding the spatial behavior of the eyes, is directly mirrored in the eye movements of the phenomenal *dream-self*. Philosophically speaking, the phenomenal dream-self is not completely disembodied, because in realizing its specific functional profile it shares part of the anatomical substrate of the waking-self. You can deliberately wake up from a lucid dream by stubbornly fixating, for example, your own hands, because you interrupt the physical mechanism of REM sleep in this way (see section 7.2.5). You can even use the correlation between phenomenal gaze shifts in the dream and physical eyeball movements to *communicate* across two very different phenomenal models of reality (LaBerge, Nagel, Dement, and Zarcone 1981a; LaBerge, Nagel, Taylor, Dement, and Zarcone 1981b). Of course, the epistemological status of psychoanalysis resembles that of a religion and it is doubtful what contribution it can make to more rational forms of theory formation concerning consciousness and the phenomenal self. But even if it is true that widespread aminergic demodulation and cholinergic autostimulation are the *triggering* causes leading to a massive change in the dreaming brain's microfunctional profile, the overall connectivity of neurons still represents a large part of the internal landscape that reflects this system's individual history. This includes its history in *waking life*. Not the stimulus, but the style of processing may actually reveal some aspects of this history.

I like to look at dreams as high-dimensional Rorschach tests, in the course of which the brain of the dreaming person assembles self-generated random figures into a complex internal narrative, by transforming them into an "internal fairy tale." This fairy tale, as a chain of concrete subjective experiences, manifests the history and the actual configuration of the system, the way in which it usually interprets the world, by trying to settle into a stable state again and again. Due to the specific functional constraints, conscious information processing is generally faulty, erratic, and highly unstable. Still, some aspects of the global internal simulation emerging may count as actual instances of *self-representation*. Even if portrayed as parts of an external reality, some aspects of phenomenal dream content will inevitably reflect properties of the *internal* neurodynamics. After all, they supervene locally and it is unwarranted to assume that they can override all of the preexisting functional architecture embodied by the dreaming brain. That is why dreams probably are not epistemically blind, empty artifacts without any biological function, but an exclusively internal type of reality-model. This model cannot be recognized *as such*. The more interesting fact, perhaps, is that dreams are fully transparent.

Yet, the phenomenal world of dreaming is much more unstable than the world of waking consciousness. This leads to a high degree of internal incoherence, the components out of which it emerges actually seeming to be chaotically dynamic, lawless entities, at least in terms of their relations to other forms of active phenomenal content. It is therefore striking that their simulational nature so rarely dawns on us. The contents of our dream experiences are constantly changing, in an unpredictable manner and frequently in a bizarre way. Properties like persistent failure in phenomenal cognition, complex hallucinations, amnesia, and hyperemotionality make the dream a state which may phenomenologically, as well as neurobiologically, provide an interesting model for a number of other altered states of consciousness. On the level of conceptual analysis it is obvious that the topic of dreams, as a philosophical interpretation of altered states of consciousness and deviant phenomenal models of reality in general, clearly has been neglected too much. In particular, it may be methodologically fruitful to introduce the dream state as a model system for fundamental aspects of "normal," nonaltered states of consciousness as well (Revonsuo 2000a). Philosophical oneirology certainly could make valuable contributions to a general theory of phenomenal representation. However, prominent philosophers of the analytical tradition in the past have sometimes even denied that dreams are conscious experiences *at all* (see Malcolm 1956, 1959; Dennett 1976; for discussion, see Metzinger 1993, p. 146*ff.*, p. 194*ff.*, p. 241*ff.*; Revonsuo 1995, p. 36*ff.*). New empirical data now have clearly falsified such purely conceptual arguments.

Interestingly, some of this new material points to the possibility of a common functional substrate of dream and waking consciousness (Llinás and Paré 1991; Llinás and Ribary 1993, 1994; Kahn et al. 1997). This line of research, from a purely methodological perspective, possesses great relevance. Why? Because dreams and waking states are the two most general, global state classes of the target phenomenon. If a common denominator on the functional level can be isolated, this will be of major importance in narrowing down the minimally sufficient neural correlates corresponding to *constraint 3*, the *globality* of phenomenal experience. For instance, global models of reality in dream and waking states may in both cases be looked upon as functional clusters or dynamical core states in terms of the original hypothesis of Edelman and Tononi (Edelman and Tononi 2000a, b; Tononi and Edelman 1998a). If two comprehensive mathematical models for each of the two global state classes were available, then a "subtraction" of one model from the other could yield a highly informative and precise description not only of the neural dynamics underlying conscious experience in general but—given a specific isomorphism assumption with regard to vehicle and content—also to a *much* more thorough analysis of the representational deep structure of phenomenal experience than the one sketched in this chapter. It is clearly too early for this. However, I have already mentioned how this line of attack leads to a beautiful phenomenological metaphor, namely, that of the ordinary waking state being a kind of *online* dreaming.[14] The constraints imposed by information flow from the sensory organs on the autonomous activity of this functional substrate during the day help to activate the phenomenal reality of waking consciousness. This view, in turn, lends credibility to the virtual reality metaphor for consciousness in general (see section 8.1), interpreting consciousness as a global phenomenal *simulation*, in which an integrated model of the world and a self within it is being generated. In some cases this global simulation is used as an instrument (i.e., a "virtual organ") in controlling behavior; in other situations this is not the case. In some situations this global simulation is fully transparent; in other situations we have a chance to make its phenomenality, the simple fact that it is just an appearance, cognitively available. As we shall see in section 7.2.5, there are also global phenomenal state classes, in which this information becomes *attentionally* available in a highly unrestricted manner.

Obviously, the most interesting feature of the global state class of dreaming for a philosophical theory is the fact that dreams are characterized by a particular *metacognitive deficit*. During normal dreams the phenomenal subject lacks any insight into the nature of the state. This is to say that the global state is itself not phenomenally represented as belonging to a certain class in terms of introspection$_2$ and introspection$_4$. A certain kind of contextual knowledge is absent during dreams, a feature called *Zustandsklarheit* in German ("state clarity"; Tholey 1984, 1987; see also Tholey 1983; Kahan and LaBerge 1994). Interestingly, we know of dreams in which the metacognitive deficit just referred to is not in existence. The transparency constraint, for this state class is not satisfied: During such dreams we have a full memory of our previous waking and dream life, and the phenomenal properties of agency, on the attentional, cognitive, and behavioral levels, are suddenly instantiated. Such states of consciousness have been called *lucid* dreams. During such dreams, the fact that it is dreaming is available to the subject of experience; it *knows* what kind of conscious state it is presently living through. Although rather rare, this additional phenomenal property of "lucidity" is of great interest for a general theory of phenomenal representation. It opens a new road to investigation and growth of knowledge toward a more differentiated understanding of phenomenal opacity and epistemological issues surrounding the notion of autoepistemic closure. In particular, the *phenomenal self* is characterized by a much higher degree of coherence and stability during the lucid dream. In order to search for a conceptually convincing analysis of such global state transitions, from which

---

14. This second phenomenological metaphor is, of course, a close relative of the first example presented in chapter 2, the notion of consciousness being an *online hallucination*.

we can then derive clear descriptions of possible explananda to be used in a search for their neural correlates, we obviously need to develop a differentiated theory of mental, as well as of *phenomenal*, self-representation. Hence, in the next chapter I again develop a number of simple conceptual tools with which this goal can be achieved.

4.3   The Concept of a Centered Phenomenal Model of Reality

In chapter 2 we opened a first conceptual tool kit. In chapter 3 we introduced a series of multilevel constraints to describe the representational deep structure of phenomenal experience and ended by introducing the working concept of a *phenomenal* mental model. All along I have been using and continuously enriching the notion of a comprehensive phenomenal "model of reality." Applying the perspectivalness constraint (*constraint 6*) to the notion of a model of reality, we naturally arrive at the concept of *subjective* experience and the notion of a *centered* type of conscious experience. All the case studies discussed so far have referred to phenomenal worlds, which were deviant in some aspects, but always centered on an experiencing self. The first defining characteristic of a centered phenomenal model of reality is that it possesses one singular, temporally stable phenomenal *self-representation*. The second defining characteristic is that this self-representation is *functionally anchored*. It has to be not only the experiential but also the *causal* core in the way in which the system emulates its own behavioral space.

However, please note that it is at least a logical possibility for representational systems to exist that operate under a *functionally* centered model of reality (e.g., by using an egocentric, internal simulation of their behavioral space in guiding their behavior) without exhibiting the phenomenal experience of selfhood or a consciously experienced first-person perspective. Somnambulism may be one example of this kind of configuration. The sleepwalker quite successfully moves around in her environment, obviously possessing an internal model of this environment having its origin in an accurate and continuously updated representation of her body. Yet she is not a subject of experience.

In order to develop a full-fledged consciously experienced first-person perspective, a third ingredient necessarily has to be added: a higher-order representation not only of the system itself but of the system *as currently interacting* with different aspects of the world (or itself). In order to arrive at a richer and more comprehensive understanding of the target phenomenon, one needs a theory of conscious self-representation and a conceptually convincing and empirically plausible theory about the representational deep structure of the phenomenal first-person perspective *itself*. In the second half of this book I make an attempt to develop such a theory. Therefore, we now have to move from the notion of a functionally centered reality-model to the truly *subjective* level of experience. We will have to start by introducing some very simple conceptual tools.

5 Tools II

5.1 Overview: Mental Self-Representation and Phenomenal Self-Consciousness

Large portions of this and the next two chapters parallel the discussions in chapters 2, 3, and 4. This chapter continues to develop a clearly structured and maximally simple set of conceptual instruments purposed to finding an answer to the problem of the phenomenal first-person perspective. After having done this, we take a closer look at the concrete representational vehicles enabling phenomenal self-consciousness. For a second time, a set of neurobiological, functional, computational, and phenomenological constraints are presented. In doing so I attempt to fill the concept of a "phenomenal self-model" with as much semantic content as is currently possible. Chapter 6 is the central chapter of this book, because the two most important theoretical entities are introduced: the "phenomenal self-model" (PSM) and the "phenomenal model of the intentionality relation" (PMIR). In chapter 7 a second set of neurophenomenological case studies are used to round off the discussion with another series of brief reality tests. Fortunately, as the general structure of the argument has already been laid out in the preceding chapters, we can now proceed at a much swifter pace.

5.2 From Mental to Phenomenal Self-Representation: Mereological Intentionality

Mental self-representation is the most interesting special case of mental representation. It is equivalent to a situation in which a system already engaged in the process of internal representation suddenly constructs an additional internal image of *itself*, as it were. It creates a new internal state—a *self-representatum*—with the help of which it generates a nonlinguistic description of itself, which at a later stage it can use to control self-directed behavior, become the object of its own attention, and cognitively refer to itself as a whole. In this case, the representandum is formed by the very system generating this mental self-representatum within itself. However, the realization of this special variant of our now well-known, three-place representational relation leads to a number of new logical, functional, representational, and phenomenal properties. To achieve a clearer understanding of these properties, it will be helpful to simply start by once again taking a look at the simple, fundamental schema of our teleorepresentational relation (box 5.1).

In comparison, let us look at the logical structure of the special case we are now considering (box 5.2). Before having a closer look at this new relative of our old friend, the three-place relation introduced in chapter 2, let me make a number of introductory remarks. Mental self-representation is a process by which some biosystems generate an internal, nonlinguistic portrayal of themselves. The states generated in this process are *internal* representations, as their content is only accessible to the respective system itself, and only in a specific manner—through a process which today we call phenomenal self-

Box 5.1

Mental Representation: Rep$_M$ (S, X, Y)

· S is an individual information-processing system.

· Y is an aspect of the current state of the world.

· X represents Y *for* S.

· X is a functionally internal system state.

· The intentional content of X can become available for introspective attention. It possesses the potential of itself becoming the representandum of *subsymbolic* higher-order representational processes.

· The intentional content of X can become available for cognitive reference. It can in turn become the representandum of *symbolic* higher-order representational processes.

· The intentional content of X can become globally available for the selective control of action.

Box 5.2

Mental Self-Representation: S-Rep$_M$ (S$_T$, X, S$_R$)

· S is an individual information-processing system.

· S$_T$ is the system as a whole, under a true teleofunctionalist description.

· S$_R$ is the system as a representandum, that is, the subset of those properties of the system which are currently accessible for its own representational capacities.

· X represents S$_R$ *for* S$_T$.

· X is a functionally internal system state.

· The intentional content of X can become available for introspection$_3$. It possesses the potential of itself becoming the representandum of *subsymbolic* higher-order self-representational processes.

· The intentional content of X can become available for introspection$_4$. It can become available for cognitive self-reference, that is, it can in turn become the representandum of *symbolic* higher-order self-representational processes.

· The intentional content of X can become available for the selective control of self-directed action.

---

consciousness. We may safely assume that this process once again is a higher-order representational process, itself only operating on physically internal properties of the system. Hence, it is important to distinguish three levels of conceptual analysis: Internality can be described as a phenomenal, functional, or physical property of certain system states.

We can now for the first time form a clearer concept of *phenomenological* internality. Phenomenological internality is the consciously experienced quality of "inwardness" accompanying bodily sensations, like a pleasant feeling of warmth; emotional states, like pleasure or sympathy; and cognitive contents, like a thought about Descartes's philosophical argument for dualism. All these forms of mental content are subjectively experienced as *inner* events and, in standard situations, as one's *own* states. Inwardness goes along with a prereflexive sense of ownership (not to be confused with phenomenal agency; see section 6.4.5). Phenomenological internality is consciously experienced "mineness." It is a characteristic feature of all contents integrated into the phenomenal level of self-representation, continuously, automatically, and independently of any high-level cognitive operations.

Internality in this sense is what certain philosophers (e.g., Frank 1991) have called "prereflexive self-intimacy." It generates the basic, nonconceptual content of self-consciousness, in which all higher-order forms of reflexive self-consciousness inevitably have to be anchored in order to avoid an infinite regression (see Bermúdez 1998; we return to this point in sections 5.4, 6.4.2, and 6.4.4). *Functional* internality, on the level of self-representation, is equivalent to the set of causal properties responsible for making the content of a self-representational process available for the conscious experience of only a single person or organism (but, see section 6.3.3). Functional internality can also be realized unconsciously. It only contributes to *experiential* internality in an indirect way. The first reading of functional internality is related to the personal level of description. There is only one individual in the universe that has the capacity to make this specific content available for conscious *self-representation* (see Nagel 1986; Metzinger 1993). Only *you* can become conscious of the content of your own, ongoing, and subpersonal process of mental self-representation as exemplifying your *own* properties. Only you possess the uniquely direct causal links, and that is what makes your self-representation an *individual* self-representation. Even if, in a science fiction scenario, the brain of another human being was hooked up to your brain so that it could directly read out the content of your current mental self-representation, this person could never—epistemically—self-represent this content as his or her *own* properties. This scenario could possibly work on the level of phenomenal content by including causal properties of your brain in the functionally internal set of properties on which this other person's self-consciousness supervenes, thereby allowing her to merely own your thoughts and feelings *phenomenally*, but this would, arguably, destroy the subject's personal identity. Nagel's problem could not be solved by making the phenomenal content of a bat available to you on the level of conscious experience—the deeper issue is what it is like to be a bat *for the bat itself*.

There is a second, subpersonal reading of functional internality. As explained in chapter 2 and in section 3.2.2 of chapter 3, it comes along with the constitution of an individual virtual window of presence. Conscious self-representational content is internal in the sense that it has been functionally defined as *temporally* internal by the system itself: it always depicts its content as the *current*, actual state of the system itself. Typically, functionally internal properties will be realized by the physically internal properties of the system. A third reading of "internality" then results from this: A phenomenal self-representatum, in an almost trivial and straightforward sense of physically simple, spatiotemporal internality, is an internal system state occurring in an individual organism or person. It supervenes locally. If all three forms of phenomenal, functional, and physical internality are simultaneously realized, the result is an embodied, individual and *present* phenomenal self.

Again, we now confront the problem of externalism and internalism, and the relationship between intentional and phenomenal content. The *intentional* content of mental self-representation can be formed by properties of the system, including all its relational and dispositional properties. Therefore it will frequently be fixed by facts external to the physical boundaries of the system and also by *possible* states of this system. However, the most fundamental level for individuating mental states subserving self-awareness is not their intentional content or the causal role they play in generating internal or external behavior (be it actual or possible). It is the level of phenomenal self-representation that counts. Whenever we speak about "*the* subject" or "*the* self" (committing the "error of phenomenological reification"), we are talking about the content of the *phenomenal self*. This is the content of an ongoing self-representational *process*. The folk psychology of self-consciousness naively, successfully, and consequentially tells us that a self simply is whatever I subjectively *experience* as myself. Arguably, the folk phenomenology of selfhood is the ultimate root of all theorizing about self-consciousness. This is why we have to start on the level of phenomenal content. Today we also know that a large amount of unconscious but functionally active, system-related information influences not only our behavior but also our thought and attention. Again, we have to answer the question of how mental and phenomenal self-representation differ from each other. Let us begin by looking at the concept of mental self-representation.

The concept of "mental self-representation" can be analyzed as a three-place relation between a single representandum (the system as a whole, in terms of those aspects that it can grasp with the help of its own representational resources) and a representatum (various, currently integrated internal states of the system) with regard to the same system (the system as a whole, under a teleofunctionalist description as embedded in a certain causal-teleological context). Self-representation is a process achieving the integrated representation of a system *for* itself by generating a singular, coherent, and appropriate internal state, functioning as the current self-representatum. Please note that on the level of *internal* (i.e., nonmental) self-representation there are likely to be many different functional modules representing a singular aspect like body temperature or blood sugar level in an isolated, nonintegrated fashion. *Mental* self-representation starts on the level of a single, integrated self-representatum tracking the system as a whole. If this structure satisfies certain additional constraints, it can become conscious.

A simple and clear way to explicate the notion of self-representation consists in introducing the notion of *emulation* while distinguishing three cases. An information-processing system S can represent a physical object in its environment. Call this process "object representation." In some cases, the object component will be another information-processing system: an information-processing system S_1 can represent another information-processing system S_2 in its environment. Call this "emulation." If $S_1 \equiv S_2$, then we have a case in which one information-processing system internally emulates *itself*. Call this process "self-representation." Ideally, the content properties of the self-representatum generated in this process would grasp the *relevant* target properties of the system. In advanced stages, this may involve representing the system *as an object*.

The "asymmetry" pertains to the second and third argument places of the relation S-Rep$_M$ (S_T, X, S_R). Again, the three-place relation of mental self-representation can be decomposed into a number of two-place relations. The relationship between S_T and X is a part-whole relation. A system S uses a physical part X of itself to achieve certain goals. This is what was meant by "mereological intentionality" in the heading of this section. The two-place relationship between S_T and S_R is the relationship of self-knowledge or, in its phenomenal variant, of self-consciousness. A system grasps epistemically or consciously experiences certain aspects of itself (namely, those accessible to its own representational resources) in order to achieve its own goals or to satisfy the adaptivity constraint on the subpersonal level. It becomes *an object for itself*, now being a subject and an object at the same time. However, this beautiful but too metaphorical way of speaking is dangerous. The relationship between X and S_R, between self-representatum and self-representandum, is an asymmetrical relationship, as explained in chapter 2. First, S_R and X are always thought of as distinct theoretical entities. Second, the relation only points in one direction; there is no situation in which it is identical with its converse relation. Third, self-representation of particular aspects of the system as a whole with the help of a distinct subsystemic part is intransitive. Therefore, we never have a situation where the system *as a whole* represents the system *as a whole*, and certainly not by *using* the system as a whole. It is a particular aspect (a subpersonal part of the system) that functions as a tool in representing a subset of the infinitely many properties the system has (i.e., a part

of these features) under a certain theoretical representation of this system (a certain set
of its aspects). It is important to note in which way the conceptual structure offered here
excludes idealistic conceptions of self-consciousness, as well as their problems. The car-
dinal problem for classical models of "reflexive" self-consciousness, for example, in
Fichte, was the problem of the identity of the subject versus its epistemicity: How could
something that was strictly identical to itself be separated into a knowledge relation? A
reflexive relation (like, e.g., similarity) is one that everything bears to itself. Please note
that the relationship between self-representatum and self-representandum, between X and
S_R in the structure proposed here is not a *reflexive*, but a *mereological* relation. It is a *part*
of the system—for example, the minimally sufficient physical correlate of the self-
representatum—which functions *for* the system as a whole by portraying, as it were, a
subset of the objective properties of this system. The two terms S_T and S_R refer to entirely
different aspects of the system: the system as a whole, theoretically described as embed
ded in a causal-teleological context versus that subset of its properties which is epistemically accessible to it by using its *own* internal resources for self-representation. Let us,
from now on, introduce the notion "S_T" for the system as a whole, possessing a true teleofunctionalist description, and "S_R" for the system as an object, that is, as potential representandum of its *own* self-representational capacities. Again, we can note that, as the
self-representatum is a physical part of the system, the system as a whole continuously
changes through the process of self-representation: it constantly generates new physical
properties within itself in order to representationally grasp a subset of its own objective
properties. There is not one rigid object (the content of self-representation), but an ongoing,
dynamical process of *self-containing*. This is a second reason why I have coined the
concept of "mereological intentionality" in the heading of this section. One aspect of the
philosophical intuition behind this way of framing the logical structure underlying mental
self-representation is that, at its core, self-consciousness is not a fully reflexive relation in
a traditional sense. Rather, it is a highly interesting kind of part-whole relation: a part of
the system functions as a representational instrument picking out certain aspects of the
system *for* the system as a whole. In almost all cases the mental content generated in this
event will be nonconceptual content.

Let me briefly point to an interesting issue, which, however, I will not pursue further
in this book. If we assume there is a kind of isomorphism underlying the representational
relation which justifies us in speaking about knowledge by *similarity* (as opposed to knowledge by truth), that is, if we assume that self-representatum and self-representandum stand
in a suitable similarity relationship to each other (which may well be founded in a complex,
higher-order, functional isomorphism; see S. E. Palmer 1978) while at the same time maintaining that the representatum doing the representing is a physical part of the system, then
obviously the process of internal self-representation turns the system into a *self-similar*

system. The interesting question is in how far this internal, representational concept of self-similarity can be related to more rigorous and formalized concepts of self-similarity, for example, in physics or mathematics.

The next step will have to consist in excluding the phenomenological fallacy (which I mentioned in chapter 2). Mental self-representation is an ongoing process. The self-representatum generated in the course of this process is a time slice, the content of the self-representational process at *t*. In principle, we could now once again commit the typical grammatical error characterizing the folk psychology of self-consciousness by treating the content of a singular time slice of the process of self-representation as an object. There is, in other words, a special variant of the phenomenological fallacy related to self-consciousness: describing the contents of phenomenal self representation as literal prop-erties of an internal and nonphysical object—namely, the *subject.*

Again, we have to differentiate two levels on which this unnoticed transition from a mental process to an imputed individual, from a sequence of events toward an indivisible mental object, could happen. The first level is constituted by *linguistic* reference to phenomenal states of self-consciousness. The second level is being formed by phenomenal self-experience *itself.* My claim is that there is an intimate connection between both of these levels and that analytical philosophy of mind should not confine itself to investigating the first level of content alone. Both phenomena are representational phenomena, and they are interdependent. The grammatical mistake mentioned above, leading to the reification of the self, is ultimately anchored in the functional architecture of our nervous system. The logical structure of conceptual self-reference is intimately connected to the deep representational structure of the phenomenal first-person perspective and the phenomenal self.[1] As we will see in the next chapter, phenomenal self-representation—and this is the *only* kind of self-representation generating content available for self-directed judgments (call this the "principle of phenomenal self-reference")—must also satisfy *constraint 2,* the presentationality of phenomenal content. Phenomenal self-representata form a class of states that are characterized by being activated within a certain window of presence. If this time window is larger than the basic neural processes leading to the activation of a coherent phenomenal self-representation, then a large amount of the fundamental, underlying processuality in the brain has, as has been explained extensively earlier, been "swallowed up." To give an example, what in bodily awareness we now experience as a

---

1. The typical philosophical mistake resulting from this interdependence of representational content is exemplified by Thomas Nagel's use of "I," when referring to what he calls the "objective self," for example, in Nagel 1986, chapter 4. As Norman Malcolm (1988) has pointed out, Nagel always uses "I" as a designator, as if referring to an object, and not as an indexical expression. Although the grammatical mistake can easily be pointed out, Nagel's conception retains phenomenological plausibility. In the next chapter we shall see why this has to be inevitably so (see sections 6.4.2 and 8.2 in particular, and Metzinger 1993, 1995a).

transtemporally stable, immediately given part of our "own" self in terms of a rather invariant and homogeneous background sensation is constituted by a functional process which systematically makes its own temporal properties unavailable for introspection₃, for attentional processing directed at one's current subpersonal self-representation (I return to this point at length in section 6.2.6). Second, the way we refer to the phenomenal content of self-consciousness using linguistic tools frequently ignores the underlying dynamics of information processing a second time. If naively we speak of *a* "content of self-consciousness" or *the* "content of *a* phenomenal self-representation," we reify the experiential content of a continuous representational process. This process is now frozen into an object, which this time is our "own" self, that is, a *subject*-object. We automatically generate a phenomenal individual and thereby run the risk of repeating the phenomenological fallacy. The core of the fallacy consists in the unjustified use of an existential quantifier within the scope of a psychological operator, this time when referring to self-consciousness. All we can justifiably say is that we are in a state which *normally* is caused by the presence of, for example, one's own body. We have seen earlier that phenomenal content is precisely that kind of content which entirely supervenes on internal and contemporaneous properties of the human nervous system. A brain in a vat, therefore, could at any time generate the full-blown phenomenal content of a conscious self-representatum. How do you *know* that you are in touch with your body? What precisely makes it *your* body? Also, in the special case of self-representation, it is true that such descriptions of phenomenal content do not refer to a privileged phenomenal individual—for example, "the self"—but only to an introspectively accessible time slice of the actual representational process—that is, to the content of this process *at t*. The vehicle carrying this content marked by a temporal indicator is what from now on I will call the self-representatum.

What is the *object*, the representandum, of self-representation? The most basic, and rather invariant, set of properties picked out by internal self-representation is obviously constituted by properties of the physical organism (see section 5.4 below). These may be properties of its internal chemical profile in particular (see, e.g., Damasio, 1999), and also of states of its internal organs, its spatial and kinesthetic properties, or relational properties with regard to other objects and agents in its environment. The representandum of S-Rep$_M$, S$_R$, is formed by *current* properties of the system.

It is at this point in our investigation that our simple conceptual tools start to yield highly interesting results for the first time. Again, we discover that one always has to presuppose a certain temporal frame of reference to be able to speak of a self-representation in "real time." Without specifying this temporal frame of reference an expression like "current state of the system" is devoid of content. Obviously, the physically realized processes of information conduction and processing in the brain will, for the process of self-representation, as for any other form of mental representation, consume a certain amount of time. Self-related information available in the central nervous system in a certain, very radical sense never is *actual* information. The simple fact of diverging conduction velocities for a host of different internal transducers—like the vestibular organ, proprioceptors in muscles and joints (like receptors in muscle spindles and Golgi tendon organs), tactile receptors (like Ruffinis corpuscle, the Racini and Meissner bodies, and Merkel cells) or visceral and pain receptors—makes it necessary for the system to define elementary ordering thresholds and windows of simultaneity in order to integrate these multiple, internal sources of information into a multimodal self-representation. We have already seen that many empirical data show how the conscious present is a *remembered* present. However, if the phenomenal Now itself is a representational construct, then the experiential *presence* of the self in the phenomenal world, the subjectively experienced actuality, "realness" and temporal immediacy integrating it into a complex multimodal scene, is itself a *virtual* kind of presence. In this more rigorous sense, the content of a conscious self-representation, on all levels (see section 6.4), is only a *possible* reality. Bodily self-modeling is not a real-time process; temporal internality in a strict analytical sense is never achieved. The ultimate realism of phenomenal self-consciousness, therefore, is generated by a possibility (the best hypothesis about the current state of the system available) being transparently represented as a reality (an immediately given fact). In short, mental self-representation is a process whose function *for* the system lies in approximatively depicting its own actual state within a certain, narrowly defined temporal frame and with a biologically sufficient degree of precision. It is not a process by which we truly are "infinitely close" to ourselves.

If a state described as self-representational fulfills a function *for* the system, we implicitly assume a context of goals and possible actions. At the beginning of this book I made teleofunctionalism one of the background assumptions for which I do not offer an explicit argument. This background assumption says that self-representational states as well possess causal properties, which are historical entities that underlie social and evolutionary constraints. They can be more or less adequate within a certain group of persons or under the selective pressure exerted by a specific biological environment. For instance, certain forms of self-representation can make successful cooperation with other human beings more or less probable, resulting in different reproduction rates. This finally leads us to a new and very unromantic, but telling, metaphor. It was first coined by Andy Clark (Clark 1989, p. 61): The phenomenal self can now be regarded as a *weapon*, developed in a cognitive arms race. Conscious selves are like instruments or abstract organs, invented and constantly optimized by biological systems. If an artificial system developed a rich and flexible form of self-representation, which, however, did not fulfill a function *for* the system, then it would not generate the kind of mental content which forms the epistemic goal of the current investigation (see section 6.2.8). However, as we have seen above, the conceptual difference between artificial and natural systems has already ceased to be an exclusive and exhaustive difference.

What about *internality*, the next defining characteristic of mental self-representation? Obviously, the intentional content of a mental self-representatum will, in many cases, include external, relational properties of the system. On the other hand, mental self-representation, in the sense intended here, generates states that are internal in a *temporal* sense. It exclusively depicts current properties of the system *for* the system. However, it only does so within a frame of reference defined by the system itself, a window of presence. The content of mental self-representation, therefore, is temporally internal content not in a strictly physical, but only in a derived functional sense related to the architecture of the system, to its self-generated "Now." Once again, we arrive at the following philosophical intuition: *Phenomenal* self-representation could be equivalent to the generation of those content properties that additionally supervene on internally realized functional properties of the system in a spatial sense. In chapter 2, our second conceptual background assumption was the local supervenience of phenomenal content on internal and contemporaneous properties of the system. For the case of higher-order self-representation this would mean that active self-representational content could only be accessed internally in a very specific manner. Phenomenal self-representation, therefore, has only currently active states of the system itself as its representandum, but achieves the goal of making system-related intentional content globally available for fast and flexible control of action, for cognition and attention.

There are now three readings of "internality," and there are now three different interpretations of the concept of a "system-world border" as well. Typically, the skin would constitute a physical system-world border. The notion of a *functional* system-world border, however, is a much more interesting issue, which may be more difficult to analyze. Let me give two examples. Utilizing the conception of "active externalism" we have seen how a system may functionally expand well across its physical boundaries, for example, by transiently establishing sensorimotor loops. A second example of a dynamic and functionally active self-world border, which is physically located *within* the system, is constituted by our immune system. The immune system operating within our bodies is constantly engaged in drawing and vigorously defending a self-world border, for example, by killing off germs or malignant cells. In doing so, it creates an immunological form of "inwardness" or "mineness." The third reading of "self-world border" is, of course, the *phenomenological* reading. Interestingly, conscious self-representation clearly seems to be a necessary precondition for the emergence of an experiential self-world border, and for the emergence of higher-order representational content like subject-object relations (see section 6.5) or genuinely cognitive self-reference (see sections 6.4.4 and 6.5.2).

We now have a whole set of conceptual constraints available, permitting us to introduce semantic differences between mental and phenomenal self-representation. As you will recall, in chapter 2 I introduced a refined version of the original Baars-Chalmers criterion of "global availability." This constraint served as a first and simple example of how multilevel constraints can be applied to the concept of mental representation to yield a very first working concept of phenomenal representation. Later, we saw that this constraint was actually a semantically "impoverished" version of *constraint 3*, the globality of phenomenal content. It turned out to be the formulation of the globality constraint on the functional level of analysis. I will now once again use this triple concept of global availability for attention, cognition, and behavioral control, *pars pro toto*, as it were, to arrive at a preliminary concept of phenomenal self-representation. The procedure is exactly the same as in chapter 2—just much shorter. In the next chapter, I apply a second set of multilevel constraints to arrive at a much richer and more realistic notion of phenomenal self-modeling.

Attentional Availability

Phenomenal self-representation generates content that can become the object of attentional processing. This type of attention is equivalent to the concept of introspection$_3$, which we formed in section 2.2, in terms of a phenomenal notion of "inner attention": the phenomenal representation of an internal system state, guided by attention, the intentional content of which now is constituted by a part of the world now represented *as internal*. Obviously, there are at least two ways in which attention can operate on an active self-representatum. During passive, process-oriented types of nonselective introspection$_3$—as, for instance, in "inner" daydreaming or effortless and exclusively introspective types of meditation—we find freely inward wandering attention, as it were, because the phenomenal property of agency, of executive consciousness related to the ongoing attentional process, is lacking. The second phenomenological state class, associated with a variable, but constantly controlled *focus* of conscious experience, does not seem to unfold spontaneously, because it is controlled by a phenomenal agent, the subject of attention. In these situations we consciously experience ourselves as deliberately pointing our attentional focus to our minds or bodies. An important phenomenal characteristic of this second set of states is that it is always accompanied by a subjective sense of effort.

Internal attentional processes, operating on an already active self-representatum, form the basis for the most basic and simple kind of phenomenal *subjectivity*. On a computational level, we introduced the notion of "functional subjectivity" in section 2.2. Subjectivity in this sense is a functional property of information active in the system, equivalent to this information only being available to the system as content of a nonphenomenal self-representatum, and in terms of uniquely direct causal links between this information and higher-order attentional or cognitive processes operating on it. The more interesting notion of "phenomenal subjectivity" arises if such links are links to the content of its *self-consciousness*. Inner attention is the simplest form of phenomenal subjectivity. It introspectively₃ represents subjective information in a way that does not lead to either external behavior ("phenomenal agency") or a mental approximation of concept formation ("*cognitive* self-consciousness"). Attention operating on a subpersonal self-representatum generates what philosophers call prereflexive self-awareness. In recent years it has become increasingly obvious that full-blown phenomenal subjectivity is rooted in such nonconceptual forms of self-awareness (e.g., see Bermúdez 1998; Metzinger 1993). Attention operating on an already active self-representatum generates precisely this form of nonconceptual mental content. Interestingly, there is also an epistemological reading of the functional notions of introspection₁ and introspection₃ to which the phenomenological notions of phenomenal objectivity ("experiential externality") and phenomenal subjectivity ("experiential inwardness") correspond. Types of prereflexive epistemic access and—in cases where cognitive availability is realized—types of conceptual self-reference correspond to the two different functional modes of presentation, in which information can be available within an individual system.

Cognitive Availability

I can only form thoughts about those aspects of myself which are given to me on the level of self-conscious experience. Call this the "principle of cognitive and phenomenal self-reference." Only information displayed on the phenomenal level of self-representation can, at a later stage, become the object of explicit cognitive self-reference and thereby initiate a process of self-directed reasoning. If there is a fundamental level of sensory self-awareness which is not cognitively available, then this level of information constitutes an aspect of myself which I can only explore in introspective₃ attention, in a meditative fashion as it were, but which can never become the object of truly concept-forming cognitive self-knowledge. It would then be ineffable self-*presentational* content (see section 5.4). Information given through self-*representation*, however, can be categorized and is available for long-term memory. It is information that can be classified, reidentified, and saved. It is the information forming the foundation of autobiographical memory. To the degree to which we approximate syntactically structured forms of mental self-representation we can be described as cognitive agents in the classic sense. Phenomenal, self-representational information is precisely that kind of information which enables deliberately initiated forms of self-directed thought. Self-initiated, explicit, and self-directed cognition can only operate on the content of an already existing self-representatum. If I want to engage in reasoning about *possible* properties of myself or about properties I have possessed in the distant past, I can only do so if I consciously simulate the exemplification of these properties *now*. It is this kind of hybrid, that is, opaque *and* transparent, self-representation that could be described as truly bridging the gulf between subpersonal and personal content.

Availability for the Control of Self-Directed Action

Phenomenal, self-representational information is characterized by enabling a specific class of highly selective behaviors: actions directed at the agent *itself*. Our autonomous nervous system constantly processes a large amount of organism-related information, for example, in regulating digestion, body temperature, and our internal chemical profile. This certainly is a kind of self-representation. However, as a large portion of this information is not available for the control of action, this form of self-representation is not *phenomenal* self-representation. In unilateral hemineglect (see sections 4.2.2 and 7.2.1) patients typically are not able to redirect attention to the left side of their body. This makes certain self-directed actions, for example, shaving the left side of their face or washing and dressing the left side of their body, impossible. It is as if the reduction of phenomenal content leads to a compression of behavioral space.

We have already seen how availability for the control of action has a lot to do with sensorimotor integration, as well as with the flexible and intelligent decoupling of sensorimotor loops. The activation of those *motor* representata and simulata preceding basic actions obviously is a kind of self-representation. It is interesting to note how *all* motor representation (be it a forward model or proprioceptive feedback) inevitably is a form of self-representation. The motor system necessarily is a part of the organism as a whole. Generally speaking, phenomenal information is information that can be directly integrated into the ongoing process of motor self-representation. What turns mental representations of ongoing bodily movements into conscious experiences? Can the criterion of availability for selective action and action termination be applied to the mental self-representation as a *currently acting* subject? Obviously the concept of "agency" will have to be differentiated and we seem to be in need of a concept of higher-order self-representation (see sections 6.4.3, 6.4.4, 6.4.5). For now, my proposal will be as follows: A mental representation of an ongoing bodily movement, a motor self-representation, is conscious if it can be *terminated*, that is, if the system as a whole can veto not only the representational process generating it but also its causal consequence, the overt action itself. In other words, and on a functional level of description, conscious action is precisely that behavior which can be vetoed or terminated at almost any point. Phenomenal self-representation of oneself as being someone who is now or currently acting makes the content of this phenomenal representation globally available for example, for the termination of this action by a higher-order form of control.

Reapplying our first, functional constraint of global availability as an example of a first constraint, we can now again formulate a preliminary, very simple concept of *phenomenal self-representation* (box 5.3). In the following two sections I develop this pre-liminary working concept further, in two directions, while gradually enriching it in content. However, one concluding epistemological remark is in order. According to the background assumptions of the current theory, internal self-representata generated by physical systems possess a property separating them from all elements of the internal model of the exter-nal *world*: in terms of content, they can never be completely empty. Remember that we have not only excluded ant colonies and stellar clouds but also angels and other non-physical beings from our intended class of systems.

Trivially, if an internal representation of the system itself exists, according to the fun-damental assumptions of any naturalist theory of mind there also has to exist a physical system which has generated it. I call this the "naturalist variant of the Cartesian *cogito*." Pathological or systematically empty self-representata may exist (see chapter 7), but their underlying existence assumption will never be false, because *some* kind of constructing system has to exist. Even if I am a brain in a vat or the dream of a Martian, from a teleofunctionalist perspective phenomenal self-representata are only given in the histori-cal context of a generating system. *Weaker* forms of phenomenal consciousness, possess-ing no true teleofunctionalist description (therefore not satisfying the adaptivity constraint; see sections 3.2.11 and 6.2.8), are, of course, interesting conceptual possibilities—for

Box 5.3

Phenomenal Self-Representation: S-Rep$_P$(S$_T$, X, S$_R$)

• S is an individual information-processing system.

• S$_T$ is the system as a whole, under a true teleofunctionalist description.

• S$_R$ is the system as a representandum, that is, the subset of those properties of the system, which are currently accessible for its own representational capacities.

• X phenomenally represents S$_R$ *for* S$_T$.

• X is a physically internal system state, which has functionally been defined as temporally internal.

• The intentional content of X *is* currently available for introspection$_3$. It is available as a representandum for *subsymbolic*, higher-order self-representational processes.

• The intentional content of X *is* currently available for introspection$_4$. It can become available for cognitive self-reference, that is, it can in turn become the representandum of *symbolic* higher-order self-representational processes.

• The intentional content of X *is* currently available for the selective control of self-directed action.

instance, when discussing machine subjectivity. But even an only weakly self-conscious machine would be justified in assuming that it possesses *some* kind of hardware. All the details of its current conscious self-representation may be false, but the underlying existence assumption is always justified. Of course, naturalism itself would have to be argued for by this machine, on independent grounds.

Mental and phenomenal models of the external world, however, can always turn out to be results of entirely misrepresentational processes or of pure, nonintended simulations. Ultimately, the system does not possess any kind of epistemic anchor in extradermal reality, preventing it from mistakenly ascribing referential character to some of its internal states. Self-representation, on the other hand, in principle possesses a higher degree of epistemic certainty and this is the modern, naturalistic formulation of the Cartesian intuition regarding the epistemic transparency of the cognitive subject to itself. As opposed to Descartes, who in the eighth paragraph of his *Second Meditation* could discover thought as inseparable from the ego, and from the perspective of the current theoretical model, the ego now *itself* becomes a thought, a very special kind of mental representation, which is functionally inseparable from the physical system unintentionally thinking *it*. It is this system, for example, the central nervous system of a biological organism, which really is the thinking thing. It generates *cogitationes* in the form of what I have called in Chapter 3 phenomenal mental models. However, as it is not able to internally represent those models *as models* (see section 6.2.6), it is not able to recognize its phenomenal ego—that is, the mental model of a *res cogitans*—as a product of its own, ongoing internal representational dynamics, but "confuses itself" with the content of this model. This leads us to discover a fundamental epistemic opacity (not to be confused with *phenomenal* opacity) underlying the generation of a phenomenal first-person perspective (see section 6.5), of what I like to call the "naive-realistic self-misunderstanding," automatically and subpersonally produced by a self-modeling physical system. In the following chapter we penetrate deeper into this core issue. However, it was necessary at this stage to point out how self-representation generates a higher degree of epistemic certainty than external-world representation. Let us now turn our attention to the logical structure of two further variants of self-directed, mental information processing. Fortunately, we can now be even briefer, as we have already encountered most of the essential issues.

5.3   From Mental to Phenomenal Self-Simulation: Self-Similarity, Autobiographical Memory, and the Design of Future Selves

Like mental self-*representata*, mental self-*simulata* are computational tools used by human brains. These tools have been used by biological systems to process as much information relevant to reproductive success and survival as possible in as fast and effective a manner as possible. However, self-simulata are precisely those instruments whose function consists in *not* achieving a high degree of covariance with the actual state of the system. Their content is formed by *possible selves*. Functionally speaking, they are system states that can be activated independently of actual, internal input and become embedded in representational states that phenomenally model possible worlds.

However, it is interesting to note one particular exception forming a further phenomenological constraint for any convincing theory of self-simulation: there are situations in which phenomenal representations of a possible self are *superimposed* onto a currently active model of the real world. For instance, while passively observing the activity of other players in a game of soccer in which you are not participating, you may constantly superimpose possible moves and complex bodily actions of yourself onto this perceptual scene, which is all the time phenomenally experienced as ultimately real. That is, there seems to be an interesting class of phenomenal self-simulations where possible selves, as it were, are not embedded in possible worlds, but in what is phenomenally taken to be the *existing* world. And as everybody knows, such processes (which resemble RBD or echopraxia) can also get out of control. Nevertheless, the paradigmatic example of mental self-simulation as the deliberate generation of counterfactual phenomenal selves is of course using them as tools in cognitive operations. They can help a system in planning its own future, in evaluating future, self-related goal states, and in generating adequate patterns of bodily action. Self-simulata also appear as agents in inner monologues, in fantasies, and in daydreams. What all these cases have in common is that they not only contain imaginary self-simulata but that the representation of a counterfactual self is only one component of a comprehensive, complex mental simulation of a possible world. On the level of phenomenal self-simulation the functional target obviously seems to be the global availability of facts about *potential* systems states, relative to certain situations. It is plausible to assume that the mental operations in question are not directly driven by proprioceptive input, but rather, for example, by the premotor cortex. Obviously, bodily events of all kinds may induce self-simulational processes, but they are not stimulus-correlated processes in the narrow sense previously introduced. Again, spontaneous self-related fantasies frequently occur when the body is resting, is engaged in routine activities, in situations in which it is not necessary to focus a large amount of attention on the current state of the body, or in which we are not directing any high-level cognitive processing at it. Let us briefly look at the new concept of mental self-simulation (box 5.4). Let us note an interesting characteristic of the process of self-simulation. Stimulus-correlated qualities of sensory awareness—like pain, the sensation of hunger, or the experience of vertigo caused by a disturbance in the vestibular system—generally cannot enter into processes of self-simulation (see also next section). It is very hard to conjure up an actual pain experience, or the fundamental, presentational aspect of hunger, or to become dizzy just by generating

Box 5.4

Mental Self-Simulation: S-Sim$_M$ (S$_T$, X, S$_R$)

· S is an individual information-processing system.

· S$_T$ is the system as a whole, possessing a true teleofunctionalist description.

· S$_R$ is a counterfactual state of the system, as available for its own simulational capacities.

· X simulates S$_R$ *for* S$_T$.

· X is a physically internal system state, which has been functionally defined as temporally external.

· The intentional content of X can become available for introspection$_3$. It possesses the potential of itself becoming the representandum of *subsymbolic* higher-order representational processes.

· The intentional content of X can become available for introspection$_4$. It can in turn become the representandum of *symbolic* higher-order representational processes.

· The intentional content of X can become globally available for the selective control of action.

---

self-related imagery alone. Again, exceptions are formed by all situations in which internal signal sources of sufficient strength confront the system. This may, for instance, be the case in dreams or other types of self-related hallucinations. Nonsensory contents of mental self-representation, however, can also be activated independently of the standard stimulus configurations, and then be employed in mental operations. They are now, as it were, not tracking the current self, but only a possible state of the system, a certain subset of its possible aspects or properties. Their content only weakly covaries with the state of the system. Self-related imagery lacks the qualitative "signaling aspect," which characterizes self-*presentata* (see next section). In subtracting the stimulus-correlated component of self-representation, we approach those aspects of system-related content that in principle can be made available *offline*. As for possible exceptions, we noted in chapter 2 that some people are eidetics by birth or have trained their brain by visualization exercises. Such people may, in nonpathological situations, be able to internally activate the full presentational aspect of an object representation, for example, with closed eyes imagine a strawberry as "really" red. There will certainly be similar cases for the capacity of phenomenal *self*-simulation. High divers or gymnasts might be able to actually *emulate* the effects of vestibular input in the phenomenal body image, when mentally simulating a series of spiral dives, somersaults, or breakneck leaps. Similar considerations may also apply to kinesthetic qualities activated by gifted dancers, mentally simulating possible moves; as we have repeatedly noted, in the highly complex domain of phenomenal experience any attempt to draw absolute conceptual lines is dangerous. Exceptions will always exist.

What makes an ongoing mental self-simulation a *phenomenal* self-simulation? Let us now apply our first standard constraint for the process of conscious experience (box 5.5). We can now see that every self-representation is simultaneously a self-*simulation*, because, epistemologically speaking, the actual state of the system presents us with at least one possible system state, one in which the representandum S_R is actually given. From the point of view created by the logical structure alone, self-simulation is the more comprehensive phenomenon, whereas self-representation is only a restricted special case. Self-representata are those kinds of self-simulata, whose function for the system consists in approximatively representing *actual* properties of the system in a sufficiently precise manner, using an adaptive frame of reference. If we integrate a genetic perspective into our investigation, self-representation turns out to be the earlier phenomenon, because only by perceiving the current state of their own body biological organisms could gradually develop those modules in the functional architecture of their nervous system which at a later stage could be used for a nonrepresentational offline activation of self-related mental states. Once again we discover how self-perception preceded attentional and cognitive self-consciousness, how perceptual phenomenal self-models were the antecedents of communicatively structured phenomenal models of the system (see section 6.3.3), how nonconceptual self-representation forms the anchor for higher-order types of abstract self-

Box 5.5

Phenomenal Self-Simulation: S-Sim$_P$ (S_T, X, S_R)

· S_R is an individual information-processing system.

· S_T is the system as a whole, possessing a true teleofunctionalist description.

· S_R is a counterfactual state of the system, as available for its own simulational capacities.

· X simulates S_R *for* S_T.

· X is a physically internal system state, which has been functionally defined as external.

· The intentional content of X *is* currently introspectively$_3$ available; that is, it is disposed to become the representandum of *subsymbolic* higher-order representational processes.

· The intentional content of X *is* currently introspectively$_4$ available for cognitive self-reference; it is disposed to become the representandum of *symbolic* higher-order representational processes.

· The intentional content of X *is* currently available for the selective control of action.

---

simulation. Only if you can feel yourself can you think, only if you can feel yourself can you have dreams about yourself and others (Cruse 1999).

Let me briefly point to an important phenomenological distinction. On a functional level of description we can easily differentiate between intended and nonintended self-simulations. There are two interesting higher-order phenomenal properties which can selectively be instantiated in the course of phenomenal self-simulations: "Mineness" and "agency" (see section 6.5). In nonpathological situations I always experience phenomenal self-simulata as my *own* states (however, see sections 7.2.1 and 7.2.2). Mineness is an interesting form of higher-order phenomenal content. When fantasizing about future selves, when fully immersed in a daydream involving childhood memories, or when automatically and internally talking to ourselves, we always experience these spontaneous phenomenal self-simulations as being our *own*. On the other hand, when consciously working on the design of a future life plan, when thinking about mistakes we made in our past love life, or when trying to generate a Nagelian objective self (Nagel 1986, chapter 4) within us, phenomenal self-simulations are accompanied by the additional experience of *agency*: Consciously we experience such self-simulations as intended, as deliberately initiated, as accompanied by a sense of effort and as executed by ourselves.

It is important to note that phenomenal self-simulations always unfold against the background of a stable and transparent phenomenal self-*representation*, against the background of a subject experienced as real, as a thinking, imagining person nevertheless continuously experienced as *present* within a world. Of course, deviant and exceptional phenomenal configurations do exist. In dreams, psychiatric disorders, and complex hallucinations, we can *lose ourselves*, because in such states the system—which we are—is only given to itself in the form of an entirely counterfactual self-model, an empty self-simulation. One of the sobering insights forced upon us by modern cognitive neuropsychology is that this critical distance toward our own inner images of ourselves can be completely annihilated by simple events on the physical level. If we lose the phenomenal anchor of embodiment (see next section) or if we drift off into the virtuality of pure phenomenal self-simulation, we "lose ourselves." Functionally speaking, our own mental images of ourselves are not our *own* images of ourselves.[2]

If we apply the transparency constraint to the process of phenomenal self-representation forming the background against which phenomenally opaque self-*simulations* can be run, we again confront the possibility that the phenomenal experience of a "simulative agent," a system deliberately initiating and causing phenomenal self-

---

2. According to Sigmund Freud's characterization of narcissistic hurts by science (Freud 1947) this is the third, namely, the *psychological* hurt. In Freud's own words, it consists in the fact of "the ego not being the master in its own house" (p. 7).

simulations, may be a functionally adequate fiction, which cannot be epistemically justified. Please note that this precisely might be a way of offering a naturalist analysis of the insight behind the Kantian concept of the transcendental unity of apperception (see also section 6.4.4).

If the intentional content of a phenomenal self-simulation is represented as temporally external, as not lying within the window of presence already functionally constituted by the system, it will be experienced as a simulation. In all other cases it will be experienced as a self-representation. Once again there is not only a functionalist but an epistemological and phenomenological reading of the concept of "self-simulation": What from a functionalist and an epistemological point of view *always* is a simulation can appear either as a self-representation or as a self-simulation on the phenomenological level of description. Taking on a strictly epistemological perspective one sees that phenomenal self-consciousness at no point brings us into a direct and immediate contact with ourselves. Self-knowledge by self-simulation always is *approximative* self-knowledge, leaping behind the real temporal dynamics characterizing the system in terms of its actual physical properties. On the level of phenomenal self-representation this fact is systematically deleted from the overall picture. Contents of noncognitive forms of consciousness (maybe with the exception of certain emotions) are always characterized by the phenomenal quality of "givenness" resulting from their transparency. Using the conceptual instruments of "self-representation" and "self-simulation" now available, we can avoid another typical variant of the phenomenological fallacy: concluding from the phenomenal immediacy of self-representation toward the *epistemic* immediacy or even "direct reference" involved in conscious self-knowledge. In the real world no such thing as direct reference exists—all there is is *phenomenally* direct self-reference. One can avoid the respective fallacy by keeping descriptive and epistemological contexts of use distinct, thereby doing justice to the obvious difference between phenomenal and epistemically justified content.

Under a teleofunctionalist analysis of phenomenal self-simulation we again discover that, for beings like ourselves, it is much easier to imagine states and activities of the system that are conducive to our survival and procreation; this is the familiar point about sexual and violent fantasies. Let us then, from a teleofunctionalist perspective, again differentiate three different types of phenomenal self-simulations: those, the proper function of which consists in generating globally available and sufficiently probable internal hypotheses about the *actual* state of the system (phenomenal self-representation); those, the function of which consists in generating globally available images and spatial portrayals of possible states of the system in action, particularly involving the constraints given by its behavioral space (e.g., pictorial self-representation and system-related imagery, forward models of the body and spatial reasoning in the planning of motor behavior, etc.); and, rarely, phenomenal self-simulations of the system as a *thinking* subject. To be able to phenomenally simulate yourself *as a thinking subject*, that is, as a system possessing rational beliefs, knowledge, and goals, I would claim, was precisely the most important building block for social cognition, that is, for the development of culture and complex societies. It was this specific kind of globally available representational content which led to conscious *inter*subjectivity. It also led to what I like to call the mental representation of the "first-person plural" (see section 6.3.3). It is only on this relatively rich and complex level of mental content that a phenomenal first-person perspective *plural* can emerge, as in the conscious experience of looking into another person's eyes and suddenly feeling that *we* understand each other right now.

Interestingly, everything I have said about the possible function of conscious experience in section 2.3—in terms of the world zero hypothesis—now also applies to the function of the transparent partition of the phenomenal self. By no means the only, but certainly a *central* evolutionarily relevant property of the interplay between self-representation and self-simulation is that it allows evaluation of the *distance* between two internal representations of states of the system itself. In order for the cognitive system not to get lost in its own self-simulations, it needs a reliable anchor on the level of self-representation. My hypothesis is that the phenomenal variant of self-representation generates exactly the anchor and the untranscendable background against which the distance between different models of the self and different routes from one possible model of the self to another can be analyzed and compared. In order to be biologically adaptive, one of the two active system representations has to be defined as the actual, as the *real* one. I will not repeat all the points made in section 2.3 but simply reiterate this hypothesis in the form of a special new variant, the "self zero hypothesis." An important factor in making the content of an ongoing self-representation the functional anchor and reference basis for concomitant phenomenal self-simulations consists in the fact that, as opposed to phenomenal self-simulata, it is not only transparent but depicted as *present* (see sections 6.2.2 and 6.2.6).

5.4 From Mental to Phenomenal Self-Presentation: Embodiment and Immediacy

By now it will be more than evident what the last two tools of the set of twelve simple conceptual instruments I have developed will be: *mental* self-presentation and *phenomenal* self-presentation. Once again, the analysis offered in chapter 2 will largely apply to this special case. However, here we will not need to take another long detour concerning the ineffability and cognitive unavailability of simple phenomenal content. Obviously, one of the beauties of the human variety of bodily self-awareness consists in its content being largely ineffable. Everything I have said, for instance, about the notions of Lewis qualia, Raffman qualia, and Metzinger qualia in section 2.4 of chapter 2 now applies as well. There will be categorizable forms of bodily sensation, as well as subtle, ineffable, "shades" and nuances in the many ways in which we perceive our own body from inside as well. And there may also be forms of simple bodily self-awareness, which are so fleeting that not only are they not available for cognition and perceptual memory but not even for self-directed *actions*. This is a first set of phenomenological constraints for every future theory.

The methodological difficulties may loom larger, however. For internally generated stimuli it will be much harder to make the difference between attentional availability and cognitive availability an empirically tractable feature. What sort of empirical experiments could we use to *precisely* delineate the discriminatory powers operating on visceral self-presentation, or on the subtleties of diffuse emotional self-experience related to mildly fluctuating hormone levels, or on the finest shadings of motion perception in proprioceptive consciousness? I am not saying such experiments are impossible. I find it hard to envision a strategy operating with the same degree of reliability that we, for instance, see in scientific research on conscious color perception or in psychophysics generally. How does one make the Raffman and Metzinger qualia constituting prereflexive *bodily* self-awareness in all its richness and elusive subtleness objects of a rigorous, empirical research strategy? Still, it seems plausible enough to assume that a very important component of human self-consciousness is constituted by a specific form or subset of nonconceptual content, which itself is strictly correlated with exclusively internal stimuli, and only rarely available for categorical perception, concept formation, and memory. It is plausible to assume that everything that has been said about Lewis qualia, Raffman qualia, and Metzinger qualia in section 2.4.4 will apply to bodily self-experience as well.

The original question remains: If we subtract the phenomenal content of a given self-*simulation* from an identical self-*representation*, what is the content component we are left with? We have seen that the teleofunctionalist and epistemological uses of the concept of "self-representation" can be reduced to that of "self-simulation." Self-representations, in both of these readings, are a subclass of self-simulations. However, on the phenomenological level of description, self-representation forms a distinct class of experiences opposed to phenomenal self-simulation. What are the elementary sensory components that can only result from a direct sensory contact to one's own body in their specific qualitative character? They are those states, whose function is to continuously signal the *actual presence* of the body (or certain of its aspects) to the system as a whole (box 5.6).

We have already seen that self-presentational content will typically be nonconceptual, cognitively unavailable, and therefore subdoxastic content. It also is *indexical* content in two interesting ways. First, in all phenomenal contexts it continuously points to the subject of experience (for a potential exception, see section 7.2.3), the conscious system itself; second, if it is a *phenomenal* form of self-presentation, it possesses the *de nunc* character already mentioned. It points to the phenomenal Now, by invariably satisfying the

Box 5.6

Mental Self-Presentation: S-Pre$_M$ (S$_T$, X, S$_P$)

· S is an individual information-processing system.

· S$_T$ is the system as a whole, under a true teleofunctionalist description.

· S$_P$ is the system as a *presentandum*, that is, an aspect of the current state of the system as available for its own *presentational* capacities.

· X presents S$_P$ *for* S$_T$

· X is a physically internal system state strictly correlated with *internally* generated stimuli.

· The intentional content of X can become available for introspection$_3$. It possesses the potential of itself becoming the representandum of *subsymbolic* higher-order self-representational processes.

· The intentional content of X *cannot* become available for introspection$_4$. It is *not* available as a representandum of symbolic higher-order self-representational processes.

· The intentional content of X can become available for the selective control of action.

---

presentationality constraint formulated at the end of chapter 2 and in section 3.2.2. However, at the present stage of our investigation it is not clear if it would be correct to say that self-presentational content is "tied to a first-person perspective." It certainly helps to *constitute* a first-person perspective, but it is as yet unclear if it can become the object of higher-order perspectival experience itself (see chapter 6). It is a narrow form of content, supervening on internal facts alone, and it is functionally grounded within the physical boundaries of the system itself. Let us again, *pars pro toto*, enrich this concept with our three standard constraints (box 5.7).

Conscious self-presentational content is interesting for a considerable number of reasons. It generates nonconceptual knowledge about the presence and current state of one's own body. This knowledge is not an episodic affair, it is permanent (as long as we are conscious), but in large portions only available for self-directed attention and self-directed action. If we are prepared to operate with the help of a narrow concept of knowledge, demanding propositional and conceptual formats for mental representation, we might (again alluding to Dretske 1969) call the continuous process of phenomenal self-presentation "nonepistemic feeling." Mental self-presentation, seen as a process, which can be either conscious or unconscious, is the most fundamental form of self-related knowledge, the most basic form of internal self-relatedness. On a functional level the generation of a self-presentatum allows a system to *feel itself* with the help of a self-generated internal state, the currently active self-presentatum.

Box 5.7

Phenomenal Self-Presentation: S-Pre$_P$ (S$_T$, X, S$_P$)

· S is an individual information-processing system.

· S$_T$ is the system as a whole, under a true teleofunctionalist description.

· S$_P$ is the system as a *presentandum*, that is, an aspect of the current state of the system as available for its own *presentational* capacities.

· X presents S$_P$ *for* S$_T$.

· X is a *functionally* internal system state strictly correlated with *internally* generated stimuli.

· The intentional content of X *is* currently introspectively$_3$ available for inward attention. It is disposed to become the representandum of *subsymbolic* higher-order self-representational processes.

· The intentional content of X is *not* currently introspectively$_4$ available for cognitive reference. It is *not* available as a representandum of symbolic higher-order self-representational processes.

· The intentional content of X *is* currently available for the selective control of action.

Self-presentata come in many different formats. As Holk Cruse (1999, p. 167) has pointed out, *tactile* self-presentation may be of particular importance in generating the self-world border. Our tactile sense, if directed to our own body, is the only sensory modality allowing for correlated and simultaneous stimulation. It also possesses a subtle affective tone. As opposed to, for example, our sense of temperature or our visceral self-perception it helps to create an accurate spatial frame of reference and a determinate border for the consciously experienced self (Cooney 1979, p. 22). Obviously, for human beings, there are also many ways in which we unconsciously, but continuously *feel ourselves* (as some readers may note, this way of putting the point is related to Antonio Damasio's concept of an unconscious "proto-self"; cf. Damasio 1999). On the preconscious, purely functional level of self-presentation we find a whole number of internal transducers, of internal sense organs transforming physically internal events within the boundaries of the system into events that are then *presented* as internal. By being presented *as internal* they gain the potential of becoming integrated into the organism's behavioral space. Information about these events may now become available for selection processes guiding self-directed behavior. As functional internality is not the same as phenomenal internality, this may not be necessarily so. It is easy to imagine configurations in which internally generated self-presentational content—to give two examples, an unpleasant sensation originating from a slipped disk or an unconscious intestinal irritation—is, on the phenomenal level, integrated into the conscious experience of *another* person, into a phenomenal person-model *as external*. We would then, transparently, experience this other person as somehow "unpleasant" or as "irritating" and would probably be searching for an explanation on the cognitive level.

If we proceed to the genuinely phenomenal level of self-presentation by introducing further constraints (like global availability for attention and action control) we are confronted with a number of hard questions: Is self-presentational content, like presentational content, *modality-specific*? Does it make sense to call the elementary phenomenal body image a supramodal or multimodal representational entity? How would we arrive at a consensus if our phenomenological descriptions of bodily self-experience turned out to be contradictory? When discussing the functional properties leading to the globality constraint in section 3.2.3 we encountered the notion of "causal density." Self-presentational content may be that partition of our conscious model of reality that (in terms of "vehicle properties") is characterized by the highest degree of causal density, and that (in terms of its "content properties") is characterized by the highest and most reliable degree of covariance with certain physical properties of the system it continuously tracks and monitors. If we look at bodily awareness as a whole, we discover two striking features: First, bodily self-perception seems to be the only kind of sensory perception which continuously possesses one and the same object only (see the philosophical notion of a "sole-object view" for bodily self-awareness, as introduced by Martin 1995, p. 273). Second, the number of interoceptors and internal transducers is *much* higher than for any other sensory modality. A large number of tactile mechanoreceptors and proprioceptors, the nociceptors underlying pain experience, visceral receptors, and the activity of the vestibular organ, as well as a whole range of specific brainstem nuclei (for details concerning their functional neuroanatomy, see Parvizi and Damasio 2001 and figure 5.1) constantly signaling the profile of the internal chemical milieu of the organism *to* the organism, all contribute to the presentational aspect of the conscious perception of one's own body (Damasio 1999, chapter 8; Damasio 2000). Marcel Kinsbourne has termed the illustrative concept of a "background 'buzz' of somatosensory input" (see Kinsbourne 1995, p. 217), which points out one important aspect of this situation. However, it is important to understand that this process is not a simple upward stream, but one that sets a stable functional context by tying the modulation of cortical activity to the ultimate physiological goal of homeostatic stability (Parvizi and Damasio 2001, p. 152). This context is an exclusively internal context. It subordinates even "higher" (e.g., cognitive) forms of processing to the goal of biological self-preservation. Bodily self-consciousness is, phenomenologically as well as functionally, the most important *source of invariance* human beings possess.

Body-directed attentional processing then makes "islands" of heightened preconceptual self-awareness emerge from this background. Trivially, whenever phenomenal self-

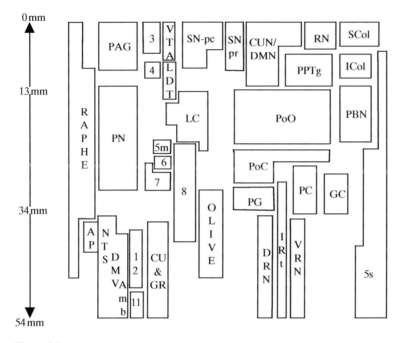

Figure 5.1
The reticular brainstem nuclei, a central aspect of the conscious self's functional and physical anchorage. The brainstem gray matter, including the region traditionally known as the reticular formation, is organized in nuclei. A nucleus is a three-dimensional collection of neurons which is usually aligned in parallel to the long axis of the brainstem. There are two sets of nuclei, one on the right and the other on the left side of the brainstem. Here, only the collection of nuclei on one side of the brainstem are shown. As the figure illustrates, each nucleus has its own idiosyncratic position within the brainstem. Some extend throughout the entire brainstem (such as the sensory trigeminal nucleus, 5s) whereas others (such as the area postrema, AP) occupy a small region and extend only a few millimeters or less. The size and the shape of the columns, as shown here, reflect the relative area of the brainstem occupied by the nucleus. For example, the size of the raphe nucleus varies according to the caudorostral extent of the brainstem. It is largest at the junction between the pons and medulla or between the pons and the midbrain. Its size is by far the least at the level of the lower pons. Abbreviations: 3, oculomotor; 4, trochlear; 5, trigeminal motor; 6, abducens; 7, facial; 8, vestibulochoclear; 12, hypoglossus; Amb, ambiguus; CU & GR, cuneate and gracile; CUN/DMN, cuneiform and deep mesencephalic; DMV, dorsal motor nucleus of vagus; DRN, dorsal medullary reticular complex, including the region of the subnucleus reticularis dorsalis; GC, gigantocellularis; ICol, inferior colliculus; Int, intercollicular; LC, locus caeruleus; LDT, laterodorsal tegmental nucleus; NTS, nucleus tractus solitarius; OLIVE, olivary complex; PAG, periaqueductal gray matter; PBN, parabrachial; PC, parvocellular; PG, paragigantocellular; PoC, pontis caudalis; PoO, pontis oralis; PPTg, pedunculopontine tegmental nucleus; RN, red nucleus; SCol, superior colliculus; SN-pc, substantia nigra pars compacta, SN pr, substantia nigra pars reticulata; TG, sensory trigeminal nucleus; VRN, ventral reticular complex. (Adapted from Parvizi and Damasio 2001, p. 143.)

consciousness emerges, the body exists as well. The body is the *only* perceptual object that is constantly given. On the philosophical level of analysis the most relevant issue is to demonstrate how the object being so experienced must be experienced by the subject as *itself* (Martin 1995, p. 283; see section 6.2.6). On the neurocomputational level it forms an important source not only of invariance but also of functional stability for the system, eventually leading to what we consciously experience as the centeredness of phenomenal space. Interestingly, there are forms of self-consciousness which completely lack bodily awareness—"Cartesian configurations" as it were (see section 7.2.2 in particular, but also 7.2.3.2). It is also important to note that in nonpathological configurations bodily self-experience will often completely recede into the background of phenomenal experience. It will be attentionally *available*, but often not attended *to* at all. Obviously, as phenomenal self-presentation constitutes the most invariant form of phenomenal content, it frequently will almost be an implicit form of content, only expressed as a subtle background presence. It seems safe to say that the phenomenal body percept, at any given time, is an integrated phenomenal whole, just like other multimodal percepts given through sensory perception of the external world (Metzinger 1995c). It is what we have termed a phenomenal mental model. Introspective attention, however, will be able to discriminate different aspects of presentational content which are integrated into this whole. This kind of introspective experience corresponds to the notion of introspection$_3$ (subsymbolic metarepresentation operating on a preexisting and coherent self-model) introduced in chapter 2. Again, introspectively discriminable self-presentational content is characterized by representational atomicity, and therefore appears as homogeneous and immediately given. Arguably, the inward feeling we have of our own body is *the* paradigmatic example of homogeneity. Phenomenal interoception truly is ultrasmooth.

The process of self-presentation realizes a unique functional property, which is of great theoretical relevance to understanding how the phenomenal self can be the center of our conscious world-model (see sections 6.5 and 6.3.1): Self-presentational content realizes a *persistent functional link*, which continuously anchors the representational vehicle (and thereby its content as well) in the system's physical basis. Persistence does not exclude dynamical structure. It is important to note how extremely fine-grained the microfunctional properties contributing to phenomenal embodiment actually are in human beings (and likely in many other animals). An important and invariant component of the physical correlate of this part of the self-model is formed by *neurohemal organs*. Neurohemal organs are those areas of the brain where it is in direct causal contact with the *molecular* dynamics of body fluids, with hormone levels, the temporal evolution of quantitative relationships between different transmitters, and so on. The enormous subtlety and the wealth of ineffable nuances involved in human self-presentation originate in the subtlety and richness of the physical world, in low-level processes of biochemical self-organization. These utterly subject-free, but self-stabilizing processes constantly modulate the internal information flow underlying the conscious self-model. It is interesting to note how all current technological attempts at creating truly embodied artificial agents, for example, in robotics, are many orders of granularity away from the *truly* bottom-up solution Mother Nature long ago found on its way to physically realized subjectivity.

In a living, evolving system something like absolute invariance never exists. However, the representational structures generating self-consciousness differ from all other phenomenal representations by possessing a persistent self-presentational core. It creates a highly invariable form of content globally available for attention and action, in turn generating the phenomenal experience of certainty about one's own existence: *I do exist, because I feel myself.* If this is true, I am committed to the prediction that experiential subjects completely unable to *feel themselves*, via globally available self-presentational content, may on the cognitive level be led to the inevitable conclusion that actually they don't exist (see section 7.2.2). This persistent functional link is one of the defining characteristics of the concept of a phenomenal self-model, to which we finally turn in the next chapter (figure 5.2). Let me point out that it may be precisely the causal link from mind to body, for which philosophers have intuitively been searching for centuries. If you would metaphorically interpret the conscious self-model of a system as its "soul," then *this* is the place where the soul is most intimately linked to the body. It is not Descartes's pineal gland, but rather the upper brainstem and the hypothalamus. Of course, from a third-person perspective, objective psychophysical correlations are something that is much more intricate and complex (see Metzinger 2000a,b). And the NCC of the phenomenal self is highly distributed. However, the structure I have described as self-presentation is the causal anchor of the *phenomenal* self in the human brain. Its content properties are intimately linked to its causal properties due to the stability achieved by the elementary bioregulatory dynamics out of which it grows.

In section 3.2.7 we discussed the notion of "phenomenal transparency," and in section 6.2.6 of chapter 6 we apply the conceptual tools now already developed to the idea of conscious self-representation. One of the centrally important aspects of phenomenal transparency is the inability of a given system to experience, that is, to consciously represent, the vehicle-content distinction *from the first-person perspective.* Transparency creates the illusion of naive realism: the inability to recognize a self-generated representation *as* a representation. At this point in our investigation it is important to draw attention to the fact that there are also important properties of the human self-model for which the vehicle-content distinction cannot be interestingly made any more, but on a *conceptual* level and *from the third-person perspective.* The persistent functional link anchoring our self-representation in our brains is the paradigmatic example of such a property: In developing an adequate, comprehensive theory about this link we have to shift from the representa-

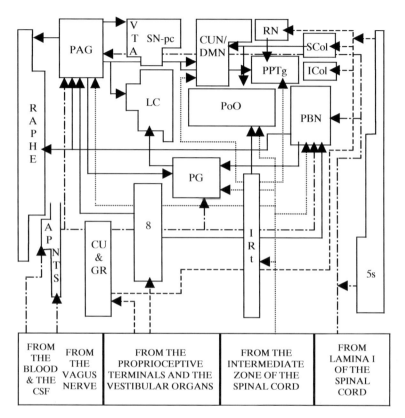

Figure 5.2
Important aspects of the persistent causal linkage generated by a continuous source of internally generated input: afferents to brainstem reticular nuclei. The brainstem reticular nuclei receive afferents from various sources. The state of the organism is portrayed in its multiple dimensions by incoming afferents signaling the current state of the internal milieu and the viscera, including the afferents from lamina I of the spinal cord (dashed-dotted lines), and the vestibular system and musculoskeletal frame (dashed lines). There are also afferents from the deeper zones of the spinal cord conveying signals about ongoing changes in the state of the organism as it interacts with an object (dotted lines). Solid lines represent the local connections within the brainstem nuclei. For abbreviations, see figure 5.1. (Adapted from Parvizi and Damasio 2001, p. 148.)

tional to the functional level of description. The conscious self, on this level, has to be understood as something that is fully integrated into the causal network constituting the physical world. In other words, there is not only a representational self-model but also a *functional* self-model. Many important properties determining the conscious experience of embodiment are not content properties, but causal properties. There will be a level of elementary bioregulation, arguably a level of molecular-level, biochemical self-organization, at which it simply is forced—from a conceptual third-person perspective—to maintain the distinction between content and vehicle. On this level mind is anchored in life, self-representation is better described as self-*regulation*, and it is much more fruitful to speak of functional self-preservation or of physical self-organization than of mental self-representation or self-simulation. Unfortunately, it is hard to decide this issue today. As soon as more empirical data are available, it will be a task for philosophy to demarcate a more fine-grained level of description on which it is plausible to assume a full match between content and causal role, that is, the *identity* of vehicle and content. On this level we may achieve a deeper understanding of the difference between experiencing ourselves *as* embodied and *being* embodied. Self-presentational content is the natural starting point for this type of enterprise.[3]

In this context, it is also interesting to note that there is one decisive part of our bodies that is self-presentationally blind. This part is the brain itself. It possesses no self-directed sensory mechanisms at all. For instance, we know from neurosurgery done on conscious patients that it is insensitive to pain. The body can feel itself with the help of the brain, but the *brain* is unable to directly feel itself. It is the blind spot of self-representation as it were. As a medium it is *functionally transparent* to the organism it supports, for instance, in functionally appropriating and owning itself with the help of a conscious self-representation. In this way, self-presentational content is safely anchored in a medium which never interferes with the generation of this content as such, because it can never become the intentional object of the presentational dynamic it generates.

---

3. Please recall the subtle residues of Cartesian dualism inherent in the vehicle-content distinction, mentioned in chapters 2 and 3. It always tempts us to reify the vehicle and the content and to conceive of them as distinct, independent entities. As noted above, any more empirically plausible model of representational content will have to describe it as an aspect of an ongoing *process* and not as some kind of abstract object. What we need is *embodied* content, as it were—an ongoing and physically realized process of *containing*, not "a" content. In a perceptual, sensorimotor loop (as in consciously seeing the book in your hands right now) the interesting point is that a perceptual object becomes *functionally internal* through the representational process of episodically "containing" it. However, it stays physically external—it is still a distinct physical element of extraorganismic reality. It is interesting to note how this second condition is not fulfilled for self-presentational content. As opposed to self-representational and self-simulational content, which can depict all sorts of relational and possible properties of the organism, the interesting subset of self-*presentational* content is best analyzed as a functional containing of properties that exclusively are functionally *and* physically internal properties of the system itself. What is eventually needed, therefore, is a mathematical model of a certain part of the neural dynamics in the brain that can be plausibly interpreted as describing an ongoing, but completely internal process of "self-containing."

Please recall that I introduced presentational content as the content of a nonconceptual indicator. Self-presentational content is the content of a continuously active analogue indicator, pointing right to the physical basis of the representational system, in any given context, thereby unequivocally determining who is the agent, who is the owner of bodily sensations, who is the representational system, and who is the experiencing subject. From the first moments of waking up till the last flicker of fading consciousness at night, we always are *embodied* experiential subjects, because the permanent source of internally generated signals forming the foundation of self-bodily consciousness is incessantly active. Functionally speaking, the set of microfunctional properties realized by the minimally sufficient neural correlate of conscious self-presentational content will not be completely invariable. Of course, bodily experience and our capacity to *feel ourselves* may, for example, undergo considerable change in the course of a lifetime, but it still has the highest internal correlation strength in comparison to all other relevant sets of microfunctional properties—at least this is one empirical prediction following from my analysis. In terms of Tononi and Edelman's "dynamical core-hypothesis" the claim is that there is one and exactly one dynamical *subcluster* with a CI-value higher than that of the overall dynamical core. Phenomenologically speaking, this reassuring, highly invariant source of body-related "nowness" leads to the phenomenal quality of *self-certainty*, of intuitively relying on the coherence, the presence, and the stability of elementary bioregulatory processes and the body in general. Consequently, any disturbances in the underlying neural functions are experienced as particularly threatening (for case studies, see sections 7.2.2 and 7.2.3).

Epistemologically speaking, however, the subjective experience of certainty transported by this kind of phenomenal content is unjustified. As we have seen, phenomenal content supervenes on internal and contemporaneous properties of the human brain. A disembodied brain in a vat, therefore, could in principle realize precisely the same degree of experiential certainty going along with our ordinary conscious experience of embodiment. The minimally sufficient neural correlate of bodily consciousness could exist without fulfilling any function *for* the system (because there *was* no system), and the indexical, nonconceptual content generated by it could point "nowhere" (because there was no extended physical basis "to" which it could point). The phenomenal self-presentatum would then possess qualitative character, but no *intentional* content. If its information flow was simulated on an artificial system, the resulting phenomenal content would only be *weakly* conscious, because it would not satisfy the adaptivity constraint formulated in section 2.3.11 (see also section 6.2.8).

In chapters 2 and 3 we encountered the phenomenal quality of "instantaneousness." For presentational content in particular it is true that the process by which it is activated and the temporal aspects of its causal history are not being phenomenally modeled. On the phenomenal level of processing this leads to a kind of mental content, which is experienced as temporally immediate, as simply given in a direct, instantaneous manner. This in turns leads to the *transparency* of phenomenal representata, which we have already used as a centrally important conceptual constraint in section 3.2.7. Phenomenal instantaneousness, immediacy, and transparency lead to an implicit epistemological assumption, namely, to naive realism. It is interesting—and of maximal theoretical relevance—to now apply these insights to consciously experienced *self-presentational* content as well.

Phenomenologically, feeling our body does not seem to be a time-consuming process. Directing our introspective attention to specific qualities of bodily experience may take a certain amount of time, but preattentive experience certainly presents them as immediately given. Self-presentational content is transparent: We are not aware of the medium in which it is activated and of the internal vehicle carrying it; we simply "look into our body." As agents, we *live* our body. Self-presentational content is like a window through which we look into the internal dynamics of our own body, while never seeing the glass of the window itself. This type of representational relation can interestingly be described as a *mereological* relation on the level of functional analysis: A *part* of the organism—the "window," chiefly realized by structures in the brainstem and hypothalamus (see, e.g., Parvizi and Damasio 2001)—functions as an epistemic instrument for the system as a *whole* in gaining nonconceptual knowledge about itself. Temporal immediacy then leads to the type of phenomenal certainty about the existence of one's own body which I have just described. Therefore, necessarily, we are caught in naive realism with regard to the presence of our own body as well. As usual, phenomenal immediacy does not imply epistemic justification. A belief that our own body actually exists cannot be justified by the internal availability of phenomenal self-presentational content. If we are a brain in a vat, this belief might be false, while an identical form of phenomenal, self-presentational content is active. Interestingly, *some* representational system has to exist according to our background assumption of the naturalized Cartesian *cogito*. Our specific belief contents about the presence and existence of our own bodies might always be false. The proper function of self-presentational content (e.g., indicating the current presence of one's own body for the organism) might not be realized anymore, the presentandum might be absent, but a more generalized existence assumption will still be justified. The only question is *how* a brain in a vat could find independent theoretical arguments justifying this assumption. How can you be a realist without being an embodied member of a scientific community? We return to the philosophical issue of the immunity to failure of misidentification in chapter 8.

Now we have a much clearer understanding of the different notions of "introspection" and "subjectivity," which were introduced in chapter 2. In addition, we have seen how the three different versions of the concepts of "global availability" and of "presentational content" can be usefully applied to the special problem of self-consciousness. We have also completed our initial set of simple conceptual instruments by introducing self-representation, self-simulation, and self-presentation, each in a mentalistic and phenomenalistic variant. Our tool kit is complete. Therefore, we are now approaching the stage at which we can begin to give more specific answers to our core question regarding a possible representationalist analysis not only of consciousness as such but of the phenomenal self and the *first-person perspective*. What we now need in order to avoid any empty, artificial scholasticism is a deeper understanding of the mechanisms by which an information-processing system can generate such structures. We need to look at the representational *deep structure* of self-consciousness and of the phenomenal first-person perspective. What is now needed is a deeper understanding of the concrete neurocomputational instrument, which is able to integrate all the three functions that I have conceptually described as self-representation, self-simulation, and self-presentation, of the actual tool which enables the human brain to transiently generate a genuine, phenomenal self. We have to form a working concept of a special virtual organ, the *phenomenal self-model*. In the next chapter, I introduce two highly interesting theoretical entities: the phenomenal self-model and the phenomenal model of the intentionality relation.

6 The Representational Deep Structure of the Phenomenal First-Person Perspective

6.1 What Is a Phenomenal Self-Model?

In chapter 3 I introduced the working concept of a phenomenal mental model. My first step in this chapter is to introduce the hypothetical notion of a phenomenal *self*-model (PSM). In order to do so, I will again, but briefly, enrich this new concept by specialized versions of the constraints already encountered in chapter 3. From section 6.5 onward I will then investigate how a PSM, integrated into a yet more complex, higher-order form of representational content, forms the central necessary condition for a conscious *first-person perspective* to emerge on the representational as well as on the functional level of description. After we have developed our two sets of basic conceptual instruments, it is now time to introduce the two central theoretical entities characterizing the current approach: the PSM and the "phenomenal model of the intentionality-relation" (PMIR). Let me start by making the concept of a PSM intuitively plausible for you by highlighting a number of its defining characteristics. The hypothetical term of a PMIR will then be defined in section 6.5.

The content of the PSM is the content of the conscious self: your current bodily sensations, your present emotional situation, plus all the contents of your phenomenally experienced cognitive processing. They are constituents of your PSM. Intuitively, and in a certain metaphorical sense, one could even say that you *are* the content of your PSM. All those properties of yourself, to which you can now direct your attention, form the content of your current PSM. Your self-directed thoughts operate on the current contents of your PSM: they *cannot* operate on anything else. When you form thoughts about your "unconscious self" (i.e., the contents of your *mental* self-model), these thoughts are always about a *conscious* representation of this "unconscious self," one that has just been integrated into your currently active PSM. If you want to initiate a goal-directed action aimed at some aspect of yourself—for example, brushing your hair or shaving yourself—you need a conscious self-model to *deliberately* initiate these actions. Of course, there is unconscious behavior like scratching or automatic self-protective behavior—for instance, when a ball suddenly comes flying toward you at high speed. We can also imagine a sleepwalker scratching himself or even avoiding a ball, or an epileptic patient with an absence automatism brushing his hair or shaving. All these are not self-directed actions, they are self-directed *behaviors*; a conscious process of goal selection does not precede them. There is no PSM. Further examples of unconscious, but functionally active regions in the self-model are the body schema (see section 7.2.3) and low-level resonance mechanisms implemented by the mirror system in many nonlinguistic creatures (see section 6.3.3). The unconscious body schema allows you to automatically keep your bodily posture, in a seemingly effortless manner. A flock of birds on the beach suddenly, as if "telepathically connected," starting to fly away in the same direction, or large schools of fish rapidly changing direction when a predator is perceived by one of them, are examples of successful and highly intelligent social cognition mediated by the unconscious self-model, therefore *not* involving any phenomenal type of goal representation.

There are also many situations in which a previously unconscious partition of the self-model suddenly *becomes* conscious, that is, globally available. This can also be a gradual process. For example, Jonathan Cole (Cole 1997, p. 470*f.*; see also Hull 1992) describes the case of a patient who went blind and for whom—due to lack of feedback, for example, by the conscious experience of other people smiling back at him—previously unconscious motor programs gradually became integrated into his conscious self-model. This patient started to become aware of his facial behavior, of the movement of his facial muscles, when smiling at other people. He now even discovered a sense of muscular effort involved in what for us is an effortless, transparent, and seemingly automatic way of social communication. In other words, facial *behavior* had now turned into goal-directed facial *action.*[1] We have seen how one illuminating way of looking at phenomenal mental-models is by analyzing them as computational or representational tools, making integrated information globally available for the system as a whole. Classes of phenomenal mental-models are classes of computational tools, in their activity subserving distinct types of phenomenal content. PSMs are a specific, and highly interesting example of such a class. Their function is to make *system-related information* globally available in an integrated fashion.

From a logical and epistemological perspective it is helpful to differentiate between simulation and emulation, in order to further enrich the concept of a PSM. We can then, in a second step, conceptually analyze the PSM as a special variant, namely, self-emulation. An information-processing system can internally *simulate* the external behavior of a target object (see section 2.3). A typical example is a computer used for meteorological prediction, generating a weather forecast by simulating the movement of clouds, temperature shifts in the atmosphere, and so on. More generally, the simulation of a target system consists in representing those of its properties that are accessible to sensory processing, and the way in which they probably develop over time. Some information-processing systems, however, form special cases in that they can also *emulate* the behavior of *another* information-processing system. They do so by internally simulating not only its observable output but also hidden aspects of its internal information processing itself. Such hidden aspects can consist in abstract properties, like its functional architecture or the software it is currently running. Abstract properties could also be content properties of certain repre-

---

1. "Nearly every time I smile, I am aware of it . . . aware of the muscular effort: not that my smiles have become more forced . . . but it has become a more or less conscious effort. It must be because there is no reinforcement . . . no returning smile . . . like sending off dead letters . . . I can feel myself smiling . . . must ask someone if it is true (17 September 1983)." (Hull 1992, quoted in Cole 1997, p. 470).

sentations currently active in the target system. For instance, in social cognition, it may even be necessary to internally emulate the way in which the content of certain goal representations in a conspecific is currently changing (see also section 6.3.3). A "clever" Turing machine pretending to be a "stupid" Turing machine, or a good human actor is an example of this type of situation. Emulation then becomes a simulation not only of observable, but also of abstract, functional, and representational properties of a given target system. It is the third possibility that is of particular interest from a philosophical perspective, the possibility of reflexive or *self-directed* emulation. Self-modeling is that special case, in which the target system and the simulating-emulating system are identical: A self-modeling information-processing system internally and continuously simulates its own observable output as well as it *emulates* abstract properties of its own internal information processing—and it does so *for* itself. Using a term from computer science, we could therefore metaphorically describe self-modeling in a conscious agent as "internal user modeling." In human beings, it is particularly interesting to note how the self-model simultaneously treats the target system "as an object" (e.g., by using proprioceptive feedback in internally simulating ongoing bodily movements) and "as a subject" (e.g., by emulating its own cognitive processing in a way that makes it available for conscious access).[2] This is what "embodiment" means, and what at the same time generates the intuitive roots of the mind-body problem: the human self-model treats the target system generating it as subject and object *at the same time*. It is interesting to note how such a self-model could either be conscious or unconscious. Only if a coherent representational structure is formed that satisfies the constraints for conscious contents, will a PSM come into existence.

Looking at the representational content transported by a PSM we discover that it integrates a large variety of different data formats. The contents of the conscious self-model of the body, for instance, are constituted by a rich, diffusely integrated mélange of bodily sensations. A host of different types of self-presentational content (see section 5.4), like visceral sensations; feelings of hunger, pain, or thirst; proprioceptive and kinesthetic formats; tactile and temperature sensations; and vestibular information are continuously integrated into a *supramodal*, conscious body image. You are never in contact with your own body—as an embodied, conscious entity you are the contents of an *image*, a dynamical image that constantly changes in a very high number of different dimensions. However, this image is at the same time a physical part of your body, as it invariably

2. This is clearly reflected in the phenomenology of self-consciousness: There is one level of phenomenal experience in which our body is *just* an object for us, part of an objective order, physically influenced by other inanimate objects, and frequently presenting considerable resistance to what we take or what is currently *being taken* to be the "true" subject of experience.

possesses a true neurobiological description. There are also, of course, a large number of self-*simulational* contents in the self-model: spontaneously occurring biographical memories or the contents of genuinely intellectual operations like future planning. Then there is self-*representational* content. This is complex relational information, like your current body position; specific, episodically occurring emotions; and the way in which you experience yourself as socially situated in a group of fellow human beings. The self-representational part of the PSM always targets the *current* state of the system as a whole. In short, a self-model is a model *of* the very representational system that is currently activating it within itself. Typically it will possess a bottom-up component driven by sensory input (self-presentation). This input perturbs or modulates the incessant activity of top-down processes, continuously generating new hypotheses about the current state of the system (self-simulation), thereby arriving at a functionally more or less adequate internal image of the system's overall, *actual* situation (self-representation). However, the pivotal question is, What justifies treating all these highly diverse kinds of information and phenomenal representational content as belonging to *one* entity?

What bundles these differing forms of phenomenal content is a higher-order phenomenal property: the property of *mineness*. Mineness is a property of a particular form of phenomenal content that, in our own case, is introspectively$_3$ accessible on the level of inner attention as well as on the level of self-directed cognition, that is, in terms of introspection$_4$. Here are some typical examples of how we, linguistically, refer to this particular, higher-order phenomenal quality in folk-psychological contexts: "I experience *my* leg subjectively as always having belonged to me"; "I always experience *my* thoughts, *my* focal attention, and *my* emotions as part of *my own* stream of consciousness"; "Voluntary acts are initiated by *myself*". In the next chapter I present a series of neurophenomenological case studies, which demonstrate that—contrary to traditional philosophical assumptions—the distribution of this property in phenomenal space may vary greatly, and that practically all of the examples just mentioned do not form necessary preconditions for phenomenal experience. Mineness comes in degrees. The phenomenal property of mineness, in bundling the wide variety of contents from which our conscious self is constructed, is closely related to the actual phenomenal target property.

This is the property of phenomenal *selfhood*. Again, let us look at some examples of how we frequently attempt to point to the phenomenal content of the internal representational states underlying this property, using linguistic tools from public space: "I am *someone*"; "I experience myself as being *identical* through time"; "The contents of my phenomenal self-consciousness form a coherent *whole*, before initiating any intellectual or attentional operations, and independently of them I am already immediately and 'directly' acquainted with the fundamental contents of my self-consciousness." What we often, naively, call "the self" in folk-psychological contexts is the *phenomenal* self, the content of self-consciousness, given in phenomenal experience. Arguably, this form of phenomenal content generated by conscious self-experience is, theoretically, the most interesting form of phenomenal content. It endows our mental space with two highly interesting structural characteristics: centeredness and perspectivalness. As long as there is a phenomenal self our conscious model of the world is a functionally *centered* model and usually tied to what in philosophy of mind is called the "first-person perspective" (see section 6.5). This notion, in turn, lies at the heart of the most difficult epistemological and metaphysical problems in the philosophy of consciousness. For instance, it generates the "epistemic asymmetry" between ascriptions of conscious states from the first-person and third-person perspectives. Obviously, you cannot have a first-person perspective without a conscious self. And, of course, for any given PSM, we can ask questions like, What is its minimally sufficient neural correlate? What are the necessary and sufficient functional and representational properties that any system activating such a self-model will have to possess?

It is important to note that a self-model is an entity spanning many different levels of description. In beings like ourselves, a PSM will have a true neurobiological description, for example, as a complex neural activation pattern with a specific temporal fine structure, undergoing kaleidoscopic changes from instant to instant. There will also be functional and computational descriptions of the self-model on different levels of granularity. Creating a computational model of the human PSM is one of the most fascinating research goals conceivable. For instance, we might describe it as an activation vector or as a trajectory through some suitable state space. One might even take on a classical cognitivist perspective. Then the self-model could be described as a *transient computational module*, episodically activated by the system in order to regulate its interaction with the environment.[3] Then there will be the representational level of description, in which the *content* of the PSM will appear as a complex integration of globally available self-representational, self-simulational, and self-presentational information (see chapter 5). In introducing the working concept of a PSM I claim that it constitutes a *distinct* theoretical entity. That is, I claim that it is not only something that can meaningfully be described on a number of different levels of description mirroring each other in a heuristically fruitful manner but that it is something that can be *found* by suitable empirical research programs. And it can be found on *every* level of description.

Let me also point out that the concept of a PSM is an excellent conceptual device for formulating research programs. It helps to mark out classes of systems as well as classes of states. Intended classes of self-modeling systems could be infants, grown-up dreamers, or psychiatric patients during a florid attack of schizophrenia, and also mice, chimpanzees,

---

3. There is a formal proof that every regulator of a complex system will automatically become a *model* of that system. Cf. Conant and Ashby 1970.

and artificial systems. From an objective third-person perspective we can principally mark out certain classes of, for example, infants, chimpanzees, and artificial systems by the kind of PSMs they use. PSMs are domain-specific entities and can be used to create flexible taxonomies. To give an example, the evolution of conscious self-models is a topic of particular interest for evolutionary psychology. The phenomenally available content of the self-model is an excellent constraint to differentiate between different phases of childhood development, certain nosological stages in psychiatric diseases, or the unfolding of social competence in the animal kingdom. If attempting to classify intended *state classes*, we will (as discussed in chapter 2) primarily have to use defining characteristics developed predominantly from the first-person perspective—at least initially. However, paying attention to the attentionally and cognitively available aspects of the PSM is an excellent way of forming a taxonomy of phenomenal state classes. We can investigate how the content of the PSM changes when making the transition from an ordinary to a lucid dream (see section 7.4.4), or what changes in content of the phenomenal self accompany senile dementia. We can, again, combine system and state classes by investigating emotional self-modeling in young human beings during a certain phase of adolescence or the dynamics of self-representation associated with ultrasound perception in bats. Most important, however, the concept of a PSM can help us to gain a new perspective on the central theoretical problem of consciousness research: It holds the promise of offering a theory about what an individual experiential perspective actually *is* in the first place. As most would agree, we urgently need a convincing theory about the *subjectivity* of subjective experience itself, and, obviously, the concept of a PSM will be able to play a central role in developing a theoretical strategy. I return to this issue in the second half of this chapter. Let us now look at possible semantic constraints for the concept of a PSM.

Again, there are numerous levels of description and analysis on which such constraints can be discovered. At our current stage, we need all of these levels. Let us have a second look at them:

• *The phenomenological level of description.* Which statements about the content and the internal structure of the phenomenal self can be made on the basis of introspective experience itself? When will such statements be heuristically fruitful? When will they be epistemically justified?

• *The representationalist level of description.* What are the specific features of the *intentional* content generated by the phenomenal variant of mental self-representation? For instance, what is the relationship between "vehicle" and content for PSMs? Are there distinct *levels* of content within the PSM?

• *The informational-computational level of description.* Which computational function does the phenomenal level of self-modeling fulfill for the organism as a whole? What is the computational goal of self-consciousness? What information is *self-conscious* information?

· *The functional level of description.* What causal properties does the physical correlate of self-consciousness have to possess in order to transiently generate the experience of being a unified self? Is there a multirealizable "functional" correlate of self-consciousness?

· *The physical-neurobiological level of description.* Here are examples of domain-specific questions: What is the role of brainstem and hypothalamus in the constitution of a phenomenal self? What is the direct *neural correlate* of phenomenal self-experience? Are there aspects of phenomenal self-consciousness which are not medium invariant?

As we now for the second time move through our checklist of the ten multilevel constraints for different types of phenomenal representational content, we will soon discover how applying it to the concept of a PSM helps to quickly enrich this new notion with substance. We can flesh it out on many different levels simultaneously. Please recall that, if not stated differently, the intended class of systems is always formed by humans in non-pathological waking states.

6.2 Multilevel Constraints for Self-Consciousness: What Turns a Neural System-Model into a *Phenomenal Self*?

6.2.1 Global Availability of System-Related Information

Let us begin with the differentiated Baars-Chalmers criterion, which we have, throughout chapters 2 and 5, used as a "placeholder," as a paradigmatic first example of one important constraint in narrowing down the concept of conscious representation.

The Phenomenology of Global Availability of System-Related Information
The contents of my phenomenal self-consciousness are directly available, it seems, to a multitude of my mental and physical capacities at the same time: I can direct introspective$_3$ attention toward a pleasurable gut sensation, a subtle background emotion quietly flickering away at the fringe of my conscious space, or at the way in which I am currently trying to cognitively frame a certain philosophical problem ("attentional availability"). I can also reason, for example, about my current mélange of background emotions. I can make a conscious attempt at finding a concept for it ("availability for phenomenal cognition"), which allows me to see them in relation to earlier emotional experiences ("availability for autobiographical memory"), and I can try to use this information in producing speech when communicating about my emotions with other human beings ("communicative availability"). I can attempt to control my visceral sensations, my background

emotions, or my capacity for clear thought, that is, by jogging, taking a hot bubble bath, or having a cold shower ("availability for the control of action"). A coherent and explicit self-representation is a necessary prerequisite of deliberately initiated self-regulatory behavior. I do experience the general global availability of the contents of my self-consciousness as my own flexibility and autonomy in dealing with these contents, and, in particular, by the subjective sense of immediacy in which they are given to me. However, it is important to point out three more specific phenomenological characteristics. First, the degree of flexibility and autonomy in dealing with the contents of self-consciousness may vary greatly: emotions and sensations of pain and hunger are much harder to influence than, for instance, the contents of the cognitive self. There is a *gradient of functional rigidity*, and the degree of rigidity itself is available for phenomenal experience.

Second, the phenomenal experience of immediacy is a graded feature as well. Typically, thoughts are something that may not even be determined in their full content before being spoken out loud or actually written down on a piece of paper, whereas bodily sensations like pain or thirst are directly given as explicit and "ready-made" elements of the phenomenal self in a much stronger sense. The self-constructed character accompanying different contents of the conscious self is highly variable (see *constraint 7*). Third, it is interesting to note that first-order states integrated into the PSM, as well as second-order attentional or cognitive states operating *on* these contents, are both characterized by the phenomenal quality of *mineness*. The conscious contents of your current body image are not experienced as *representational* contents, but endowed with a phenomenal sense of ownership: at any given time, it is your *own* body. While consciously reasoning about the current state of your body, you will typically be well aware of the representational character of the cognitive constructs emerging in the process while at the same time such thoughts about your current bodily state are characterized by the conscious experience of "mineness," by just the same immediate sense of ownership. This is the way in which beings like ourselves experience a representational structure as *integrated* into the PSM.

From a purely philosophical perspective, availability for self-directed, phenomenal cognition may be the most interesting feature of all information integrated into the PSM (see section 6.4.4). Conscious human beings do not direct their attention to bodily sensations alone, they can also form thoughts *de se*. The content of *de se* thoughts is formed by *my own cognitive states* about *myself*. It is interesting to note how in some cases the generation of these thoughts will be accompanied by a sense of effort and phenomenal agency, whereas in others, for example, in spontaneous, briefly occurring episodes of reflexive self-consciousness or in daydreaming about oneself, this will not be the case. Reflexive, conceptually mediated self-consciousness makes system-related information cognitively available, and it obviously does so by generating a higher-order form of phenomenal content. This content, however, does not appear as an isolated entity, but is recursively *embedded* in the same, unified phenomenal hole, in the self-model. A related observation can be made for introspective₃ self-directed attention. The existence of a coherent PSM generates a preattentive self-world border and thereby realizes the central necessary condition for the development of genuine *intro*spection, on the representational as well as the phenomenological level of description. Self-related information is now available for higher-order processes that do not approximate a quasi-conceptual, syntactically structured format of mental representation, but which are much more fluid, serving predominantly to highlight a specific and already existing aspect of the phenomenal self by locally increasing processing capacity. Again, phenomenal introspection₃ can be accompanied by a sense of effort and attentional agency; it can also be experienced as effortlessly wandering or even resting in a certain region of the PSM. This difference has to be explained. Again, it is interesting to note how the phenomenal quality of mineness in such cases of attentional access pertains to first-order and to higher-order content: It is *my own attention*, which is directed toward an aspect of *myself*. Attentional processing directed at the phenomenal self generates a recursively embedded and higher-order form of conscious content, while always preserving the overall coherence of the PSM. The deliberate conscious act of introspection itself may be the paradigmatic example of intentional action in its purest form (Jack and Shallice 2001, p. 170). The theoretical problem consists in achieving a homunculus-free representationalist-functionalist analysis of the *phenomenal* target property of attentional agency, without simply introducing something like "the brain's chief executive officer (CEO)," that is, a metaphorical, personal-level entity which exercises "the ultimate high-level decisionary control over the flow of attention" (Kilmer 2001, p. 279). Research into developmental shifts concerning the ability for bodily, emotional, and behavioral self-regulation may supply us with a tractable behavioral model of how a young human being can gain not only control of her own behavior, but *mental* control in guiding attention as well (Posner and Rothbart 1998). For instance, it is interesting to note how adults possessing better capacities for guiding and focusing attention, at the same time report experiencing less negative emotional content.

I have already noted that the constraint of "global availability" actually is only a restricted functional aspect of *constraint 3*, the globality constraint for phenomenal content. Phenomenologically, self-related information is only one subset of globally available information because, although itself highly differentiated and at any point in time forming an integrated whole, it is itself bound into a highly differentiated, but at any point in time integrated *highest-order* phenomenal whole. In short, the phenomenal self is always embedded in a phenomenal world, seamlessly and preattentively. Being self-conscious is being-in-a-world.

Global Availability of Self-Representational Content

The existence of a coherent self-representatum for the first time introduces a self-world border into the system's model of reality. For the first time, system-related information now becomes globally available *as system-related* information. On the other hand, environment-related information can now be referred to as *non-self*. Objectivity emerges together with subjectivity. The importance of this way of generating a very fundamental partitioning of representational content into two very general classes lies in the way in which it forms a necessary precondition for the activation of more complex forms of phenomenal content: *Relations* between the organism and varying objects in its environment can now for the first time be consciously represented. A system that does not possess a coherent, stable self-representatum is unable to internally represent all those aspects of reality associated with self-world, self-object, and, importantly, self-self and self-other relations. A basic form of self-representational content is a necessary precondition for the internal processing of information about perceptual and social relationships. Let us call this the "principle of phenomenal intentionality-modeling": complex information pertaining to dynamical subject-object relations can only be extracted from reality and used for selective and flexible further processing if a conscious self-model is in existence.

Informational-Computational Availability of System-Related Information
Self-related phenomenal information is equivalent to globally available system-related information. One of the fascinating features of the human self-model is that this information ranges from the molecular to the social. For instance, the PSM is important in processing internal information relevant to elementary bioregulation (Damasio 1999). It is also important in making information about the fact that the system itself is constantly engaged in information processing and reality-modeling (including *other-agent modeling*) available to a large number of different *metarepresentational* processes (see above).

Global Availability of Self-Related Information as a Functional Property
Under a functionalist analysis, a PSM is a discrete, coherent set of causal relations. In chapter 3 we saw that, when looking at the system as a whole, the possession of phenomenal states clearly increases the flexibility of its behavioral profile by adding context sensitivity and choice. Now we can see that a PSM not only allows the system to make choices about itself but also adds an *internal context* to the overall conscious model of reality under which a system operates. First, self-representation is an important tool for optimizing homeostasis and elementary bioregulation, by offering system-related information to a large variety of other functional modules, which can now react to sudden challenges presented by the internal context in a differentiated manner. Elementary bioregulation may simply *be* self-representation, because, as Conant and Ashby (1970) pointed out, every regulator of a complex system will automatically and by necessity become a *model* of that system. I like to look at this elementary form of self-modeling as "internal output management": It came into existence because the organism's own internal production of specific molecules (hormones, neurotransmitters, etc.) had to be fine-

tuned. Output management is an important capacity on the level of molecular microbe-havior as well as on the level of overt, motor macrobehavior.

A PSM also exerts an important causal influence, not only in differentiating but also by *integrating* the behavioral profile of an organism. As one's own bodily movements for the first time become globally available as one's *own* movements, the foundations for agency and autonomy are laid. A specific subset of events perceived in the world can now for the first time be treated as systematically correlated *self-generated* events. The fact that there can be events in the world that are simultaneously self-generated and self-directed can be discovered and made globally available. To put the point simply: By generating a coher-ent self-model, a system for the first time becomes a distinct entity within its own behav-ioral space, and thereby for the first time becomes a part of its own reality. We shall return to this and related points repeatedly. Now it is only important to note that the most central aspect of the causal role played by a PSM may consist in later enabling the system to become and treat itself as a second-order intentional system (Dennett 1978b, pp. 273–284; 1995), thereby turning it from a behaving system into an *agent*. On the functional level of description, Dennett may clearly have isolated an important conceptual condition of personhood. Readers may not be surprised, however, that my own interest consists in shed-ding light on the issue of what a second-order *phenomenal* system would be, a system that consciously *experiences* itself as being endowed with conscious experience.

Neural Correlates for the Global Availability of System-Related Information
Almost nothing is currently known about the necessary neural correlates for the mental self-model, as well as about sufficient correlates for the *phenomenal* mental self-model. A number of contributing subsystems, like the somatosensory and prefrontal cortex, hypo-thalamus, and upper brainstem, are known, but it is essentially unknown at which level of processing functional integration takes place and how high the degree of holism and dis-tribution is on this level. We do not possess any good neurobiological theory about the relationship between coherent, unconscious self-representation and its relationship to the *phenomenal* partition of the human self-model. However, there are a number of promis-ing hypotheses and speculative ideas regarding possible empirical research programs. One typical example may be the difference between the proto-self and the core self as intro-duced by Damasio (Damasio 1999). I claim that the conscious self is the phenomenal correlate of a distinct representational entity[4] characterized by a specific set of func-tional properties. I also claim that the self-model is a correlative notion in that self-

4. The distinctness of this entity is constituted by the distinctness of its intentional object (the system *as a whole*), and, of course, it does not exclude the actual representational format being of a widely distributed and dynami-cal nature. Also, it is a *theoretical* entity on the representational level of description, not a metaphysical entity in terms of philosophical ontology. The conscious self is not a substance.

consciousness always implies being-in-a-world. In terms of, for example, the dynamical core hypothesis advanced by Tononi and Edelman (Tononi and Edelman 1998a; Edelman and Tononi 2000a, b), this leads to the prediction that within the global functional cluster described by a set of neural elements with a CI value higher than 1, there will typically exist one and only one *subcluster* describing the self-model. SMT (the self-model theory of subjectivity), the current theory, predicts that in humans this subcluster will itself possess an area of highest invariance, which in turn is correlated with functional activity in the upper brainstem and hypothalamus. If what I have said about the persistent functional link anchoring the PSM in the brain is true, this subcluster will likely have a CI value that is even *higher* than that of the global dynamical core. It, too, will at the same time exhibit high values of complexity and internal differentiation while constituting its own functional border *within* the phenomenal world-model. At the same time it will be highly integrated with information internal to the self-model, that is, causally coupled to itself in a stronger sense than to other elements of the global functional cluster. This, of course, does not mean that the self-model is an isolated island—like a localized, automatic subroutine that has dropped out of the organism's phenomenal reality and lost a large amount of its context sensitivity and global availability. One must conceive of it as an entity that is still *embedded* in the global functional cluster, continuously exchanging information with it. Nevertheless, at any given moment it will only be the group of neurons belonging to the functional subcluster just described which *directly* contribute to the contents of self-consciousness.

6.2.2   Situatedness and Virtual Self-Presence

The presentationality constraint, the necessary condition of conscious contents always being activated within a virtual window of presence, was introduced in chapter 3 (section 3.2.2). However, if we apply it to the concept of a self-model, it yields a number of interesting new aspects. Some of these aspects have a distinct philosophical flavor.

Treated as a first-person, phenomenological constraint, presentationality again proves to be a necessary condition: Whatever I experience as the content of my phenomenal self-consciousness, I experience *now*. It is not only that a world is present; it is that I am a *present self* within this world. My own existence possesses temporal immediacy: a sense of being in touch with myself in an absolutely direct and nonmediated way, which cannot be bracketed. If it were possible to subtract the content now at issue, I would simply cease to exist on the level of subjective experience: I could not represent myself *as* carrying out this subtraction, because I would then not be a present self in my own model of reality anymore. I would cease to exist as a psychological subject and I would not be *present* for myself and others as such. Only because the fundamental content of my phenomenal self invariably is content *de nunc* can I experience myself as now being present within a world.

Phenomenology of Self-Presence and Temporal Situatedness

Phenomenal experience not only consists in "being present"; it also consists in "being present *as a self.*" As we saw earlier, the generation of a self-model leads to the emergence of a self-world border in the phenomenal model of reality. There now are two kinds of events: internal and external events. Interestingly, there is now a more specific sense of "internality"—that is, *temporal* internality—that overlaps with the more general sense of internality constituted by the notion of self-representation. Phenomenologically speaking, I am not only *someone* but also someone who is *situated in a temporal order*. From the first-person perspective, I simply experience this overlap of two different kinds of representational content (self-representation plus temporal internality) as my own presence in reality. If I happen to be a being that is not only capable of self representation but also of self-simulation in terms of autobiographical memory and the internal construction of potential and future selves, then a completely new dimension of phenomenal experience becomes available to me. It is the historicity of my own person: the conscious experience of being a self having a past and a future while being currently localized at a specific point on a given temporal order.

We have seen that the phenomenal experience of time is constituted through a series of achievements, that is, the representation of temporal identity, difference, seriality, wholeness, and permanence (see section 3.2.2). The same will now be true of all events defined as *inner* events in terms of the PSM. An internal Now, an internal psychological *moment* emerges when singular events constituting the representational dynamics of the self-model are integrated into temporal gestalts. If such internal events are not only represented as successive but are integrated into temporal figures, they then generate an internal context, and form a whole. Sequences of conscious thoughts or the unfolding of different nuances belonging to one and the same emotional reaction is an example of such temporal gestalts. In each of these bound sets of singular events we experience ourselves as present, for example, as subjects of experience existing *now*. If (as noted earlier) it is true that phenomenal experience, in its core, may precisely be the generation of an island of presence in the continuous flow of physical time, then we can now say that *subjective* phenomenal consciousness starts when a self-modeling system operating under the presentationality constraint we are currently discussing generates an island of *self*-presence in the continuous flow of physical time. Phenomenologically speaking, if the specious present of a psychological moment is integrated with a self-representation, then it will (all other necessary constraints being satisfied) lead to the conscious experience of *someone's existence*. As soon as one has a theory about what a first-person perspective is and how a full-blown phenomenal self emerges, one will be able to understand how this becomes the content of *my own existence*.

In section 3.2.2 we noted that what makes phenomenal time experience so hard to analyze on a conceptual level is the fact that the river of experienced succession is not only flowing around the island of the Now emerging from it, but actually *through* the island, as if the Now were a continuously superimposed entity in this flow. For the special case of self-consciousness this means that there is an invariant background of self-presence (typically exemplified by bodily self-experience and the more invariant parameters of conscious somatosensory perception) that is *permeated* by the conscious experience of the temporal evolution of more short-lived elements of the phenomenal self (as in constantly changing perceptual states, thought episodes, or quick emotional reactions).

De Nunc Character of the PSM

Again, everything that has been said in section 3.2.2 applies, but in a slightly different manner. Even when carrying out a phenomenal self-simulation, for example, when making plans about my own distant future, or when spontaneously simulating past states of myself, for example, when being haunted by spontaneous autobiographical memories, it is always clear that I am making these plans *now* and that I am having these memories *now*. Interestingly, our capacity for mental time travel is never complete. In standard situations, the presentational component of the self-model functions as a stable anchor for self-simulational processes of different kinds. Temporarily, our attention may be fully absorbed by simulational content generating future selves or recreating the legend of a putative past self, but there is a subtle phenomenal presence of bodily awareness, which is never entirely lost. It anchors us within the phenomenal window of presence generated by the system which we are. In fact, this may be one of the greatest achievements of the human self-model: It *integrates* the representational content constituted by basic, bioregulatory information processing currently carried out in order to keep the physical condition of the body stable, with higher-order cognitive contents simulating possible states of the organism. It is the self-model, as it were, which bridges the gulf from the actual to the possible, from the bodily to the cognitive. It links self-representations and self-simulations by the common phenomenal property of mineness. In doing so, the PSM allows the organism to continuously feel its own existence and temporal situatedness while simultaneously *owning* the process by which it remembers past events and designs self. It is important to note how this combination of different and highly specific forms of representational contents presents a highly advanced level of intelligence.

Self-Presence as an Informational-Computational Property

At this point I have to return to my old favorite, the virtual reality metaphor. For any system using a self-generated virtual reality to guide its own behavior, it will be optimal if the model of the agent itself is *fully immersed* in this virtual reality (see also next section). We have already seen how, from an epistemological point of view, every self-representation must also be a self-simulation, because from a third-person perspective it never truly models or "grasps" the current physical state of the system. However, if it approximates the target properties forming the intentional content of its simulation in a functionally adequate manner, if it simulates its own physical dynamics in a good enough way, it may treat such contents as temporally internal. In doing so it can behave as if it were actually fully immersed in the reality that it is simulating.

Self-Presence as a Functional Property

A system continuously modeling itself in a window of presence thereby gains a number of new functional properties. It generates a reference basis for phenomenal self-simulations. For example, autobiographical memories can now be compared and related to the current status of the system. In the context of the self-zero hypothesis we have already seen how, from a teleofunctionalist perspective, self-simulations not covarying with actual properties of the system can only be turned into helpful tools (e.g., in forward-modeling motor behavior or in making future plans) if a representation of the current state of the system *as* the current state of this system is in existence. Self-modeling within a window of presence achieves precisely this. Second, the existence of a preattentive self-world border and a coherent self-representation as *now* holding enable the generation of higher-order forms of attentional or cognitive self-representation operating on them. For instance, the fact of the system being currently part of an objective order onto which, however, it has an individual perspective becomes cognitively available. As soon as the system is internally represented as perceiving the world from a special, constantly changing point on a linear time order, its own historicity becomes *cognitively* available. The principle of presentationality, applied to the self-model, yields a necessary precondition for the development of an autobiographical memory: Autobiographical memory can only function against the background of a present self. Obviously, such functional properties will be highly adaptive in many biological environments (see section 6.2.8).

Neural Correlates of Self-Presence

To my knowledge, so little can be said about this point that I will simply skip it.

6.2.3   Being-in-a-World: Full Immersion

A self-model precisely emerges from drawing a self-world boundary. If this boundary is conflated with the boundary of the world-model, phenomenal properties like mineness, selfhood, and perspectivalness will disappear. However (remaining with the standard case for now), phenomenal events integrated into the self-model will, interestingly, at the same time be experienced as taking place *in a world* and *within my own self*. Phenomenologically speaking, they are bound into a global situational context as well as into an internal, psychological context. Phenomenal selves are situated selves, and their contents inherit this characteristic by not only being tied to a phenomenal subject but to a phenomenal subject-in-a-world. From a third-person perspective we can say that any system embedding a PSM into its phenomenal model of reality not only experiences a world but also that it is a *part* of this world. It is now a system to which this very fact is cognitively available and that can use this fact in selectively controlling its own actions.

It is interesting to note how the self-model becomes a world-within-a-world, a subjective universe embedded in an objective universe. The second fact that becomes cognitively available for a phenomenally situated being is that some states of reality are parts of the world *and* at the same time parts of the self. Therefore, two general classes of binding problems have to be solved in order to understand the globality constraint on the level of self-representation. First, how are conscious contents integrated into the PSM? Second, how is the PSM integrated into the currently active world-model?

The Phenomenology of Subjective, Nonepistemic Situatedness
If an integrated PSM is embedded in a comprehensive, highest-order representational state, this puts the phenomenal quality of "mineness" characterizing its contents into a new, global context. The experiential model of reality is now characterized by a fundamental dichotomy of "me" and "other." As the global state itself is pervasively characterized by autoepistemic closure, by the fact that the system cannot recognize this representation *as* a representation, the transparency constraint, the fundamental subject self-world dichotomy, is characterized by the same phenomenological feature. The existence of a boundary between self and world, as well as the accompanying part-whole relationship between self and world, is experienced in the mode of naive realism. In other words, for beings like ourselves the fact that there is an irrevocable boundary between ourselves and our environment, while at the same time we are prior to any cognitive activities seamlessly embedded in this environment, is simply a fundamental feature of reality itself, about which to have doubts seems fruitless. It is a phenomenal necessity. In the chapter 7 we will see how it would be just another phenomenological fallacy to conclude that this has to be a necessary feature of all conscious experience.

Again, the fact that a system experiences itself as nonepistemically situated in the way described above does not automatically entail that this fact is also attentionally or cognitively available to it. Probably many of our biological ancestors lived their lives in transparent reality-models characterized by a fundamental self-world dichotomy, without being able to either deliberately direct a stable form of introspective, high-level attention or even cognition to this feature of their reality. Given our now existing catalogue of constraints, it is possible to imagine a stage at which biological systems just simply *functioned* under this dichotomy, making it globally available for enriching their behavioral profile, while not yet being able to deliberately direct their attention to it. And it seems highly likely that only human primates started to make the subject-object dichotomy cognitively available, by eventually turning it into the object of explicit intellectual operations.

The Subject-Object Dichotomy as a Representational Property

On the representational level of description we need to achieve a better understanding of three fundamental steps. First, a coherent PSM has to be constructed, possessing a transtemporal identity and unequivocally being characterized as the *self*-model. As for its coherence, plausible empirical models of feature binding are already in existence, and in section 5.4 we have seen how the self-model is exclusively marked out by being the only phenomenal model that is anchored in a constant stream of presentational content possessing a highly invariant core. Second, a stable self-world boundary has to be defined. And third, a part-whole relationship between the currently active self-representation and the overall model of reality has to be achieved. The last point seems to call for a dynamical and continuous integration of the self-model into the world model. On the representationalist level of analysis all three steps are equivalent to generating a new form of representational *content*.

It is easy to see how a subjectively experienced, numerical identity of the self can emerge from a high degree of internal coherence. As I have pointed out earlier, the empirical project consists in searching for the right kind of mechanism that can achieve the continuous integration of self-representational content. As for the subjectively experienced *transtemporal* identity of the self, obviously, two factors are of principle importance: transtemporal *continuity* and the invariance of returning contents of self-consciousness (e.g., the experience of agency), and the emergence of autobiographical *memory*. At this point, it is important not to confuse the theoretical issue of the transtemporal identity of persons with the neurophenomenological issue of how the actual *experience* of possessing such an identity is generated—veridical or not. Phenomenal personhood could exist in a world without persons. In chapter 7 we look at a number of interesting configurations in which the respective kind of phenomenal content has been lost.

It is also interesting to note that what appears as the self-world dichotomy on the phenomenological level of description has to rest on the most fundamental partitioning of representational space conceivable. For beings like ourselves, the representation of a self-world boundary is the most fundamental characteristic of our representational state space: all other forms of representational content always belong to at least one of those two categories, which, in standard situations, form an exhaustive distinction within reality itself. Everything belongs either to the self or to the world. A third fundamental category is not given—indeed, the underlying partitioning of our representational space is so fundamental and rigid that it is very hard to even *conceive* of anything else. It is simply very hard for us to run corresponding mental simulations.

However, there are many representational contents which *simultaneously* belong to the world and to the self. The conceptual distinction introduced above is exhaustive, but not exclusive. The philosophically most important example of a representational content bridging the gulf between subject and object in phenomenal experience is formed by the different varieties of the PMIR, the conscious model of the intentionality relation (see section 6.5). A simple example is given by visual attention: If you visually attend to the book in your hands as a perceptual object, the process of attention is itself modeled on the level of conscious experience. It is like a nonverbal arrow pointing from you to the book, uniting subject and object as it were. It is important to note that what you are experiencing is not attention "as such," but a specific form of representational *content*, the way in which ongoing attentional processing is modeled on the phenomenal level.

There is a second way in which the distinction between self states and world states is exhaustive, but not exclusive. This is given by what I have earlier called the mereological relation between different forms of representational content. Interestingly, if we ask whether *all* contents of the phenomenal self at the same time are experienced as also being in the world, we confront strongly diverging philosophical intuitions. There is an honorable philosophical tradition which says that a certain part of ourselves, that part which possesses only temporal but no spatial characteristics ("the thinking self"), precisely is *not* embedded in the world. Self-conscious thought, one might think, is precisely that part of the phenomenal self that is not embedded in the world-model. In section 6.3 I explain why this classic Cartesian intuition *necessarily* has to appear with beings possessing a representational architecture like ourselves.

In conclusion, if we want to model a centered version of *constraint 3* within a particular class of representational systems, for example, within an embodied, situated, and connectionist model, the three major goals to be achieved would consist in (1) modeling the activation of a coherent self-model possessing an invariant core of internally generated input, and an element corresponding to the psychological notion of autobiographical memory; (2) a partitioning of state space mapping the self-world dichotomy; and (3) implementing a part-whole relationship between the self-model and overall representational state.

The Generation of a Self in a World as Informational-Computational Strategy

Again, many of the observations made in section 3.2.3 once more apply. Generating a single and coherent self-model is a strategy for reducing ambiguity. The amount of information that is globally available for introspective attention, self-directed cognition, and action is minimized and thereby the computational load for all mechanisms operating *on* the PSM is reduced. Consequently, if mechanisms exist for selecting already active representata and embedding them in the conscious self-model, the selectivity and flexibility with which the system can now react to the new type of *self-related* information is increased. If, for example, the organism is suddenly afflicted with an injury and automatically generates a fast and predominantly rigid reaction to this injury—for instance, by generating a swift protective limb movement or guiding low-level attention to the injured body part—it may not be necessary for the functionally relevant information already active within the system to also be a component of its conscious self-model. The *final* result of the unconsciously initiated motor response or shift in attention, however, may well be consciously available. If this information about a new state of the system has to simultaneously and permanently be available to a multitude of mechanisms, then it will be a strategic advantage to make it a content of the conscious self.

It is important to note that the introduction of a self-world boundary, while not automatically realizing them, is a necessary precondition for a large number of higher-order computational functions. Higher-order forms of self-representation, in turn being a precondition for social cognition, now become possible. All information having to do with system-world *interactions* can now for the first time be processed, including relationships to other agents. As noted earlier, the internal simulation of possible selves now has a firm reference basis, because a central part of the overall internal self-representation—namely, the transparent partition of the PSM—is irrevocably defined as being a part of the actual world.

Phenomenal Self-Modeling as a Functional Property

The activation of a PSM generates so many new functional properties and possibilities that it would take a book of its own to investigate them. Let us look at a simple, first example. A standard working definition of self-consciousness in the primate literature is what, in the context of the current theory, would be called attentional availability of a coherent self-model (e.g., see Gallup 1970, 1991, 1997; Kitchen, Denton, and Brent 1996). Self-consciousness is *the capacity to become the object of one's own attention*. As soon as a coherent self-model exists, mirror self-recognition becomes possible. On the representationalist level of description the sufficient condition consists in the ability to embed a visual representation of the body as an external object in the multimodal PSM. As I have argued elsewhere (Metzinger 1994, p.49*f*.), the precise moment of mirror self-recognition occurs when a partial relational homomorphy between temporal and spatial dynamics of a visual percept (the seen mirror image) and certain proprioceptive and kinesthetic aspects of the self-model simultaneously active is discovered by the system, leading to a transient integration of something that previously was only a component of the phenomenal world-model ([another chimpanzee moving back and forth in front of me]) into the transparent self-model ([*myself*]). The object-representational content can now become a new element for an ongoing subject-representational containing. Mirror image and self-model merge. A certain "goodness of fit" between two simultaneously active data structures is discovered, leading not only to a transient subject-object relation (see section 6.5) but actually to a phenomenal "subject-subject relation" with the content of the visual percept now becoming an actual component of *myself.* After a chimpanzee has discovered itself in a mirror, it frequently starts inspecting and manipulating parts of its body which were hitherto visually inaccessible, like the lower back or teeth. Obviously, attentional availability leads to a number of new functional properties, some of which may possess a high survival value. For instance, it is now conceivable how an attentionally available self-model could be used for predicting one's own future states of consciousness or for the development of social strategies.

In a similar sense, for beings capable of mental concept formation and speech, the phenomenal segregation of a coherent self-model against a background of a world-model enables self-directed cognition as well as the utterance of self-referential statements in a public language. *Cognitive availability* of integrated, coherent, and system-related information can therefore become realized as reflexive self-consciousness (see section 6.4.4). The global availability of system-related information for speech processing generates what I have earlier called "communicative availability," and can be realized as introspectively$_4$ *reporting* about the current content of one's self-model to other human beings (see section 6.3.3). It leads us to another large set of new functional properties. This set is not generated by making a coherent self-model as such available for higher-order operations, but by making the fact that the self-model is seamlessly *integrated* into a comprehensive world-model available for such operations. The system can now explicitly represent itself as standing in certain *relations* to external objects. Simple motor behavior, for example, a grasping movement directed at a visually perceived object, can now be internally represented as a *goal-directed* movement, and actions can now be internally represented as relations to objects in the external world. In turn, objects themselves can be coded in terms of possible motor trajectories (see Gallese 2001).

If a representation of its own movement as being essentially goal-directed in terms of establishing a relation to an external object or a set of such objects becomes attentionally or cognitively available, the representational foundations for cognitive agency have been laid (see section 6.4.5). Importantly, the same is true for perceptual objects. The difference between a perceived object and the subjective experience *of* this object can only become cognitively or attentionally available if a coherent self-model and a stable self-world boundary exist. An object will be a coherent, preattentively integrated set of perceived features. The experience of this object is a representation of the perceptual *process*, which has been integrated into the self-model. The difference between the perceptual object and the perturbance in the perceptual states of the system itself allows for *internally* attributing a causal relation between both events, the appearance of a perceptual object and the change within the self-model. The first functional property resulting from this is attentional availability: the object can now be made more salient by focusing attention on it. Second, however, the overall relation between object and perceiving system can now be made globally available, thereby becoming a potential object for higher-order processes operating on it. This is functionally relevant, because the difference between the external object and the internal representational activity *related* to the object can now not only be cognitively grasped but also used in the control of action. A simple way of using this new distinction in the control of action is by trying to "get a better take" on the object, by improving sensory perception itself. A more interesting way of making use of this newly available distinction is by presupposing it in other conspecifics (see section 6.3.3).

Let me point out a third essential change in the global functional profile of systems embedding a self-model into their model of reality. In section 5.4 we saw that the PSM is privileged relative to all other forms of phenomenal content active in the system by its possessing a persistent functional link to a specific part of its physical basis. The PSM is firmly anchored in the brainstem and hypothalamus by a constant source of what I have called "self-presentational content." The functional level of description leads to an important feature of our phenomenal model of the world: it is a "centered" model of reality. It is not simply that the self-world border constitutes a fundamental way of partitioning our representational space. The deeper point is that one section of representational space, the one occupied with constantly processing system-related information, is functionally privileged by being locked to a source of maximal invariance, the body. The self-model, by being a transparent, body-anchored, and indexical representation, achieves *context binding* for the system generating it: it ties the system into its own conscious model of reality, allowing it to live *in* as well as *with* this model (for a related perspective, see also Brinck and Gärdenfors 1999). In short, we are beings that have developed a highly relevant global feature of the way in which we process information: We consciously operate under *egocentric* models of reality.

This is not to say that a large number of our most successful mental simulations do not take place in subspaces possessing an allocentric coding. To give an example, it might be that we discover the goals and intentions behind the perceived behavior of fellow human beings by automatically running an unconscious simulation of their motor behavior. We might simultaneously produce a "retrodiction" of their mental states by generating an abstract, allocentric goal representation related to this perceived behavior, which we, as it were, first "enact" in terms of an unconscious, egocentric motor simulation (e.g., see Gallese and Goldman 1998; see also section 6.3.3). Another example of mentally simulating a noncentered model of reality is found in Thomas Nagel's *The View from Nowhere* (Nagel 1986, chapter 4; Metzinger 1993, 1995c; Malcolm 1988; Lycan 1987). The condition of possibility for all these intended simulations is that they take place against the background of a centered model of reality. Developing and operating under an egocentric model of reality may first have turned out to be adaptive simply because our behavioral, as well as our perceptual space, *is* centered. Trivially, we are beings concentrating all our sensors and effectors in a very narrow region of our interaction domain. We have one single body. As José Luis Bermúdez (1997, p. 464*f.*; 1998) has pointed out, *ultimately*, first-person thought and linguistic self-reference are essentially grounded in the continuity of a single path through space time. Moreover, the spatiotemporal continuity of a single, enduring body forms not only an important part of the content of perception but causally underlies the point of origin expressed in the internal coherence of perceptually based states. Of course this is not a logical necessity, but it makes certain forms of reality modeling more practical than others. Ultimately, on a higher level, however, it is an important step toward establishing a genuine first-person perspective in terms of phenomenally modeling the intentionality relation *itself*. I return to this issue in section 6.5.

Neural Correlates of Full Immersion
Today, we possess some first speculative ideas about the necessary neural correlates for specific contents making up the human self-model, like emotion or proprioception (see e.g., Damasio 1999, chapter 8). However, almost nothing is known about sufficient correlates or the necessary integrative mechanism grouping these different contents into a coherent, phenomenal self-representation. All that can plausibly be assumed is that they will be widely *distributed* in the brain.

6.2.4   Convolved Holism of the Phenomenal Self

The space of our conscious experience possesses a holistic character, and this holism is pervasive, because it also holds for the many different forms of ever-changing phenomenal content of which it is composed. This is also true of that subregion that is phenomenally experienced *as internal*, the region constituting the self-model. The conscious self is the paradigmatic case of a phenomenal holon. In chapter 3 we touched upon the point that every phenomenal holon can be analyzed as a functional window causally mediating between parts of the organism's internal structure and the rest of the universe, allowing these parts to act as a unit. In 1967 Arthur Koestler, who introduced the notion of a holon, wrote: "Every holon has a dual tendency to preserve and assert its individuality as a quasi-autonomous whole; and to function as an integrated part of (an existing or evolving) larger whole" (p. 343). This statement, although made in a different context, obviously is true of the phenomenal self-model too. However, the content active in this specific region of state space is not only holistic but also exhibits a variable degree of internal coherence plus a rich and dynamic internal structure.

Convolved Holism as a Phenomenal Feature of Self-Consciousness
An important factor in generating the *subjectivity* of phenomenal experience consists in the untranscendable presence of a self within a world. The phenomenal self constitutes a subglobal whole (a "world within the world"), and information displayed within and inte-

grated into this whole is globally available for system-directed cognition, attention, and control of action. The overall holism of the phenomenal self results from the fact that introspectively discriminable aspects of experience formed by it cannot adequately be described as isolated elements of a set. They are not individual components of a class, but constitute a mereological relationship between parts and a whole. Excluding special situations like florid schizophrenia (see section 7.2.2), it is always true that decontextualized phenomenal atoms never exist within the conscious self. The self *is* the context determining their meaning, by binding them into a comprehensive representation of the system as a whole. What an atomistic analysis can never grasp is the subjectively experienced *strength* by which the different aspects of our phenomenal self are integrated. A second phenomenological constraint is the *variability* of this strength. Different aspects of our phenomenal self display varying degrees of relative interconnectedness, for instance, in cognitive versus emotional self-representation—the value we ascribe to ourselves as thinking subjects may be quite isolated from the respective emotional relationship we have with ourselves. This variability of coherence is itself a content of subjective experience. Therefore, it is an explanandum as well.

Again, the unknown subpersonal mechanism automatically and continuously constituting the phenomenal self is much stronger than the mechanism underlying the formation of classes or mental predications, as we find them, for instance, in cognitive processes. The possession of a phenomenal self is a necessary precondition for cognition and not its result. The phenomenal first-person perspective, genetically as well as conceptually, precedes the cognitive first-person perspective (see section 6.4.4). To *experience* selfhood is different from thinking a self or *conceiving of* one's self as a subject. A self composed of discrete building blocks could form a unity, but never become a phenomenal whole. All parts of myself are seamlessly integrated into a phenomenal gestalt—as a matter of etymological fact, the German word *Gestalt* originated on the *personal* level of description. The phenomenal self, on a subglobal level of phenomenal granularity, possesses an organic structure and its contents are linked in the manner of a subtle network, producing a quasi-liquid dynamics, including fast and smooth transitions in their content. We all can direct our introspective attention to this feature of our phenomenal self. At this point it also becomes inevitable to note that the target object internally modeled by the phenomenal self possesses an organic structure (because it *is* an organism). The neural elements in its brain are linked in the manner of a subtle network (because its brain *is* a network) and not only the informational dynamics in the organism's brain but the biochemical level of information–processing going on in terms of hormone or blood sugar levels, and so on in all of the organism's internal fluids is a liquid dynamics in an even more literal sense (because all of it *is* ultimately embedded in body fluids). The fine-grained, elegant, and smooth way in which changes in our self-consciousness take place may actually reflect objective physical properties of our bodies on many levels, and in a much more literal sense than we have ever thought. It is fascinating to note how such properties may even "spill over" or infect the way we internally model the *external* world. After all, at least the phenomenal content of our internal *world*-model supervenes entirely on synchronous and internal properties of our body.

The mechanism leading to this flexible subsymbolic dynamics, however, cannot be penetrated cognitively and it is available neither for attention nor for direct volitional interventions. For instance, I am not able to deliberately split or dissolve my phenomenal self. Have you ever tried it? On the other hand, conscious self-representational content itself is highly selective, and by guiding introspective attention I can highlight the most different aspects of my current self-consciousness. Its content can be modulated, enhanced, or repressed. I can also deliberately add new content to it, that is, by running phenomenal self-simulations of different sorts. Interestingly, the degree to which attentional availability is actually realized can vary greatly: Attention is typically attracted by sudden changes in the emotional landscape or in cognitive content, whereas most people hardly ever pay attention to the most invariant regions in their PSM, that is, to those very stable features of bodily self-awareness, for instance, constituted by proprioception, the sense of balance, and visceral sensitivity. Phenomenologically, the body itself may at many times only be given as a quietly flickering background presence or in the form of shifting, but isolated "attentional islands." The wandering of such attentional islands could, for instance, be conceived as being systematically attracted by domains in which the difference between sensory input and the actual output of the self-model is large (Cruse 1999, p. 168*f.*). Still, even when we are in a relaxed and static state (i.e., when the body model is appropriate because the difference between its output and its sensory input is zero) our bodily self-awareness *as such* does not simply disappear. The attentional landscape may be flat, but we certainly don't feel disembodied. This is a further phenomenological constraint for computational modeling: there seems to be a basic and functionally autonomous level in the PSM that is active independently of attentional or cognitive processing operating on it.

Why is the holism of the self-model a *convolved* kind of holism? The concrete wholeness of my own self, as is apparent in conscious experience, is characterized by a multitude of internal part-whole relationships. These relationships are dynamical relationships (*constraint 5*): they may undergo swift and kaleidoscopic changes. Not only the overall phenomenal model of reality, but the self-model as well is not composed out of a bag containing atomic elements, but emerges out of an ordered hierarchy of part-whole relationships. However, any realistic phenomenology will have to do justice to the fact that this hierarchy is a highly flexible, "liquid" hierarchy. Viewed as a perceptual object, the phenomenal body image integrates a number of very different properties such as felt temperature, emotional content, spatial and motion perception, and so on, into an integrated whole. It constitutes something like an internal scene, a stage, an exclusively *internal* multimodal situational context. Against this unified background many different forms of experiential content can continuously be segregated. Another way to look at the phenomenal self is not as a perceptual, but as a cognitive object (see section 6.4.4), which, however, is also anchored in this constant phenomenological subcontext. Although it takes very careful introspection to discover that even cognitive activity possesses experiential motor aspects, and even though cognitive activity does not seem to possess any sensory or spatial components, it is continuously bound into the background of the bodily self generating the phenomenal quality of "mineness," which I already mentioned. Feelings of temperature or thirstiness, different emotions, as well as the results of reasoning and other purely intellectual activities, are all experienced as my *own* states. Even as the constant phenomenal experience of the actual body state is superimposed by intended phenomenal simulations of possible selves it is always clear that these fantasies and future plans are my *own* in the same sense my current bodily sensations are. As the focus of my introspective attention wanders, the overarching wholeness is never threatened. What continuously changes, however, is the way in which bodily, emotional, and cognitive contents of experience are nested into each other.

Convolved Holism as a Property of Self-Representation

The question of the unity of consciousness is closely related to the question of the unity of self-consciousness. Can the first exist without the second? The difficulty is on the level of intuition: We cannot phenomenally simulate a situation in which there would be a unified consciousness without the unity of self-consciousness. For beings like ourselves, such a configuration is *phenomenally impossible* and many philosophers have drawn the dubious conclusion that the presence of a unified self somehow presents a *conceptual necessity*. But how is the unity of the self constituted? If our phenomenological analysis of the conscious model of reality as displaying the abstract feature of convolved holism is correct, it must be possible to discover a corresponding feature on the level of representational deep structure, and on the level of underlying functional structure (see section 3.2.4). The same must be true of the phenomenal model of the self. As soon as we have narrowed down the minimally sufficient neural correlate for the phenomenal self—which will no doubt be highly distributed—we have to seek a set of abstract properties explaining the features mentioned above. This could, for instance, take place on the level of mathematical models describing the relevant portions of neural dynamics. Obviously, it is much too early to be able to make any clear statements in this direction. All we can do at present is formulate two important representational constraints: A representational analysis of the phenomenal self will have to offer, first, a candidate for the *specific* integrational function generating the phenomenal quality of "mineness," characterizing all features bound by the self-model, and, second, a comprehensive theory describing the multitude of internal, dynamical part-whole relations.

Convolved Holism as an Informational-Computational Strategy for Self-Representation

Again, many of the observations made in chapter 2 apply. System-related information represented in a holistic format is coherent information. System-related, phenomenal information is that kind of information available to the system as a *single* possible object of intended cognition and focal attention. At the same time, information integrated into a convolved holistic self-model generates an *internal* kind of interdependence. As single features, for example, background emotions and cognitive states, directly influence each other within this model, it provides a new way of representing the complex causal structure governing the internal dynamics of the system itself.

Convolved Holism in Self-Representation as a Functional Property

Obviously, it is a major advantage to have all those properties of the system that have to be constantly monitored in one integrated format, because the system has to be able to react to them in a fast and flexible manner. Such an integrated data format for self-presentation, self-representation, and self-simulation might precisely be the most relevant factor in understanding the computational role of the PSM. If it is true that the convolved character of phenomenal content given in the mode of self-modeling is reflected on the functional level, then it should be possible to directly access aspects of its own internal causal structure for the system. For instance, when running an intended self-simulation of certain possible cognitive states, the system could attempt to directly "read out" how its own emotional state would probably have changed in this situation. ("How would it feel to be convinced of *this*?") That is, during phenomenal self-simulations the system can make use of the fact that all the components of a phenomenal self-simulatum can be updated in a fast, flexible, and context-sensitive manner, depending on the content of other self-representational parts which may be either currently active or laid down as implicit features inherent in the system's functional landscape.

Neural Correlates of Convolved Holism in Self-Representation

Again, it is true that almost nothing is currently known about possible neural correlates for the phenomenological features and the subpersonal constraints I have just described.

6.2.5   Dynamics of the Phenomenal Self

There is an essential part of the PSM, the function of which is to generate stability and invariance (see section 5.4). However, many forms of self-representational content, resulting from active constructive processes, undergo frequent changes. We are not only perceiving, attending, and thinking subjects but *agents* as well. As cognitive, attentional, and volitional agents we continuously generate changes in the content of phenomenal self-consciousness. As embodied agents moving through the world we continuously generate proprioceptive and kinesthetic feedback. Changes in our PSM are tied to an internal time order, which—as we sometimes experience when engaged in very pleasurable activities or during an emergency—can divert greatly from what we subjectively experience as "external" or "physical" time. In short, the temporal evolution of the conscious self is a richly textured phenomenon.

Phenomenology of the Dynamic Self

Whatever my true nature is, I am an entity that undergoes changes. Some of these changes, like pangs of jealousy, are very fast. Others are almost too slow to be noticed. Thus, certain emotional nuances or subjective "energy levels" in the background of bodily awareness undergo slow transformations, which are subtle and can last for many decades. I can introspectively discover all of the phenomenological aspects of time experience, described extensively in section 3.2.5, in myself: the simultaneity of bodily sensations; succession and seriality as paradigmatically experienced in conscious reasoning; experiencing myself as a part of and in touch with reality by being a *present* self; and, finally, the phenomenology of self-consciousness characterized by a strong element of duration. This last aspect is particularly interesting, because the coherence and duration of the phenomenal self is, as a matter of trivial fact, highly discontinuous, for instance, in being repeatedly and reliably interrupted by phases of deep and dream sleep. It is the invariance of bodily self-awareness, of agency, and autobiographical memory which constitutes the conscious experience of an enduring self. The conceptual reification of what actually is a very unstable and episodic process is then reiterated by the phenomenological fallacy pervading almost all folk-psychological and a large portion of philosophical discourse on self-consciousness. But it is even phenomenologically false: we are not things, but processes.

The aspect of *lived* experience, what in the German tradition of philosophical phenomenology is termed *Erleben*, becomes most salient on the level of the phenomenal self: I am a *living* person, not a machine constructed out of atomistic elements, but a holistic being generating a phenomenal biography by being a context-bound, active subject. In order to again avoid the classical phenomenological fallacy it is important to point out that no conceptual necessity is involved in this description. You do not have to experience yourself as a *living* person to be conscious. There are neuropsychiatric disorders in which patients have lost just this, and only this, aspect of their phenomenal self without losing conscious experience or the first-person perspective altogether. In Cotard's syndrome, patients experience themselves as dead, as not being living entities anymore (see section 7.2.2). Such patients form the firm and persisting belief of not being a living person anymore, and they consciously experience this very fact. In severe forms of depersonalization, the patient will typically come to see a psychiatrist because he experiences himself as turning into a machine or into a remote-controlled puppet. One of the greatest dangers in philosophy of mind and in traditional theories of subjectivity in particular has been to underestimate the richness and complexity of the target phenomenon, for instance, by making absurd claims about necessary features a priori. Many different kinds of deviant phenomenal self-modeling do exist (see chapter 7). They do not even have to be pathological. As we all know, the degree to which we experience ourselves as real and fully present is another aspect of dynamic self-consciousness, which can vary greatly—even in nonpathological situations. Just imagine being completely absorbed in a game of chess or the "unreal" feeling you may have during an accident or in a dream. In meditation, after all cognitive activity has effortlessly come to an end and attention has settled into a stable, globalized state, specific aspects of phenomenal self-consciousness—like autobiographical memory, cognitive and attentional agency, and emotional self-modeling—can be temporarily suspended. Phenomenologically, this can lead to a marked loss in terms of constraint satisfaction for dynamicity, while at the same time creating an experience of heightened and maximally integrated bodily presence. These examples show how the convolved holism of phenomenal self-consciousness expands into the temporal dimension by simply constructing and *re*constructing particular aspects of the conscious self from a network of dynamical part-whole relationships. They also demonstrate the richness of phenomenal self-modeling: Obviously, even the subclinical variability involved in the temporal properties of conscious self-modeling is very high.

Dynamicity as a Property of Phenomenal Self-Representation

One important aspect in understanding what a PSM actually is consists in analyzing it as a representational tool allowing a system to *predict its own behavior*. Not only the brain but the whole, behaving organism as well can be described as a nonlinear dynamical system. Adaptive behavior results from the continuous interaction between *three dynamical* systems possessing a rich, complex, and highly structured dynamics: nervous system, body, and environment (Chiel and Beer 1997).

The nervous system, according to this conceptual frame of reference, is not issuing commands to the body, but makes "proposals" to the physics of the system which in turn generates its own functional structure. The nervous system, and this will be true for the particular case of self-representation as well, is not so much a top-down controller, but more a system whose task consists in generating adequate *patterns* within this overall dynamics. Interestingly, new behavioral patterns now are properties of this threefold, coupled system. Our behavioral profile is rich and flexible and minimal changes in initial conditions can lead to dramatic changes in the overt patterns of our behavior. For infants or young children it is hard to know what they will do next: They are frequently surprised by their own behavioral reactions and are not yet capable of any long-term planning for their own behavior. As adults, we are to a much higher degree capable of predicting our own future actions, thereby achieving biographical consistency and laying the foundations for stable social relationships. In general, it is easy to see that the ability to predict one's own behavior possesses a high adaptive value and why it is a necessary precondition for conceiving of oneself as an agent.

In principle, there are two important classes of predictive strategies for complex nonlinear systems. The first class operates from an external, third person perspective. For instance, we might develop a theoretical approach and use certain mathematical tools to make the behavior of the system formally tractable. Mathematical modeling probably is the best example of such an external strategy. However, *mentally* modeling the behavioral dynamics of a certain target system is another, equally valid, third-person strategy to achieve the same goal. Individual systems, if they possess the necessary and sufficient representational resources to activate mental models (see section 3.3.1), can internally model the behavior of another individual system. If they meet the necessary and sufficient conditions for generating *phenomenal* mental models (see section 3.3.2), they may even develop the conscious experience of attempting to mentally predict the behavior of, for example, a fellow human being. In other words, they might develop *phenomenal* simulations of the likely future behavior of another system.

Importantly, there is a second class of strategies for predicting the behavior of a highly complex, nonlinear dynamical system with the help of a phenomenal model—but this time from the first-person perspective. It consists in *internally* modeling the future behavior of the system by the very system *itself*—by activating an internal self-model and using it as a tool to predict one's own behavior. Again, if such a system meets the necessary and sufficient conditions for developing a conscious self-model, it now has the capability to subjectively experience itself as a being that makes attempts at predicting its own future behavior. The continuous attempt to develop a coherent, temporally structured, and well-integrated sequence of behaviors extending into the future is now a property of the system, which has become globally available. The fact, that this very system *makes* predictions about its own future behavior in turn becomes available for self-directed attention and cognition. Obviously, the representational structure just described is a central necessary condition for the emergence of that higher-order phenomenal property we usually call "agency" (see section 6.4.5).

Moreover, if an internal self-model is to be a successful instrument in predicting the future behavioral dynamics of an individual system, it must in some way mirror or reflect important functional characteristics of precisely that part of its *internal* dynamics, which in the end will cause the overt actions in question. In this way it becomes obvious how many of the remarks about the dynamicity of phenomenal representations offered in section 3.2.5 now apply to the PSM as well. One of the important ideas inherent in dynamicist cognitive science is not to conceive of intentionality as a rigid, abstract relation pointing from a subject to an intentional object, but as a dynamical physical process. In the same way, *reflexivity* will now not be a rigid, abstract relation in which a subject stands to itself, but a constructive, dynamical physical process generating a constantly updated self-model, which can, as we have just seen, be extended into the fourth dimension. Both points are particularly relevant to describing the phenomenal content that actually underlies the emergence of a strong cognitive subject and the conscious model of the intentionality relation (see sections 6.4.4 and 6.5). Both forms must satisfy the dynamicity constraint.

Dynamicity as an Informational-Computational Strategy for Self-Representation
The coherent self-model leads to the most fundamental segmentation of representational space, by generating a preattentive self-world border. Hence, it allows a system to view its behavioral space, its domain of direct causal interaction with the physical world, from a new perspective. In particular, self-directed behavior now becomes possible: System-related information can be made globally available for the control of action. The second point, now repeatedly encountered, is that one can plausibly assume that the biological value of consciousness in part consists in increasing the *flexibility* of the behavioral repertoire of an organism. Obviously, one important factor in achieving this feature must have consisted in modeling the temporal structure of the causal interaction domain and of ongoing sensorimotor loops in a more precise manner. This is especially true for that part of the behavioral repertoire constituted by self-directed actions: the biological system *itself* can sometimes be characterized by sudden, and sometimes even unpredictable changes. This dynamism will, therefore, have to be reflected in the relational properties and the fine temporal structure of the PSM. In short, a self-model will only be a good computational instrument if it successfully mimics the relevant aspects of the physical dynamics characterizing the system in which it is generated.

Furthermore, it is interesting to note that the actual representational covariance with the physical world established through the self-model may be highly variable, and that this fact might be directly reflected in certain contents fluctuating in and out of the *conscious* PSM. As Jun Tani (1999) has pointed out, an interesting way of conceiving of the PSM under a dynamicist perspective is as an entity that possesses grounded as well as ungrounded components and which, from time to time, more or less "takes off" by departing from its coupling to the current state of the body. A fully grounded self-model would simply disappear.[5] In principle, phenomenal selfhood emerges as long as there is a conflict or incoherence between bottom-up and top-down processes, between expectancy and actual perception. According to this model, self-consciousness is substantially diminished during steady phases, demanding no additional attentional processing (Tani 1999, p. 172; see also Cruse 1999). It is a phenomenon which arises in an open dynamical system interacting with the external world. In the course of its own temporal evolution goal-directedness functions as a source of stability for this system, while the physical embodiment presents constant perturbations and instabilities. A conscious self emerges precisely in those moments when incoherence arises and has to be resolved by processing on the level of global availability.

Dynamicity as a Functional Property of Conscious Self-Representation

One of the most beautiful properties of a human being is that it can surprise itself. As we saw, young children are a constant surprise to themselves. As their self-model develops, their capacities for self-prediction grow as well. It is interesting to note how the capacity to deliberately surprise *others* will have been a highly advantageous property from an evolutionary perspective. For animals continuously facing the threat of predators, the generation of chaos and unpredictability will be of maximal importance. A rabbit being chased by a hawk will create the best chances for its own survival and for the survival of its offspring if it can generate *chaotic* motor behavior, a way of running that is unpredictable and cannot be *learned* from observation. From a teleofunctionalist perspective, therefore, it will be highly adaptive if a self-model allows for the generation of unpredictable motor output in certain situations. Dynamicity can be interpreted as a content property of the self-model, for example, assessing temporal properties of the self-modeling system. It is interesting to view it as a functional property of the vehicle of self-modeling as well. It realizes a certain causal role—for example, by making coherent, system-related information globally available in a virtual window of presence—in a very specific manner. First, it mimics the temporal profile of certain aspects of the system itself. Second, as a physically realized vehicle of representational content, it is, of course, causally embedded in the very physical system dynamics, certain aspects of which it is internally modeling *for* the system.

Neurodynamics of Phenomenal Self-Representation

At the time of this writing, hardly anything is known about the concrete neurodynamics underlying the process of phenomenal self-modeling.

---

5. This view may actually be too extreme, because it overlooks the autonomous activity of self-presentational content (see section 5.4.). To take an example, the phenomenology of meditation—viewed as a fully grounded state without any cognitive contents in the PSM or a focused attentional PMIR—seems to show that a certain level of autonomous, residual self-modeling is preserved. Bodily awareness is never fully lost.

6.2.6   Transparency: From System-Model to Phenomenal Self

In chapter 3, introducing our original set of ten multilevel constraints, in section 3.2.6, we discussed the perspectivalness constraint. Because perspectivalness is itself the major component in understanding the representational deep structure of the phenomenal first-person perspective, I will now *skip* the corresponding section and turn to this specific issue in detail at the end of this chapter (section 6.5). However, let me note at the outset that there is a highly specific and relevant sense in which the original perspectivalness constraint (*constraint 6*) *can* be satisfied by the self-model, and not only by the world-model. If we attend to ourselves or think about ourselves, a second-order process of self-modeling is directed at an already existing self-model. It is as if the first-person perspective is drawn inward, its target object now an aspect of the *subject* itself. I discuss these higher-order self-representational structures in the second half of this chapter. First, we must understand how they are *possible*. They are possible because one decisive partition of the self-model invariably remains transparent.

At the very beginning of this chapter, I identified three phenomenal target properties: "mineness," "selfhood," and "perspectivalness." A while ago, in section 3.2.7 of chapter 3, we developed the transparency constraint for phenomenal representata. Applying this constraint to the concept of a conscious self-model is the decisive step in understanding how the second of our target properties—the conscious experience of *selfhood*—can be reductively explained, using the representationalist level of description as a starting point.

When it comes to selfhood, the antireductionist reply to the representationalist-functionalist strategy developed here is obvious and straightforward. There simply is no conceptually necessary connection, the opponent will argue, from the functional and representational constraints so far developed to the phenomenal target property of selfhood. The representational process of mental self-modeling within a coherent world-model and a virtual window of presence, holism and dynamics conceded as well, does not *necessarily* lead to the existence of a full-blown phenomenal self. It is conceivable, a typical property dualist might argue, that biological information-processing systems open functionally centered representational spaces and always embed a model of themselves in the model of reality active within this space—without thereby automatically generating a phenomenal self. An active, dynamical "self-model," upon closer inspection, is just a representation of the system; it is a *system-model*, and certainly not a self. A particularly malicious opponent might even argue that by introducing the concept of a "self-model," I have actually cheated, by installing an intuition pump, which ultimately rests on an equivocation smuggled in with the help of the concept of "self." A system-model simply is not a *self*-model. Any machine can do this, and, in fact, many machines do this today. The facts that the system-model is an internal model, and even the identity of the target and

emulating system and the satisfaction of our three minimal constraints for any type of phenomenal representation (presentationality plus globality plus transparency) do not determine that a *genuine* experience of *being someone*, of phenomenal selfhood, will come into
existence. What is needed—by conceptual necessity—to take the step from the functional
property of centeredness and the representational property of self-modeling to the consciously experienced phenomenal property of selfhood?

My claim in this section is that what in philosophy of mind is called the "phenomenal
self" and what in scientific or folk-psychological contexts frequently is simply referred to
as "the self" is the content of a *phenomenally transparent self-model*. As we have already
seen, there are other necessary conditions for an unconscious, merely *mental* self-model
to become a conscious self, a PSM. However, I think that the transparency constraint, for
a number of reasons, is the decisive defining characteristic. In chapter 3, I pointed out that
the concept of transparency is by no means new, and has recently become popular with a
large number of philosophers in the current debate. Previously, as readers may remember,
I introduced my own, slightly refined concept of transparency, explicitly not making any
direct connections to other current uses. Before proceeding to our four levels of description, let us apply the central insight to the concept of a self-model: A phenomenal self-
representatum, then, is equivalent to one that cannot be recognized *as such* by the system
activating it within itself. We do not experience the contents of our self-consciousness as
the contents of a representational process, and we do not experience them as some sort of
causally active internal placeholder *of* the system *in* the system's all-inclusive model of
reality, but simply as *ourselves, living in the world right now.*

The Phenomenology of Transparent Self-Modeling

The transparency of the self-model is a special form of inner darkness. It consists in the
fact that the representational character of the contents of self-consciousness is not accessible to subjective experience. This statement refers to all the different sensory modalities, constituting the internal sources of information out of which the PSM is generated:
visceral sensitivity, kinesthetic and proprioceptive, tactile and haptic, and even vestibular
stimuli. However, it is also true of self-directed visual, auditory, externally tactile, olfactory, and gustatory experience, of self-perception through extradermal sources of information. In particular, it is true of the integrated phenomenal model of the organism as a
whole: The *instrument* of self-representation is not globally available as such and this
is also the reason why the experiencing system, by necessity, becomes entangled in a
naive realism with regard to the contents of its own mental self-representation. For many
forms of conscious self-representation, earlier processing stages are not attentionally available. Through a contingent property of its representational architecture, such a system
simply *has* to experience itself as being in direct contact with the contents of its self-

consciousness. The fact, which is inaccessible to the system using its on-board representational resources, is that its self-experience takes place within a *medium*. Completely transparent self-representation is characterized by the fact that the mechanisms which have led to its activation and the additional fact that a concrete internal state exists, which functions as the carrier of their content, cannot be recognized anymore. Therefore, the phenomenology of transparent self-modeling is the phenomenology of selfhood. It is the phenomenology of a system caught in a *naive-realistic self-misunderstanding*.

Again, *opaque* phenomenal self-representation does exist. Intended phenomenal simulations, certain emotions, and consciously experienced cognitive processes in particular are standard examples of ongoing processes of self-modeling being experienced *as a representational process*. Cognitive self-modeling generally is opaque, although it always possesses a transparent component. Because the question of how full-blown cognitive, reflexive self-consciousness can be anchored in nonconceptual forms of self-awareness possesses great relevance for philosophical discussion, I have devoted a number of special sections to this problem and can safely skip the issue of opaque self-modeling at this point (see sections 6.4.1, 6.4.4, and 6.5.2). At this point, to do justice to the phenomenology of transparent self-modeling, it is only important to point out the two most interesting aspects. First, there is a subtle *continuum* from transparent to opaque content in self-consciousness. There are aspects of ourselves, for example, the concreteness and immediacy of bodily presence and some elementary emotions, which we never experience as *mental* (in the sense of them resulting from an essentially representational-simulational activity). There are other forms of self-representation in which it starts to dawn on us that we might actually be *misrepresenting* reality, in particular our social environment. However, sometimes we suddenly become aware that our emotional response might actually be inappropriate to our current social environment. Take jealousy as an example. We may suddenly realize the representational character of our own jealousy if we become aware of the fact that all this actually might be a *misrepresentation*—for instance, of those persons in our social environment of whom we are jealous. In emotions we frequently oscillate between certainty and uncertainty, between the immediacy of an obvious perception and doubts. At the beginning of jealousy it may well be experienced as something indubitable, concrete, and directly given, as a direct perception of how your husband or wife currently behaves. As time progresses, you may well find yourself experiencing your own emotional state, a certain partition of your PSM, *as* a mere representation, which might, as a matter of fact, be false. What was a property of another person suddenly is a property of yourself. The medium becomes visible, as it were. Jealousy, by the way, is a good example of how phenomenal misrepresentation can possess a true teleofunctionalist description: obviously, to suffer from jealous paranoia is highly advantageous from a biological perspective.

Then there are sections of the PSM that are always opaque. Whereas higher-order forms of self-modeling, like self-directed attention, may still be fully caught in a naive-realistic self-misunderstanding—you simply "look at" or "feel into" that part of yourself, with which you believe you are in direct contact with anyway—self-directed *cognition* is typically characterized by the phenomenology of insight. You simply seem to know that all this is an ongoing process of self-representation, while at the same time you are certain that you are the initiator of this process *yourself*. This is, of course, Descartes's classical intuition, and I return to the question later, to what extent is it simply another version of the phenomenological fallacy—the unjustified use of an existential quantifier within a psychological operator.

A second phenomenological characteristic is important. There are large classes of phenomenal states in which our self-model is completely transparent and we do not think or engage in higher-order processes of self-modeling like self-directed attention and cognition. If we are not jealous, or fully immersed in physical activities, there will be phases in which our PSM is devoid of any opaque content. In a certain, equally important, sense we are "one with ourselves" in such situations. We do not *distance* us from ourselves by generating higher-order self-representational content, as it were, and the philosophical mind-body problem would never occur to us. Phenomenal self-transparency can exist without opaque components. Many animals and most human infants may be in this stage. However, phenomenologically, the opposite situation never exists: there simply are no phenomenal state classes in which we experience ourselves as pure, disembodied spirits, not possessing any location in physical or behavioral space (see section 7.2.3.2). The thinking subject needs the bodily self, and this situation is clearly mirrored on the level of phenomenal self-modeling. There simply is no conscious self-representation characterized by opaque content in its entirety; cognitive self-reference always takes place against the background of transparent, preconceptual self-modeling. More about this later.

Phenomenological constraints are first-person constraints. By now it should have become obvious how the existence of a transparent self-model is one of the central conditions necessary to explain what we actually *mean* by a concept like "first-person constraint". In section 6.5, I return to this issue, and we may then also arrive at a deeper understanding of the nature of the corresponding conceptual constraints themselves.

Transparency as a Property of Self-Representation

A phenomenal self-representation is transparent, because the content seems to be fixed in all possible contexts: the hands that you are now using to hold the book you are reading are always going to remain your *own* hands, parts of yourself, no matter how much your internal or external perceptual situation shifts. Of course, this belief is epistemically unjustified. In chapter 7 we consider a series of neurophenomenological case studies, which demonstrate how precisely this phenomenal quality of "mineness" or bodily "selfhood" is by no means a *necessary* precondition of conscious experience and how the distribution of these properties in phenomenal space possesses considerable variance. However, leaving deviant phenomenal models of the self aside for now, what you currently experience is not an "active body emulator" that has just been integrated into your global model of reality, but simply the *content* of the underlying self-representational process. What you feel are simply your *own hands* as integrated parts of yourself, effortlessly given in the Here and Now. Your tactile sensations, the subtle sense of muscular effort, the almost implicit information about your body's position in space, and the almost unconscious sensation of the temperature of your hands (to which, however, you can at any time direct your attention) are as immediate as they are concrete. They are an integrated form of presentational content, which—phenomenologically—has nothing representational, inferential, or cognitive about it. Let us, once more, make a distinction between the vehicle and the content of a self-representation.

The representational vehicle of your conscious hand experience is a certain process in your brain, a complex neural activation pattern. This process of bodily self-representation—which may fulfill its function by abstract, higher-order isomorphisms and may, therefore, not possess anything "booklike" in any concrete manner—is not consciously experienced by you. It is not globally available for attention and it is transparent in the sense of you currently looking through it. However, in this special case, what you are looking through to is *yourself*: What you are looking and feeling *onto* is its self-representational content, the existence of your hands, here and now, given through a multitude of internal as well as external sensory channels. This content is an abstract property of the concrete self-representational state, of the currently active self-representatum in your head.

Please recall that there are at least two kinds of mental content. The *intentional* content of the state in your head depends on the fact of your hands really existing or on the state being a reliable instrument for gaining knowledge about yourself in general. If the self-representational vehicle (e.g., the "neuromatrix of the body image"; see, e.g., Melzack et al. 1997, and section 7.2.3.1) currently is a good and reliably functioning instrument of self-knowledge, then it allows you, precisely due to its transparency, to directly look and feel "through it," onto your own hands. It makes the information carried by it globally available in an integrated fashion without you having to care about how this actually happens. The *phenomenal* content of your hand representation, however, is one component which stays invariant, regardless of whether your hands exist or not (for real-life examples of such state classes, see sections 7.2.3.1, 7.2.3.2, and 7.2.5). It does not matter if all this is a dream or an out-of-body experience, or if you are using two phantom limbs to hold a hallucinated book right now, because the phenomenal content of your bodily self-representation can in principle stay the same. A bodiless brain in a vat, could certainly enjoy the *phenomenal* experience of holding a book like this one in its *own* hands right now. The phenomenal content of your bodily self-representation is entirely determined by internal properties of your brain. If, while reading these sentences, you actually *are* a brain in a vat, you are, as it were, not anymore "intentionally" or "epistemically" looking through a state in your head onto your hands, but only onto this state itself—without *this* fact being globally available to you on the level of phenomenal representation. As the phenomenology of phantom limbs clearly shows, a special characteristic of phenomenal self-representation is that this aspect of its content will be maximally concrete, absolutely unequivocal, directly and immediately given, even if the fact that it actually results from a process of *mis*representation or afunctional simulation is cognitively available. It is subpersonal, and automatic. A transparent phenomenal self-representation, again, is characterized by the fact that we are unable to discover the difference between self-representational content and self-representational vehicle on the level of phenomenal representation itself.

Can you imagine suddenly realizing that your own body simply is a *thought*? Philosophically, this may turn out to be an attractive strategy: Is your body actually a *fixed thought*, a transparent form of something that ultimately has to be analyzed as a form of *cognitive* content, something like an *automatic* thought—like a prejudice that you have long ago forgotten? Is embodiment a philosophical prejudice? It is easy to imagine a situation in which your hands holding the book right now might actually be hallucinated hands, and in which this hallucination would suddenly shift into a pseudohallucination: Your phenomenal hand representation would suddenly become *opaque*, because the information that the hands are the result of an internal, misrepresentational state, which currently is not a good instrument for gaining self-knowledge, suddenly becomes globally available. Your phenomenal hands might well lose their transparency. Proprioception and the ongoing neural simulation of your current limb position and their kinematic geometry, for instance, in the superior parietal lobule (area PE) and parts of the rostrally adjacent cortex surrounding the anteriormost part of the intraparietal sulcus (area PF) in your brain (see Bonda, Petrides, Frey, and Evans 1995, p. 11180*ff.*) might simply turn out to be highly unreliable. But if you then realize that not only the book and your hands but your whole current reality takes place in a dream, what would happen if you suddenly became *lucid* (see section 7.2.5)? Would it be possible to realize that your body, in its entirety, is a misrepresentation, to which nothing in the world corresponds? It seems impossible to imagine such a situation. There is always self-*presentational* content, there are always emotions and gut feelings, for instance, and presentational content is always fully transparent. How could your phenomenal body image, in its entirety, ever become opaque? Is it possible to lose *internal* sensory transparency? Obviously, it is possible for a brain in a vat to generate a full-blown body image without there being any body, or hands, or any guts, for that matter. But what would it mean for an ordinary human being, like the reader of this book, to make the fact globally available that she is currently a self-modeling system caught in a naive-realistic misunderstanding, not only cognitively in terms of introspection$_4$ but also attentionally in terms of introspection$_3$? What would it mean to be able to make the fact that the contents of your conscious self, in their entirety, are the contents of an integrated self-simulation available for the control of action, for higher-order cognitive processing, and for guidance of attention? This is a situation which you simply cannot imagine.

Please recall how phenomenal possibility (or impossibility) does not imply logical or nomological possibility (or impossibility). There is a reason why *you* cannot imagine a situation in which the transparency of your self-model has altogether dissolved. The current theory makes a clear prediction for this class of phenomenal configurations: the phenomenal property of "selfhood" would vanish. The fact that *you* cannot imagine a self-less global phenomenal state does not mean that such state classes or system classes are inconceivable or neurobiologically impossible. The fact that completely opaque, phenomenal processes of self-modeling are not a phenomenal possibility for you right now does not imply that they are logically or nomologically impossible. Once again, this would just be another case of what Daniel Dennett has called philosopher's syndrome: mistaking a failure of imagination for an insight into necessity.

In particular, given the conceptual instruments now at hand, we can clearly envision the possibility of systems that *functionally* operate under an egocentric frame of reference (centered on a model of the body as the origin of object and behavioral space), while at the same time *phenomenally* operating under a nemocentric[6] reality model (centered on a globally available, but fully opaque self-model embedded in the current virtual window of presence). A nemocentric reality model is one that satisfies a sufficiently rich set of constraints for conscious experience (see section 3.2.7), while at the same time not exemplifying phenomenal selfhood. It may be functionally egocentric, but it is phenomenologically selfless. It would, while still being a functionally centered representational structure, not be accompanied by the phenomenal experience of *being someone*. Please note how such a model of reality would also be richer in informational content than "ordinary" conscious experience, because it would make *more* information globally available, that is, information about earlier processing stages of the self-model (see section 3.2.7). For any phenomenal representation, its degree of phenomenal opacity is given by the degree of attentional availability of earlier processing stages.

We will now formulate the first main argument of this book: If all other necessary and sufficient constraints for the emergence of phenomenal experience are satisfied by a given

---

6. Grush 2000, p. 80, to my knowledge, first introduced the specific notion of a nemocentric representation: one that is centered on nobody.

representational system, the addition of a transparent self-model will by necessity lead to the emergence of a phenomenal self. Phenomenal selfhood results from autoepistemic closure in a self-representing system; it is a lack of information. The prereflexive, preattentive experience of *being someone* results directly from the contents of the currently active self-model being transparent. Any system acting under a transparent self-model will, if all other necessary conditions for the emergence of phenomenal experience in the domain constituted by this class of systems are realized, *by necessity* experience itself as being in direct and immediate contact with itself. The phenomenal property of selfhood is constituted by transparent, nonepistemic self-representation, and it is on this level of representationalist analysis that the refutation of the corresponding phenomenological fallacy becomes truly radical, because it has a straightforward ontological interpretation: no such things as selves exist in the world. Under a general principle of ontological parsimony it is not necessary (or rational) to assume the existence of selves, because as theoretical entities they fulfill no indispensable explanatory function. What exists are information-processing systems engaged in the transparent process of phenomenal self-modeling. All that can be explained by the phenomenological notion of a "self" can also be explained using the representationalist notion of a transparent self-*model*.

Transparent Self-Modeling as an Informational-Computational Strategy

Earlier we had made a slightly metaphoric use of Dretske's useful conceptual distinction between nonepistemic (transparent) and epistemic (opaque) seeing, for instance, when developing the new concept of "nonepistemic situatedness" (see section 3.2.3). Correspondingly, we may now describe the process of transparent self-modeling as nonepistemic self-consciousness. Thus, it is important to note that even if this nonpropositional form of phenomenal self-representation has not generated truth and falsity, it certainly presents an overwhelming amount of *information* to the system. The phenomenal self, computationally speaking, is an exceptionally rich structure in terms of the information it makes globally available to the system. What precisely is the information carried by a conscious self-model? A PSM makes system-related information globally available for attention, cognition, and action control. It does so within a window of presence—self-related information is displayed as being *de nunc*—and as a PSM it is embedded in the global model of the world as an integrated, coherent structure. The information integrated into the *transparent* partitions of the self-model, again (see section 3.2.7), systematically lacks *contextual* information about its own internal causal history. In terms of autoepistemic closure, it is now possible to offer a more precise formulation: not only subjective experience in general but the *subjectivity* of this experience, the way in which it is tied to a phenomenal self, has not evolved in pursuing the classical philosophical ideal of maximizing self-knowledge. Evolutionarily speaking, it was a strategy, which, for a certain period, proved to be successful, for example, by differentiating representational space and enabling a more flexible form of self-directed action and cognition. Apparently, conscious self-modeling greatly constrains the possibilities of a system to gain knowledge about itself by "on-board" resources. It is only the opaque, epistemic form of phenomenal self-modeling which eventually opens the door to social cognition, to the formation of scientific communities and theory construction. However, as we shall see, the transparent process of self-modeling is a necessary condition of possibility for higher-order, cognitive forms of self-modeling.

Obviously, viewed as a computational strategy, transparent self-modeling drastically reduces computational load. In particular, it prevents the system from being caught up in an infinite regress of self-modeling. Why? It is important to note that self-modeling, in terms of its logical structure, is an infinite process: A system that would model itself as currently modeling itself would thereby start generating a chain of nested system-related mental content, an endless progression of "self-containing," of conscious self-modeling, which would quickly devour all its computational resources and paralyze it for all practical purposes. I call this the "principle of necessary self-reification": Any self-modeling system, operating under real-world constraints and evolutionary pressures, will have to constantly minimize the computational resources needed to make system-related information available on the level of conscious experience. Because, as I have just pointed out, self-modeling possesses a potentially infinite and circular logical structure, it has to find an efficient way to break the reflexive loop. One simple and efficient way to interrupt a circular structure is by introducing an untranscendable *object*. My hypothesis is that the phenomenon of *transparent* self-modeling developed as an evolutionary viable strategy because it constituted a reliable way of making system-related information available without entangling the system in endless internal loops of higher-order self-modeling. Any biological system on the path to self-awareness must find a solution to this problem, or it will greatly diminish its reproductive success. One reason philosophers do not have many children may be that they think too much about themselves. In any case, what the self-reification argument proposes is that what we experience as our phenomenal self on the most fundamental level is precisely the transparent representational object that blocks the self-representational loop. Interestingly, this process, on closer inspection, has not resulted in object formation, but in *subject* formation (see section 6.5). In short, transparent self-modeling viewed as a computational strategy generates a simply structured and safely closed user surface for those parts of an organism's nervous system that are engaged in processing information about this organism *itself*.

Second, as we have already noted when introducing the world-zero hypothesis and the self-zero hypothesis, the generation of a transparent PSM is an efficient and elegant means of creating a reference model for the planning of future system states. What I have called the naive-realistic self-misunderstanding is a necessary precondition for the comparison of possible selves to an *actual* self. In saying this, it is important to note that a transparent self-model cannot only function as an *internal* frame of reference but will also be a necessary precondition for successful social cognition. For instance, in the schizophrenic patient (see section 7.2.2), a conscious representation of the social environment will frequently be pathologically enriched by heard voices and inserted thoughts, because the ongoing process of cognitive self-simulation cannot be integrated into the background of the transparent self-model any more. Social cognition is continuously distorted by social *hallucinations* in these patients. In order to develop and sustain social intelligence, you need a "who" system (see Georgieff and Jeannerod 1998) allowing you to understand who the current thinker is and who the current agent actually is. You need to know who *you* are: Action perceptions and internal simulations of ongoing thought processes have to be successfully bound to models of agents and models of thinkers. In order to achieve this, you need a transparent self-model.

Transparent Self-Modeling as a Functional Property
If a system meets all other necessary constraints for conscious experience, it will instantiate the phenomenal property of selfhood as soon as it possesses a transparent self-model. Obviously, the functional profile of a system is greatly enriched if it possesses a persisting, globally available source of system-related information (see section 6.2.1). Here, I want only to point out a more general aspect of this development: Systems operating under a transparent self-model constantly assume their own existence as an individual, coherent entity. They generate the self as a fictitious fixed point in their flexible, internal ontology (see also Blau 1986). They become *realists—naive realists—*about themselves, and this will obviously have functional consequences. I like to express this point by saying that the possession of a transparent PSM makes a system maximally *egotistic*. The newly introduced difference between the system and its environment, as well as the difference between the system and *other* agents in its environment, now becomes an irrevocable, ultimately real difference. Because the transparency of the self-model can, in standard situations, not be transcended, the representational segregation of the system from its physical as well as from its social environment is a preattentionally, precognitively fixed structural feature of its model of reality. It will therefore be characterized by maximal causal efficacy. Representational segregation leads to functional segregation. Transparent self-modeling turns us into mentally isolated, individual beings on the level of conscious experience. It is precisely opaque, cognitive self-representation that much later enables philosophical doubts about the irrevocable nature or the subject-object dichotomy or phenomena like social cognition and solidarity. More about this later.

When introducing the notion of phenomenal transparency in section 3.2.7, we identified three different possible misunderstandings: transparency as an *epistemic* characteristic of the mind in general and of self-consciousness in particular (the Cartesian intuition that turned out to be epistemically unjustified, but phenomenologically adequate); the *semantic* notion of transparency as a property of extensional contexts (not applying to nonlinguistic entities like phenomenal states, but involving a similar kind of existence assumption); and the notion of transparency as a property of *media* (as used in the theory of telecommunication). It is, in terms of new functional properties brought about by a transparent self-model, highly interesting in noting that (a) the self-model is an entity entirely located on the subpersonal level of description, while at the same time (b) it is the decisive link in enabling personal-level communication between human beings and within larger groups. You *become* a person by having the right kind of subpersonal self-model, one that functionally allows you to enter mutual relationships of acknowledging each other's personhood in a social context. Just as in the e-mail example given in section 3.2.7, personal-level communication and intersubjective information processing in societies takes place in a seemingly effortless and direct manner, while being facilitated by a transparent subpersonal mechanism. As a functional property, the transparency of large portions in our self-model was important, because the self-model could become the *medium* through which human beings could become causally linked in cultural contexts.

Neural Correlates of Transparent Self-Modeling
Again, not much is presently known about the neural underpinnings of the transparent self-model in humans. We return to this issue in section 6.3.1, and we study a number of neurological deficits leading to deviant forms of transparent, phenomenal self-modeling in chapter 7. However, let me briefly point out that the concept of a transparent PSM bears at least some similarity to Antonio Damasio's notion of the "core-self" (see Damasio 1999, 2000).

6.2.7   Virtual Phenomenal Selves

Just as there are transparent and opaque partitions of the human self-model complementing each other, there also exists a permanent online component along with more or less transient forms of self-*simulational* content. These are activated offline. The human self-model not only targets the current state of the organism but *possible* selves as well. Biographical memories are perfect examples of such phenomenal self-simulations, as are sexual fantasies or thoughts about life after death. Clearly, viewed from an epistemological perspective, every PSM is a simulation; in all its internal complexity it is merely a hypothesis about the current state of the system, which itself is never in absolute contact with its own current physical reality. However, starting from the phenomenological level of description, a number of further and interesting constraints for the concept of a PSM can now be developed, utilizing the well-known conceptual instruments introduced in chapter 5.

The Phenomenology of Phenomenal Self-Simulation

There are basically two kinds of phenomenal self-simulations: those accompanied by the higher-order phenomenal property of agency (see sections 6.4.3, 6.4.4, and 6.4.5) and those which appear as spontaneously happening on the level of conscious experience. What is common to both classes of phenomenological processes is that they experientially *distance us from ourselves*. We now have a clear conceptual understanding of why it makes good sense to employ this metaphor: There actually *is* a distance created within the global model of reality currently activated by the system, namely, the representational distance between the current self-representatum and the current self-simulatum, which are both integrated into one singular PSM (see section 3.2.8). As representational entities, they could both be described as activation vectors in a neural net, and their distance could be precisely described in terms of trajectories connecting both points in state space or in terms of an angle holding between them. Although their representational content can be compared, they are nevertheless functionally integrated because the neural activity described by one vector (the self-simulatum) is bound into the ongoing activity of the larger portion described by the other vector (the self-representatum). Both vectors causally overlap, and a similarity relationship can be objectively described between the nonoverlapping portions (and introspectively detected in some types of systems). Although the phenomenal self still forms a single, integrated structure, as can be seen from the fact that self-representational, as well as self-simulational content, is integrated by the overarching phenomenal property of "mineness," there is an increasing portion of the self-model, which does not representationally covary with or functionally track the current state of the organism. Let us look at some examples.

If, while riding on a train and gazing out the window in a deeply relaxed state, you suddenly drift off into pleasant childhood memories, the focus of your attention is now bound by a spontaneous process of reconstructing past phenomenal selves. Your current bodily self remains globally available for attention and cognition, but this availability is presently not realized. Subtle self-representational content is always active in the background, constituting your phenomenal body image, but the most comprehensive part of your PSM is now constituted by the reconstruction of the emotions you had that day when granddad took you out fishing and you caught your first pike. You may relive a considerable part of the emotional experience, but find it hard to feel yourself into the actual vibrating sensations the fishing rod caused in your hand while battling with the big fish, of which you had not yet had a glimpse, and which was fighting down there in the deep. The conductor, suddenly entering your compartment, disturbs your reverie, and you suddenly find yourself in the present—firmly locked to your body while busily searching for your ticket. Embarrassed, you now start to run an *intended* simulation: What exactly were my next actions after I picked up the ticket I received from the clerk in the train station? Did I leave it in the telephone booth?

There is an interesting difference between intended and nonintended phenomenal simulations: Subjectively, they may be accompanied by a conscious sense of effort, as when deliberately constructing the sequence of changes in the phenomenal self following the purchase of the ticket. Or they can come about in a seemingly effortless manner, without the phenomenal quality of cognitive agency or goal-directedness. Interestingly, there is a preattentive, precognitive property shared by *all* phenomenal self-simulations: they are your *own* images about yourself.

Phenomenal Self-Simulation as a Representational Property

In standard situations, a PSM integrates self-presentational, self-representational, and self-simulational content. What is special about self-simulational content, activated at the level of conscious experience? As we have already seen, phenomenal simulations endow an organism with a competence for counterfactuality and allow it to distance itself from whatever it experiences as the immediate present. In this way the appearance-reality distinction becomes available (on the level of subjective experience); the difference between actuality and potentiality, the difference between what is real and what is only possible, is itself introduced into the organism's model of reality. The possibility of misrepresentation becomes available for the first time. The real trick however, consists in the fact that in standard situations the phenomenal simulation of possible worlds or situations is always firmly *anchored* in a comprehensive, transparent model of the world.

If we apply these general insights to the special case of phenomenal self-simulation, we can start to see why it is such a highly interesting phenomenon. Because intended phenomenal simulations are always integrated into a preexisting, transparent PSM—which is not recognized *as* a model by the system—they can be *owned* by this very system. What does this mean? For intended phenomenal self-simulations we always find two transparent phenomenal properties, namely, mineness and agency, which lead to an overall state in which the content of these states is clearly marked out as my *own* mental activity, which has been deliberately created by *myself*. Thoughts about the future of this organism now unequivocally become *my own* thoughts about *my own* future. Mental images, rising about those fabulous fishing trips with granddad that I enjoyed so much in the distant past, can be *owned* by myself. They can become represented as parts of an integrated biography, which is *my own*. This, certainly, is a new achievement. It allows any system capable of it to not only endow some of the results of internal information processing with the property of global availability, it will for the first time allow it to conceive of itself *as* a persisting *cognitive agent* (see section 6.4.4).

However, self-related dreaming is not the same as cognitive agency. It is important to note that at least three essential factors are involved in reaching the level of a truly intended phenomenal self-simulation: first, a generation of possible phenomenal selves as such (which could also take place in a simple dream); second, the embedding of these opaque self-simulations in the background of an already existing transparent self-model (as in gazing out the train window, slowly drifting away into childhood memories, which are owned but experienced as occurring spontaneously); and third, a self-model including a representation of the actual process of *selecting* certain mental images for attentional processing as opposed to others (as in full cognitive agency, when deliberately trying to remember when you saw your train ticket for the last time; see also sections 6.4.3 and 6.4.4).

Phenomenal Self-Simulation as an Informational-Computational Strategy

Globally available self-simulations make new forms of knowledge possible, for instance, by allowing a system to conceive of the difference between self-representation and self-misrepresentation. They permit the use of new sources of, for example, biographical information, by making it globally accessible, and thereby increase the overall intelligence of the system. It is interesting to note how the transparent process of self-modeling underlying self-simulational episodes experienced as effortless and spontaneous turns out to be highly robust in a psychological sense, whereas genuinely cognitive information processing in the sense just sketched, for beings like us, is an episodic enterprise, experienced as effortful and unreliable, and in general turns out to be much more fragile. This is a clear indicator of the relative evolutionary age and elementary relevance to survival corresponding to these processes. Conscious thought is an expensive luxury. For beings like us, opaque self-modeling seems to be much more demanding on the computational resources our central nervous system has to offer.

Intended Phenomenal Self-Simulations as Functional States

The causal role of phenomenal self-simulations possesses two essential characteristics, both of which we have already encountered. Self-simulations can be activated independently of the persistent functional link to the physical basis of the system that is characteristically generated by self-*presentational* content. However, second, they are always integrated into the background of a preexisting, transparent self-model. From a teleo-functionalist perspective, obviously, the advantages of conscious self-simulation have been that they make self-related information, which is not information about the *current* state of the system, globally available for guiding attention, for cognition, and for the control of external behavior. In particular, they not only generate cognitive agency but can eventually make the fact *that* one is currently a cognitive agent globally available. Obviously, there are many situations—for example, in social cognition and "theory of mind" tasks—in which this new functional property serves to increase reproductive success.

Neural Correlates of Phenomenal Self-Simulation

We are now witnessing an intensification of the search for physiological correlates to the phenomenal content activated by conscious, intended self-simulations. For instance, on the level of the emotional self-model, recent scanning data show what kinds of subcortical and cortical brain activity correspond to the conscious feeling of self-generated emotions (Damasio, Grabowski, Bechara, Damasio, Ponto, Parvizi, and Hichwa 2000; see section 6.3.1 for further examples). But let us proceed to the question of how a system can use a conscious self-model in satisfying the adaptivity constraint, the last of the ten constraints developed in chapter 3. Please note that at this point I am also skipping issues of how intensities in self-presentational content and the homogeneity of "attentionally atomic" self-representational content contribute to the overall profile of the self-model. I do this simply because I am convinced that what has been said in sections 3.2.9 and 3.2.10 already suffices for my present purposes.

6.2.8   Adaptivity: The Self-Model as a Tool and as a Weapon

Let us conclude the first part of this chapter by looking at some defining characteristics for the concept of a PSM which can be developed from a third-person perspective. What insights can be gained from treating PSMs as historical entities that have developed in the course of a biological evolution? What functions can be fulfilled by PSMs during different stages of ontogenetic development? Applying our teleofunctionalist background assumption to the concept of a conscious self-model serves to further enrich this concept: Self-models are neurocognitive tools which can be discovered and sharpened, which can function in isolation, or, like instruments in a large social orchestra, form coherent ensembles. They are new kinds of virtual organs, and certain aspects of their content can even be passed on to future generations. In a certain context, they can fulfill a function *for* the organism. If we want to take them seriously, as psychologically real cognitive capacities, we must accept what José Luis Bermúdez has called the "acquisition constraint": There must be an explanation of how it is possible for an individual human being in the normal course of her development to acquire the capacity for conscious self-modeling (Bermúdez 1998, p. 19*ff.*).

Let us start with the stimulus-correlated part of the self-model. Transparent self-presentational content (see section 5.4) allows an organism to *feel* itself as itself. As a physical system continuously engaged in the process of self-organization and self-regulation, the organism has to maintain a robust functional boundary with its environment and keep a large number of internal parameters stable and invariant. A large section of self-presentational content precisely generates a continuous flow of information about the degree of invariance that is currently being achieved. One of the merits of Antonio Damasio's empirical investigations concerning the physical basis and function of the phenomenal self has been to highlight the way in which this flow is very likely rooted in elementary bioregulatory processes, those processes concerned with keeping the internal chemical milieu of the body stable in a continuously changing environment. Here is a brief passage pointing out how higher-order self-modeling has likely grown out of elementary homeostatic dynamics. It also gives an idea of how the most fundamental content in the self-model may supervene on an exclusively *internal* causal role, and is intimately connected to the ongoing attempt to stay alive.

The specifications for survival that I am describing include: A boundary; an internal structure; a dispositional arrangement for the regulation of internal states that subsumes a mandate to maintain life, a narrow range of variability of internal states so that those states are relatively stable. Now consider these specifications. Am I describing *just* a list of specifications for the survival of a simple living organism, or could it be that I am also describing some of the biological antecedents of the sense of self—the sense of a single, bounded, living organism bent on maintaining stability to maintain its life? I would say that I might be describing either. It is intriguing to think that the constancy of the internal milieu is essential to maintain life *and* that it might be a blueprint and anchor for what will eventually become a self in the mind. (Damasio 1999, p. 136)

If self-modeling could contribute to the elementary life-managing functions, as they are, for instance, realized in certain brainstem structures (see section 6.3.1), this would obviously be an evolutionary advantage that may have been selected. Conscious self-presentational content pointing to the internal state of the body and supplying information about hunger, thirst, hormone and transmitter levels, intestinal states, and skin temperature does precisely this: It integrates a large number of continuous signals into a unified structure and makes its content *globally available* for attention, cognition, and, in particular, for self-directed action. The *inter*oceptive component of conscious self-perception allows us to make threats to the integrity of the overall functional structure constituted by the intricate network of underlying bioregulatory mechanisms immediately available not only for introspective attention but for a whole range of other processing mechanisms. This information now is globally available for a *flexible* kind of control. If self-presentational information is available for cognition, it can be categorized and compared to earlier experiences of the same kind represented in autobiographical memory. *Internal* behavior can now be selected from a large variety of different possibilities in order to maintain stability and return to an optimal internal state. Viewed in this way, conscious self-presentational content simply is a new strategy for controlling the dynamics of the internal chemical milieu, for keeping the flow of elementary biological dynamics as smooth as possible. Obviously, there are precursors to this achievement on the level of unconscious processing. For example, what in my terminology is mental or merely internal (i.e., necessarily nonphenomenal) self-presentation bears a close resemblance to Damasio's concept of the unconscious proto-self (e.g., Damasio 1999, p. 153*ff.*).

It is important to see how unconscious self-modeling is a continuous process, guiding the organism through phases like deep sleep when it is not a phenomenal subject. What exactly the phenomenal level of representation adds can now be derived from the constraints developed in chapter 3: It makes a merely neural collection of patterns continuously mapping the state of the organism globally available *for* the organism; it allows the organism to conceive of these states as *present* states; as part of a more comprehensive *reality*, in which the organism owning these states is itself embedded; it integrates information from many different sources into a multidimensional whole, while still allowing for a certain degree of differentiation. It permits the organism to direct its attention to the *convolved* nature of its own internal body states, that is, to their dynamic, temporal profile and interplay. If the organism is capable of focal attention and intended cognition, it makes these states available from a higher-order first-person perspective directed onto them as apparently simple, first-order self-states; by presenting them to the organism in a *transparent* manner, it, importantly, makes them appear as absolutely real and directly given; and although there will be a fundamental level of representational atomicity generating the characteristic feature of the homogeneity and grainless "ultrasmoothness" of simple bodily sensations, it offers the important possibility of representing *intensities* for individual parameters. Obviously, different classes of conscious systems will satisfy these constraints to differing degrees. But it is now plausible to assume that even the most elementary form of conscious self-modeling will have possessed an obvious biological advantage. And realizing how the most fundamental forms of human self-consciousness satisfy the adaptivity constraint in a strong sense possesses a deeper philosophical flavor: For beings like ourselves, more complex forms of *being someone* are inextricably interwoven with the actual struggle of *preserving existence*. This is where we come from. It is interesting to note how for artificial or postbiotic systems not meeting the adaptivity constraint in terms of their self-models, a completely different kind of phenomenal identity could arise.

One interesting way of looking at brains is as systems predicting *reward events* in the future. The PSM will be an important and essential computational tool for any such system. Why? It is now well-known that the dopaminergic system is a part of the brain that continuously produces input into the self-model by labeling certain events as being more or less rewarding. What the PSM adds is the integration of this information into the context of the organism as a whole, making them reward events for the system *itself*. The dopaminergic system functions as an economic evaluator and as a decision-maker. As a very old system (already in existence in the honeybee) it diffusely projects into the prefrontal cortex. It modulates cognitive processing and selection processes, such as decisions on certain behavioral patterns. Therefore, the brain may in part not only be conceived of as a correlation-representing system but as a system producing predictions about the environment by representing events in terms of their *self-rewarding potential*. It is plausible to assume a high adaptive value for such a mechanism, particularly if it makes the above-mentioned type of information globally available, if it brings additional autobiographical knowledge about *past* self-rewarding events online, and so on. The possession of a PSM will be necessary and crucial to realizing or further developing such a mechanism.

Let us look at another example, this time on the level of self-*re*presentation, the level of consciously representing complex, relational features of the current state of the organism. Obviously, for moving, hunting, fleeing, mating organisms it must have been of great relevance to possess a good representation of their own body—for instance, in planning motor behavior, but also, more simply, to perceive their own boundaries. Any organism carrying out complex movements in an environment where it would pay a high price for making mistakes needs an online representation of not only the internal state of its own body but also of its current shape, momentum, and velocity, of its "collision properties," and so forth. To give an example, one highly speculative, but interesting hypothesis in primatology (Povinelli and Cant 1995) proposes that an integrated self-conception originally developed from the arboreal clambering of orangutans. Because of their bodily weight and the great height at which orangutans climb through trees, it may have been necessary for them to maintain an integrated and continuously updated body-model to successfully coordinate their behavior. Obviously, it is only a *conscious* body-model that could make the current state of the body as a whole available, in terms of constituting a potential object of attention and fast learning processes. Whatever the merits of this specific theory, Povinelli and Cant interestingly point out that the metabolic price to be paid for self-consciousness and the amount of neural hardware needed is very likely large. Therefore, if no corresponding reproductive advantage would result from possessing this feature, it would very likely disappear through genetic drift, and in a short period of time. After orangutans leave the trees they have to either find a new, for example, a *social*, function for their rudimentary self-model or they will be in permanent danger of losing it. And this is a further important teleofunctionalist constraint on the development of conscious self-models: Either you use it or you lose it. Gorillas may have already lost the capacity for self-modeling, because they developed different social structures and are not making use of it any more. Chimpanzees may currently be *in the process* of losing it, while human beings have focused on this new virtual organ in making it a source of their own superb intelligence. (However, it is important to note that the use of conscious self-models in social cognition is just one way of expressing intelligence. In terms of overall information density and computational performance, the noncognitive, bodily self-model of, say, a dolphin might display a comparably superb form of intelligence—one that was fine-tuned to another niche and therefore had invested all of the available neurocomputational power into another "format.") Gordon Gallup (1997) argues that orangutans may have developed the first online-model of the self as an agent, including a certain degree of control over their own actions, because they were forced to develop *nonstereotyped patterns* of climbing through high trees. Again, we see that the step from nonconscious to conscious representation is the step from rigidity to flexibility: A conscious self- or body-model is needed if bodily behavior has to transcend a certain threshold of flexibility. As Gallup points out, only 50% of all chimpanzees show convincing signs of mirror self-recognition. They might therefore actually be in the process of losing certain self-representational abilities. It is interesting to note how some species developed by focusing on competition, while others (e.g., social insects) focused on cooperation. There must be an optimal combination of both strategies, and this may have been a prime reason for a more developed self-model to become an advantageous instrument: It enabled introspectively accessing simulations of the experiences and intentional states of *other* beings.

Possessing an integrated, conscious self-model also allows you to discover isomorphisms between your own movement and shapes and movements perceived in the external environment. This may, for instance, be important in recognizing a conspecific as currently imitating your behavior or a predator following your trajectory. More abstractly, we may conceive of this capacity as dynamic pattern matching in the domain of kinematic geometry. However, there is a special case of this ability that has received wide attention since Gordon Gallup's original 1970 paper: the capacity of some, but not all primates to recognize themselves in a mirror (Gallup 1970, see also Metzinger 1994). What precisely is the moment of mirror self-recognition, according to the theory proposed here? A successful representationalist theory of the conscious first-person perspective must be able to point to this moment in terms of a new kind of representational *content* appearing in the mind of the subject. It also has to do justice to the dynamic nature of the overall process. What kind of *containing* exclusively characterizes this moment? It is the moment when the visual phenomenal mental model of a conspecific moving back and forth in front of me is *embedded* in the currently active, multimodal self-model. The first stage of this situation consists of a transparent self-model, which is currently integrated with a transparent, visual model of a conspecific depicted as external: [Myself now looking at another member of my own species] (see also section 6.5). In this phase an animal will typically display social behavior, then disinterest. In the second stage the system discovers a *partial* relational homomorphy between the moving object component in the external model of reality, given through vision and the multidimensional dynamics of its own kinematic geometry, as accessed through different channels of proprioception. The moment of mirror self-recognition is precisely the moment at which the system suddenly realizes that it can successfully *embed* the "external" model in the currently active self-model: it can *identify* itself with the phenomenal content given in the mode of external perception. *Self-containing* is possible. In a very literal sense, this integration of representational content leads, transiently, to the instantiation of the phenomenal property of "mineness," which I introduced as one of our explanatory target properties at the beginning of this chapter. At this very moment, the content of conscious experience is: ["This is *myself* moving!"]. I had first proposed this representationalist analysis for the phenomenal correlate of mirror self-recognition in 1994 (p. 49*f.*). Now we begin to see evidence demonstrating that the relevant parts of the monkey self-model are bimodally coded by somatosensory and visual neurons in the monkey intraparietal cortex, which possesses multimodal representations of the body and peripersonal space utilized in the motor planning of goal-directed actions, which in turn can extend, for example, to a video image of the monkey's hand by rearranging its visual receptive field around the image of the hand seen on the video screen (Iriki, Tanaka, Obayashi, and Iwamura 2001). Through training, monkeys learned to recognize the image of their body parts in the video monitor as a part of their own body. The neural correlate of this type of self-recognition in an "electronic mirror" can now plausibly be hypothesized as a transient shift in certain visual receptive fields, functionally *integrating* them with a previously active multimodal self-representation dominated by somatosensory input. It is also interesting to see how the above-mentioned investigators are led to propose a PSM by these data, namely, the concept of a "subjective self-image" (p. 170).

Please note that the PSM of human beings can even *extend* to the visual representation of one's own mirror-image as well, for instance, when feeling the tactile sensations accompanying the process of shaving *in* the visually perceived mirror image. Have your ever tried this? The fact that chimpanzees are also able to recognize themselves in mirrors that produce distorted or multiplied self-images demonstrates that they do not do so by recognizing single properties, but very likely because of the temporal *contiguity* of volition, proprioception, and visual representation (Kitchen et al. 1996). What they do is exploit the convolved holism of their reality-model. Obviously, then, an integrated multimodal body model displaying the temporal characteristics of certain movements and possibly even realizing the higher-order property of phenomenal agency is a necessary precondition for primates to be able to recognize themselves in mirrors. In humans, candidates for a distinct neural correlate of conscious mirror self-recognition of one's own face have recently been discovered (see Kircher, Senior, Phillips, Rabe-Hesketh, Benson, Bullmore, Brammer, Simmons, Bartels, and David 2001). However, I am offering a brief *representationalist* analysis of the target capacity here because I take it to be a much more universal, hardware-independent feature of certain classes of self-conscious systems. Eventually what is needed is a computational-representational model of mirror self-recognition to complement these data. Neuroanatomical substrates may be highly variable. To give an example, there is now robust evidence for the existence of mirror self-recognition in a cetacean, namely, the bottle-nosed dolphin (Reiss and Marino 2001). Dolphins and chimpanzees are phylogenetically distant and their cortical cytoarchitecture differs considerably, because cetacean and primate ancestral lines diverged at least 65 to 70 million years ago (Reiss and Marino 2001, p. 5942). Therefore, a more abstract level of analysis is needed. Else we cannot describe the evolutionary *convergence* as a convergence toward *one* cognitive capacity. Although from an evolutionary perspective the advantage gained by this specific capacity may be rather small, it is also of interest to see how this new representational ability immediately enriches the internal as well as the external behavioral profile of the chimpanzee and the bottlenosed dolphin. The chimpanzee is now able to attend to its body parts, and to engage in self-directed behavior toward these body parts of which it was previously unaware, as can be seen when it inspects its teeth, its nostrils, or the lower part of its back in front of the mirror. A dolphin sham-marked on its right pectoral fin may exhibit a continuous sequence of twelve dorsal-to-ventral body flips in front of a reflecting surface so as to bring the right pectoral fin into close viewing range or, upon being marked for the first time on the tongue, immediately swim to a mirror and engage in a mouth opening-and-closing sequence (ibid., p. 5941). New system-related information has become globally available; the phenomenal model of reality has been expanded.

An *unconscious* body image is an important neurocomputational tool for sensorimotor integration: The body simply *is* the place where perceptual states and motor responses come together. A rudimentary, innate image of your own body may also have been what enabled you to recognize yourself in the mirror of your mother's face. Newborn infants are able to imitate the facial expressions and head movements of grown-ups hours after birth, sometimes even as soon as 40 minutes after birth (Berlucchi and Aglioti 1997). An infant has never seen its own face, nor would it be capable of mirror self-recognition. It has to translate a visually perceived facial gesture into a motoric simulation of the same movements by its own facial muscles. Again, an isomorphism has to be generated and sustained across modalities. I am saying that an integrated self-model is the representational tool needed to achieve this goal. The ability to establish a firm emotional contact with your parents soon after birth, creating an interpersonal bond, is another example of the adaptive value a coherent self-representation can possess at a very early stage of life. However, while the possession of an innate body schema enabling early social communication and intermodal integration of information is clearly of high value from a teleofunctionalist perspective, this does not guarantee the existence of a PSM at this early stage. Obviously, since the autobiographical self-model only emerges at the age of 2 years, we have no introspective access to the these early phases of our lives and therefore no kind of first-person knowledge of the existence of first-person experience at this point. Gallagher and Meltzoff (1996) presented two independent lines of argument for an innate body image. I return to their proposals concerning phantom limbs in section 7.2.3. In our present context it is highly interesting to note how these authors point out the possibility that a *phenomenal* connection between self and others could actually exist from birth onward. As we have seen, a number of new studies on the imitative behavior of newborn infants support the conclusion that a computational model transforming visual information into motor commands must be in existence at birth. Interestingly, if mouth movements are temporarily suppressed by pacifiers, even temporarily delayed imitations of facial gestures are possible. This may justify the conclusion that infants not only possess an innate body image but also a globally available, that is, a *conscious*, proprioceptive self-model of their own face which they can hold in working memory. Meltzoff and Moore had earlier introduced the notion of a *supramodal* perceptual system, an idea that is obviously closely related to the theory proposed here. The concept of such a supramodal code means that visual and motor systems speak the same "language" right from birth (Gallagher and Meltzoff 1996, p. 225). This language is the language of the self-model. Gallagher and Meltzoff speculate that body image and the proprioceptive self-model may therefore be coupled to those of other human beings right from birth in, as it were, offering a common *format* or window for interpersonal communication. This, of course, would be a discovery of the highest philosophical interest, but it seems that further, careful empirical investigations are necessary to firmly establish the idea. Against Merleau-Ponty, Gallagher and Meltzoff write:

In contrast, the conception of an already-accomplished, innate, supramodal visual-motor/ proprioceptive link suggests that the transgression is immediate and that *experientially*, and not just objectively, we are born into a world of others. (Gallagher and Meltzoff 1996, p. 226)

I return to the role self-models have played in making the transition from biological to cultural evolution at a later stage. At this point, it is only important to note how possession of a conscious self-model will, very obviously, have been adaptive in enabling social cognition and the construction of interpersonal relationships.

In conclusion let me mention two more aspects of the PSM that obviously possess great adaptive value and that could fulfill a large range of functions *for* an organism. The generation of *virtual selves*, as discussed in sections 5.3 and 6.2.7, opens a whole new universe: the universe of planning one's own behavior and remembering one's own past. This will start on the level of simulating bodily movement, thereby minimizing mismatching errors, supporting learning processes, and enabling a whole range of internally simulated alternatives. For instance, the process of intended phenomenal self-simulation on the level of the spatial model of one's own body allows for *forward models* that simulate the development from motion to perception: Which proprioceptive perception would be caused by this movement of the body? It would also enable *inverse models*, simulating the development from perception to motion: Which motion would lead to the perception of a certain, desired body position? Good computational models for sensorimotor integration internally simulating the causal flow of a motor command and anticipating sensory feedback already exist (see, e.g., Wolpert et al. 1995; Wolpert and Ghahramani 2000). It is obvious what the advantage of elevating such computational processes to the phenomenal level of representation would be. They would become available for attentional processing, continuous refinement, and immediate stopping by inserting a "veto." It is obvious how more abstract and refined versions of such original simulations utilizing the bodily self-model, for example, when simulating the "grasping" of a concept (see Gallese 2001; Rizzolatti and Arbib 1998; and section 6.3.3), would have constituted a major evolutionary advantage, by enabling higher cognition, language use, and the emergence of complex societies. I will not go deeper into these issues at this point. Rather, I want to point out that one of the most important biological functions of the human self-model consists in *integrating* all the different capacities that developed in the course of its long biological history. It not only allows an organism to "own" certain mental representations and simulations activated by its central nervous system, it also achieves a coupling of higher, genuinely cognitive forms of self-simulation—for example, reasoning and the mental simulation of symbol use—to the elementary bioregulatory processes, that is, the *presentational* self anchored in interoception and elementary homeostasis which was mentioned at the beginning of this section. Conscious creation of virtual selves, therefore, is always ultimately tied to the physical needs and the low-level functional self-organization of the organism in which it emerges. In this way the integrative function of the human self-model achieves another adaptive advantage. It consists in tying all processes of self-representation and self-simulation into the logic of survival, by putting them in an emotional context, and by imposing an implicit, normative structure (a "valence axis") on all processes of self-representation and self-simulation. All levels of phenomenal self-representation are, therefore, ultimately grounded in bodily self-management and the self-regulation of the underlying life process. Another quotation from Antonio Damasio will illustrate this point:

Creatures with consciousness have some advantages over those that do not have consciousness. They can establish a link between the world of automatic regulation (the world of basic homeostasis that is interwoven with the proto-self) and the world of imagination (the world in which images of different modalities can be combined to produce novel images of situations that have not yet happened). The world of imaginary creations—the world of planning, the world of formulation of scenarios and prediction of outcomes—is linked to the world of the proto-self. The sense of self links forethought, on the one hand, to preexisting automation, on the other.

Consciousness is not the sole means of generating adequate responses to an environment and thus achieving homeostasis. Consciousness is just the latest and most sophisticated means of doing so,
. . .

I would say that consciousness, as currently designed, constrains the world of imagination to be first and foremost about the individual, about an individual organism, about the self in the broad sense of the term. I would say that the effectiveness of consciousness comes from its unabashed connection to the nonconscious proto-self. This is the connection that guarantees that proper attention is paid to the matters of individual life by creating a *concern*. (Damasio 1999, p. 303 *ff.*)

6.3   Descriptive Levels of the Human Self-Model

The application of the constraints developed for the concept of phenomenal representation in chapter 3 now has yielded another helpful working concept, the concept of a PSM. Let us now strictly limit the intended class of systems to human beings in non-pathological waking states. The conscious self-model of human beings, conceptually, is an entity that can simultaneously be described on multiple subpersonal levels of description. Phenomenal content supervenes on internal system properties. Therefore, to further flesh out the notion of a PSM, to put it to work in interdisciplinary cooperation between philosophy and neuroscience, it is important to look for neural correlates of the conscious self.

6.3.1   Neural Correlates

Arguably, the conscious self-model constitutes the most complex form of individual phenomenal content we know. This makes the search for neural correlates of phenomenal self-consciousness extremely difficult, because, for a number of theoretical and empirical reasons, it has to be assumed that, at any given moment, the neural correlate of self-consciousness (NCSC) will be highly distributed. Strategically, there are at least two important ways to cope with this general obstacle: first, focus on the invariant partitions of the self-model, namely, precisely those aspects which are self-*presentational* in terms of being directly correlated with internal stimuli; second, concentrate on very specific forms of mental self-modeling while keeping constant as many other functional factors as possible. Still, the general task is of overwhelming difficulty and will doubtlessly remain a major target for neuroscience for many decades. However, let me point out that there is a positive aspect to the empirical search for the NCSC as well.

The search for the neural correlate of consciousness (NCC) has only just begun at the beginning of this millennium (see, e.g., Metzinger 2000). As will become obvious at the end of this chapter, a very large class of active phenomenal states can be *defined* precisely by the fact that they become episodically integrated with the current self-model on a very small time scale as attention, volitional selection mechanisms, and cognition wander around in representational space and create transient phenomenal representations of *subject-object relations*. This is one straightforward empirical prediction, following from the theoretical considerations developed in this chapter. Global availability of information always means availability for transient, dynamical integration with the currently active self-model. The self-model theory of subjectivity developed here can serve as a valuable tool to mark out a specific, and arguably the most interesting class of NCCs: those conscious experiences explicitly bound to a first-person perspective. And that is why the search for the NCSC, even though we are at the very beginning of this arduous task, is of high methodological relevance. Only if we find the neural and functional correlates of what philosophers call the "phenomenal self," will we be able to discover a more *general* theoretical framework into which all data can fit. Eventually, it is only this empirical project, which will allow us to understand what it means precisely that our target phenomenon, phenomenal experience, is a *subjective* phenomenon. Let us call this the "principle of perspectival integration" (PPI). I return to it in section 6.5.

What are the most invariant parts of the conscious model of reality? The answer is now evident: It is phenomenal content constituted by the presentational part of the bodily self-model. The most invariant part of the conscious model of reality is, in standard situations, identical with the most invariant part of the self-model. This part possesses a phenomenal as well as an unconscious, nonphenomenal partition. According to the conceptual tools developed in chapter 2 and in section 5.4 of chapter 5 in particular, there is mental as well as phenomenal self-presentation. You may recall that according to the simple terminology used here there are basically three different kinds of content-bearing structures: *internal* representations (which are never conscious), *mental* representations (which *sometimes* can become conscious), and *phenomenal* representations (which *always* are conscious). The human self-model is unique in that it creates a highly invariant and persisting functional link between phenomenal, mental, and internal self-presentation. Phenomenal self-presentation is anchored in mental self-presentation, which in turn is rooted in purely internal, self-regulatory states of a merely functional nature. Therefore, we have to search for all those processes that, first, generate strictly stimulus-correlated representational content; second, that intrinsically process only system-related information; and that, third, can be marked out by different levels of global availability for attentional processing.

For example, in terms of concrete candidates for focal points within what undoubtedly is a complex and distributed network, there is an unconscious component of the process of permanently mapping body signals. Damasio proposes three different brain structures to implement this elementary level of self-modeling (which, in his terminology, constitute the "proto-self"): Certain *brainstem nuclei*, the *hypothalamus*, and the *basal forebrain*, and a certain part of the somatosensory cortices, namely, the *insular cortex*, *S2*, and the *medial parietal cortices* located behind the splenium of the corpus callosum (Damasio 1999, p. 155*ff.*). Functionally, these brain regions serve to regulate body states and constantly signal the overall current body state. In particular, their function consists in presenting aspects of the internal milieu, as, for instance, hormone or ion concentrations, pH value, nutrient levels, and so on, and invariant aspects of the musculoskeletal frame.

According to the current model, the conscious component is formed by a subset of the ongoing activity of these structures, which is integrated into the window of presence and the global model of the world. For example, elements of this subset will be all neural processes that functionally penetrate working memory.

In section 6.5, we look at a third characteristic of the PSM, which holds in almost all classes of conscious experience: it is bound into a phenomenal subject-object relation. Damasio also offers three neuroanatomical candidates for major components contributing to the complex and ever-changing network, which may underlie the internal representation of this organism-object relation. They subserve what, in his own terminology, would be the process of "second-order mapping": the cingulate cortex, certain thalamic nuclei, and the superior colliculi (Damasio 1999, p. 260ff.) The cingulate, while being involved in attentional processing and emotion, contributes to the generation of complex behavior while simultaneously being a massively somatosensory structure, driven by inputs from many different sources, including signals caused by the musculoskeletal aspects of the body, the viscera, and the internal milieu. The superior colliculi may play an important role in integrating activity related to orienting movements involved in attending to the source of a visual or auditory stimulus. The thalamus, finally, could serve to implicitly signify object-organism relationships (Damasio 1999, p. 265) and cause the emergence of more explicit neural patterns in cingulate cortices and somatosensory cortices. Interestingly, there is evidence from metabolic imaging data (Chugani 1999) suggesting that four structures constituting something like a bridge from the core of the mental to the *PSM*—namely, the brainstem and hypothalamus, the somatosensory cortices, and the cingulate—functionally precede the development of the neural correlates for higher-order forms of self-representational content. Conducting neural imaging research with the help of positron emission tomography (PET) scans on newborn infants, researchers found precisely these structures that are already characterized by strong activity at birth.

A second important theory concerning neural correlates for the bodily self, especially for phenomenal self-representation in terms of spatial properties, is Ronald Melzack's neuromatrix theory (see Melzack 1989, 1992; Katz and Melzack 1990; Melzack et al. 1997). Results stemming from research on pain experience in phantom limbs may, as a matter of fact, point to the existence of a genetically determined neuromatrix, the *input-independent* autonomous activation pattern which could form the functional basis of the most invariant partitions of the phenomenal body image (i.e., the "phylomatrix of the body schema"). Please note that now we are not talking about the self-regulation of the internal milieu constituted by the body but about an issue concerning *spatial representation*. How does the body represent itself as a spatial entity, using its own brain? Is there an *innate* component of the self-model, an inbuilt image of the organism as a whole, occupying a specific region within a spatial frame of reference?

Many investigators may be inclined to think that the elementary body percept is only consolidated in social interactions after birth or during early motor behavior in the womb.[7] On the other hand, a persistent functional link between regions of primary somatosensory cortex and certain regions in the bodily self-model has been proved by direct electrical stimulation during neurosurgical operations under local anesthesia. In the somatosensory cortex, regions of the body that are capable of making finer discriminations of touch (e.g., palm of hand and mouth) have a larger area of representation than areas that are capable of gross discrimination only (such as the back or feet). Electrical stimulation of any of these regions results in the conscious sensation of being touched on the represented body part. Of course, sensory body and motor maps are highly plastic and subject to the influence of experience, even in the adult organism. And, of course, one has to see on theoretical grounds that there is probably no such thing as *absolute* invariance or functional rigidity in highly complex, dynamical systems like the human brain. However, there is interesting evidence for some kind of innate or at least partially genetically determined "body prototype." We have already encountered Meltzoff's work on imitation behavior in newborn infants, which definitely points in that direction. Another line of evidence results from phantom sensations reported by children who are born without one or more limbs (phocomelia). I return to phantom limbs at length in section 7.2.3. For now, let me only point out that well-documented data today show that even people *born* without limbs develop complex bodily self-models which *include those limbs*—even if there never was a source of input in the first place. For example, Melzack and colleagues, in a series of recent (1997) case studies, provide convincing evidence that phantom limbs are experienced by at least 20% of congenitally limb-deficient subjects, and by 50% who underwent amputations before the age of 6 years. If *all* of these congenital cases would fail to have phantom experiences, it would be plausible that *all* bodily self-modeling is only experientially based, but taken together with the fact that some of these patients do not lose the relevant parts of their PSM even as adults, this seems to constitute plausible evidence that the neural correlate of the spatial model of the self is partly immune to local neural plasticity in the somatosensory cortex. Taken together, these data seem to show that a continuous flow of peripheral input is not necessary to activate a phenomenal model of certain body parts, that an innate component within a highly distributed network may actually exist, and that it is highly unlikely that the material now existing in terms of experiential reports given by patients, in its entirety, results from confabulations. Another interesting detail, as pointed out by Melzack, originates in the experience of neurosurgeons. There exist numerous cases in which an excision of the somatosensory cortex did

7. I am greatly indebted to Toemme Noesselt for a number of very helpful discussions of this issue.

not prevent the reappearance of a phantom limb at follow-up (Gybels and Sweet 1989, quoted in Melzack et al. 1997, p. 1619). Here is how Melzack formulates the core idea:

In essence, I postulate that the brain contains a neuromatrix, or network of neurons, that, in addition to responding to sensory stimulation, continuously generates a characteristic pattern of impulses indicating that the body is intact and unequivocally one's own. I call this pattern a neurosignature. If such a matrix operated in the absence of sensory inputs from the periphery of the body, it would create the impression of having a limb even when that limb has been removed. (Melzack 1992, p. 123)

The idea behind neuromatrix theory is that a large part of the phenomenal body-self simply is the output of the autonomous activity of this neuromatrix. Of course such a matrix will be plastic—there will be an *ontomatrix* that changes in the course of an individual's life experience, and there will be something like a *phylomatrix*, an elementary aspect of the body self-model that is, with small variations, shared by all members of a species. There are three concrete components which have so far been named in the context of understanding conscious pain experience located in phantom limbs (for a recent, careful review of the phenomenology and literature on potential mechanisms, see, e.g., Hill 1999): the sensory pathway that travels through the thalamus to the somatosensory cortex, the pathway that goes through the reticular formation to the limbic system, and the parietal lobe (damage to which leads to typical deficits in the PSM, as we will see in chapter 7). However, neuromatrix theory has been criticized because the postulated neural entity extends over such a large and diffuse area of the brain that "the proposed mechanisms are almost impossible to operationalize and test" (Hill 1999, p. 130). Of course, it is not the fault of the theory if the theoretical entity it sees itself as forced to propose, according to current methodologies, cannot be operationalized or easily broken down into isolatable functional subcomponents. It may well be that the search for the NCSC will turn out to be a highly difficult task, precisely because of the hard-to-satisfy phenomenological and representational constraints of "convolved holism," which were introduced earlier. Even the core of the more invariant parts of the PSM could be so densely nested that any straightforward mechanistic strategy of reductive explanation would simply turn out to be not feasible for technical reasons.

Let us now turn to some "higher" levels of content in the PSM. Donald Stuss (1991) pointed out that different representations of self will be related to particular brain structures or regions and that frontal systems appear to be important for those higher levels of self-representation (see also Stuss and Benson 1986). He observed that the ability to maintain and organize information in meaningful sequences, as well as the ability to initiate and drive behavior, seems to have its anatomical basis in the posterior dorsolateral and medial frontal regions (Stuss 1991, p. 258; for further discussion, see also Vogeley,

Kurthen, Falkai, and Maier 1999; Vogeley 2000). Two more important self-related functions can be found in the frontal cortex: executive control and conscious metacognition, the ability to be aware of one's self and one's relation to the environment while possessing the reflective ability to "know about knowing." In cognitive neuropsychiatry, the prefrontal cortex has long been a candidate for disorders related to deficits in executive and monitoring functions of the self-model.

Some studies, however, give us ideas about what the correlates of transient, high-level contents integrated into the PSM could be. Particularly interesting is the ongoing phenomenal experience of *agency*: the volitional self-model, which is generated by briefly integrating a specific phenomenal content, namely, the object component of a "volitional act" (see section 6.4.5). Patrick Haggard and Martin Eimer have investigated the relationship between brain potentials and the awareness of voluntary movements. They replicated classic studies (Libet, Gleason, Wright, and Pearl 1983), trying to pin down neural events corresponding to the perceived time of voluntary actions or the perceived time of initiating those actions. Subjects reported the moment at which a certain representational content within the previously unconscious self-model became globally available for introspective attention—the time when they first "felt the urge" to make a freely willed and endogenous movement (Haggard and Eimer 1999, p. 128.). On average, awareness of this urge to move occurred 296 ms prior to the onset of electromyographic activity. Haggard and Eimer, however, measured *lateralized* readiness potentials as an additional indicator of movement selection and then investigated its temporal relation to actual verbal reports of the subjects which *could*, obviously, only be based on the phenomenal content of their self-models.[8] Haggard and Eimer replicated the temporal patterns in the data produced by the earlier Libet studies, but their studies have the advantage that they allow assumptions about the *content* that is reported in the self-directed judgments of subjects. This issue is of philosophical interest: What is the mental content forming the object component at which a volitional act is "intentionally directed?"

The interesting question, of course, is precisely which component of the rather extended readiness potential directly correlates with the phenomenal content of the urge or will to move. More recent research seems to show that the actual awareness of movement initiation must be based on a transparent phenomenal self-*simulation*, that is, on the content of an internal *prediction* of the state of the system to be expected (see Frith, Blakemore, and Wolpert 2000, p. 1776; Haggard, Newman, and Magno 1999, p. 302; Haggard and

---

8. Please note how, should it turn out that such verbal behavior was actually triggered by the *unconscious* dynamics of the self-model, they could no longer count as *reports* about a mental property that was previously cognitively available. They would not be verbal reports "based on" or "about" the current conscious content of the self-model, but simply complex patterns of motor behavior *caused by* the functional dynamics of the nonphenomenal self-model in the brain.

Magno 1999).[9] The phenomenal content of movement initiation is not determined by signals arising from the actual physical movement of the limb, but by the current state of certain predictors that calculate the potential *consequences* of a specific motor output. It is now plausible to conclude that what we are aware of is an ongoing simulation of a particular, specified movement simulation (an "inverse model"; see Wolpert and Ghahramani 2000). However, this movement simulation is always integrated into the background of an ongoing representation of the system as a whole. More important, however, this type of functional architecture constitutes another highly instructive example of what phenomenal transparency, as functionally constraining the process of conscious self-modeling, actually is. A possibility is portrayed as a reality on the phenomenal level of representation; what subpersonally is only a model of *potential* proprioceptive feedback becomes the subjective experience of [*myself* currently and actually initiating this arm movement]. This transition is achieved by integration into the PSM, and the underlying change in properties of the system can now be reported using personal-level predicates.

A new study suggests that what the self-model gives us access to are only those stages of premotor processes occurring *after* the state of actual movement selection (Haggard and Eimer 1999, p. 132). In other words, what we can report by directing internal attention to the content of our current self-model are not the abstract higher levels of premotor processing preceding the selection of an actual movement, but the actual phenomenal content that later is activated by the functional process of preparing a *specific* bodily movement. It is, of course, an interesting question, whether the abstract, normally unconscious processing stages preceding volitional and phenomenally self-modeled movement selection can already count as *egocentric* representations, or whether this is precisely the step at which those computations are integrated into a self-representation, which also *makes* them conscious.

---

9. Concerning earlier studies of phenomenal volition (e.g., see Libet et al. 1983), Haggard and Magno write: "These findings may specify the timing of *motor awareness* (i.e., the consciously perceived time of a specified motor event). However, they do not specify its *contents*. That is, they do not reveal what motor awareness is an awareness *of*." (Haggard and Magno 1999, p. 102). From this statement it is clear that Haggard and Magno aim at delineating the intentional content of a certain neural representation, a content that currently also is *phenomenal* content, because it is consciously experienced. However, what their own research ingeniously does is something else—namely, narrowing down the minimally sufficient neural correlate for what they call consciously experienced "judgments of reaction time." Viewed as a conscious, reportable form of representational *content* transiently integrated into the PSM, these "judgments of reaction time" are elements of a complex self-representation, a representation of the system *as a whole*. The intentional object of this conscious self-model is not an isolated subpersonal process (e.g., it is not a phenomenal representation of "premotor processes occurring prior to the activation of primary motor cortex" *as such*) (Haggard and Magno 1999, p. 107). The target is the system as a whole, as currently initiating a movement. What transcranial magnetic stimulation can do is delay the integration of certain subpersonal contents into the PSM. Haggard and Magno's experiments are valuable because they produce significant evidence not so much of what "motor awareness" is a conscious representation *of*, but what processing stages it actually supervenes *on*.

In any case it now seems plausible to assume that what gets integrated into the PSM of the organism *as* a now deliberating subject is a determinate, single, and concrete representation of a specific behavior. The authors point out how lateralized readiness potentials may well bear a causal relation to the report about the current content of the PSM, but that it is, at the same time, a rather late event in the chain of physiological happenings leading to the action. I return to the question of free will later. However, let me briefly point out what seems to be the core issue from a philosophical perspective: There will certainly be a minimally sufficient neural correlate for the activation of a specific kind of conscious content, which, when embedded in the transparent self-model, is reported by subjects as their "*own* conscious volition." There will, obviously, also exist a minimally sufficient neural correlate causing the subsequent external action. Both minimally sufficient neural correlates may, although overlapping, greatly diverge if more closely investigated from an objective, third-person perspective and it is precisely the kind of research Haggard and Eimer have conducted which will generate progress on these issues. However, folk psychology usually treats the conscious experience of volition, that is, the phenomenal representation of a specific selection process transiently integrated into the PSM and thereby made available for public report, as the sole and direct *cause* of the observed behavior. It is important to note how this reflects the way in which things are transparently represented on the level of the PSM. This attribution of a causal link is now becoming untenable, and it is not only that folk psychology is false—it is the content of the conscious self-model that actually attributes a causal relation between two events represented within it. However, what is false or hallucination from a rigorous, scientific third-person perspective may be functionally adequate for a biological organism. More about this later.

Let us now take a brief look at possible correlates for the process of phenomenal self-simulation, as realized by the conscious awareness of episodic *memory* retrieval. Düzel and colleagues have conducted a study concerning event-related brain potential correlates of two differing states of conscious awareness in memory tasks. (Düzel et al. 1997). They differentiate between autonoetic awareness (remembering) and noetic awareness (knowing). Autonoetic awareness is a kind of conscious experience characterizing the mental "reliving" of happenings from one's personal past, a capacity that these authors also call the "traveling back in time" in their own minds, well-known to all healthy people. Obviously, this is precisely what was called phenomenal self-simulation earlier: the active, globally available simulation of past system states in an egocentric frame of reference. Noetic awareness is allocentric and more abstract, it expands to the general knowledge laid down in semantic memory. In a true-and-false recognition task, as to be expected, false-positive responses to newly presented items were produced by subjects. The authors point out how it is a well-known and reliable finding that perfectly normal and intelligent people frequently claim not only that they know that false targets were in the study list presented but also that they actually *remember* the events of the false targets' appearance (Düzel et al. 1997, p. 5974). In other words, phenomenal self-simulations of the memory retrieval type can occur with *and* without intentional content. They can be *misrepresentations*. A consciously relived memory episode can be empty, or it can refer to an actual event in the past biography of the subject. Two important assumptions underlying the logic of the experiment were that the subjects' autonoetic awareness correlated with judgments of remembering is the same for true and false targets and that the brain activity correlated with autonoetic awareness and retrieval is essentially the same regardless of whether it is elicited by a true target or a false one. In other words, the study attempted to isolate the intentional from the phenomenal content of the targeted type of phenomenal self-simulation, and made an attempt at finding sufficient neural correlates for the common *phenomenal* aspects of both kinds of processes. One result of the study was that two distinct types of phenomenal content associated with memory retrieval—a phenomenal self-*simulation* causing a conscious experience of "remembering" an actual biographical event as opposed to a phenomenal self-*representation* causing a conscious experience of now "knowing" a presented item—first, possessed different neural correlates, and second, were not sensitive to the differences in the preceding causal history within the system, that is, in the preretrieval processing of presented versus not-presented targets. In the first case the electrophysiological correlate consisted in a late, widespread, bifrontal and temporoparietal positivity in the time window of 600 to 1000 ms, whereas in the second case the correlate was a frontal central negativity in the same time window, preceded by a bilateral temporoparietal positivity in the time window of 300 to 600 ms (Düzel et al. 1997, p. 5977). This study serves as an excellent example of how we are presently taking our first steps in narrowing down the neural correlates of *specific* aspects of conscious self-modeling, in this case with regard to the phenomenon of self-*simulation*.

6.3.2 Cognitive Correlates

The search for neural correlates of phenomenal self-consciousness has to be usefully complemented by a search for the *computational* correlates of phenomenal self-consciousness (Atkinson, Thomas, and Cleeremans 2000). More generally, the NCC may be paralleled by a computational correlate of consciousness (CCC) in that it may possess a purely abstract and merely functional-level description which turns out to be highly relevant to understanding what conscious experience actually is. Computational correlates, it must be noted first, are not correlates in a strict sense, because they are multiply realizable: they are much more abstract descriptions, lacking the domain-specificity that comes along with implementational details. Therefore, any mapping from CCCs to NCCs (or physical correlates in general) will be a one-to-many mapping, and not a one-to-one mapping. A second important aspect consists in combining an investigation of *causal roles* with an investigation of *representational contents*. In more broadly speaking of the "cognitive correlates" of the phenomenal self one unites the two levels of description which have been most important in the past: the conceptual levels of functionalist and representationalist analysis. Both of them are the domain of a more classically conceived cognitive science, and in this sense the search for the cognitive correlates of the PSM means demanding a *cognitive science approach to self-consciousness*.

Philosophers are traditionally attracted by the project of a hardware-independent, universal theory of mind. The most recent fruit of this attraction was philosophical machine functionalism, employing the notion of a Turing machine table as a model for analyzing mental states (Putnam 1975). Philosophers typically are also interested in maximizing conceptual precision and the degree of generality at the same time. For them, more abstract levels of description are more *relevant* levels of description—as long as they can still count as informative. This is also one reason why I have focused on representationalist and functionalist levels of description in developing constraints for the notions of "conscious experience" and "phenomenal self-modeling" in sections 3.2 and 6.1. Therefore, I can be very brief at this point, because much that needed to be said has already been said, particularly in the preceding sections of this chapter. In short, what is needed is a computational model of phenomenal self-consciousness that directly correlates with the specific *content* and the specific *causal role* played by this content for the system, at the same time. Although it is presently unclear what that level will be in a specific domain like conscious human beings, this description will also define the appropriate level of description for neural activity as such, in terms of a certain level of organization in the brain (Revonsuo 2000a).

6.3.3   Social Correlates

Have you ever seen a child, who has just learned to walk, run toward a set of two or three stairs much too fast and then fall on its face in an unprotected way, which might have caused considerable injury had it been an adult? The child, now lying face down, lifts its head, turns around, and searches for its mother. It does so with a completely empty facial expression, showing no kind of emotional response. It looks into its mother's face to find out how *it* is actually now feeling *itself*. How bad was it really? Should I cry or should I laugh?

We have all encountered this situation. What it shows is that the phenomenal content of the toddler's self-model, of its emotional self-model in particular, is not yet fixed. It does not yet know how it should *feel itself*. Therefore, it looks into its mother's face in order to define the emotional content of its own conscious self-experience. It is interesting to note, that, from a third-person perspective, we have two biological systems that used to be *one*, which have been physically separated for many months, but are still intimately coupled on the *functional* level of self-modeling. Their self-models drive each other. And for adults, as Merleau-Ponty pointed out, a similar principle frequently holds: I live in the face of the other. Proceeding from the perceptual to the emotional level, social cognition is accompanied by what could be termed an "affective dissolution of the self."[10] Obviously, subtle discoveries like this are not a matter of philosophical phenomenology alone, but they will have to be reflected in any serious neurocomputational theory of the conscious first-person perspective or of the *second*-person perspective, the phenomenal representation of the *you*. There exist considerable and highly relevant portions of the human self-model, which are, in standard situations, driven by the perception of fellow human beings as cognitive agents, as subjects of attention, and so on. There are kinds of self-consciousness, which an *isolated* human being could never have. Into certain partitions of phenomenal state space we can only enter with the help of other human beings. It is important to note that this does not touch the principle of the phenomenal content of self-representation locally supervening on internal properties of the nervous system. The transition in the toddler's PSM when it looks into its mother's face and starts to smile in relief, suddenly discovering that nothing really hurts and that the only thing that really happened was a big surprise, could, of course, in principle be generated by an evil scientist manipulating a brain in the vat. The *phenomenal* experience of interpersonal connectedness or shared attention could always be a hallucination—it could take place without the existence of any other human beings in the world; it could even take place without the existence of a body or of sense organs. In other words, there will be a minimally sufficient neural correlate even for phenomenal intersubjectivity, for the kinds of conscious experiences we

10. There are, as Evan Thompson (personal communication, 2001) has pointed out, important higher-order variants of empathic, social cognition. The respective forms of phenomenal content will be a necessary target for any full-blown theory doing justice to consciously experienced, human intersubjectivity. For instance, in empathy, I typically also grasp the ongoing or at least potential empathic simulation *of myself by the other* as being a "lived body" just like himself. That is, in my mental emulation of another human agent, I typically grasp his property of at any time being capable of mentally simulating himself *as being in my place* as well. Technically speaking, I activate a PMIR. The object component of this PMIR is formed by a *subject*, modeled as potentially possessing an internal PMIR with *myself* as the object component *as emulating subject*. As in the cases of mirror self-recognition of chimpanzees discussed in section 6.2.8, a homomorphy in mental content can now be discovered: there is a structural similarity in both internal models of reality. In both reality models the phenomenal first-person perspective has transiently been transformed into a phenomenal *second-person* perspective, with the respective subject and object components finding a precise match in the other agent's phenomenal reality. It is important to note that the phenomenal content of this subjective experience of mutual empathy, of course, supervenes locally and may at any time turn out to be *hallucinatory* content. The intentional or epistemic content of *successful* intersubjectivity, however, seems to be in need of a unified representational vehicle of what Thompson interestingly calls an "interpersonal body schema" realizing a "groundfloor core of empathy." Obviously, there exists a physical coupling, a bidirectional causal link between two agents "driving" each other's brains during successful episodes of social cognition. The interesting question is whether the physical link transiently holding between two agents successfully mirroring each other, taken together with their respective minimally sufficient neural correlates, can count as *one* representational structure mediating the higher-order content just mentioned.

individually have when we suddenly understand somebody else's argument or when, in the fraction of a second, we suddenly discover the sparkle in another human being's eyes, which tells us that he actually likes us. However, in order to understand how these specific, high-level contents generated in the process of mutual, social self-modeling could come about and what function they fulfill *for* systems like us one has to look at the standard conditions of their appearance. In order to expand our understanding to further levels of description, we must assume a corresponding kind of *intentional* content as well. There really are those situations in which they are caused by their social correlates. Normally, they constitute knowledge, and not only experience. Additionally, a teleofunctionalist analysis—employing the adaptivity constraint introduced in sections 3.2.11 and 6.2.8— will have to assume that they are processes with a long biological history.

Let us look at a number of examples in which the content of the PSM is driven by social correlates. On the lowest level of phenomenology, conscious bodily sensations may be directly caused by conspecifics, as in fighting, grooming, or mating behavior. As a matter of fact, it has been shown that even emotions recognized from visually presented facial expressions not only engage the visual system but also significant portions of the somatosensory cortex plus additional regions linking the two. Conscious social cognition is therefore likely to be anchored in the spatially coded layers of the PSM, which functions as the decisive link in a "composite visuosomatic system" (Adolphs, Damasio, Tranel, Cooper, and Damasio 2000, p. 2689). Frequently, shifts in the conscious focus and content of perception can be caused by other conscious agents. There are also important classes of presentational content integrated into the conscious self-model that are *typically* caused by conspecifics: being fed, stroking, grooming, and so on are examples of such phenomenal state classes. Then there are a large number of emotions that, in our own case, simply cannot be felt without the presence of another human being triggering them. Furthermore, if a child does not learn to activate the corresponding parts of its emotional self-model during a certain, decisive period of its psychological development, it will not be able to have these feelings later as an adult. During such a formative period for the emotional self-model the presence of certain social correlates triggering the relevant states is essential, or the corresponding partitions of the space of conscious experience may remain forever closed to this child. There seems to be an important functional principle underlying many of the examples just given. The emotional layers of the self-model are representational windows through which an internal (e.g., metabolic) context can interact with an external (e.g., interpersonal) context. Most interesting, however, are all situations in which the self-model is employed as an instrument in explicit, genuine social cognition.

All situations in which it is necessary to represent goals and intentions of another agent can lead to the emergence of particularly interesting forms of self-representational content. Here are some examples: [Myself in the act of understanding another human being's goal],

[Myself in the act of understanding that another human being has understood my *own* goal], [Myself in the act of discovering that another human being is trying to deceive me; i.e., currently attempting to install a false belief in me], [Myself in the act of attempting to prevent another human being from discovering the true content of my current conscious self-model]. One could extend this list almost ad infinitum.

Such states are interesting for a number of reasons. First, they present us with complex, nested forms of intentional content, which are vital to understanding intersubjectivity and the logic underlying social cognition. They are a paradigmatic example of intelligence in the social domain. Second, they have a clear reflection in the PSM. They are accompanied by distinct classes of conscious experiences. These experiences are interesting, because they do not satisfy the transparency constraint. When thinking about the mental states of fellow human beings in this manner we subjectively experience ourselves as manipulating mental *representations*. On the other hand, all this activity is integrated into the transparent background of a phenomenal self, as embodied and as being the initiator of these cognitive activities. In addition (as, e.g., investigations into virtual reality interestingly show; see Heeter 1992), a phenomenal reality as such becomes the more *real*— in terms of the subjective experience of presence—the more agents recognizing one and interacting with one are contained in this reality. Phenomenologically, ongoing social cognition enhances both this reality and the self in their degree of "realness." Third, it is interesting to note that there is a basic underlying content common to all such states. In alluding to the work of Martin Buber, we could call this the phenomenal "I-Thou structure": the conscious experience of currently being confronted with *another* conscious agent, the phenomenal representation of currently interacting with a being possessing a genuine phenomenal first-person perspective *itself*—thereby constituting a first-person *plural* perspective.

There are many situations in which this type of experience is purely hallucinatory. For instance, we just cannot help attributing a conscious first-person perspective to a patient in a persistent vegetative state (PVS; cf. Jennett and Plum 1972; for three case studies demonstrating stereotyped, but coordinated behavior in chronically unconscious persons, see Plum, Schiff, Ribary, and Llinás 1998). We all know how children and some members of non-Western cultures sometimes attribute conscious experience and an inward perspective to inanimate objects in their environment, and all of us, during states of stress or intoxication, in the dream state, while suffering from psychiatric diseases including hallucinatory episodes, can drift off into a "magical worldview," a phenomenal model of reality in which we just cannot help perceiving objects in our surroundings as possessing psychological properties, as having their own intentions, and as possessing a conscious first-person perspective of their own. The I-Thou structure could be based on or form a specific aspect of an innate mechanism (frequently called the "theory-of-mind module"), which can conceivably get out of control and display an autonomous function in situations where it is functionally inadequate.

In normal situations, an interesting possibility is that it is the *unconscious* self-model that possesses social correlates and actually subserves the conscious experience of being a self, "immediately" understanding the goals and attentions of other selves. To develop successful social strategies, one has to internally model those properties of the social environment, those properties of other beings that are not available "online," that is, through sensory perception. Because the epistemic target is the content of the self-model of another agent, the task is not only simulation but also *emulation* (see section 6.1). During a second stage it is necessary to attribute this very representational activity to oneself. Because what needs to be represented is *oneself* in the act of emulating; target emulation and self-emulation have to go hand in hand. The most elegant solution would be one that uses the same anatomical substrates while never confounding both sources of information and both forms of representational content.[11] However, it may be that the first part of this process starts on the unconscious level and that phenomenal states driven by the phenomenal states of other individuals are only the final stage of a rather complicated causal chain.

Giacomo Rizzolatti, Vittorio Gallese, and their coworkers described two different, interesting classes of neurons in area F5 of the ventral premotor area of the monkey (Rizzolatti, Fadiga, Fogassi, and Gallese 2002). These neurons code movements in an abstract way, not as commands to individual groups of neurons, but as relations between an agent and the object of his action. A particularly interesting new concept in this context is that of a "motor vocabulary" consisting of whole action representations, including their temporal and teleofunctional aspects (e.g., "grasp," "precision grip," and "aperture phase"). Neurocomputationally, such a system makes good sense: developing an action vocabulary reduces the space of possibility for actions to a small set of stereotypes, which, for instance, allow realizing the same grasping movement again in a certain situation. It is also interesting to note that the motor system of the embryo develops long before the sensory organs do. Rizzolatti and colleagues call the class of neurons just mentioned "canonical" neurons. They are characterized by responding to classes of visually perceived three-dimensional objects, by coding them according to what Gibson might have called their "affordance"

---

11. Therefore, it is vital to clearly separate logical and genetic levels of analysis. When introducing the concept of a "self-model" at the beginning of this chapter, I distinguished three logical steps: simulation, emulation, and simulation plus emulation under the condition of an *identity* of target system and representing system. The *genetic* hypothesis I am now proposing says that step 3 preceded step 2. In order to successfully mirror another human being in terms of using an internal, unconscious simulation of his behavior to guide an emulation of his *intentions* (i.e., for "retrodictive mind reading") on the conscious level you need a basic self-model to be already in place. It is the preexisting anatomical structure subserving ongoing motor self-simulations to control the agent's own body which is later exploited and put to a new use in social cognition.

(e.g., of a specific grasping movement), that is, *in relation to the effect of interaction with an agent.* However, there exists a second class of premotor neurons, which was discovered some time ago. These neurons have been dubbed "mirror neurons." Mirror neurons are localized in the same brain region and their motor profile is similar to that of canonical neurons. Interestingly, on the functional level of description, they are only visually activated when another *agent* is observed acting in a purposeful way upon objects, for example, with his hand or mouth. In many mirror neurons we find a strict congruence between the particular action that is being *observed* and the executed action effective in driving exactly the same motor response that has been observed. Mirror neurons, therefore, have been hypothesized to constitute the neural correlate of an observation/execution matching system that, in turn, may underlie the mind-reading abilities of human beings which are also found in some nonhuman primates (Gallese and Goldman 1998). The interesting question is whether something like a "mirror vocabulary" could exist as well, defining the space of representational possibility that allows an organism to internally reflect the degree of goal-directedness in an externally observed action.

Frequently we encountered the fact that an important part of the human self-model seems to consist in running motor simulations, as in generating internal models of possible motor behavior on which selection processes can then operate. The hypothesis, convincingly presented by Gallese and Goldman, is that the capacity to use simulative processes to recognize the mental states of other individuals has, in humans, developed from a preexisting system to observe and match actions, the neural correlate of which is formed by a certain class of neurons in premotor cortex. Please note that these neurons will, first, necessarily be a component of the self-model (because they represent a certain aspect of our own motor abilities), and, second, that they are elements of the *unconscious* partition of the self-model (while observing other humans engaging in motor behavior in our environment we never consciously experience these automatic simulations taking place in us all the time). Scanning data supporting the direct matching hypothesis exist (e.g., see Iacoboni, Woods, Brass, Bekkering, Mazziotta, and Rizzolatti 1999). They point to potential mechanisms and neural correlates of human imitation. However, the deeper and more interesting question is how a human individual preserves the sense of self during action observation, given the shared motor representation between the actor producing the initial pattern of movement and the imitator (ibid., p. 2527). The answer can now be given, using the conceptual instruments developed earlier: The phenomenal property of selfhood (the consciously experienced "sense of self") supervenes on the globally available partition of the human self-model. Therefore, the motor representation embedded in this partition, due to the transparency of the PSM (see section 6.2.6), underlies the conscious experience of *being a self in the act of imitating.* The motor representation *not* embedded in the PSM is neither opaque nor transparent. It is a functional property, possibly not even directly reflected on the level of phenomenal experience. It is a part of the unconscious self-model which, however, is currently used as a model of a certain part of external reality, of the social environment, namely, as an *other* self-model. The reason that it can be used in this way is a commonality in the functional architecture holding between conspecifics. In short, the hypothesis is that—within the emulator or imitator's brain—one motor representation is integrated into the PSM during imitative behavior, whereas an efferent copy is fed into an unconscious mind-reading mechanism, or, alternatively, into a perceptually driven and consciously experienced "actor model." It is important to be clear about the notion of "shared motor representation": two different *representational* structures within one and the same brain can share the same content through integrating copies of one and the same internal motor representation. On the other hand, two different *individuals* (or representational *systems*) can share the same kind of goal representation through a functional coupling of their mirror systems.

Mirror neurons, as we have already seen, are not only correlated with contractions in individual muscle groups but create an equivalence with specific motor acts and thereby constitute what has been called a "motor vocabulary" (Rizzolatti and Gentilucci 1988). Obviously, a lot of data on imitation behavior (e.g., Meltzoff and Moore 1977) and simple facts like infants being able to smile at the age of 3 months, long before being able to recognize themselves in a mirror, have predicted the existence of a functional level in the self-model that achieves this mapping from visual input to imitative motor output and also facilitates all those learning procedures which are rooted in the ability to imitate, the ability to run intended, motor self-simulations. However, in applying an extended teleofunctionalist analysis to this newly discovered system, an interesting hypothesis says that it is a rudimentary element of precisely the same mechanism that later enabled us to possess a folk psychology and develop social cognition. This also has a direct bearing on philosophical theories about what it actually means to possess something like a folk psychology. The "theory-theory" of folk psychology analyzes our capacity to understand the mental states of others as a theoretical activity, which applies theoretical inferences and concepts while being detached from the embodied subject, that is, as a purely cognitive activity. On the other hand, the simulation theory of folk psychology—which very obviously would have to be the variant favored by the theoretical model proposed here—posits that the understanding of the mental states of fellow human beings is anchored in an unconscious self-simulation, an internal, nonintended imitation, which brings about a real "embodiment" of the mental states and behavioral goals that form the target of this kind of representational activity. I call this process a "meta-emulation": An information-processing biosystem emulates itself *as* currently emulating another agent. The prediction associated with this new concept of meta-emulation is that the physical substrate and the necessary computational tool for this new representational achievement are identical to specific partitions of the human self-model. The fact that such a mental imitation of other cognitive subjects by the process of internal self-simulation actually exists is, as Gallese and Goldman have pointed out, a prediction of the simulation theory, but not of the theory-theory (Gallese and Goldman 1998, p. 497). That part of the human self-model implemented by the mirror system in a way that is mostly unconscious and automatic activates a state in the human observer that matches that of the observed agent, constituting an internal type of imitative behavior on the functional level, aptly described as a (subpersonal[12]) "attempt to replicate, mimic, or impersonate the mental life of the target agent" (ibid.). Externally driven activity of this part of the non-PSM could therefore serve the goal of "retrodicting" the mental state of a target person by not only activating a motor self-simulation in the observing subject but at the same time, an active goal representation. Please note that a functional reading of the convolved holism constraint discussed in sections 3.2.4 and 6.2.4 makes such an assumption plausible.

What is an action, as opposed to a behavior, in terms of the self-model theory? An action is a behavior caused by an internal, motor self-simulation, which is additionally accompanied by an abstract goal representation presented in, first, a nonegocentric frame of reference, and, second, a representation of an actual selection process for a *specific* movement (e.g., Haggard and Eimer 1999), which is then integrated into the PSM, thereby becoming "my *own* intention to act." The functional link, which is shared by both parts of the conscious motor self-model, by canonical neurons as well as by mirror neurons, is that they are easily linked to allocentric goal representations. The goal of another agent is recognized by the observer in mapping it onto a shared motor representation. In this vein, what is actually happening when we consciously understand the intention of another perceived agent could consist in discovering an abstract property, namely, a "motor equivalence." If this is true, the degree to which the functional structure of self-models between two classes of systems are similar also determines the degree to which successful social cognition, successful *intersubjectivity*, can take place between them. The mirror neuron theory of simulative mind reading is valuable because it opens a completely new interpretation of the function of this part of the human self-model, namely, as an "intentionality detector." It helps a system to recognize stimuli as volitional by detecting their goal in terms of an internal self-simulation (Gallese 2001; figure 6.1). One further interesting

---

12. A philosophically interesting point, which I am skipping, is whether the minimally sufficient social correlates for the kind of high-level self-modeling discussed here are formed exclusively by *subpersonal* properties of other agents, such as specific motor patterns, which may or may not be intention-driven. While it is clear that the principle of local supervenience holds for consciously experienced intersubjectivity as well—hallucinated, purely phenomenal intersubjectivity could certainly be realized by a brain in a vat—it is much less clear what precisely constitutes the *intentional* content of successful social cognition in real-life situations. Is the motor equivalence read out by the mirror system and coded as "understanding another agent's intention" on the level of conscious self-modeling a *personal* or a *subpersonal* property of this other agent?

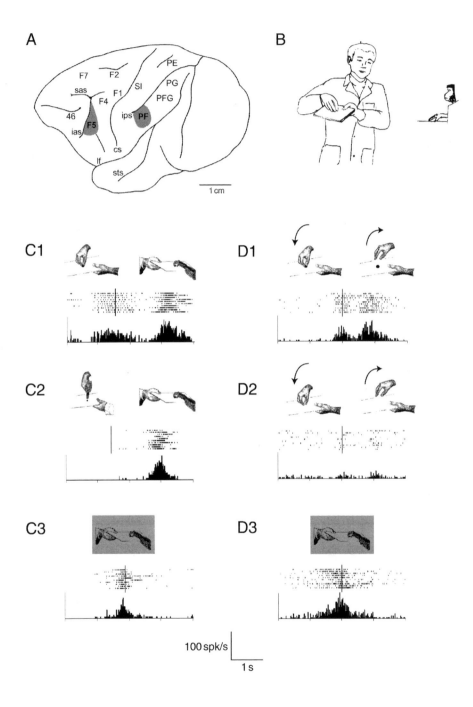

100 spk/s

1 s

aspect of this line of thought is that most functional aspects of the human self-model enabling *intersubjectivity* and social consciousness are clearly nonconceptual, prerational, and pretheoretical, a particular kind of simulational-representational content embodied by the egocentric aspects of the motor vocabulary. Those parts of the human self-model which can be described as a set of motor schemata allow for the transformation of external knowledge (constituted by the observations of motor behavior in other individuals) into internal knowledge (the conscious discovery that, in oneself, this kind of behavior would usually be driven by a certain kind of goal) and thereby generate globally available knowledge about internal aspects of those parts of external reality that are actually constituted by other agents. This knowledge is knowledge by embodied metaemulation.

It is important to note how the conscious experience of being someone who understands the current intention and goals of fellow human beings will only result if the internally represented action goal is then successfully attributed to the external, currently observed agent and if this, rather complex, kind of mental content is made globally available. It is, for instance, conceivable that a particularly sensitive or hyperactive "agent-detection device" could lead to the conscious experience of the presence of an invisible agent

Figure 6.1
Mind reading with the help of a preexisting internal self-model: A macaque monkey using parts of its own motor system to mentally simulate a human agent as currently being directed to a concrete action goal. *A*, Lateral view of macaque monkey cerebral cortex showing frontal and parietal areas. Frontal agranular cortical areas are classified according to Matelli et al. (1985). The posterior parietal areas are classified according to Von Bonin and Bailey (1947). Shaded areas indicate the cortical sectors where mirror neurons were recorded. Abbreviations: cs, central sulcus; ias, inferior arcuate sulcus; ips, intraparietal sulcus; lf, lateral fissure; SI, primary somatosensory area; sas, superior arcuate sulcus; sts, superior temporal sulcus. *B*, Illustration of the experimental situation for testing the visual properties of mirror neurons. (Modified from diPellegrino et al. 1992.) *C*, Example of the visual and motor responses of a F5 mirror neuron. The behavioral situation during which the neural activity was recorded is illustrated schematically in the upper part of each panel. In the lower part rasters and the relative peristimulus response histograms are shown. *C1*, A tray with a piece of food placed on it was presented to the monkey; the experimenter grasped the food and then moved the tray with the food toward the monkey, which grasped it. A strong activation was present during observation of the experimenter's grasping movements and while the same action was performed by the monkey. Note that the neural discharge was absent when the food was presented and moved toward the monkey. *C2*, As in *C1*, except that the experimenter grasped the food with pliers. Note the absence of response when the observed action was performed with a tool. *C3*, The monkey grasped the food in the dark. Rasters and histograms are aligned (vertical bar) with the moment in which the experimenter (*C1* and *C2*), or the monkey (*C3*), touched the food. Abscissae: time. Ordinate: spikes/s. Bin width: 20 ms. (Modified from Rizzolatti et al. 1996.) (*D*) Example of the visual and motor responses of a prefrontal mirror neuron. *D1*, A tray with a piece of food placed on it was presented to the monkey; the experimenter grasped the food and subsequently released it, moving the hand away from the food. Note the strong response during observation of both the experimenter's grasping and releasing actions. The neuron did not respond during the presentation of the food on the tray. *D2*, The same action as in *D1* was mimed. Note that in this condition the neural response was virtually absent. *D3*, The monkey grasped the food in the dark. Rasters and histograms are aligned (vertical bar) with the moment in which the monkey (*D3*) or the experimenter touched the food (*D1*) or the tray (*D2*). All other conventions as in figure *C2*. (Modified from Gallese et al. 2002.)

(Barrett 2000).[13] An important question, of course, is whether self-models possessing the necessary functional properties of leading to low-level motor resonance and imitative behavior in groups of biological organisms could exist *without* the conscious capacity of mind reading.

Have you ever seen a group of deer all turn their heads after one of them has suddenly and attentively looked in a certain direction, for instance, after discovering that it is being seen by *you*? An interesting question is whether those deer actually "share attention" in terms of being aware that the first animal, triggering the group behavior, had a certain mental state directed at a specific intentional object and they are all simultaneously aware of the *content* of each others' attentional state. The fact that many species monitor and respond to visual attention in conspecifics does not mean that they actually attribute the presence of intentional content to them. Conceivably, the motor aspects of the self-model could (in other species as well as in human infants) implement a gaze-following system, achieving the important property of making systems look at the same object in unison under certain conditions. The fact that humans, great apes, and macaques possess the ability to follow the gaze of conspecifics is important, because it suggests that essential mechanisms for the development of mind-reading abilities are shared by all these primate species and may allow us to describe a *continuous* evolutionary path leading onward to strong social cognition, for example, via shared mechanisms of action control, action representation, and finally *intention* representation (Gallese, Ferrari, Kohler, and Fogassi 2002; Gallese 2001). But, as Daniel Povinelli and Christopher Prince (1998, p. 59*ff.*) have pointed out, *joint* attention does not ensure *shared* attention. Povinelli and Prince review data suggesting that human infants only at some point in their second year develop a self-model which enables them to interpret the actions of others in terms of an attentional state, whereas human children have already developed a rudimentary gaze-following system that allows them to track where, for instance, their mother is currently looking (if the object is contained within their own perceptual field). It is only at the age of 18 months that their self-model allows them to create what Povinelli calls a "mentalistic notion of attention," that is, the capacity to represent an external agent as "possessing" the same intentional object also constituting the focus of their *own* visual attention if they imitate his gazing behavior.

---

13. Such a misattribution could, for instance, be a frequent correlate of schizophrenic delusion (see section 7.7.2) or of certain types of religious experiences. As Barrett writes in a recent review, discussing the so-called "hyperactive agent-detection device (HADD)" hypothesis: "Thus, people are particularly sensitive to the presence of intentional agency and seem biased to overattribute intentional action as the cause of a given state of affairs when data is ambiguous or sketchy. These observations suggest that whatever cognitive mechanism people have for detecting agency might be extremely sensitive; in other words people can be said to possess hyperactive agent-detection devices (HADD). According to Guthrie, such a biased perceptual device would have been quite adaptive in our evolutionary past, for the consequences of failing to detect an agent are potentially much graver than mistakenly detecting an agent that is not there" (Barrett 2000, p. 31).

We can now clearly distinguish between different forms of representational content that may or may not be present in a certain biological species. In order to be an attentional subject (see section 6.4.3), the self-model has to be integrated with an object component. This may result in an *attentional* first-person perspective, a transient phenomenal representation of a subsymbolic subject-object relation (see section 6.5.1). The second level is given if an organism is able to represent *another* animal as currently possessing such an attentional first-person perspective. If this involves observable, overt behavior in the other agent, as in the case of gazing behavior, then it is entirely plausible that the motor partitions of the self-model in the *first* animal mediate the kind of automatic metaemulation described before. A prime candidate for the anatomical substrate would consist in the mirror neurons discovered by Rizzolatti and collegues. However, for the third step in new functional properties and new representational content we must at least differentiate two possible cases. First, just as there is low-level attention, there might be something like a low-level resonance mechanism: what is mirrored are only *movements* without a goal representation, in terms of the *object component* in the subject-object relation of visual attention currently modeled on the level of conscious experience. Second, a high-level "attentional resonance mechanism" could serve to actually lock the first animal into the same internal model of the intentionality relation (see section 6.5), including the same object component. However, it is possible that even this form of shared representational content on the level of the object component is not accompanied by a globally available model of the other attentional agent *as* having changed its own internal representation of self and world accordingly. In chimpanzees it turns out that there are actually indicators for the provocative or at least counterintuitive interpretation that gaze-following behavior does not take place with any accompanying phenomenal understanding of the same mental state of attention that is simultaneously present in the first animal.

Do chimpanzees understand the intentional aspect of seeing? One of the central issues in this context is the question of how it could be possible for nonhumans to share so many behavioral patterns with us, patterns which, in humans, clearly go along with a successful metaemulation of other agents (a "mentalistic representation" of them in Povinelli and Prince's terminology). An important explanatory target is the radical incongruence between the similarity of human-chimpanzee behavioral patterns and the dissimilarity in theory-of-mind abilities (Povinelli and Prince 1998, p. 81). The notion of a self-model now allows us to differentiate different stages in the evolution of subjectivity and intersubjectivity as stages in representational content. The functional self-model can be driven by social stimuli in low-level resonance situations, and this may be followed by a corresponding shift of content in the PSM. This does not mean that a phenomenal model of the intentionality relation (PMIR; see section 6.5) is present nor does it lend itself to the conclusion of a globally available meta-emulation, a full-blown, conscious representation of a goal representation being currently active in another agent. However, if the prime substrate for the emulative processes underlying the evolution of the "self-other psychology" is formed by *motor* structures constituting the self-model, then it is plausible to assume that self-modeling *preceded* intentionality modeling and the evolution of theory-of-mind task capacities. If this is true, this first step may have taken place in isolation in another biological species. Therefore, on the level of representational analysis it is a plausible assumption that some animals on our planet represent social interactions only as forms of behavior, and not as forms of behavior *plus* an invisible mind. Data from developmental psychology also seem to show clearly how self-knowledge is not a sufficient condition for ascribing complex social properties (Povinelli 1993, p. 503). Children between the age of 18 and 24 months clearly have a capacity of self-knowledge while not yet understanding the mental states of other human beings. In chimpanzees, it might also be the case that during cooperative behavior they do not mentally represent the *goals* of other chimpanzees. Human beings, however, may possess a system to interpret behavioral homologues in a way that actually involves the mental simulation of a strictly nonobservable property in the other agent: her *intention*.

Recent imaging studies demonstrate that when humans observe specific goal-directed behaviors carried out with mouth, hand, or foot (such as biting an apple and chewing, grasping a little cup, or kicking a ball), specific and different sectors of their premotor cortex are activated (Buccino, Binkofski, Fink, Fadiga, Fogassi, Gallese, Seitz, Zilles, Rizzolatti, and Freund 2001). Perceived actions are representationally mapped onto the corresponding motor region of the frontal lobe, and target objects are mapped onto effector-related representations in the parietal lobe. Therefore, the same neuroanatomical structures that would normally be involved in the *actual*, voluntary execution of the same action are now recruited for what, according to our conceptual tools, is a nonphenomenal self-simulation. Only the final result of this event is made globally available on the level of the PSM: we consciously experience *understanding* another agent's intention. An interesting general point is that the variability of representational architectures in the animal kingdom may be higher than, for instance, many philosophers, assuming a linear development toward the final goal of human psychology, have imagined. As Povinelli (1993) points out, a typical mistake in comparative psychology consists in looking for one single "ladder," a phylogenetic scale in representational properties, while overlooking the fact that this development was "part of the radiation of animals outward in all directions" (Povinelli 1993, p. 193). Obviously, you can have a self-model without having a *conscious* self-model. Obviously, you can put a self-model to use in a low-level resonance mechanism without having the conscious form of metaemulation and intentionality detection described. And to have a PSM of yourself *as currently metaemulating another conscious being* may be confined to human beings. However, it is important to note how the possession of an integrated self-model is a necessary precondition for all these different stages.

The discussion of these issues in primatology is still highly controversial, but as Povinelli and Prince conclude, there is in general little evidence that nonhuman primates reason about other mental states any more than they do about attention. Though chimpanzees clearly noticed and responded to gaze direction in a number of experiments, there seems to be no firm basis for the conclusion that they actually understood how certain bodily postures were connected to an internal state of attention. Interestingly, this kind of research in our close relatives is so difficult because any more hard-headed analysis of the actual functional properties possessed by chimpanzees is constantly interfered with by what Povinelli and Prince call the "unavoidable subjective impression" (ibid., p. 72), that some kind of "attentional glue" between the conscious subject and an object actually exists. Not only is the notion of "attentional glue" itself interesting from a philosophical perspective (see section 6.5.2) but it is also instructive in terms of investigator phenomenology. Like all phenomenal content, "immediately perceived attentional glue" may always be *hallucinatory* content. This subjective impression, of course, is constituted by automatic functional mechanisms underlying the activation of the conscious self-model in the human *scientist* (who may certainly possess a high degree of "motor equivalence" in relation to the self-model of the observed chimpanzee), and the impression is unavoidable, because the human self-model satisfies the transparency constraint. However, there are many examples of groups of animals in which obviously non–goal-directed behaviors are automatically mirrored by a large number of conspecifics with great speed and accuracy—just think about schools of fish or flocks of birds. In humans, the same is true of behaviors like yawning and laughing. Often a group will burst into laughter before actually having conscious access to what it is that is being laughed *about*.

Obviously a functional and cognitive continuity among human beings, nonhuman primates, and other animals not only exists in the domain of ascribing intentional states to other agents, the anatomical substrate of which are mirror neurons, but also in automatic, unconscious patterns of mutual self-simulation *not* accompanied by phenomenally represented goals or intentions. There seem to be functionally active partitions of the self-model which are driven by social stimuli, but nevertheless do not lead to explicit metaemulation and social cognition reflected on the conscious level of the self-model. Rizzolatti and colleagues (Rizzolatti et al. 2002) hypothesized that an evolutionarily old resonance mechanism exists, which maps visual representations of perceived behavior directly onto motor representations of the observer. In this case the posited isomorphism and the functional congruence would not hold between observed and executed actions, but only between observed and executed *movements*, that is, behaviors without the accompanying goal representation mentioned above. It is precisely this kind of low-level resonance that could explain how newborn infants, at a very early stage, are able to imitate facial expressions and hand movements. High-level resonance, however, would be responsible for genuinely cognitive emulation implemented in the self-model and "real" imitative behavior. Results of brain imaging experiments suggest that the neural correlates of low-level and high-level resonance mechanisms implemented by the self-model do not coincide (e.g., see Decety, Grèzes, Costes, Perani, Jeannerod, Procyk, Grassi, and Fazio 1997; Grèzes, Costes, and Decety 1998). As Rizzolatti and colleagues speculate, the high-level resonance mechanism could describe the goal of an action, while at a later state attention may become focused on the *form* of the action—the repetition of which, if it takes place, is mediated by the circuit involved in the low-level resonance mechanism.

The general picture emerging from recent research in this area throws light on a whole range of issues relating to social correlates of the PSM in humans. For instance, it allows us to understand certain well-known psychiatric disturbances like echopraxia and compulsory imitation behavior. The development of a capacity to *control* the mirror system, that is, to successfully decouple it from the actual executive structures in the motor system, is a necessary precondition for achieving voluntary control (see also Rizzolatti and Arbib 1998, p. 191*ff.*). Any person suffering from a disinhibition of that part of her unconscious self-model implemented by the low-level resonance mechanism will be forced to imitate visually observed behavior in her social environment. Echopraxia is a disturbance found in a range of psychiatric disorders, for instance, in autism. In fact, one way to interpret configurations of this type is as one in which a previously nonexisting PSM is "mirrored" in or "projected" onto the patient. That is, such patients would have their *unconscious* self-model driven by another human being in their environment, and only then activate a *conscious* self-model matching their current, involuntary behavior. But whose behavior is it? Who is the agent? One such patient describes her own phenomenology:

Another disturbance in looking at people was that being echopraxic, taking on their postures and facial expressions unintentionally, disturbed me and sometimes disturbed them. . . . It disturbed me because I just wanted to keep my own body connectedness intact and not to have it trail off like that, like a wild horse. Sometimes others had more control over my body than I did and I did not like to experience that, when I realized I had slipped into involuntarily mimicking them.[14]

14. Cf. Williams 1992, 1994, quoted in Cole 1997, p. 478. Given the current context it is also interesting to note how this patient describes her desperate attempts to keep her self-model globally available, to prevent it from dropping out of the global model of reality: "At home I would spend hours in front of the mirror, staring into my own eyes and whispering my name . . . frightened at losing my ability to feel myself" (ibid., p. 477). Social contacts could make all such attempts fail, because, as Jonathan Cole aptly puts it, they "would engulf her fragile sense of selfhood in a flood of 'other' " (p. 478). As the current theory would predict, any person who has problems stabilizing her self-model on the level of global availability will also have problems in establishing an enduring phenomenal first-person perspective (a PMIR; see section 6.5) and, a fortiori, a phenomenal *second*-person perspective. "Once, as an adolescent, she met a boy, 'He kissed me—or perhaps I should say that he kissed my face, as I wasn't in at the time.' To become too close was to be overwhelmed by the 'otherness' of that person, and to risk losing all connection to the fragile sense of 'self.' " (p. 477)

Obviously, the PSM is the computational tool to achieve "body connectedness" for the organism. It is also central in establishing—or interrupting—personal-level processes of social cognition. It may well be that the process of conscious self-modeling is what is needed to make such processes globally available for control by the system as a whole, for example, by actually stopping and suppressing their behavioral consequences. However, it may also be plausible to assume an additional low-level, "inverted mirror system" on the level of the spinal cord (in fact, the mirror system might act differently at cortical and spinal levels, with even two different mechanisms at the spinal level, a "subthreshold preparation to move and a superimposed suppression of overt movement"; see Baldissera, Cavallari, Craighero, and Fadiga 2001, p. 193). Such a system could complement conscious control on the unconscious and subpersonal levels of processing. It would prevent us from echopraxia, that is, from having to act out every behavior we perceive. As we have already seen, nonphenomenal self-modeling is a process that is not globally available for attention, cognition, and self-directed control. Agency only starts on the phenomenal level, and the mirror system may play a decisive part in making this transition (Gallese 2000, 2001; Metzinger and Gallese 2003). It may, in this expanded context, also be interesting to note how new insights in developmental psychology show theory-of-mind capacities emerging simultaneously with capacities for action control during the fourth year. Mind-reading abilities emerge simultaneously with the capacity to suppress spontaneous actions (Perner and Lang 1999). It is also interesting to note how both capacities are simultaneously disturbed in autism and schizophrenia. Both situations are characterized by the need to successfully represent the fact of actions being causally mediated by internal representations active in another agent.[15]

The functional link between motor representation and motor behavior may have been broken for the first time. This made three classes of new content available: motor simulations, motor self-simulations, and motor self-simulations used as a new computational tool in social cognition. On the level of representational analysis, the content of such states is always constituted by *possible* actions. On the level of neural implementation, the fact that the neural systems in question can be activated by the visual system, as well as by the motor system, is an empirical argument for them representing *potential* actions. It is interesting to note that such internal action simulations could conceptually be analyzed as extremely *weak* actions in a way that may prove to be heuristically fruitful. Running mental motor simulations is a kind of internal behavior not currently coupled to

---

15. As Perner and Lang write: "We have shown that there is increasingly clear evidence of a specific developmental link between theory-of-mind development and improved self-control around the age of 4 yrs. The available evidence shows that the observed correlations go beyond common methodological features of the assessment tasks, and points to a functional interdependence of ToM [theory of mind] and EF [executive function]. Better understanding one's own mind provides better insights into how to exert self-control, and the exercise of self-control is one of the main grounds for building such an understanding." See Perner and Lang 1999, p. 343.

the effector system. By coupling an ongoing self-simulation to the motor system a covert action can become an overt action. Imitation, then, is a borderline case of mental simulation with the help of a metaemulatory self-model. The underlying computational problem is how to generate a motor emulation of the dynamics of a bodily action from a purely visual perception of the kinematics of this action. If a supramodal level of action representation exists, for instance, in terms of Meltzoff's "active intermodal matching" hypothesis, this might help to solve the problem. I propose that the human self-model provides us with precisely this supramodal level of computing action representations. The next question is whether such an embodied comprehension system could be turned into an embodied communication system by supplying a common neural substrate for imitation and *language*.

The line of research now experiencing such a forceful renaissance looks back to a long tradition of philosophical attempts to analyze what empathy really is (e.g., Lipps 1903), as well as to numerous attempts in experimental psychology at the end of the nineteenth and during the first half of the twentieth century to achieve a better understanding of "ideomotor" effects and phenomena (Carpenter 1875; for a review, see Richter 1957). In 1903, Theodor Lipps, in a paper on empathy, inner imitation, and organ sensations, analyzed the representational content of empathy ("*Einfühlung*") as not sensing something in your own body, but as *feeling yourself in an object* (p. 202). For him, interestingly, objects could be perceived human movements or body postures, but also architectural forms. Only decades ago, concepts like "motor mimicry," "virtual body movements," and "motor infection" were already under discussion in social psychology. Today, a particularly interesting aspect consists in discovering that communication, as well as reasoning, may be a highly refined version of motor behavior (for an earlier motor theory of language, see Libermann and Mattingly 1985). According to current proposals it consists of abstract, allocentric representations of goals and intentions embedded in a conscious partition of the human self-model, thereby generating the emergence of a cognitive subject (see section 6.4.4). However, cognitive and linguistic subjectivity may be more intimately connected than previously thought. As Rizzolatti and Arbib (1998) pointed out, an observation or execution matching system could provide a bridge from "doing" to "communicating." A highly interesting, commonly shared interpretation is that the rostral part of the monkey ventral premotor cortex is a homologue of Broca's area 44 in the human brain (for references, see Rizzolatti and Arbib 1998, p. 189). In humans, Broca's area is viewed as an area responsible for speech, whereas F5 is frequently considered as being responsible for hand movements that have a somatotopical structure, with one part representing hand movements and another part representing mouth and larynx movement. Interestingly, Broca's area in humans, as recent PET data have shown, not only relates to speech but is also involved in mental imagery of hand grasping movements.

What is a mentally imagined hand grasping movement? It is an intended, phenomenal self-simulation. In particular, it is a self-simulation involving *making an external object your own*. At this point it is intriguing to recall how the Latin notion of *concipere*, of taking something and firmly holding it together, is the etymological root of our present-day notion of forming a concept, that is, of *cognitively* appropriating it under a single and integrated representation. Rizzolatti and Arbib also point to the fact that Broca's area becomes active in patients recovering from subcortical infarctions when they are asked to use their paralyzed hand. In short, a number of empirical data show that the direct neural correlates of those parts of the human self-model that functionally enable the execution and recognition of observed actions *overlap* with those parts involved in linguistic competence, that is, in representing oneself as an individual currently comprehending certain concepts. I will not go into details about theories concerning the development of speech production here. What I want to point out is that the two elements of the PSM, which obviously possess overlapping physical correlates, could, of course, represent two successive stages of psychological evolution. This discovery would shed new light on ancient questions shared by scientists and philosophers interested in the social correlates of self-consciousness. It gives a completely new and rich meaning not only to the concept of "grasping" and the concept of "mentally grasping the intention of another human being" but, importantly, also to the concept of "grasping a *concept*."

6.4   Levels of Content within the Human Self-Model

In 1911 Edward Titchener, evaluating a set of reports produced by Cornell graduates who had received an unusually thorough training in "systematic experimental introspection," arrived at the conclusion that "self-consciousness is, in many cases, an intermittent and even a rare experience" (Titchener 1911, p. 550). This is an important phenomenological constraint. The human self-model is constituted by many different layers of representational content. These layers are accessed by different readout mechanisms in a task-dependent manner, and therefore their degree of phenomenal explicitness may vary considerably. Titchener's phenomenological constraint is still valid today, and conceptual confusions can only be avoided if one stops making broad claims referring to "the self" in a naive-realistic way.

In the following five sections I will briefly continue to enrich the concept of a PSM by pointing out five different levels of system-related information, which are made globally available by the conscious self-model and which in turn constitute five different classes of phenomenal content. Of course, many other classifications are possible. Any full-blown neurophenomenology of phenomenal self-consciousness will have to develop them in detail and in a much more systematic manner. I will, however, only sketch a limited

number of additional distinctions, because they possess particular relevance with respect
to traditional philosophical issues related to the phenomenal first-person perspective.

6.4.1   Spatial and Nonspatial Content

Why is it that Descartes's distinction between *res extensa* as extended, material objects
and *res cogitans* as nonspatial, thinking subjects, after centuries of philosophical criticism
and an endless series of counterarguments, has never lost a certain intuitive attractiveness?
Why is it so hard to uproot the classical Cartesian intuition of our minds, in some important sense, not being located in physical space? The answer can be found in the internal
structure of the human self-model. The conscious self-model, that part of our internal self-
representation about which we can reason and report because it is introspectively$_4$ available, actually possesses two parts—one part that is coded *as* possessing spatial properties
and another part that is coded as *not* possessing spatial properties. Human subjectivity is
embodied subjectivity, because it always unfolds against the background of a stable bodily
model of the self. In phenomenal self-consciousness we are functionally rooted in interoception and in the continuous activity of the neuromatrix of the body image. More recent
forms of cognitive self-simulation, under standard conditions, are always accompanied by
the spatial model of the self. However, step by step, they become less and less spatial. Our
highest and most abstract cognitive operations are only characterized by a sequential, temporal "orderedness." Human beings only represent intellectual operations in the modus of
seriality—one *after* the other—on the level of conscious experience, but not in the mode
of spatial distribution and localization—one *next* to the other. This fact, in our own case,
creates what I call the "pre-philosophical mind-body problem."

The pre-philosophical mind-body problem rests on an intuitive dissonance inherent in
our conscious self-experience, which in turn lets us feel the relevance of the *theoretical*
problem of psychophysical causality. It has its root in a "technical" problem associated
with the process of human self-modeling: How does a human brain manage to integrate
self-generated phenomenal mental models without spatial properties (e.g., the conscious
thought "I am a thinking thing") into a self-model which, for reasons of its biological
origin, developed from a *spatial* model of the system? And how can it internally simulate
causal relations between such purely cognitive events and bodily transitions inevitably
coded *as* taking place within a spatial frame of reference? Descartes's distinction between
thinking and extended substances is, I would claim, a plausible conceptual distinction for
us human beings, because it is mirrored in the representational structure of our self-models.

The distinction between phenomenal, nomological, and logical possibility introduced
in chapter 2 will now help to clarify this point. Cartesianism is philosophically attractive,
because it is intuitively plausible. It is intuitively plausible, for beings like ourselves,
because it is easy for us to run the phenomenal self-simulations corresponding to the

philosophical claim. Cartesian dualism, for beings with self-models like ours, certainly is *conceivable*. What has been frequently overlooked in the philosophical tradition is that, because implications do not hold between phenomenal simulations and propositions, the *phenomenal* possibility of disembodied existence does not entail any modal claims whatsoever. What is the root of the intuitive dissonance between spatial and nonspatial content in the PSM? We are systems which have to explain to themselves how it was possible that we can carry out abstract, cognitive operations using nonsensory, second-order simulata. We achieve this goal by generating what one might call a metacognitive self-model: We generate a mental model of ourselves *as beings producing thoughts and conceptual knowledge* (see section 6.4.4). The thinking self is born. It introduces a fundamental chasm in the conscious self, because it is a continuous source of fragmentation. What makes it a highly successful new virtual organ is the fact that it possesses an entirely different function *for* the system than the bodily model of the self: It has to make those cognitive processes that need to be constantly monitored available for self-directed attention and higher-order cognition. Before, this partition of the unconscious self-model (see Crick and Koch 2000) cannot directly be connected with the phenomenal image of our body on the level of conscious experience and therefore the organism cannot *own* it. If a certain thought leads us to raise our arm, the causal relationship between those elements of the self-model so readily attributed by folk psychology is something that we cannot introspectively observe *in* ourselves. Interestingly, this widely neglected phenomenological feature of the impossibility of introspecting$_3$ the actual modus operandi of mental, top-down causation as it is portrayed by the conscious self-model finds a direct reflection in the difficulties of Descartes's own attempt to solve the mind-body problem he had just created. Descartes's own model of psychophysical interaction in the pineal gland fails on logical grounds. Something without any spatial properties cannot causally interact with something possessing spatial properties *at a specific location*. If Descartes had taken his own premises seriously, he could never have come up with this solution, which is so obviously false. If the mind truly is an entity not present in physical space, it would be absurd to look for a *locus* of interaction in the human brain. It is interesting to note how a number of classical philosophical confusions result from the naive realism regarding the content of our self-consciousness caused by the transparency of the human self-model, which we discussed in section 6.2.6. Specifically, the spatial character of bodily experience is taken for granted, as if it were not a representational construct but something to which we had direct and immediate epistemic access. The same mistake is then made with regard to phenomenal cognition, the internal representation of certain cognitive processes on the level of conscious self-simulation. Even the best of today's still living Cartesians (see, e.g., McGinn 1995) systematically equivocate between "space" and "the phenomenal experience of spatiality," then swiftly proceed to the usual conclusions.

In order to do justice to the phenomenology of localization one has to admit that phenomenal localization is not an all-or-nothing phenomenon. Those contents of conscious experience that are bundled by the subjective quality of "mineness" exhibit differing *degrees* of localization in the phenomenal body image. Tactile sensations or surface pain usually possesses a narrowly confined location at which it is felt. As we shall see in the next chapter (see section 7.2.3.2), new research on pain in phantom limbs and cortical remapping phenomena following the amputation of a limb demonstrate how plastic the mechanisms underlying the phenomenal referral of certain sensations to certain parts of the conscious self-model can be. Some amputees feel corns or wedding rings 30 years after surgical amputation of a limb. These cases provide examples of simple sensory content, integrated into the self-model, possessing a narrow and specific phenomenal localization. Interoceptive sensations like the diffuse feelings sometimes associated with the digestive process or a stomachache are much more ambiguous. For those inner states that have been developed early on, it is true from a phylogenetic perspective that they can be integrated into the spatial self-model quite easily. In particular, this is true of emotions: The conscious feeling of gratitude can be *heartfelt*, a sudden negative experience can *shake us to the core*, and thinking about our political leadership may *turn your stomach*. Emotions are always my *own* emotions, because they are diffusely localized in the body image. For thoughts, we know of pathological phenomenologies, for example, in schizophrenia (see chapter 7), in which integration into the self-model fails and "introspectively alienated" conscious thoughts are experienced which do not possess the quality of "mineness" anymore. For emotions this seems to be impossible; we know of no psychiatric disturbance in which emotions are not experienced as the normal patient's *own* emotion anymore. In fact, Antonio Damasio has made a compelling case demonstrating that while low-level attention and wakefulness can actually be separated from consciousness, consciousness and emotion are inseparable (Damasio 1999, p. 15; chapters 2, 3, and 4). It seems that emotions are accompanied by local somatic states of arousal (e.g., the depletion of epinephrine or by visceral activity), which are in part made globally available by being represented in the conscious self-model. Emotional content is always spatial content.

The emotional self-model can be analyzed as the integrated class of all those representational states modeling the overall state of affairs of the interests of the system. As opposed to other forms of representational content they are structured along a *valence axis*. They contain a *normative* element, and this element is, for instance, expressed as affective tone. What is nonconceptually represented by this affective valence or tone will in many cases be the *survival value* of a specific state of affairs. What the adaptivity constraint (see section 3.2.11) is from a third-person perspective greatly resembles the role played by emotions from the first-person perspective. It is important to note how this emotional self-model has a long evolutionary history. For example, and from our own mammalian perspective, the "reptile self" will be something deprived of all genuine friendliness, something lacking all the rich emotional content that only entered the world through child care, grooming, and so on. Reptile sexuality will strike us as cold and alien, something that can only be related to sadism, to dominance and submission in human terms. Conscious feelings are historical entities. For every type of emotional self-consciousness there will be a time in the evolutionary history of our planet when it was (or *will be*) exemplified for the first time. Emotional states integrated into the PSM will frequently possess a true teleofunctionalist description, a "proper function" of some sort (Millikan 1989). In terms of phenomenal localization they constitute a bridge between elementary bodily sensations and those purely "cognitive operations" Descartes used in laying the foundation of his epistemology. An interesting feature they share with the bodily self is their rigidity: It is very hard to effectively influence the content of your emotional self-model by "higher," deliberately induced cognitive operations. Emotions come and go; they are functionally removed from the control of the psychological subject to a high degree.

Empathy certainly does exist, but for human beings it is hard to take their emotional self-model offline, deliberately using it as an emulator for possible situations. In particular, emotional self-simulations are very hard to carry out, as are the intended simulation of elementary bodily sensations. It is hard to deliberately conjure up the conscious sensation of heartfelt gratitude in yourself if this is not mirrored by the real profile of your overall interests and actual social relationships. It is even more difficult to deliberately activate the self-representational content, for example, supplied by your vestibular system, which you would have when practicing a somersault or jumping off a 10 m jumping board into a swimming pool. Spatial content integrated into the PSM cannot be easily manipulated on the level of intended simulations. It is strongly correlated with internal stimulus sources and covaries with actual body properties. Emotions, in particular, confront the phenomenal self with its fundamentally biological nature.[16] Emotions cannot freely be triggered by external stimuli; they need an internal context and a preexisting goal hierarchy to be activated. Biological systems, when subpersonally modeling their own current state and comparing it with certain internally defined goal states, can be confronted with rigid

16. For many years, the most popular counterargument against the possibility of machine consciousness has always run as follows: "But an artificial system will never have *emotions*!" The intuition underlying this counterargument rests on the observation that nonbiological systems, to date, do not find themselves in a genuinely competitive situation. (In other words, they do not satisfy the adaptivity constraint.) Such a genuinely competitive situation, for example, in terms of scarcity of resources, would automatically fixate their fundamental interests (e.g., survival and procreation). For this reason, present-day artificial systems only possess "goal variables" installed by a programmer, but not the subjective *experience* of the determined and rigid nature of certain internal states simultaneously covarying with the current overall state of their interests and ultimately the "logic of survival," which has shaped the history of their species.

and hard-to-control forms of phenomenal content like panic, jealousy, or falling in love. The sudden occurrence of this kind of content in the conscious self-model, if it is cognitively available, demonstrates how it is bound by certain biological imperatives like the fight for survival and procreation, that is, how strongly it is *determined* in terms of its functional architecture. By possessing a conscious, emotional self-model we are not only given to ourselves as spatially extended beings, but as beings possessing interests and goals, which, to a considerable degree, are fixed. However low the degree of phenomenal plasticity associated with our emotional self-experience may be, it allows us to *feel* the degree of our own functional rigidity.

However, we are much more than beings possessing a body and biological interests. We are information-processing systems internally operating with higher-order, nonsensory representata. We extract prototypes from perceptual models, we cognitively form classes out of objects given through the sensory modules, we mentally represent relations between such classes, and we generate mental models of propositions and of sentences in public languages. We exhibit a large number of abstract cognitive activities, which can, at times, be integrated into the PSM and constitute important elements of our conscious self-experience. For example, Keith Oatley (1988, p. 383*ff.*) has argued that one of the central functions of the self-model consists in organizing and structuring the goal hierarchy of a system. Common to all these genuinely cognitive components of the self-model is that they are *not* coded as spatial. For some people such conscious reasoning is a process diffusely localized inside their head in terms of a vague sense of effort, but for most people it does not possess any localization at all. There is a simple explanation for this phenomenological characteristic. Higher cognitive processes are implemented by neural processes which in turn operate only on patterns of activity "upstream" from sensory processing, on representations which themselves are only implemented by complicated sequences of events *in the central nervous system*. If there is a common computational principle underlying all kinds of phenomenal object formation (see Singer 2000), then conscious cognition will simply result from processes which iterate representational principles already found at the level of perceptual processing. However, it is important to recall how the central nervous system itself is devoid of any sensory sensitivity—the brain itself is insensitive to pain. This may be the fundamental architectural reason why some conscious states do not possess any phenomenal localization in the phenomenal body image, while still being fully integrated into the self-model and displaying the higher-order quality of "mineness." They are not integrated into the spatial frame of reference of *perceptual* or of *behavioral* space, and in this sense they are functionally "disembodied" and "nonsituated" or "unworldly" forms of processing. Possibly, this observation also possesses relevance to understanding the difference between phenomenally opaque and phenomenally transparent content (see next section).

Phenomenal spatiality of self-representational content is not an all-or-nothing matter, because what we actually find is a continuum from nonspatial to fully determinate spatial content with a high degree of interindividual variability. It is also interesting to note how the genetically recent cognitive partition of the self-model will automatically acquire a quality of nonworldliness, because of its nonspatial nature. The phenomenal model of the external world is a spatial model through and through. It is only our own intentions and higher cognitive states, and those of other human beings, that do not possess this spatial, sensory-mediated character. Obviously, any philosophical interpretation of these phenomena taking the naive realism inherent in our conscious model of the world and the self as its starting point will inevitably act from deep-rooted intuitions that our mental life *must* be something that, in an important sense, is not an element of objective reality or even of the world as a whole. The intuitive sense of impossibility, however, is only *phenomenal* impossibility, not a conceptually interesting variant. As we can now see, the basic fundamental structure of our own self-model lies at the heart of those philosophical intuitions, that, for instance, classical German idealism attempted to explicate. Unfortunately, as we have already seen, phenomenal necessity does not imply conceptual necessity.

A large part of the human self-model functions as a tool for processing and storing geometrical information, while a much smaller and evolutionarily more recent part is used to process and store more abstract, nonspatial information. On the level of phenomenal experience this leads to a continuum of self-representational contents, along a spectrum from spatial content to content that is experienced as only possessing temporal properties. This observation provides us with a further constraint for any empirically minded (e.g., connectionist or dynamicist) attempt to model the internal structure of the conscious human self-model. It will have to *reflect* this structural characteristic.

Before closing, let us look at the question of how self-*presentational* content is distributed over the PSM. Are what we used to simply call "qualia" (see section 2.4) phenomena which only exist in association with the phenomenal model of the body as a spatially extended entity, for example, as in tactile experiences or in consciously felt pain? Or do "intellectual qualia" exist as well? As almost all philosophers know, there are very concrete phenomenal qualities accompanying successful intellectual operations—for instance, "aha experiences." Phenomenologically, such experiential transitions are maximally simple and concrete. Adopting a dynamical stance, we might say the following: If a system like the human brain, after taking a long and winding path through its state space, all of a sudden finds itself dropping into a stable state, this transition, if globally available, can be accompanied by the conscious experience of sudden relaxation, of a salient and concrete "intellectual quale." However, it would be inadequate to introduce the notion of a phenomenal "aha presentatum," because, obviously, what we experience is not a stimulus-correlated state, but an abstract property of the ongoing system dynamics. What *can* be said is that a representationally atomic state, which is not correlated to any external stimulus but to a highly specific event in the internal dynamics of the cognitive system, is integrated into the PSM and, taking on a supplementary teleofunctionalist perspective, now fulfills an important function *for* the system by signaling a sudden drop in what, introducing a thermodynamic metaphor, would be the current energy level of the relevant cognitive subsystem. Phenomenal self-presentational content (as introduced in section 5.4) does not only possess the *de nunc* characteristic of all forms of presentational content. By contributing to the preconceptual experience of embodiment it is also content *de se*, and it always possesses a spatial component, because it is integrated into the geometrical self-model.

6.4.2   Transparent and Opaque Content

In chapter 3 (section 3.2.7) I introduced the transparency constraint for phenomenal representata in general, and in section 6.2.6 above we saw how this constraint, if applied to the concept of a PSM, leads to a decisive argument concerning the conditions under which a conscious self will, by necessity, emerge in a self-modeling system. Obviously, transparency itself is not a *sufficient* condition to turn the content of an internal system model into the content of a conscious self. However, if all other conditions and constraints for the activation of representational states with phenomenal content are satisfied, it will play precisely this role.

To avoid potential misunderstandings it is important to emphasize that the notions of "phenomenal transparency" and "phenomenal opacity" are only indirectly related to the well-known distinction between intensional and extensional contexts in epistemology and semantics. An intensional context is a referentially opaque context. An extensional context is a referentially transparent context. These contexts are constituted by different types of sentences and epistemic background situations. Phenomenal experience is not constituted by sentences at all, but by representations activated in a nonpropositional format. A sentence can constitute an extensional context if coreferring expressions in this sentence can be substituted for one another while preserving its truth-value. Phenomenal representations, viewed *as* carriers of phenomenal content do not possess truth-values. I will make no claims about the issue if the intentional content at the same time carried by some phenomenal representata possesses truth-values. The second condition for sentences constituting a referentially transparent or extensional context is that they entail the *existence* of the entities they speak about, whereas the first property of sentences constituting extensional contexts may be called intersubstitutivity *salva veritate*. The second constraint is supporting existential quantification. This, however, is a feature that (on the level of nonpropositional content) can be ascribed to transparent conscious contents as well: It forces the system experiencing this content to assume the existence of whatever is portrayed by this content. At least this is true of systems exhibiting no cognitive states. For sentences constituting *intensional* contexts—typically sentences expressing propositional attitudes like believing that *p* or desiring that *p*—neither of these criteria hold: the entities about which such sentences speak do not have to exist, and coreferring expressions cannot be substituted for one another. In a first-order approximation, and in trying to understand the difference between the referential and phenomenal versions of opacity and transparency it may be helpful to recall another technical term, namely, the "intensional fallacy." This fallacy consists in treating an intensional context as an extensional context. One possible variant is of particular importance, namely the automatic inferral of the existence of entities mentioned in an intensional context as if it were an extensional context. What I am saying, when I claim that the largest part of the conscious human self-model is transparent is simply that the human brain is a system that, on a subsymbolic and nonlinguistic level of representation, continuously commits something structurally resembling this variant of the intensional fallacy with regard to its own, internally generated self-model.

A transparent representation is characterized by the fact that the only properties accessible to introspective attention are their content properties. This is a strong claim to make about the representational architecture in which these states occur. It does not allow for the representation of a vehicle-content distinction using on-board resources. If we apply these thoughts to the idea that the human self-model possesses a transparent and an opaque component, we can gain a clearer picture of what this means in terms of global availability for self-directed attention. The transparent partition of the conscious human self-model is constituted by those of its parts for which it is true that introspective attention cannot make the difference between the content and the vehicle of self-representation globally available. In particular, what is not available are earlier processing stages. As I pointed out earlier, transparency is a special form of darkness. It is a lack of information. For the system operating under a PSM, transparency generates a specific kind of *internal* darkness, a systematic lack of access to system-related information. This time it is not that we don't see the window, but only the bird flying by; this time it is that we don't see the mirror, but just ourselves. What links this notion of *phenomenal* transparency to the well-established philosophical notion of *referential* transparency is that, for the system operating under this type of representational structure, it automatically entails the existence of the entity forming its content. "Entailment" is not a logical relation, but a phenomenological consequence. In the special case of phenomenal self-modeling, transparency means that, for the system operating under this self-model, it automatically and inevitably entails the existence of *itself*. What widely differs between the case of an extensional context and the internal, subsymbolic context constituted by the process of transparent, phenomenal self-modeling is the format and the epistemological properties of the kinds of representations involved.

What does it mean to say that a certain partition of the conscious human self-model is, in the phenomenological sense, opaque? If I engage in typical cognitive activities like reasoning, and if I then direct my introspective attention to this process as it unfolds, I experience myself as operating with internal representations that I am deliberately constructing myself. They do not imply the existence of their simulanda, and they might be coreferential with other mental representations of myself without me knowing this very fact. Self-directed attention to this part of the conscious self-model makes a difference between vehicle and content globally available. In other words, there is a certain partition of the conscious self-model for which introspective access, that is, access by the higher-order mechanism of self-directed attention, is *not* exhausted by its representational content properties. What is available are earlier processing stages (see section 3.2.7). For my own thoughts a reality-appearance distinction exists: I assume their existence *as* self-generated simulata, but what I do not know is if they actually are *representata*, in terms of possessing a representandum in the real world.

Again, in order to do justice to the real phenomenology, one has to admit that the property of phenomenal transparency at issue is not an all-or-nothing phenomenon, but may be distributed across varying parts of the human self-model to differing degrees. In general, the bodily self-model is fully transparent, while high-level cognitive processes like reasoning are phenomenally opaque. However, one of the particularly interesting features about the phenomenology of human self-consciousness is that there are aspects, for example, certain emotional processes, which on the level of subjective experience may *oscillate* between transparency and opacity multiple times. This is particularly evident in social relationships. Subjective experiences of trust, jealousy, and mild paranoia are interesting examples. In section 3.2.7 we saw how the phenomenology of transparent experience is the phenomenology of not only knowing but of also knowing *that* you *know* while you know; opaque experience is the experience of knowing while also (nonconceptually, attentionally) knowing that you may be *wrong*. In trusting another human being, a certain part of your emotional self-model has a direct and perception-like quality: You just *know* that you know that a certain fellow human being is trustworthy and this conscious experience is accompanied by a maximal sense of certainty. If that person disappoints you, not only does your phenomenal model of that person suddenly change but at the same time a certain internal decoherence or disassociation in your own self-model is created: You realize that your emotional state of trust was just a *representation* of social reality, and in this case a misrepresentation. It becomes opaque. In jealousy, we may oscillate between the transparent, perception-like character of an emotional state, for example, the state caused by, as it were, immediately perceiving another person as not being faithful, and the accompanying emotional experience of suspicion. Sudden, frequently repeated discoveries of this part of your emotional self-model being the result of an ongoing *mis*representation, an empty simulation determined in an unfortunate way by internal factors like your own biological or individual history, and not by real facts in your social environment, may again lead to an internal fragmentation of the conscious self. It hurts. A vehicle-content distinction is introduced where there previously was none. Again, we find that the emotional level of self-representation takes a middle position between the extremes. Emotional experiences vary in their degree of phenomenal opacity, just as they vary in the degree to which they are localized in the spatial model of the self.

The transparent partition of the conscious self-model is of particular importance in generating the phenomenal property of selfhood, in making processes of sensorimotor integration globally available, and in generating an internal user surface for motor control. However, if it had not been for the opaque partition of my self model, I could not have written this book. But is it *my* self-model? It is precisely the ability to internally model ourselves as thinking subjects, as systems actively generating abstract mental *representations* of the world (see section 6.4.4), that opens a window into the world of extended social cognition and genuine theoretical activity. For any system operating under a conscious, fully transparent self-model it would be impossible to *discover* this very fact, let alone form a theory or write a book about it. Very likely many animals on our planet are in precisely this kind of state. If they satisfy the necessary and sufficient constraints for phenomenal experience, they are minimally conscious (see section 3.2.7). If, in addition, they possess a transparent self-model, they are self-conscious—they instantiate the phenomenal property of selfhood. If such animals possess mechanisms of action control in terms of executive selection mechanisms for different behavioral patterns and if they possess attentional mechanisms, the globally available parts of their transparent self-model will be available for self-directed action and self-directed attention. Such animals might also possess a nonconceptual first-person perspective in terms of realizing a transparent model of the intentionality relation (see section 6.5). However, such animals would never, with regard to their conscious self-model, be able to make an appearance-reality distinction or develop the concept of misrepresentation. In other words, the principle of *autoepistemic closure* would characterize their psychological life in its entirety. Epistemologically, such systems would not have a chance of escaping what I have previously called the naive-realistic self-misunderstanding. Obviously, the same line of argument could be used to mark out a class of possible artificial systems.

What makes the conscious self-model of human beings so unique, and so enormously successful as a representational link between biological and cultural evolution is the fact that it violates the principle of autoepistemic closure. The fact of us possessing an opaque part of our self-model allows us to *conceive of* the possibility of an appearance-reality distinction not only for our own perceptual states but for the contents of self-consciousness as well. It allows us to distance us from ourselves by critically assessing the content of any PSM and—by opaque simulation—it allows us to conceive of certain possibilities, for instance, the epistemological possibility that every phenomenal representation might actually be a *simulation* if viewed from an objective third-person perspective (see chapter 2). It also allows us, for the first time, to conceive of the possibility that every phenomenal *self*-representation might actually be a self-*simulation*. Such cognitive discoveries, of course, do not yet change the fundamental architecture of our phenomenal space. But they allow us to break through the principle of autoepistemic closure that in our biological past governed the dynamics of phenomenal experience in our ancestors, and to employ external means of information processing—for example, in forming scientific communities, in constructing empirical theories about the basis of mind, and so on. Transparency is not a logical necessity, only an epistemic deficit. One of the most remarkable features of the human self-model is the fact that this epistemic deficit is only a *partial* deficit. We return to this issue soon.

If these observations point in the right direction, a further constraint for any future theory of phenomenal self-consciousness naturally flows from them. What has to be described, for example, on the level of computational or dynamicist modeling, is how, first, a continuum ranging from phenomenally transparent to phenomenally opaque content can be realized by an information-processing system like the human brain. The second constraint for any future theory of phenomenal self-modeling is a solution to what I want to term the "integration problem for cognitive subjectivity": How does a conscious self-modeling system manage to *integrate* phenomenally opaque mental content into an already existing transparent self-model? This issue may turn out to be closely related to the question of spatial versus nonspatial encoding touched upon in the previous section. What we need is an empirically plausible story about how such a capacity could be gradually achieved under biologically realistic conditions. I believe that both theoretical problems are of highest importance for any theory about the emergence of genuinely cognitive subjects. However, I admit that I do not possess even the very first conceptual tools that are needed to take initial steps toward a solution of these two problems.

6.4.3 The Attentional Subject

A particularly interesting type of phenomenal content is of the form "myself in the act of attending to an object." It has a subject component (*myself*), an object component (e.g., the book in your hands), and it portrays both components as standing in a certain, asymmetrical relation to each other (the "arrow of attention"). Also, the functional constraint of global availability for attention now reappears on the first-person level of conscious contents itself. In understanding the conscious experience of attention, the concept of a PSM is helpful in at least two ways. First, it can help us understand why the content of attentional processing is always experienced as the content of my *own* attention. Second, it can help us to grasp what it means to take on a nonconceptual first-person perspective toward *oneself.* Attentional availability is one central constraint for the concept of conscious representation. Phenomenal representata are characterized by the fact that we can always attend to their content. Obviously, this is not true of unconscious representational structures. In order to understand attention and object awareness, the theoretical framework now has to be expanded, using a component of self-representation. A plausible hypothesis is that an experience only becomes *my own* experience when it is simultaneously activated with those cortical regions corresponding to the body landscape or integrated with cognitive-style memories of certain autobiographical episodes (D. LaBerge 1997; see also D. LaBerge 1995). If the process of attention is itself represented on the level of conscious experience, it is, interestingly, inevitably integrated with the self-model. Phenomenologically, we know of no such thing as "objective attention," of a consciously experienced process of attending which is not fundamentally my own. A potential exception to the rule is likely to be presented by certain types of meditative or spiritual experience.

However, an important conceptual distinction has to be introduced. While, phenomenologically, clearly all representations of ongoing attentional processing are endowed with the phenomenal quality of "mineness," the experience of internal agency accompanied by the sense of effort in directing one's attention can either be present or absent. In low-level attention the process of focusing on an object is initiated on the unconscious level. We are surprised by our own head suddenly moving and our gaze fixating a particular object. However, the final result of this kind of event, triggered on a purely functional level, is a conscious representation of *a self in the act of attending* to a certain object. The second phenomenological variety is focal attention. In these cases we experience ourselves as initiating, controlling, and sustaining the shift in the direction of attention toward a certain object. Therefore, we have to differentiate between the passive attentional subject—a transparent self-model of involuntarily attending to a certain perceptual object or mental contents, while not having initiated the preceding shift in attention—and *attentional agency*, that is, the existence of a transparent self-model as *causing* shifts in attention and deliberately holding a certain object in its focus. Both classes of phenomenal states are interesting, because they transparently represent the system as standing in a certain *relation* to an object component. What the three different forms of high-level phenomenal content, which we will be discussing in this and the following two sections—namely, the attentional subject, the cognitive subject, and the subjective experience of agency—have in common is that they are instances of what, in section 6.5, I will introduce as the "phenomenal model of the intentionality relation" (PMIR). They represent a subject *as standing in a specific relationship* to a certain object, for example, as attending to it, thinking about it, or acting on it. What already is a frequently neglected, deeper phenomenological truth about perception—the content of a perceptual state really is *not* a part of the environment, but a *relation* holding to this part—is something that can be rediscovered on higher levels of self-consciousness: Full-blown, phenomenal self-consciousness always involves a relation between the self and an object component. However, what varies in these different forms of phenomenal self-modeling is the nature of the object component and the manner in which the phenomenal property of transparency is distributed across the overall content.

Consider focal attention. In standard situations, the object component will be transparent. If you visually attend to the cover of the book you are now holding in your hands, the experience is not one of attending to a phenomenal model of a book, but simply one of attending to a book. If you attend to the tactile sensations in your fingers, while holding the book or turning it around to have a closer look at its cover, your conscious experience is not one of attending to a part of your PSM, but simply one of highlighting, as it were, certain bodily sensations in your fingertips. *Attentional agency*, the conscious experience of initiating the shift of attention and holding its focus fixed on a certain aspect of reality, is fully transparent as well. The content of your conscious experience is not one of self-representation or an ongoing process of self-modeling, of depicting yourself as a causal agent in certain shifts of "zoom factor," "resolving power," or "resource allocation," and so on, but simply of *yourself* selecting a new object for attention. There is an interesting additional aspect, namely, the phenomenally experienced "arrow of intentionality." It consists in the fact that the relation between attentional subject and attended object clearly is represented as asymmetrical: attention *points* from subject to object. We return to this issue later. For now it is only important to point out that this feature of phenomenally represented attention is transparent as well—it is not experienced *as* a representation of some sort of asymmetrical relation currently holding, for example, between yourself and the visually attended-to book cover. It simply is there.

In low-level attention we do not experience the phenomenon of attentional agency. More precisely, we may experience ourselves as *holding* attention to a certain object, but the shift to the new attentional object is experienced as being forced upon the phenomenal self, which is passive. If while reading this sentence you suddenly hear the sound of glass shattering behind you, the sudden turn of your head, the process of visual search immediately following the event, and the sudden discovery of, let's say, a soccer ball, which has been kicked through your window by neighborhood children, then this is a chain of phenomenal states lacking the property of attentional agency. You experience this series of events as having been caused unconsciously. The cascade of physical events mirrored in the quickly changing contents of your transparent self-model is simply triggered by events in the objective order. You have not initiated it yourself. But at the *end* of this process you are an attentional subject. At the beginning you were not. An empirically very plausible way of conceiving of this type of representational shift consists in analyzing it as a perturbation of the unconscious self-model by a newly activated percept (e.g., the auditory representation of glass shattering), which then triggers the emergence of an integrated representation of the system *as* currently being perturbed by a new perceptual object, thereby generating a more salient phenomenal mental model of the object itself, as well as integrating a new model of the relation between self and object into the conscious model of reality (see Damasio 1999, chapter 6).[17]

What is different about this process of generating a phenomenal, attentional subject as opposed to focal attention? Attention here is a process that can be described as *saliency-driven*. Functionally speaking, it is driven by a sudden change in the external environment, triggering a sudden shift in the subpersonal mechanisms of attentional processing. What is lacking is a phenomenal representation of the *selection process* by which the object component of the attentional relation is integrated with the subsequently activated PSM. Attentional agency therefore is a transparent, phenomenal representation *of* these selection processes preceding focal attention on the level of self-modeling. Above, I claimed that, in its core, the theoretical problem consists in achieving a homunculus-free representationalist-functionalist analysis of the *phenomenal* target property of attentional agency, without simply introducing a metaphorical–personal-level entity which exercises some sort of ultimate high-level decisional control in shifting attention. My answer now is that there is no *ultimate* stage, causally speaking, but just a *phenomenal* stage of an ongoing dynamic process of self-organization, involving multiple loops and a highly recurrent form of information processing. Some stages are conscious, some are unconscious. As a whole, this process displays an extremely high degree of flexibility and short-term adaptability, involving the explicit internal simulation of alternative objects for attentional processing. We like to call this "selectivity," but there is no little attentional homunculus in the brain *doing* the selecting. What there is, in the sort of phenomenal agency involved in focal attention, is a globally available representation of the process in which different alternatives are matched against each other and the system settles on a single solution. Because this representation is part of the PSM, it is part of a representation of the system as a whole. It stands in a certain representational context that also is a *functional* context.

---

17. Cf. Damasio 1999, for instance, figure 6.1, p. 178. The "map of object X," is what, according to my representationalist analysis, is an unconscious neural activation pattern caused by the auditory input, which in turn is caused by the glass shattering. What, in Damasio's terminology, would be the "map of the proto-self at inaugural instant" would be the mental self-representatum (the content of the ongoing process of unconscious self-modeling at *t*), which is then functionally affected by the shift in perceptual dynamics and integrated into a globally available model of the intentionality relation (see section 6.5, this chapter). This process is the representationalist and functionalist description of what, in Damasio's conception, would be the "assembly of a second-order map," in turn leading to increased saliency in the object component of that map. However, the philosophical issue here is to mark out those cases in which this process is accompanied by the property of "attentional agency."

Subpersonal selection and sustaining processes for attention represented in the PSM are those which, within certain limits, can be *terminated* by the system as a whole.

Are there exceptions to this principle with regard to the special case of self-directed attention? A sudden pain in your foot may force your attention to this part of the phenomenal self, but the overall process does not lose any of its transparency. You simply experience your *own* attention as suddenly being forced to shift to a pain in your *own* foot. Phenomenologically, the same is true when deliberately directing attention to other aspects of your body. The sense of attentional agency is fully realized on the level of conscious experience, and the partition of your PSM, on which attentional processing now starts to operate, is not experienced as a model—it is simply *yourself*, your *own foot*, you are attending to. An interesting case, however, confronts us when investigating those classes of phenomenal states in which the object component of the attentional relation is formed by *opaque* sections of the PSM. What precisely does it mean to direct introspective$_3$ attention to the process of activating opaque cognitive representations, for example, when carefully attending to your own conscious experience of reasoning?

Let me first point out an interesting phenomenological feature of this process, which, however, I will not discuss further at this point. As practitioners of meditation from highly diverging cultural backgrounds have consistently reported over centuries, effortlessly attending to the flow of your own cognitive processes is an efficient means to *end* these processes. Attention is a means to make the flow of conscious thought eventually cease. Naturally, the conscious experience of deliberately attending to your own thought processes is a metarepresentational activity that is then reintegrated into the PSM, that is, the ongoing activity of focusing on and representing *phenomenally* opaque states with the help of phenomenally *transparent* states. Again, what remains transparent and phenomenally immediate is the subject component: the experience of a *self* having selected a certain kind of attentional object and "staying with it" for a certain time. The object component is formed by a dynamic chain of mental representations, intended simulations, which are represented as *representations*, as something that could in principle be false. One empirical speculation concerning this feature consists in proposing that the more *central* neural correlates of certain representational states are—in terms of being functionally distant from the sensory input layers of the human brain—the easier it is for attentional processing to access properties of the representational "vehicle." Transparency means that introspective$_1$ access to a phenomenal mental model is limited to its content properties. Opaque phenomenal models, for example, those making reasoning processes globally available for the system, would therefore be formed by a subclass of structures for which vehicle properties are introspectively accessible as well, therefore enabling the system to depict a difference between form and content, and to make a reality-appearance distinction with regard to these states globally available. Phenomenally experienced cognition seems to be precisely this kind of process. Its content is abstract, removed from sensory processing, and closely associated with activities in prefrontal cortex. Attending to your own conscious thought, then, is a situation where certain aspects of the ongoing dynamics in the opaque partitions of the conscious self-model are monitored by the system. The result of this monitoring process then is continuously integrated into the transparent part of the conscious self-model. The final result is the conscious experience of *yourself* attending to your own deliberately activated mental representations. The important point to note is that the subject component resulting from the self-attribution of causal efficacy, the phenomenal property of attentional and cognitive "agency," is fully transparent. In order to better understand this interesting type of representational structure, let us now look at yet another higher-order form of consciously experienced, self-representational content.

6.4.4   The Cognitive Subject

A conscious cognitive subject is generated as soon as a globally available representation of the system currently generating or operating on quasi-linguistic, opaque mental representations is integrated into the already existing transparent self-model. It is vital to arrive at a convincing analysis of this form of phenomenal content, because this provides us with an understanding of what it means to possess a *cognitive* first-person perspective, as opposed to a merely *phenomenal* first-person perspective. A phenomenal first-person perspective could already be realized by an animal or a primitive artificial system operating under a fully transparent mechanism of attentional processing, as described in the previous section. The attentional first-person perspective is the more fundamental phenomenon, on top of which higher levels emerge. One of the many advantages of the self-model theory of subjectivity (SMT) is that it offers a deeper understanding of what—representationally—cognitive self-reference actually is and of what—epistemically—is special about propositional attitudes *de se* (Chisholm 1981; D. K. Lewis 1979). In a nutshell, a central part of the answer is that both result from an integrated interaction of transparent and opaque content mediated by one and the same representational vehicle. I will try to illustrate the issue by drawing on an example from the recent philosophical discussion.

In an important and helpful paper (Baker 1998) Lynne Baker pointed out how a convincing conception of the cognitive first-person perspective will constitute a test for any robust version of naturalism. Baker differentiates between two classes of first-person phenomena. Weak first-person phenomena are those in which, for instance, animals can be conceived of as operating under an egocentric world-model forming the center of their own universe and the origin of their own perspective. As Baker points out, all sentient beings are conscious subjects of experience, but not all of them have first-person *concepts* of themselves. For Baker, only those who do are fully self-conscious in an interesting sense

(Baker 1998, p. 328).[18] Given the conceptual tools introduced in section 6.2 it is clear what such a description amounts to: Such animals would use an integrated, global, and transparent model of the world functionally centered by a transparent self-model in order to regulate their own behavior. They minimally satisfy the presentationality constraint, the globality constraint, the transparency constraint, and the perspectivalness constraint. As Baker correctly points out, such organisms could be said to be solving problems by employing perspectival attitudes, while not yet possessing a concept of themselves *as a subject.*

First-person phenomena in a stronger and more interesting sense, however, are not only characterized by the necessary condition of possessing a self-world-boundary and being able to differentiate between the first and third person but also by the capacity to possess this distinction on a *conceptual* level and actually use it. In the terminology so far introduced, this means that the existence of a preattentive self-world boundary and the difference between first- and third-person attributions is cognitively available. As Baker points out it is not only necessary to have thoughts that can be expressed using "I." What is necessary is the possession of a concept of oneself as the *thinker* of these thoughts, as the *owner* of a subjective point of view. In short, what is needed is not only reference from the first-person point of view but the capacity to mentally "ascribe" this act of reference *to* oneself while it is taking place. Here is how Baker makes the point:

> A conscious being that exhibits strong first-person phenomena not only is able to recognize herself from a first-person point of view . . . but also is able to think of herself as herself. For strong first-person phenomena, it is not enough to *distinguish* between first-person and third-person; also one must be able to *conceptualize* the distinction, to conceive of oneself as oneself. To be able to conceive of oneself as oneself is to be able to conceive of oneself independently of a name, or description or third-person demonstrative. It is to be able to conceptualize the distinction between oneself and everything else there is. It is not just to have thoughts expressible by means of "I," but also to conceive of oneself as the bearer of those thoughts. . . . But merely having a perspective, or a subjective point of view, is not enough for strong first-person-phenomena. Rather one must also be able to conceive of oneself as having a perspective, or a subjective point of view. (Baker 1998, p. 329 *ff.*)

This conceptual distinction is important for cognitive science in general, and also for the philosophical notion of a true cognitive subject. As Baker notes, this capacity may also be important for so-called theory-of-mind tasks: Only if one is able to think about oneself as

18. Here is how Lynne Baker characterizes weak first-person phenomena: "Two points should be noted about weak first-person phenomena: (i) They are exhibited by sentient organisms, who solve problems by means of perspectival attitudes; these attitudes then explain the problem-solving behavior. (This point is independent of any theory of how, or whether, attitudes are explicitly represented in the brain.) (ii) No first-person concept is needed to bind belief-desire-behavior to a single organism. . . . Although such an animal has beliefs and desires, he has no conception of belief or desire, nor of himself as the subject or bearer of beliefs and desires" (Baker 1998, p. 328).

being the thinker and the subject of first-person thoughts, is one also able to form the concept of *other* subjects of first-person thoughts. The capacity at issue would also enable one to conceive of one's own desires and wishes *as one's own*—for instance, in terms of second-order volitional acts in the sense of Harry Frankfurt (Frankfurt 1971).

In the light of the theoretical model proposed here it is quite clear what Baker is really demanding. The representational architecture needed for cognitive subjectivity is not only a self-representation, including certain cognitive activities as one's own, plus a mental representation of oneself being the initiator of these internal events, that is, a cognitive agent. What is really needed is a representational structure which makes this very fact *globally available for higher-order cognition*.

It is important to note that the concept of a phenomenal self-model proposed here achieves precisely this capacity. If a system integrates its own operations with opaque mental representations, that is, with mental *simulations* of propositional structures that could be true or false, into its already existing transparent self-model while simultaneously attributing the causal role of generating these representational states to itself, the system as a whole—all other necessary constraints for phenomenal representation being satisfied—will not only possess the conscious experience of cognitive agency, of being the thinker and the subject of its *own* thought; it will also make this new phenomenal content available for higher-order cognitive processing: it now possesses the additional capacity to form a concept of itself *as* a cognitive agent. What previously was a subpersonal representational process is now *appropriated* on the whole-system level, by using a transparent representation of the system as a whole. One advantage of the self-model theory of subjectivity therefore is that it offers a more detailed and empirically tractable understanding of what a propositional attitude *de se* actually could be (D. K. Lewis 1979; Chisholm 1981). However, as Baker writes:

If I attribute first-person reference to myself, my sentence cannot be adequately paraphrased by any sentence that fails to attribute first-person reference to me: The attribution of first-person reference to one's self seems to be ineliminable. (Baker 1998, p. 331)

I disagree. Here is where I offer an alternative. First, no such things as selves exist in the world; all that exists are conscious systems operating under transparent self-*models*. Second, we need to differentiate between the contents of linguistic and of mental representations. Linguistic self-reference always refers to the phenomenal content of the self-model, typically to its transparent portion (as the PSM is what functionally *enables* linguistic self-reference in the first place). Because this transparent portion cannot be experienced *as* a form of representational content, the fact that a linguistic content refers to a mental content cannot be consciously experienced. This fact, however, must be reflected in our theory of self-consciousness. One way of paraphrasing this sentence according to the current model would be as follows: "This system currently uses a sentence in a public language to refer to a certain capacity, namely, the capacity to access the content of certain opaque, cognitive simulations integrated into an already existing transparent self-model by higher-order cognitive operations, which then in turn can be integrated into this self-model." Let me explain.

According to Baker, to possess a first-person perspective in the more interesting sense consists in possessing a certain *capacity*. It is the capacity of forming I*-sentences or I*-thoughts (the asterisk is used here following the common notation introduced by Hector-Neri Castañeda 1966).[19] As Baker correctly adds, a complete mastery of "I" includes this capacity. She writes:

The first-person perspective is a necessary condition for any form of self-consciousness, and a sufficient condition for one form of self-consciousness as well. (Baker 1998, p. 333)

Baker then goes on to illustrate her point, using a particularly beautiful example:

For example, there is no third-person way to express the Cartesian thought, "I am certain that I* exist." The certainty that Descartes claimed was certainty that he* existed, not certainty that Descartes existed. (Baker 1998, p. 336)

What really was the reason for Descartes's certainty about his own existence? He possessed a transparent self-model that turned him into an "autoepistemically closed" being: the representational nature of a considerable portion of his self-model was in principle unavailable to him, that is, he could not gain *introspective₃* knowledge about it. Autoepistemic closure, as represented by the phenomenal transparency constraint being maximally satisfied for large partitions of the human self-model, must by necessity lead to the prereflexive phenomenal property of "selfhood," which simply *is* the certainty about one's own existence (including all other properties transparently represented). Therefore, any representational system satisfying the constraints for conscious experience while operating under a transparent self-model *has* to be certain of its own existence. This is a conceptual necessity for the class of representational systems described, in all possible worlds. The linguistic expression "I*" invariably refers to this content of the conscious, current transparent model of the self.

Baker is, of course, right in pointing out that Descartes's claim did not refer to any third-person representation of the person Descartes. What he referred to was a representation of Descartes "in the mode of selfhood," under a "phenomenal EGO-mode of presentation" as

19. "An ability to conceive of oneself as oneself* in the sense just described is both necessary and sufficient for the strong grade of first-person phenomena: An individual who is the locus of strong first-person phenomena can conceive of herself as a bearer of first-person thoughts. She manifests an ability not only to make first-person reference, but also to attribute to herself first-person reference" (Baker 1998, p. 331).

it were (see, e.g., Newen 1997). This mode of presentation is the subsymbolic, nonconceptual mode of internal, transparent self-modeling. It leads to the phenomenal experience of possessing a transtemporal identity, but it does not presuppose any linguistic self-identification. The content of this transparent self-model, in particular the phenomenological characteristic of this content as being given in a seemingly direct and immediate manner, of being "infinitely close" to oneself, is cognitively available. If so, then, obviously, *higher-order* cognitive content referring to this very fact can also be formed. If this content, in turn, is embedded in the already existing phenomenal self-representation, then the relevant conscious experience of *having* this thought will automatically ensue. An additional and nonconceptual sense of ownership will emerge as a new form of active, higher-order phenomenal content. This thought is Baker's I*-thought. Its content is:

[I am certain that I exist]*

From now on, I refer to active phenomenal content by using square brackets (as above), and to linguistic expressions referring *to* active phenomenal content by using pointed brackets. The *linguistic* expression ⟨I⟩ refers to the fact that this current conscious thought is a component of the speaker's self-model. However, this fact is simultaneously available to cognitive introspection operating on the self-model in terms of introspection$_4$. It is phenomenally represented as the experience of being the *thinker* of this thought (more below). ⟨I*⟩, on the other hand, refers to the transparent partition of this self-model. The certainty predicated of the phenomenal self, and in particular the existence assumption invariably going along with it, refers to a globally available mental representation of the phenomenal quality of "infinite proximity," the indubitable (i.e., *phenomenally* necessary) experience of selfhood, of direct givenness-to-oneself caused by the transparency of the self-model.[20]

   The *sentence* ⟨I am certain that I* exist⟩ therefore refers to a complex, integrated, and globally available form of phenomenal mental content, namely, to the currently active PSM of the respective person. Given the necessary output device, it could be uttered by a brain in a vat, as this content locally supervenes. The content of this self-model is: *[I am certain that I* exist]*. From now on I will only be concerned with the phenomenal mental content and not with the linguistic expression that, as Lynne Baker puts it, "indicates" the existence of this content. However, please note the fascinating architecture of this structure: We are confronted with a form of metarepresentation crossing the linguistic-phenomenal divide between propositional and nonconceptual content, a metarepresentation meeting the

---

20. Let me illustrate this point. Baker convincingly criticizes Flanagan (1992, p. 194*ff.*) by pointing out that one has to analyze "thinking about one's model of one's self" as thinking about one's model of oneself as oneself and not just as thinking of a model of someone-who-is-in-fact-oneself (Baker 1998, p. 342). The current proposal achieves this by introducing the transparency constraint.

additional condition *that it is not experienced as such* by the representing system. An internal, locally supervening form of phenomenal content becomes the content of a *linguistic* representation in public space, with the speaker being unaware of this very fact due to the transparency of the first-order mental content. Let us take a closer look.

The issue I want to draw attention to is that the content of this self-model possesses a phenomenally transparent and a phenomenally opaque component. The degree of attentional availability of earlier processing stages varies. The transparent component of the self-model (e.g., the content of the body-model) is experienced as directly and immediately given. The opaque component is often but not necessarily experienced as deliberately constructed, for instance, as one's own thought. *Both* forms of content are subsymbolic content. The opaque component, if not consisting of pictorial imagery and suchlike, approximates constituent structure, propositional modularity (Ramsey, Stich, and Garon 1991), and so on to a sufficient degree to be able to be interpreted as a quasilinguistic form of mental content on the level of external autophenomenological reports. However, let us stay with the phenomenal content itself and begin with the transparent component of Baker's Cartesian thought.

[I]*

is the content of the transparent self-model. This content is activated under the "principle of autoepistemic closure" mentioned above. Any conscious system operating under a transparent self-model will by necessity instantiate a phenomenal self to which, linguistically, it *must* refer using $\langle I^* \rangle$. It is autoepistemically closed against earlier processing stages of its own self-model, because it cannot introspectively₃ discover its *representational* nature. In other words, in Baker's example, the I*-thought is being constituted by the content of the transparent self-model, by a subset of its content properties. Please note how a natural background assumption is that the system already satisfies all other constraints sufficient for at least a minimal degree of conscious experience.

[I exist]*

denotes the decisive property of the transparent self-model (in this context). What are general constitutive conditions for the phenomenal experience of "existence?" Let us define a *minimal* notion of self-consciousness: the content of the self-model has to be embedded in the currently active world-model; it has to be activated within a virtual window of presence; and it has to be transparent. Therefore not only the fact that the world-model is a *model* but also the fact that the temporal internality of the contents of the window of presence is an internal *construct* is not introspectively₃ available to the subject. Then there is the special case of phenomenal *self-presence*, the subjective experience of *Anwesenheit*: the fact that the self-model is a *model* and that the temporal internality of its content as integrated into the current window of presence is an internal *construct*, again, is not available to the system as a whole. This property is a microfunctional property (attentional unavailability of earlier processing stages, i.e., of certain vehicle properties), not a content property.

[I]

⟨I⟩ refers to the speaker of a sentence; [I] is the phenomenal content of the *opaque* component of the current self-model, the thinker of this thought. The fact that the current cognitive content is only a mental *representation* is introspectively available for attention as well as for cognition. In addition, we also have the structural characteristic of cognitive agency: I experience myself as the *thinker* of the I* thought. The opaque component of the self-model represents the respective subject as a being, which *deliberately* generates the mental content in question within itself. Therefore, [I] internally models the system as a whole, including the content of the opaque component, which has already been *embedded* in the continuously active background of the transparent self-model. The content of [I] is the thinker, currently representing herself as operating with mental representations. Please note that the content here referred to, like all phenomenal content, cannot count as epistemically justified content.

[am certain that]

is the subsymbolic equivalent of what would be an "attitude specificator" (believing that *p*, wanting that *p*, being certain that *p*, etc.) of a propositional attitude. It is the relation between self and cognitive content as it is currently *phenomenally* represented. What are constitutive conditions for phenomenally experienced certainty? Let me name the two defining characteristics: the object component of the phenomenal first-person perspective is transparent and the respective person is, therefore, on the level of phenomenal experience, forced into an (epistemically unjustified) existence assumption with respect to the intentional content of the object component. The same is true of the subject component. The second defining characteristic is the transparency of the self-model, yielding a phenomenal self depicted as *being* certain. Please note how a phenomenal first-person perspective now reveals itself as the ongoing conscious representation of dynamic subject-object relations: to see an object, to feel a pain, to selectively "make a thought your own," to chose a potential action goal, or, to be *certain* of oneself, as currently existing.[21]

21. This certainty can be lost for contingent reasons, for instance, in patients suffering from Cotard's delusion. It may be interesting to note that this form of phenomenal content is not a necessary feature of all conscious experience. There is phenomenal consciousness in combination with the absolutely certain belief of already being dead, or of even not existing at all. Anecdotal reports say that some of the patients just mentioned will even stop using the pronoun "I." See section 7.2.2.

Being phenomenally certain about *oneself*, again, is a special case. It appears if the object component of the phenomenal first-person perspective is formed by a transparent *self-representation*; for instance, by a phenomenal model of the respective person *as* a now-existing subject. Please note how the object component of a phenomenal first-person perspective will typically be transparent, because this precisely is what *makes* it an object—something that cannot be experienced as a representation anymore. So we are confronted with a consciously experienced form of second-order self-representation. It is important to note that what we used to call the "vehicles" of representation are not distinct entities: If, for heuristic reasons, one wants to hold on to the vehicle-content distinction one always has to keep in mind that from an empirical point of view the neural carriers very likely are not distinct states anymore, but are characterized by a part-whole relationship within a dynamical process.

On the representational level of description, strong first-person phenomena and Cartesian I*-thoughts can now be analyzed as the *integration* of an opaque self-model into a preexisting, transparent self-model. What we are unable to consciously experience during cognitive self-reference is the fact that, even in this situation, we are referring to the content of a *representation* that is "in ourselves" (in terms of locally supervening on brain properties). This is a necessary consequence of the transparency constraint for the subsymbolic self-model. Cognitive self-reference, therefore, on the phenomenal level is necessarily experienced as direct and immediate, because it is not mediated through any sensory channel (it takes place in a supramodal format) and because of the fact that it is a *second-order* process of phenomenal representation, is not introspectively available (naive realism). Therefore, the possibility that the first-order component might be a *mis-representation* is not available to us on the level of attentional introspection$_3$.

Let us now return to the level of linguistic self-reference. The overall sentence ⟨I am certain that I* exist⟩ indicates that a certain form of phenomenal content is currently active. From a third-person perspective, this linguistic content can be analyzed as follows:

⟨The speaker of this sentence currently activates a PSM in which second-order, opaque self-representations have been embedded. These representations are characterized by three properties:

First, they possess a quasi-conceptual format (e.g., through a connectionist emulation of constituent-structure, etc.);

second, their content is exclusively formed by operations on the transparent partitions of the currently active PSM;

third, the resulting relation between the system as a whole and content is phenomenally modeled as a relation of certainty.⟩

Now we can see how it is the internal model of the relation between system and content, which, in this case, generates the cognitive first-person perspective. This cognitive first-person perspective, however, can now always be reduced to a special case of the *phenomenal* first-person perspective and, as such, all corresponding belief states are not epistemically justified. Therefore, all beliefs about *what* it is that is being mentally represented—that is, beliefs about the intentional or epistemic content of strong first-person phenomena and Cartesian I*-thoughts—are themselves not epistemically justified in any way. In particular, this is true of the belief that it is a *self* that carries out the respective act of cognitive self-reference.

One further interesting consequence of this short representationalist analysis of strong first-person phenomena in the sense of Lynne Baker is that the phenomenal first-person perspective is a condition of possibility for the emergence of a *cognitive* first-person perspective. Cognitive self-reference always is reference to the phenomenal content of a transparent self-model. More precisely, it is a *second-order* variant of phenomenal self-modeling, which, however, is mediated by *one and the same* integrated vehicle of representation. The capacity to conceive of oneself as oneself* consists in being able to activate a dynamic, "hybrid" self-model: Phenomenally opaque, quasi-symbolic, and second-order representations of a preexisting phenomenally transparent self-model are being activated and continuously reembedded in it. This process is the process of introspection$_4$. In this process, not the conscious reality-model, but the *self-model* suddenly satisfies the perspectivalness constraint: Reflexive self-consciousness consists in establishing a subject-object relation *within* the PSM.

What, then, can be said about the concept of a conscious cognitive subject? The transparent, subsymbolic self-model is a tool used by an information-processing system to make a certain type of information *cognitively available*. It does so by enabling opaque mental self-simulations. Such self-simulations can be phenomenally expressed as conscious I*-thoughts or, linguistically, as I*-sentences, that is, they can lead to the cognitive or linguistic self-attribution of a prereflexive first-person perspective. Cognitive self-reference is a process of phenomenally modeling certain aspects of the content of a preexisting transparent self-model, which, from a conceptual third-person perspective, can be interpreted as the capacity of conceiving of oneself as oneself*.

Baker is perfectly right in pointing out that the postulation of a mental symbol functionally playing the role of ⟨I*⟩ only renames the problem without solving it. She thinks what is truly necessary is the possession of a particular capacity, the capacity to conceive of oneself as oneself*, a capacity beyond having self-localizing beliefs à la Perry (J. Perry 1979). The capacity she is looking for is the capacity to operate under a phenomenally transparent self-model that is globally available, not only for self-directed attention and selective action control but for mental *concept formation* as well. It is the capacity to apply introspection$_4$ to a preexisting transparent self-model. In human beings, natural evolution on our planet has already brought about this capacity—as can be seen from the writings of René Descartes. However, cognitive agency, conceptually mediated self-consciousness, and strong first-person phenomena in Baker's sense do not constitute an insurmountable obstacle to naturalism. It is possible to accommodate these phenomena in an empirically plausible theory of mental representation. The deeper philosophical issue, however, is that the implicitly presupposed *epistemic* content of cognitive self-reference can now in principle always be reduced to a purely *phenomenal* kind of mental content. Cognitive self-consciousness and the form of self-reference discussed here are in need of an independent epistemic justification.

However, let me point out one important caveat. As Baker points out, any robust reductive naturalism has to offer an analysis of the constitutive conditions of the above-mentioned capacity in terms of nonintentional and nonsemantic concepts. I have therefore offered an analysis in terms of *phenomenological* concepts. Self-representational phenomenal content is a special sort of intentional content, one that *locally supervenes* on brain properties—and as such it is open to naturalization. If it is true that phenomenal content locally supervenes, then there may even be a nomologically coextensive physical property for every phenomenal property; that is, empirical research programs might discover domain-specific identities for every individual form of phenomenal content. This will also be true of the phenomenal content of cognitive self-reference. On the other hand, if, as many philosophers today believe, phenomenal content is just a special variant of intentional content, the model sketched here will eventually have to be supplemented by a full-blown naturalist theory of intentional content, a theory that additionally allows us to understand the *relation* between phenomenal and intentional content. We are very far from this goal. Today, it only seems safe to say two things: Phenomenal content as such is not epistemically justified content, and it locally supervenes on brain properties. A brain in a vat could generate the conscious experience of thinking *[I am certain that I* exist]*. Cotard's syndrome patients can generate the conscious experience of thinking *[I am certain that I* do not exist]*. It is therefore plausible to assume that a minimally sufficient neural correlate for the phenomenal content characterizing the specific conscious experience of thinking *[I am certain that I* exist]* does exist. The phenomenal content will supervene on or even be identical to this physical correlate. But will there not be many cases in which this content is typically and reliably correlated with *intentional*, epistemically justifiable content? It is interesting to note how even under naturalistic background assumptions *some* kind of representational system has to exist, because, trivially, transparent self-models are conceptually introduced as being realized by physical vehicles. If this background assumption possesses an independent epistemic justification, then any conscious system is justified in thinking the I*-thought that at least some physical representational system exists, which right now carries out the act of cognitive self-reference. What is not clear is if this system actually is a *self*.

What, then, can be said about the concept of a conscious cognitive subject? The transparent, subsymbolic self-model is a tool that can be used by an information-processing system to make a certain type of information *cognitively available*. It does so by enabling opaque mental self-simulations. Such self-simulations can be expressed as I*-thoughts or, linguistically, as I*-sentences, that is, they can lead to the phenomenal or linguistic self-attribution of a prereflexive first-person perspective. Cognitive self-reference is a process of phenomenally modeling certain aspects of the content of a preexisting transparent self-model, which in turn can be interpreted as the capacity of conceiving of oneself as oneself*. In short, the phenomenal first person perspective is the central necessary condition for possessing a *cognitive* first-person perspective. And again, in order to achieve phenomenological plausibility and avoid the introduction of theoretical artifacts into computational or neurobiological modeling, it is important not to assume yet another principled dualism between two forms of mental content. As we have seen in section 6.4.2, there actually is a *continuum* from transparent to opaque content in the human self-model. Empirically speaking, this will be reflected in the way in which reflexive self-consciousness is functionally anchored in emotions and in the bodily model of the self as well.

6.4.5 Agency

As we have seen, the phenomenal experience of being an attentional subject can be accompanied by the experience of phenomenal agency. It can also unfold without this property. In low-level attention we do not experience ourselves as voluntarily causing the sudden shift in conscious content. After the shift has taken place, however, we are attentional subjects. A transparent self-model of the system *in the act of attending* exists. The crucial difference seems to consist in the integration of a representation of the *selection process for the object component*. In focal attention we experience ourselves as deliberately selecting a certain part of reality, that is, of our transparent phenomenal model of reality, and then focusing on that part. For instance, you could now focus your attention first on the blackness of the letters on the paper in front of you, then on the slight sensation of pressure in your fingertips. A representation of the final stages of the selection process is integrated into the self-model and thereby, on the level of phenomenal experience, it becomes our *own* selection. You are initiating the shift from the blackness of the letters to the pressure in your fingers *yourself*. In high-level attention, an automatic attribution of causal agency immediately goes along with this selection process. However, this process itself is a *subpersonal* process. It is a selfless, subjectless, and homunculus-free process of dynamical self-organization in the brain.

A similar principle seems to hold when we turn into conscious thinking subjects. There are processes, for example, in daydreaming or in freely associating cognitive contents in a subjectively effortless manner, in which opaque content is automatically made our *own* by being integrated into the PSM, while we do not experience this content as deliberately selected and enhanced. Dreaming away in a boring lecture, we experience the effortless flow of thoughts and mental images as being an autonomously unfolding representational activity, as belonging to ourselves, but the agency component is missing in these types of states. Cognitive agency, on the level of conscious experience, results when a process of *selecting cognitive contents for further processing* is represented and integrated into the PSM. Choosing the right words, as it were, thinking thoughts in a logical manner, implementing logical relations of implication into mental relations of temporal succession, and so on are accompanied by the quality of agency, and certainly not experienced as effortless mental activity. Thinking clearly is hard. In short, there is spontaneous cognitive behavior and there is cognitive agency, with the distinguishing phenomenological characteristics being a globally available representation of the selection process and a certain sense of effort.

However, most people would typically associate the question of agency with overt motor behavior and the control of external actions. Conscious human beings are "mobile points of view" (Brinck and Gärdenfors 1999, p. 101). We are not only modeling object-object relations in conscious perception, but we *actively* create new subject-object relations, not only by functionally interacting with our environment but also by restructuring our phenomenal model of reality accordingly. Let us therefore now turn to the question of how the conscious experience of being an *acting* subject can be analyzed in terms of the current theoretical model. As a flood of neuropsychological data show (for a selection of case studies, see chapter 7), the phenomenal property of agency is determined by subpersonal properties on the neurobiological level of description. Phenomenal agency locally supervenes on brain properties: we can lose the ability to experience ourselves as agents as a direct consequence of narrowly circumscribed neurobiological deficits. Attentional agency is something we lose every night, during phases of REM-sleep dreaming, and *cognitive agency*, as well as the sense of motor agency, can get lost in psychiatric disorders like schizophrenia. Conversely, a fact that many antinaturalist philosophers stubbornly try to ignore, phenomenal volition is something that can be *hallucinated* as well (see Wegner and Wheatley 1999 and section 7.2.3). Sobering as these and many other empirical data certainly are, they encourage an attempt to analyze the relevant phenomenal properties on the representationalist and functionalist levels of description more clearly.

What is the object component in the phenomenal experience of being an agent? A number of different phenomenological aspects seem to be involved. First, an allocentric goal simulation must exist. As Joëlle Proust has pointed out, the final stage, the goal event related to an action, includes the object with regard to which one acts, as well as the final state of the organism in relation to this object (Proust 2000). From an empirical point of view, phenomenal simulations of goal-achieving states, "goal representations," are typically described as allocentric; they are not localized in an egocentric frame of reference (Gallese 2000). Obviously, multiple simulations of possible action goals can be active in a given system. There will also be multiple motor trajectories, for example, in a simple grasping movement, which would all achieve the same final stage. Therefore, multiple and parallel action simulations may also be simultaneously active in a system preceding a concrete action. The concrete experience of agency, however, will only result if two further representational states are activated. The first will consist in a representation of the selection process itself, directed at one of the possible actions leading to the goal, all of which are currently being mentally simulated. Please note that it is *not* a necessary condition for all of these targets of the selection process to be conscious themselves. The second component will be of a more proprioceptive and kinesthetic kind, being constituted by *feedback* informing the system about the progress of its own ongoing motor behavior. Two kinds of system-related information must be bound into the self-model: information about an ongoing selection process and information about ensuing changes in body state. Therefore, the bodily self-model, as well as what we called the cognitive subject in the preceding section, will be involved in generating the phenomenal experience of full-blown agency.

There are basically two kinds of phenomenal content we have to understand in order to describe what the conscious experience of being an acting subject is on the representational level of analysis. *Phenomenal volition* is the conscious representation of a selection process. *Agency* is an experience involving the body, and motor content in particular. It is what Proust called "sensorimotor awareness," the form of awareness that identifies an action through its dynamics, that is, via the spatial and temporal properties of the bodily movement involved in the action (Proust 2000). A full-blown neurophenomenological analysis of agency would doubtlessly have to be more complex, introducing further conceptual distinctions. However, for our present purposes let us attempt to describe the conscious correlates of a typical action, using only the conceptual resources now at hand. Phenomenal volition, the first step, consists in activating a rather abstract goal representation, in an allocentric frame of reference. Please note that this process in itself does not have to be conscious and that its object component—as empirical data show—is likely to be self-other neutral. However, the abstract, nonegocentric representation of the action goal may be precisely what we use in individuating actions by their *intentional* content. This would open the teleofunctionalist level of analysis, categorizing actions according to their adaptive value and the function they play for a system (in Proust's terminology this would be "goal awareness"). Phenomenologically, however, this may simply be described as the content of an experienced motive or desire. The second step would then consist in making this potential motive or desire *my own*. It consists in integrating the already active goal representation into the current self-model. Whereas the first step could be analyzed as a subject-object relation, the second step could more aptly be described as the *embodiment* of a goal. In the first step, the object component present in the relation is an action goal, not yet existing in an egocentric frame of reference. The subject component is formed by the content of the currently active self-model, the phenomenal self. It generates the experience of *wanting* a certain goal, of standing in a "practical intentionality relation" (see next section) toward the possible outcome of an action. The second step consists in fully integrating the currently active goal representation into a centered model of reality. It is important to note that an extended planning stage can mediate the transition from step 1 to step 2: After a goal has been identified, it may be important to run forward models of possible bodily action—intended self-simulations—in order to compare them and arrive at the most efficient way to realize the goal, that is, make the opaque representation of a *possible* state of the world a component of the centered, transparent model of reality—of *my own world*. In other words, agency consists in the attempt to make a possible self-state an irrevocable part of *your reality*.

Not all mental simulata are sensory structures. Human beings generate motor simulations as well, and it is important to keep our epistemological principle in mind, according to which every motor representation also is a motor *simulation*. Due to the time lags involved, what is accessible to the process of conscious experience, even during concretely realized, ongoing actions, is always a *possible* state of the body, the best current hypothesis about its dynamics and kinematics. Phenomenologically, there is a sudden shift from phenomenal motor self-simulation to phenomenal motor *self-representation* as soon as one of the currently active forward models tested by the system is selected and embodied. Something that was opaque now becomes transparent. Thought becomes reality. Functionally, an embodied motor simulation is one that is currently causally coupled to the effectors. As we have already seen, there are cases in which an *involuntary* embodiment of spontaneously induced or externally driven motor simulations takes place, for example, in REM-sleep behavioral disorder or in echopraxia. The phenomenal property of agency, therefore, is exemplified at precisely the moment when an internal motor simulation, the representation of a possible behavior, "becomes real." In standard situations it "becomes real" because a specific action simulation leading to the previously activated representation of the goal state is selected, then coupled to the effector system, and immediately leads to proprioceptive and kinesthetic feedback confirming that the action is *actually* being carried out *right now*. As we will see in section 7.2.2, there are identity disorders in which phenomenal volition cannot be realized anymore, because the system is not able to make a goal its own, to integrate a goal representation into its current self-model (a situation in which the most parsimonious explanation for the system itself will be that behavior is driven by someone else's goals), and where agency cannot be realized because the process monitoring proprioceptive feedback is disturbed, thereby making the phenomenal embodiment of an intended action impossible. It is also important to note that the experience of volition, as well as the experience of agency, can be *hallucinated*. As we will see in section 7.2.3.3 the proper setting of perceptual parameters in a social and perceptual environment can lead a person to experience passive body movements as willed actions.

When considering the special level of content realized by the PSM of a voluntary agent, it becomes obvious how the perspectivalness of phenomenal space not only is a property of sensory consciousness and of perception but a property of *behavioral* space as well. The first-person perspective structuring this space possesses passive, receptive aspects as well as active, productive characteristics. The concept of a behavioral space doubtlessly has been neglected too much in the past. For instance, it can be shown that important parts of the monkey motor cortex do not code individual muscles or joints, but coordinates of workspace (Cruse, Dean, and Ritter 1998, p. 106). In action, the functional levels of the self-model are integrated into the currently active model of reality. What is common to all sensory modalities is the possession of a common spatial element: they are integrated into an internal *simulation of behavioral space* (Grush 1998, p. 188). Behavioral space may be interestingly conceived of as a "supra-empirical neurocognitive resource" (Grush, unpublished manuscript). The egocentric space, in which beings like ourselves operate, may be the representation of a highly specific manifold, a manifold in which sensory perceptions and motor simulations have been coordinated in a coherent and adequate way by generating systematic relations between them. The internally simulated behavioral space of a system could then be conceived of as being generated from continuities between stabilized manifolds, for instance, of tactile and visual space (Grush 2000, p. 66*ff*.). It is therefore important to understand that the levels of content in the PSM referring to perception and action are not *separate* levels. A PSM—just like the simulated space in which it is embedded—is a supramodal, virtual entity. The functional role of the self-model as the center of representational space results precisely from this integration of sensory and motor states: we are simultaneously perceiving *and* acting subjects. In establishing a stable region of continuity between motor and sensory manifolds, we generate an internal space, which is now an *egocentric* space. The conscious self is that partition of this space in which current processing going on in the relevant region of continuity is made globally available for attention, cognition, and selective motor control.

A further important point flows from applying the concept of cognitive subjectivity to that of agency. Once a transparent self-model of being a volitional subject and a bodily agent is in place, new information becomes globally available. In particular, this new information becomes *cognitively* available. The information that the system is capable of activating abstract goal-representations,[22] of simulating possible actions to achieve the goal states represented by them, and finally of *selecting* and embodying a specific motor simulation is now itself available for further cognitive processing. The system, therefore, is able to form a concept of itself *as an agent.* This step of generating higher-order, self-representational content, however, is an obvious necessity for the development of a theory of mind. The phenomenal self is not a loose bundle of volitional and cognitive aspects; it is characterized by a complete *integration* of both types of representational content.

Consciously experiencing oneself as a volitional subject, as an agent that is also able to *ascribe* this very property to itself on a conceptual level, is the central prerequisite of the development of moral subjectivity. As noted earlier, in the early philosophy of consciousness, *conscientia* was taken to necessarily involve moral conscience. It is this level of phenomenal self-consciousness that opens the ethical dimension, as it were. It forces us to move upward to the personal level of description. Moral agents certainly are *persons.*

For beings that cannot only consciously experience themselves as agents but are also able to represent the actions of others *as* actions, a new class of problems to be solved emerges: Such creatures continuously have to differentiate between those actions which are their own, and those which are actions of others. As action is one of the main channels used for communication between individuals; reliably determining the agent of an action contributes to differentiating the self from others and is a central factor in generating stronger versions of self-consciousness (Jeannerod 1999; Proust 2000). For the fast and flexible control of social interactions, attributions of agency—the content of what Proust called "agency judgments"—have to be made globally available. It is on this level of representational content that the human self-model can finally be used as a tool for generating complex and coherent social behavior. The conscious experience of agency in self and others may have been the decisive step in the transition from biological to cultural evolution.

---

22. Why do we need something like goal representations in the first place? Why would it be adaptive to *presuppose* the existence of entities of this type, in ourselves as well as in other agents? An acting system possessing intentional states does not react to identical situations with physically identical movements, but always generates the same *effects.* A system with intentional states is an *intelligent* system. The cause of its intelligent behavior invariably is an internal one, but we cannot explain obviously maladaptive behavior in terms of dispositions alone. We need an analysis in terms of representation and *mis*representation. However, increasing behavioral complexity forces us to assume ever-new representational states and ever-new laws governing them. We can minimize the number of these laws by using *action goals* as conceptual tools in classifying such states. This may be true on the level of theoretical analysis as well as for biological systems operating under the pressure of evolutionary mechanisms. Ascribing *goals* to yourself and others may be an extremely elegant and parsimonious way of representing a domain characterized by almost intractable causal complexity. For an interesting analytical discussion, see Beckermann 1996.

6.5 Perspectivalness: The Phenomenal Model of the Intentionality Relation

At the beginning of this chapter I introduced an important theoretical entity, the "phenomenal self-model." My claim was that this entity is something that actually *exists*, not only as a distinct *theoretical* entity but something that will be *empirically* discovered in the future—for instance, as a specific stage of the global neural dynamics in the human brain, characterized by a discrete and unitary functional role. I now introduce a second theoretical entity, which also possesses central importance in understanding the representational deep structure of the phenomenal first-person perspective. It is the concept of "the phenomenal model of the intentionality relation," which we have encountered a number of times in the preceding three sections. The concept of a PMIR will, finally, give us a more precise understanding of *constraint 6*, the perspectivalness constraint for conscious processing which was developed in section 3.2.6. Together with the idea of a transparent global model of the world, as activated within a window of presence, this third major theoretical entity will, at the end of this chapter, allow us to offer a more informative version of the minimal concept of *subjective* consciousness. It will help us to develop a very first representationalist and functionalist analysis of *perspectival* experience, of the fact that consciousness is, under standard conditions, always tied to an individual first-person perspective.

What is the phenomenal model of the intentionality relation? It is a conscious mental model, and its content is an ongoing, episodic *subject-object relation*. Here are some examples, in terms of typical phenomenological descriptions of the class of phenomenal states at issue: "I am someone, who is currently visually attending to the color of the book in my hands"; "I am someone currently grasping the content of the sentence I am reading"; "I am someone currently hearing the sound of the refrigerator behind me"; "I am someone now deciding to get up and get some more juice." The first defining characteristic of phenomenal models of the intentionality relation is that they depict a certain *relationship* as currently holding between the system, as transparently represented to itself, and an object component. This class of phenomenal mental models is particularly rich, because, first, the number of possible object components is almost infinitely large. Let us look at our examples from a third-person, representationalist stance and see how the object component can vary.

In the first situation the object component is formed by a perceptual object, given through the visual and tactile modalities. The representational content could be described as [A self in the act of attending to a book in its hands]. An important characteristic, demonstrated by the second example, is that the object component can also be formed by an *opaque* kind of conscious content, as in cases of cognitive self-modeling. In the second example the representational content could be described as [A self in the act of understanding the semantic content of the sentence it is currently reading]. Looking at this second example, we can point out the third defining characteristic for the class of phenomenal mental models of the intentionality relation: The subject component, formed by the currently active self-model, is *always* transparent, although it *may* possess additional opaque partitions. What the second example also shows is how different phenomenal mental models of the intentionality relation make different *types* of relationships between subject and object globally available, for example, attending, thinking, willing, and so on. Of course, all this is not propositional attitude psychology, as the underlying theory of mental representation is of a much more empirically plausible kind, following connectionist and dynamicist background assumptions. However, it may be helpful to note that just as in the conceptual analysis of propositional attitudes we have something like a *content specificator* (the object component), a *person specificator* (the transparent model of the system as a whole), and an *attitude specificator* (the kind of relation between subject and object as represented on the level of conscious experience). This will become more evident when we consider our next two examples.

In low-level attention, the phenomenally modeled self-object relation is suddenly popping up, as it were, without the accompanying phenomenal quality of agency. Compare our third example: [A self in the act of suddenly noticing the sound of the refrigerator behind him]. Here we have a transparent self-model, a transparent object-model, and the relationship between them appears as entirely "unconstructed," as immediately given, as effortlessly and naturally appearing in the conscious model of the world, as it were. Of course, there is a complex chain of unconscious neural events preceding the sudden activation of this model. The type of relationship consciously experienced is not [deliberately attending], as in the book case, but [finding yourself forced to automatically attend]. What is missing is attentional agency, a transparent representation of the process of selecting the object component for attention, as integrated into the self-model. However, there is not only a cognitive and an attentional first-person perspective but also a *volitional first-person perspective*. Interestingly, the object component can now also be constituted by phenomenal simulata, for example, by the conscious representation of possible actions. From a third-person, representationalist point of view, the fourth and last example can be analyzed as [A self in the act of selecting a certain possible action, e.g., walking over to the refrigerator and getting another drink]. What typically follows the activation of this kind of representational content is the real *embodiment* of the action, the running of a complex motor self-simulation, which is now coupled to the effectors. The event before consisted in phenomenally simulating a number of possible actions and then, as it were, "reaching out" for one of them, making one of them *your own*. This is the moment of integrating the currently active, transparent self-model with an opaque action simulation, or an allocentric, as yet self-other neutral goal representation, thereby generating a phenomenal model of the *practical* intentionality relation.[23] A conscious, volitional first-person perspective emerges if a phenomenal model of the system as a whole as standing in relation to a potential *volitional* object component is activated. In passively desiring a certain object, for example, the juice to be found in the refrigerator, we have a nonvolitional kind of relationship being consciously modeled, and the object component is not formed by a possible action—as in the genuinely volitional perspective—but only by a possible action *goal*. In short, phenomenal models of the intentionality relation consist of a transparent subject component and varying object components, which can be transparent as well as opaque, transiently being integrated into an overarching, comprehensive representation of the system as standing in a specific relation to a certain part of the world. The overall picture that emerges is that of the human self-model continuously integrating the mechanisms of attentional, cognitive, and volitional availability against a stable background formed by the transparent representation of the bodily self.

Please note how the PMIR has a phenomenally experienced *direction*: PMIRs are like arrows pointing from self-model to object component. In being phenomenal representations of an asymmetrical two-place relation, they resemble the asymmetrical relationship between representata and representanda as *conceptually* introduced in chapter 2. As soon as one has understood the arrow-like nature of the PMIR, two special cases can be much more clearly described. First, the arrow cannot only point outward, but also *downward* (phenomenologically speaking: *inward*). In cases where the object component is formed by the PSM itself (as in attending to or consciously thinking about oneself) the PMIR *internally* models a system-system relationship instead of a system-object relationship. Second, in consciously experienced *social* cognition the object component can be either formed by a phenomenal model of another agent or an arrow *in* the other agent's head (as in observing another human being observing another human being). It is important to always remember that we are only speaking about phenomenal content when discussing a particular PMIR. The experiential content locally supervenes on brain properties. A brain in a vat, kept alive by machine intelligence long after the last forms of biological or conscious intelligence have vanished from the universe, could enjoy reflexive self-consciousness just as well as vivid forms of phenomenal intersubjectivity.

23. In classical conceptions of intentionality there are two basic types of intentionality: *theoretical* and *practical* intentionality. Theoretical intentionality is aimed at gaining knowledge about the world. In terms of the propositional attitude framework, theoretical intentionality is realized by cognitive attitudes, possessing content specificators exhibiting truth values—as in thinking, believing, and so on. Practical intentionality, however, is realized by the class of volitive attitudes, for example, in wishing, desiring, and so on. In these cases the content specificator only possesses *fulfillment conditions* and it points to a certain action goal, in terms of a changed state of affairs in the world. A consciously perceived volitional first-person perspective emerges precisely if the second class of object components and relations is phenomenally modeled in accordance with the current background assumptions.

In other words, the philosophical step just taken consists in *phenomenalizing intentionality*. Phenomenalizing intentionality, I would submit, may be a necessary detour, an indispensable first step in the project of *naturalizing* intentionality *tout court*. Meaning and the conscious experience of meaningfulness may have to be separated. Generally speaking, mental representations possess two kinds of content: phenomenal content and intentional content. Phenomenal content supervenes locally. Intentional content, in many cases, is determined by external and nonlocal factors. As noted above, intentionality as such is not an epistemic target within the scope of this book. However, it is important to note how intentionality (on a prerational level, probably starting with the motor system and early levels of attentional processing) is *itself* depicted on the level of phenomenal content. And it is precisely this kind of conscious content that has guided theoreticians for centuries in developing their own, now classic theories of intentionality. Due to the principle of local supervenience it has today become highly plausible that *this* aspect of intentionality can be naturalized. The *phenomenal* experience of being an intentional agent, of being a perceiving, attending, and cognizing subject, can be naturalized. Of course, this in no way precludes the possibility that intentional content *as such* can never, and maybe even for principled reasons, be naturalized. But getting the first obstacle out of the way may greatly help in gaining fresh access to intentionality *as such*, because it frees us from the burden of false intuitions generated by our own transparent model of reality and it helps us to set aside the issue of how we come to consciously *experience* our mental states as meaningful and directed toward an object component. We can separate the issue of consciously experienced intentionality from the more general problem of how something like representational content could evolve in the minds of human beings and other animals *at all*. If we succeed in anchoring our concept of the PMIR on the functional and neurobiological levels of description, then the notion could even survive a dynamicist revolution. If some day it turns out that, strictly speaking, something like mental content does not even exist (because it *never* existed in the first place), if what is now the most important level of analysis—the "representational stance"—should eventually be abandoned by a science of the mind advanced beyond anything imaginable today, then we would still possess building blooks for a theory about how it was possible, and necessary, for beings like ourselves to consciously experience themselves as possessing "contentful" intentional states as described by classical theories of mind.

It is interesting to note how the genuinely philosophical concept of a conscious model of the intentionality relationship currently surfaces at a number of places in the cognitive neurosciences. Jean Delacour, in an excellent review of current ideas about possible neural correlates of conscious experience, explicitly introduces the notion of an "intentionality-modeling structure" (Delacour 1997, p. 138). LaBerge (D. LeBerge 1997, pp. 150, 172*ff*.) points out how important an understanding of the self-representational component present in attentional processing will have to be for a full-blown theory of conscious attention. Craik and colleagues point out how episodic memory, of course, is a process of *recon-*structing what was here termed a PMIR, because one necessary constituent of memory retrieval is not simply the simulation of a past event, but an association of this simulation with a *self-*representation (Craik, Moroz, Moscovitch, Stuss, Winocur, Tulving, and Kapur 1999, p. 26). This helps to pin down the first candidates for some of the necessary neural correlates, for example, in the right frontal lobe. Building an autobiographical memory is a process of self-related encoding, and conscious, episodic memory retrieval is a process necessarily involving the self-model, because reactivating a PMIR inevitably means reactivating a PSM. Most notable, of course, is Antonio Damasio's conception of a "juxtaposition" of self and object (see Damasio and Damasio 1996a, p. 172; 1996b, p. 24 *ff.*) and the general framework of a fully embodied "self in the act of knowing" (Damasio 1994, 1999). In philosophy of mind, on the other hand, it is hard to find the idea of Brentano's ([1874] 1973) concept of intentionality as *itself forming the content of an internal, transparent representation* (but see Loar 2003).

After having looked at some first defining characteristics for our working concept of the PMIR on the phenomenological and representational level, let me again point out how, like every form of phenomenal content, this class of phenomenal states supervenes on internal and contemporaneous functional properties of the human brain. Neither the object component nor the physical body carrying the human brain has to exist, in principle, to phenomenally experience yourself as being related to certain external or virtual objects. Strictly speaking, *any* physical structure functionally isomorphic to the minimally sufficient neural correlate of the overall reality-model structured by the PMIR will realize first-person phenomenology. A brain in a vat, of course, could—if approximately stimulated—activate the conscious experience of being a self in attending to the color of the book in its hands, in currently understanding the semantic contents of the sentences being read, or in selecting a particular, phenomenally simulated action like walking to the refrigerator. Even the proprioceptive and kinesthetic feedback, which would have to result from an "embodiment" of a specific chosen pattern of bodily action, could, in principle, be brought about by the minimally sufficient neural correlate for the somatosensory, phenomenal content. In fact, candidates for contributing elements to the neural correlate of the PMIR are already under discussion (e.g., the cingulate gyrus, certain thalamic nuclei, and the superior colliculi; cf. Damasio 1999, p. 260*ff.*) What the discovery of the correlates of the PMIR could never help us decide is the question of how the brain in a vat could ever *know* that it is in this situation—or how *you* could know that you are now *not* this brain.

Note that the theory is mute about the question whether anything like "real" intentionality exists. Of course, a highly interesting speculation is that philosophical models of the intentionality of the mental have ultimately resulted from a naive-realistic interpretation of the process of visual attention, of the phenomenal self directing its gaze at a visual object, thereby making it more salient, and simply elevating this interpretation to the level of epistemology. The concept of the intentionality of the mental may simply be a mistaken attempt to theoretically model epistemic relations in accordance with the consciously experienced model of the intentionality relation. Pursuing this point is outside the scope of this book. But let me at least briefly point to two interesting issues of considerable philosophical interest.

As Gerhard Roth (personal communication, 1998) has pointed out, the phenomenal self is a virtual agent, perceiving and acting on virtual objects in a virtual world. This agent does not know that she possesses a visual cortex, and she does not know what electromagnetic radiation is: she just sees "with her own eyes," by, as it were, effortlessly directing her visual attention. Of course, the phenomenal model of how knowledge enters the system is a greatly simplified model, a kind of shorthand glossing over the myriad intricate details of information processing actually going on on the neural level. The virtual agent does not know that it possesses a motor system which, for instance, needs an internal emulator for fast, goal-driven reaching movements: it just acts "with its own hands." It does not know what a sensorimotor loop is: it just effortlessly enjoys what researchers in the field of virtual reality design call "full immersion"—what for them is still a distant goal. This global effect is achieved by continuously activating dynamic and transparent representations of a subject-object relation, which episodically integrates the self-model and those perceptual, cognitive or volitional objects, which cause the changes in its content, by telling an internal story about how these changes came about. This story does not have to be the true story. It may well be a greatly simplified confabulation, which has proved to be functionally adequate. It is a high-level feature of what I have called the internal "user surface" the system has created for itself. It is interesting to note that if the phenomenal model of, for example, one's own perceptual states, contains a transparent representation of their causal history (e.g., as seeing "through" the eyes), then convolved global states will result which can only truthfully be described by the system itself as, for example, "I myself (the content of a transparent self-model) am now seeing this object (the content of a transparent object-model), I am seeing it *now* (the perceptual content is integrated into a virtual window of presence), and I am seeing it *with my own eyes* (the simple story about immediate sensory perception, which sufficed for the brain's evolutionary purpose)."

Of particular interest is the fact that the brain models the relationship between subject and object as an asymmetrical relationship. It is the consciously experienced "arrow of intentionality," paradigmatically experienced in having the feeling of "projecting" visual attention outward, as it were, or in attentionally "tracking" objects in the environment. *Intendere arcum*, to bend the bow of the mind and point the arrow of knowledge toward parts of the world, is an intuitively plausible and popular philosophical metaphor, in particular in combination with the idea of "direct," magical intentionality. We can now understand why such an idea strikes beings like us as intuitively plausible: it is *phenomenally* possible, because there is a directly corresponding structural element in our conscious model of reality. Many theoretical models of the representational relationship are implicitly oriented at the phenomenal experience of visual attention, of the *directedness* inherent in the phenomenal model of the intentionality relation. Frequently, the theoretical model we design about ourselves as cognitive agents is one of organisms, which, ad libitum direct the beam of their "epistemic flashlight" at parts of the world or their own internal lives, as beings, which generate the representational relation *as subjects of experience*. This can lead to the kind of fallacy, which Daniel Dennett has described as "Cartesian materialism."[24] A related hypothesis is that philosophical theorizing about the intentionality relation has generally been influenced by that aspect of our phenomenal model of reality that is generated by our strongest sensory modality: If the process of mental representation in general is modeled in accordance with our dominant sensory modality (namely, vision), we will automatically generate *distal objects*, just as we do in our transparent, visual model of reality. If the object component of a PMIR is of an opaque nature, as in genuinely cognitive contents or in goal representation, a philosophical interpretation of these mental contents as *nonphysical*, "intentionally inexistent" objects becomes inevitable.

Returning to the project of developing an empirically plausible conception, we have to ask: Are there situations which can exclusively be explained by using the first theoretical entity, the PSM, without bringing into play the second theoretical entity, the PMIR? Obviously the existence of the PMIR is what generates full-blown consciousness, and it is precisely this feature of the deep representational structure of our conscious model of reality which appears as of highest relevance to most of us. Full-blown conscious experience is more than the existence of a conscious self, and it is much more than the mere presence of a world. It results form the dynamic interplay between this self and the world, in a lived, embodied present.

Bilateral anterior damage to the cingulate gyrus and bilateral medial parietal damage lead to a situation which can be described by, first, the absence of the PMIR, while, second,

---

24. Cf. Dennett 1991, p. 333. As Dennett has pointed out, many of the different forms of Cartesian materialism, the assumption of a final inner stage, can also be generated in the context of representationalist theories of mind by mistakenly transporting what he called the "intentional stance" (Dennett 1987a) into the system; cf. Dennett 1991, p. 458. The model proposed here, of course, does not make this mistake; it is much more closely related to the idea of a "second-order intentional system," a system that applies the intentional stance to itself—but in a phenomenally transparent manner. Thomas Nagel has pointed out that Dennett's own strategy of "heterophenomenology" implicitly has to rely on the first-person perspective if it does not want to fall back into a trivial version of behaviorism. Cf. Nagel 1991.

a coherent conscious model of the world centered by a phenomenal self is retained. Antonio Damasio has introduced a useful conceptual distinction, which is simple and straightforward: Such patients exhibit wakefulness, but not what he calls "core consciousness." Core consciousness is the minimal form of phenomenal experience constituted by what he calls a "second-order mapping" and what *is* the basic phenomenal model of the intentionality relation in terms of the representationalist analysis proposed by the current theory. Let us look at how Damasio describes such cases:

> Just as is the case with patients with bilateral cingulate damage, patients with bilateral medial parietal damage are awake in the usual sense of the term: their eyes can be open, and their muscles have proper tone; they can sit or even walk with assistance; but they will not look at you or at any object *with any semblance of intention* [emphasis added]; and their eyes may stare vacantly or orient toward objects with no discernible motive. These patients cannot help themselves. They volunteer nothing about their situation and they fail to respond to virtually all the examiners' requests. Attempts to engage them in conversation are rarely successful, the results being erratic at best. We can coax them into looking briefly at an object, but the request will not engender anything else in terms of productive reaction. These patients react no differently to friends and family than they do to physicians and nurses. The notion of zombie-like behavior could perfectly well have come from the description of these patients, although it did not. (Damasio 1999, p. 263)

This well-documented condition is akinetic mutism, the absence of volition following ventromedial damage or the bilateral anterior lesions of the cingulate just mentioned. A number of diverging etiologies exist. It is a silent immobility, the only behavioral manifestation being gaze following relative to the examiner's movements and, in some cases, monosyllabic speech (for three further cases studies, plus a brief review of the literature, see Ure, Faccio, Videla, Caccuri, Giudice, Ollari and Diez 1998). Phenomenal volition can deviate in two directions. There is hypervolitionalism as, for instance, in obsessive-compulsive disorder. There are also hypovolitional states, in which the ability to generate the experience of conscious will is greatly diminished. Akinetic mutism is a state of wakefulness, combined with the absence of speech, emotional expression, and movement. Obviously, for such patients there is an integrated functional self-model, because they are able to briefly track objects, pull a bedcover, or, if forced, say their own name (for a brief case study, see Damasio 1999, p. 101*ff.*). Obviously, these patients still have an integrated self-representation, making self-related information globally available for the control of action or guided attention. However, there is no *volitional subject* that could exert control. As these examples show, the use of globally available system-related information can be forced or triggered from the outside to a limited degree, but what is missing is an *autonomous* phenomenal representation of a self in relation to possible action goals. The integration of the subject component with what has earlier been described as volitional objects—abstract, allocentric goal representations or mental simulations of possible, concrete actions in an egocentric frame of reference—is missing. The model of reality of such patients is still functionally centered; they are awake and embodied selves, but what they do not possess is precisely a phenomenal first-person perspective. They certainly have phenomenal experience, but no conscious representation of the arrow of intentionality. Their phenomenal states do not satisfy *constraint 6*. They are phenomenally embodied beings, but their conscious reality is not an *enacted*, *lived* reality in the full sense of the term. They are not *directed*. What the outside observer experiences as a vacuous stare or emotional neutrality is the complete absence of any willed action or communicative intention, the absence of a globally available model of subject-object relations (and, as can be seen in lacking the desire to talk, of subject-*subject* relations as well). Functionally centered, but phenomenologically aperspectival and self-including models of reality, therefore, are not only conceptual possibilities but, in some tragic cases, actually occurring representational configurations. They very clearly demonstrate what it means to say that the phenomenal first-person perspective is the decisive factor in turning a mere biological organism into an agent, into a willing subject.

Epileptic absence automatisms are another class of states in which complex behavior may result, in which low-level attention and wakefulness are preserved, while the whole episode as such will not be integrated into autobiographical memory. In addition, an astonishingly high degree of intellectual complexity can be found in some cases of psychomotor automatisms.[25] The brief explosions of complex motor behavior sometimes following an absence seizure in certain cases of epilepsy can be conceived of as complex motor artifacts, which, however, have not been initiated by a system operating under a model of itself as a conscious volitional subject. A complex bodily self-model must certainly be in place, because otherwise there would be no way of understanding the overall coherence

25. Brian Cooney (1979, p. 28*ff.*) presents the case study of Dr. *Z* originally reported by Hughlings Jackson (Taylor 1958, p. 405*f.*). Dr. *Z* correctly diagnosed a patient with lung problems in a completely unconscious state following a seizure, which began just as he started examining the patient: "I remember taking out my stethoscope and turning away a little to avoid conversation. The next thing I recollect is that I was sitting at a writing table in the same room, speaking to another person, and as my consciousness became more complete, recollected my patient, but he was not in the room. I had . . . an opportunity an hour later of seeing him in bed, with the notice of a diagnosis I had made of 'pneumonia of the left base.'" Cooney points out how psychomotor automatisms typically go along with a loss of flexibility, an "inability to re-evaluate or to choose a substantially different course of action. . . . ," that is, the inability to select another action goal as the object of the PMIR. As the author puts it, "It is as if the goal of the project intended before the seizure now is the only possible motive for the automaton" (ibid.,). According to this view, such patients do not lack intellectual capacities as such, but the ability to "divert intact intellectual functions of the neocortex toward any object other than the one chosen when the limbic system was last functional" (p. 29). Case studies of this type are important because they demonstrate, first, how a phenomenally experienced first-person perspective is not necessary for complex and successful cognitive processing, and, second, how it *is* necessary to functionally elevate us from the status of deterministic automatons to that of systems achieving a much higher degree of flexibility by increasing their selectivity for internal, self-generated goal representations. See also Crick and Koch 2000 for a related discussion.

of the motor behavior ensuing and the successful sensorimotor integration achieved by those patients, if only for a brief period. Low-level attentional processes can be externally triggered during such episodes, but focal attention (the attentional subject described in section 6.4.3) is fully absent. What is entirely absent in epileptic absence automatisms, as well as in akinetic mutism, is long-term future planning and the generation of elaborate behavioral strategies. These observations are valuable, because they demonstrate what a phenomenal first-person perspective is probably *good* for.

6.5.1 Global Availability of Transient Subject-Object Relations

Drawing on a number of the conceptual constraints introduced earlier, we can now formulate what, from a teleofunctionalist perspective, the advantage of possessing a phenomenal first-person perspective actually consists of. Phenomenal mental models are instruments used to make a certain subset of information currently active in the system globally available for the control of action, for focal attention, and for cognitive processing. A phenomenal model of subject-object relations makes an enormous amount of new information available *for* the system: all information related to the fact that it is currently perturbed by perceptual objects, that certain cognitive states are currently occurring in itself (see section 6.4.4), for example, that certain abstract goal representations are currently active, that there are a number of concrete self-simulations connecting the current system state with the state the system *would* have if this goal state would be realized; and allowing for selective behavior and the information that it is a system capable of manipulating its own sensory input, for example, by turning its head and directing its gaze to a specific visual object. A first-person perspective allows a system to conceive of itself as being part of an independent objective order, while at the same time being anchored in it and able to act *on* it as a subject (see, e.g., Grush 2000). In the earlier sections on the attentional, cognitive, and volitional subject, I described how this newly available information leads to dramatic changes in the behavior available to the system.

Let me now mention one particular application of this representational principle, which, although lying outside of the scope of this book, is of utmost relevance. Once a system is capable of representing transient subject-object relations in a globally available manner, it becomes possible for the object component in the underlying representational structure to be formed by the *intentions of other beings*. A phenomenal first-person perspective allows for the mental representation of a phenomenal *second-person* perspective. The PMIR is what builds the bridge to the social dimension. Once a full-blown subjective perspective has been established, *inter*subjectivity can follow. If a functional mechanism for discovering and phenomenally representing the unobservable goal states of conspecifics is in place, the observed behavior of *other* systems in the organism's environment can lead to an activation of a goal representation, which in turn can be represented as belonging to someone *else*. As we have seen, it is empirically plausible that such a mechanism, possibly based on mirror neurons and the discovery of "motor equivalences," is actually in place in human beings. Therefore, representations of the intentions of external agents can now become the object component of the phenomenal model of the intentionality relation as well. If this happens on the level of conscious experience, a completely new and highly interesting form of information becomes globally available for the system: the information of actually *standing in certain relations to the goals of other conspecifics*. I would claim that it is precisely the conscious availability of this type of information which turned human beings from acting, attending, and thinking selves into social subjects. If the fact that you are constantly not only standing in perceptual and behavioral relation to your environment but that you are frequently realizing *subject-subject relationships* becomes globally available, it also becomes available for cognition. This, in turn, will allow those systems capable of concept formation to mentally model social relations from a third-person perspective. Such beings can mentally represent social relationships between other individuals depicted as intentional agents, even if they are not involved themselves. I will not pursue this point at length here, but it is obvious how this representational ability is of great relevance to social cognition and the pooling of cognitive resources.

Proceeding from representationalist and teleofunctionalist levels of description to the phenomenological changes inherent in the emergence of a full-blown phenomenal first-person perspective, it is easy to see how, for the first time, it allows a system to consciously experience itself as being not only a part of the world but of being fully immersed in it through a dense network of causal, perceptual, cognitive, attentional, and agentive relations. I have described these relations at length in the preceding sections and therefore conclude this chapter by highlighting only two phenomenological characteristics, those that seem to be of greatest relevance.

6.5.2 Phenomenal Presence of a Knowing Self

Let us subsume the notions of a conscious, attentional subject and of a conscious, cognitive subject under the unitary heading of a "knowing self." A knowing self by necessity emerges, because in all the different classes of phenomenal mental models of the intentionality relation, a major portion of the subject component is inevitably represented in a transparent manner. The introspectively accessible properties of even these kinds of higher-order self-modeling are exhausted by their content properties. Attention and cognition are always integrated into the transparent background of the bodily self-model, generating the pervasive structural feature described as the naive-realistic self-misunderstanding in section 6.2.6. We also have to do justice to the fact that the whole structure just described is not only integrated into a global model of the world but also into the window of presence described in section 3.2.2. We can now see how a specific, high-level form of phenomenal content will necessarily emerge, if all the constraints so far mentioned are satisfied. It is the content that allows a system to experience itself as *[being a knowing self, present in a world]*. As the phenomenal model of *theoretical* subject-object relations will necessarily be characterized by the constraints of globality and presence, we can now see how a global, convolved representational state will emerge which, due to its underlying transparency, can only be truthfully described by the system itself (if it possesses linguistic abilities) as, for example: ⟨I, *myself*, (= the content of the currently active transparent self-model) am present (= the *de nunc* character of all representational content activated within the virtual window of presence) in a *world* (= the transparent, global model of reality), and I am currently (= the *de nunc* character of the phenomenal model of the intentionality relation) perceiving or attending to or thinking about (= the transparent representation of the *type* of relation integrating subject and object in the currently active model of the intentionality relation) the book in my hands (= a particular example of one possible *object component*, as portrayed in the phenomenal model of the intentionality relation)⟩.

6.5.3   Phenomenal Presence of an Agent

A parallel analysis is possible for the phenomenological properties of *volitional* subjectivity and agency. Conscious volition is generated by integrating abstract goal representations or concrete self-simulations into the current model of the phenomenal intentionality relation as object components, in a process of decision or selection. However, let us differentiate a number of cases. If we contemplate a certain action goal, for example, when we ask ourselves whether we should get up and walk over to the refrigerator, we experience ourselves as cognitive subjects. This kind of phenomenally represented subject-object relationship can be analyzed in accordance with the model presented in the last section, the only difference being that the object component now is opaque. We know that we take a certain attitude toward a self-generated *representation* of a goal. A completely different situation ensues if we integrate a goal representation into the self-model, thereby making it a part of ourselves by *identifying* with it. Obviously, goal representations and goal hierarchies are important components of self-models that are not based on transient subject-object relations, but on enduring internal reorganizations of the self-model, of its emotional and motivational structure, and so on, and which can possibly last for a lifetime. A *volitional first-person* perspective—the phenomenal experience of practical intentionality—emerges if two conditions are satisfied. First, the object component must be constituted by a particular self-simulatum, by a mental simulation of a concrete behavioral pattern, for example, like getting up and walking toward the refrigerator. Second, the relationship depicted on the level of conscious experience is one of *currently selecting* this particular behavioral pattern, as simulated. Again, it is useful to speak about representational identification. The moment following volition, the moment at which concrete bodily behavior actually ensues, is the moment at which the already active motor simulation is *integrated* into the currently active bodily self-model, and thereby causally coupled to the rest of the motor system and the effectors. It is precisely the moment at which we *identify* with a particular action, transforming it from a possible into an actual pattern of behavior and thereby functionally, as well as phenomenologically, *embody* it. Embodiment leads to enacting. Interestingly, the moment of agency seems to be the moment when the phenomenal model of the intentionality relation *collapses*. We can now describe the experience of being a volitional subject and the experience of being an agent more precisely, using the simple tools already introduced (see also Metzinger 2004).

Phenomenal volition is a form of phenomenal content, which can be analyzed as *representational* content as follows: [I *myself* (= the currently active transparent model of the self) am currently (= the *de nunc* character of the overall phenomenal model of the intentionality relation as integrated into the virtual window of presence) present in a world (= the transparent, global model of reality currently active) and I am just about to select (= the type of relation depicted in the phenomenal model of the intentionality relation) a possible way to walk around the chairs toward the refrigerator (= the object-component, constituted by an *opaque* simulation of a possible motor pattern in an egocentric frame of reference)]. The experience of agency follows at the moment in which the internal "distance" created between phenomenal self-representation and phenomenal self-simulation in the previously mentioned structure collapses to zero: I *realize* a possible self by enacting it. As I experience myself walking around the chairs and toward the refrigerator, proprioceptive and kinesthetic feedback allows me to feel the degrees to which I have already *identified* with the sequence of bodily movements I have selected in the previous moment. Remember that transparent representations are precisely those representations the existence of whose content we cannot doubt. They are those we experience as real, whereas opaque representations are those we experience as thoughts, as imagination, or as being hallucinated. *Realizing* a simulated self means devising a strategy of making it the content of a transparent self-model, of a self that really exists—on the level of phenomenal experience. Ongoing agency, the conscious experience of sustained executive control, can therefore be representationally analyzed according to the following pattern: [I myself (the content of the transparent self-model) am currently (= the *de nunc* character of the phenomenal model of the intentionality relationship as integrated into the virtual window of presence) present in a world (= the transparent, global model of reality) and I am currently experiencing myself as carrying out (= continuously integrating into the transparent self-model) an action which I have previously imagined and selected (the opaque self-simulation forming the object component, which is now step by step assimilated into the *subject component*)]. Of course, there are all sorts of functional and representational complications, for example, if the proprioceptive and kinesthetic feedback integrated into the internal emulator of the body does not match the forward model still held active in working memory. In any case, it is interesting to see how agency conceived of as executive consciousness (*Vollzugsbewusstsein* in the sense of Karl Jaspers) can be analyzed as an ongoing representational dynamics *collapsing* a phenomenal model of the practical intentionality relationship into a new transparent self-model. Again, as the whole structure is embedded in what in section 3.2.2 was described as a virtual window of presence, the transparent, untranscendable experiential state for the system itself is one of being a full-blown volitional subject, currently being present in a world and acting in it.

Let us close this section by looking at an interesting special case, namely, the possibility of *subpersonal* goal directedness. It may serve as an introduction to the case studies following in chapter 7, while—from a different angle—vividly illustrating how the phenomenal self-model is the decisive tool for transforming subpersonal properties of a conscious system into personal-level features. A widespread philosophical assumption is that the ascription of goals and goal representations is the hallmark of *personal-level* analysis, because having goals and actions guided by explicit goal representations clearly seems to be a characteristic found on the whole-system level only. *Persons* have goals, but not brains, self-models, or other functional modules of the organism as a whole. Unfortunately, the philosophical intuition underlying this assumption is false on empirical grounds: In human beings explicit goal-directed behavior can appear on a modular level, and without the formation of a corresponding PMIR. One particularly salient example is the alien or anarchic hand syndrome.

Alien hand syndrome (first described by Goldstein 1908; Sweet 1941; the term introduced by Brion and Jedynak 1972; Goldberg, Mayer, and Toglia 1981; for an important new conceptual distinction, see Marchetti and Della Sala 1998) is characterized by a global experiential state in which the patient typically is well aware of complex, observable movements carried out by the nondominant hand, while at the same time experiencing no corresponding volitional acts. Subjectively (as well as functionally) the arm is "out of control," with a sense of intermanual conflict. For example, a patient may pick up a pencil and begin scribbling with the right hand, but react with dismay when her attention is directed to this fact. Then she will immediately withdraw the pencil, pull the right hand to her side with the left hand, and indicate that she had not *herself* initiated the original action (Goldberg et al. 1981, p. 684). In another case, the patient's left hand will grope for and grasp nearby objects, pick and pull at her clothes, and even grasp at her throat during sleep to the point that she will, while not denying bodily ownership, refer to her limb as an *autonomous entity* (case 1 in Banks, Short, Martinez, Latchaw, Ratcliff, and Boller 1989, p. 456). Not only is there no explicit goal representation associated with the conscious self-model, and no phenomenal sense of volitional ownership, but we even find an attribution of quasi-personhood in terms of agency and autonomy of the patient to one of her body parts. Such part-whole conflicts can also extend to the level of conscious *cognitive* activity, for instance, when in playing checkers, the patient's left hand (i.e., the body part not functionally appropriated under a volitional PMIR) makes a move he did not wish to make, after which he (i.e., the system as a whole operating under its PSM) corrects the move with his right hand, and the functional module then reacts, to the patient's frustration, by repeating the false move (case 2 in Banks et al. 1989, p. 457).

The central point is that many such arm movements clearly seem to be goal-directed actions, although no such goal representation is available either on the phenomenal level in general or on the level of conscious self-representation. The underlying goal representations are not phenomenally owned, and therefore are not *functionally appropriated*. Therefore, they may also be open to causal influences from the environment. Geschwind and colleagues offered a case report of a 68-year-old woman suffering from a stroke-caused transient alien hand syndrome, with the lesion being limited to the middle and posterior portions of the body of the corpus callosum:

On postoperative day 11, she was noted by nursing staff to have left-sided weakness and difficulty walking. According to her family, she had complained of loss of control of her left hand for the previous 3 days, as if the hand were performing on its own. She awoke several times with her left hand choking her, and while she was awake, her left hand would unbutton her gown, crush cups on her tray, and fight with the right hand while she was answering the phone. To keep her left hand from doing mischief, she would subdue it with the right hand. She described this unpleasant situation as if someone "from the moon" were controlling her hand. (Geschwind, Iacoboni, Mega, Zaidel, Clughesy, and Zaidel, 1995, p. 803)

In this case the functional correlate of representational shift is likely to have been an inter-hemispheric motor disconnection, whereas the neural correlate of this functional deficit was a rather circumscribed lesion in the midbody of the corpus callosum. In general, the necessary or sufficient sets of lesions determining this syndrome are presently unclear. On the representational level we see that the triggering events leading to a certain subset of contradictory—but impressively complex and very obviously goal-directed—patterns of motor behavior that cannot be depicted as *my own* volitional acts anymore. In other words, the information about these events taking place within the system cannot be integrated into the phenomenal self-model or appropriated under a PMIR. This insight, however, now leads us to an important conclusion about what the *function* of a conscious, volitional first-person perspective actually is. From a control-theoretic perspective (see Frith, Blakemore, and Wolpert 2000, p. 1777*f*.) the patient suffering from alien hand sign has the problem that his movement specification mechanism is driven by visually perceived objects in the immediate environment, by *affordances* taking the causal role of explicit goal representations. With an impaired selection mechanism these affordances can now causally "take over" part of his body. What I have termed the PMIR, therefore, is the phenomenal reflectance of a successful selection process operating on sets of possible behaviors or goal states. More precisely, it is the final stage of this process, made globally available for the system as a whole. It is interesting to note the intuitive plausibility of the picture now emerging: The stronger and more stable your conscious first-person perspective, the lesser the degree to which you can actually be driven by the affordances of your immediate environment.

It is important to note that at least two different kinds of ownership will be involved in any accurate description of the phenomenology: ownership for the resulting body movements, and ownership for the corresponding volitional act, for example, the conscious representation of the selection process preceding the actual behavior. Phenomenal ownership for bodily motion is achieved by the PSM. The conscious representation of a volitional act consists in the construction of a PMIR, that is, a representation of the system as a whole now being directed at a certain, selected goal state. The self-model theory of subjectivity predicts that one could exist without the other. One could lose ownership of a body part that sometimes even makes movements, as in hemisomatagnosia. This would mean that the body part was not represented in the PSM anymore. But one could also have ownership for this body part, an intact bodily self-model, but be unable to construct a PMIR corresponding to its movements. One would not have a *volitional* self-model. The second possibility is that bodily behavior is phenomenally owned, but cannot be owned as an *action* of one's own. I would submit that the first representational possibility may correspond to what, since Brion and Jedynak (1972), has been called "alien hand syndrome"; the second possibility may be what Della Sala, Marchetti, and Spinnler (1991, 1994) termed "anarchic hand sign." Anarchic hand sign is defined by the occurrence of goal-directed and complex upper limb movements, which are being experienced as nonintended although the body part is phenomenally owned. To experience an event as nonintended is synonymous to not possessing a phenomenal model of the intentionality relation for this event.

In the patient suffering from anarchic hand sign, there exists no globally available information about the goal-selection process, neither as a property of the world nor as a property of the system itself. Therefore these action-generating events are—from the patient's perspective—not part of *her* phenomenal biography anymore. Only the visually and proprioceptively represented anarchic arm movements themselves are endowed with phenomenal subjectivity in the sense of ownership. They are, however, *not* subjective in the sense of phenomenal agenthood, because a volitional PMIR cannot be constructed. Again, what is missing is a certain integrative capacity: the capacity to integrate a representation of the causal history of certain motor commands into the phenomenal self-model.[26]

---

26. Note the implicit parallels to the discussions of schizophrenia in Daprati, Franck, Georgieff, Proust, Pacherie, Dalery, and Jeannerod 1997 or Georgieff and Jeannerod 1998. On the functional level this loss is possibly mirrored in the loss of interhemispheric integration of motor and supplementary motor areas. See, for example, Geschwind et al. 1995, p. 807; but see also Marchetti and Della Sala 1998.

6.6   The Self-Model Theory of Subjectivity

At the end of chapter 3 we used *constraint 2* (presentationality), *constraint 3* (globality), and *constraint 6* (transparency) to formulate a minimal concept of conscious experience. It was a concept of conscious experience as *the activation of a transparent, global model of reality within a window of presence*. Possibly this concept could be enriched by further empirical constraints to describe certain phenomenal state classes like mystical experiences, full depersonalization, persistent vegetative state, and other potential forms of non-perspectival consciousness. However, what this concept did not allow us to do was to describe *subjective* experience.

Subjectivity, in the theoretically interesting sense of being bound to an individual, consciously experienced first-person perspective, is something that can only be conceptually analyzed and turned into an *empirically* tractable feature of consciousness by introducing the two new theoretical entities I presented in this chapter, namely, the transparent PSM and the transparent PMIR. We can now see how full-blown subjective consciousness evolves through three major levels: the generation of a world-model, the generation of a self-model, and the transient integration of certain aspects of the world-model *with* the self-model. What follows is a minimal working concept of subjective experience: *Phenomenally subjective* experience consists in transparently modeling the intentionality relation within a global, coherent model of the world embedded in a virtual window of presence. Call this the "self-model theory of subjectivity" (SMT; see also Metzinger 1993). We will now proceed to test the SMT and our new working concept of conscious subjectivity against some real-world data, using it to analyze deviant phenomenal models of the self. Let us, in chapter 7, look at a second set of neurophenomenological case studies.

7 Neurophenomenological Case Studies II

7.1 Impossible Egos

There are many states of phenomenal self-consciousness which healthy persons—for good reasons—never experience, because healthy persons are constitutionally unable to run the respective self-simulations. The corresponding regions of phenomenal state space are, as it were, forbidden territory for beings like ourselves. Therefore, it is hard for us to even imagine what the internal landscape of these regions, defined as "off-limits" by psychological evolution, actually looks like. In this second set of case studies my investigation pursues the question of whether the conceptual tools, which are now completely developed and in our hands, possess the necessary strength and precision to describe a larger variety of nonstandard cases of conscious self-experience. From a methodological and argumentative point of view, they function as a *test* of the theory just formulated. If this theory can deal successfully with pathological cases by submitting them to a functionalist-representationalist analysis, then this will be a major advantage. Again, such case studies are of particular importance for philosophy of mind because they point to the defects in existing theories and prevent failures of imagination to be interpreted as insights into conceptual necessities. Many classic theories of mind, from Descartes to Kant, will have to count as having been refuted, even after consideration of the very first example. The reason for this unfortunate state of affairs is that all the theories operate under the "epistemic transparency" assumption of self-consciousness: they assume that within the self the light of knowledge shines through and through, thereby making unnoticed errors about the content of one's own mind logically impossible.

7.2 Deviant Phenomenal Models of the Self

7.2.1 Anosognosia

Anosognosia consists in the loss of higher-order insight into an existing deficit. As this deficit is always a deficit of the person herself, anosognosia is equivalent to a lack of information on the level of *self*-representation, typically in terms of attentional or cognitive availability. The paradigmatic case is blindness denial (Anton's syndrome). Patients suffering from cortical blindness following bilateral injury of the occipital lobes are unable to phenomenally process visual information, and they behave in a similar fashion to someone who suffers peripheral blindness (Anton 1898, 1899; Benson and Greenberg 1969). They bump into furniture and show all the functional signs of blindness. However, some of these patients deny their blindness and attempt to behave as if they have vision. They confabulate visual experiences, acting as if the subjective disappearance of the visual world is not something they are currently conscious of, while at the same time telling stories about nonexistent phenomenal worlds, which they seem to believe, and denying any functional deficit with regard to their own visual abilities.

Many patients with Anton's syndrome have associated parietal lobe lesions and sensory neglect. On the phenomenological level of description, denial of blindness can be analyzed as a second-order deficit: the fact that something is not phenomenally experienced anymore is itself not available from the first-person perspective. Under the present theoretical model, there are two possible routes of interpretation. Either the object component of the second-order, cognitive phenomenal model of the intentionality relation (PMIR) (in this case, the transparent model of oneself *as a person no longer seeing*) is simply absent. Information concerning the deficit simply does not exist. This could happen when it is impossible for the postlesional brain to *update* its phenomenal self-model (PSM). However, there exists a second possibility. There could exist an updated self-model in the patient's brain, but this new model could functionally not be *globally available for attention*. Deficit-related information would then be active within the system as a whole, but it could never become subjective information, because, for functional reasons, it cannot be represented under a PMIR. In the context of the current theory it is interesting to note how Anton himself tried to develop a terminology for the syndrome he had discovered. In a lecture he gave to the Society of Physicians in Styria (Austria) on 20 December 1879 he described his patients as *seelenblind für ihre Blindheit*, "soul-blind for their own blindness" (reprinted in Anton 1898, p. 227). If one substitutes the concept of "soul" (*Seele*) with the concept of a PSM, the concept of "soul-blindness" (*Seelenblindheit*) with the inability to internally represent something *under* a PSM, and takes "blindness" to be that something, namely, the dramatic shift in functional properties going along with cerebral blindness, one arrives at a very similar hypothesis: Anton's syndrome is the inability to use a PSM in making a certain functional loss globally available for conscious experience. Anton also investigated a number of cases of deafness denial, and described those patients as "soul-deaf for their own deafness" (*seelentaub für ihre Taubheit*; cf. Anton 1899, p. 119). For example, he describes a 69-year-old woman, who was completely deaf for typical stimuli such as clapping, whistling, and shouting:

In conversations as well she never became conscious of the fact that she was not hearing or understanding the questions posed to her; her replies were nothing but a continuation of her current sequence of thoughts. Repeatedly she was asked in writing if she could hear anything, and guilelessly and indifferently she gave assurances that she was hearing well. One time the following question was written down for her: "Mrs. Hochrieser, are you hearing well?" The patient read this aloud, continuously repeating her name, saying, "Yes. That's how I am called, that's my name," and could in no way be made to answer the question. (Anton 1899, p. 107; English translation by T.M.)

Anton also pointed out how deafness denial results not only from attentional but also from *cognitive* unavailability. He wrote that an aspect particularly hard to understand is the indifference of the patient, her inability to draw conclusions or consequences from her deficit. He wrote: "Therefore, all respective thought formations had been eliminated as well, as if everything acoustical had been deleted from her soul. Not only had the raw material of acoustic sensation ceased to exist after this deficit but also the mental images [*Vorstellungen*] and combinations in the soul [*seelische Combinationen*], which are tied to it" (Anton 1899, p. 229; English translation by T.M.).

Interestingly, there is also a mirror image of the denial of cortical blindness, "inverse Anton's syndrome" (Walsh and Hoyt 1969; for a recent case study, see Hartmann and Wolz 1991). Such patients show that the conscious identification of a percept may not be necessary for the activation of associated semantic knowledge. If shown a moving object, like a moving cloth in the area of spared vision, they resolutely deny visual perception while correctly describing the target event. They do not possess a conscious self-model of themselves as seeing persons, but rather give autophenomenological reports of the following kind: "I feel it," "I feel something is there," "it clicks," or "I feel it in my mind" (Hartmann and Wolz 1991, p. 33). The authors hypothesized that in this configuration cognitive availability is achieved without *attentional* availability, that is, that "a semantic activator bypasses attentional systems and is processed at the semantic level" (ibid., p. 38). Although able to correctly name objects, colors, famous faces, read individual words, and recognize facially expressed emotions, such patients do not construct a PMIR for the respective part of the visual domain: They do experience shifts in their self-model, but the causal *relation* holding between perceptual object and this shift cannot be explicitly represented as being a visual one.

Anton's syndrome is a form of anosognosia. This concept was first introduced to refer to the loss of awareness or recognition sometimes associated with hemiplegia (Babinski 1914). There is a weaker form of this type of disorder, sometimes described as *anosodiaphoria* (Critchley 1953; for a brief study of a case oscillating between anosognosia and anosodiaphoria in Anton's syndrome, see T. Feinberg 2001, p. 28*f*.). Patients suffering from anosodiaphoria display a partial form of insight, by verbally acknowledging that they have a certain disability or deficit while on an emotional and motivational level being quite unconcerned about their current situation. Another reason why the extensive and well-documented class of restricted self-consciousness presented by the blindness denial in Anton's syndrome is theoretically relevant consists in falsifying an assumption on which many classic theories of subjectivity have been based. I call it the "epistemic transparency" assumption (not to be confused with the notion of *phenomenal* transparency distinguished earlier). Descartes is the paradigmatic example of a philosopher making this assumption in following the intuition that *I cannot be wrong about the contents of my own consciousness*. As the empirical material clearly shows, unnoticed and in principle unnotice*able* forms of self-misrepresentation do exist, because large partitions of our subsymbolic self-model are cognitively impenetrable. Let us look at a first example:

"Mrs. M, when were your admitted to the hospital?"

"I was admitted on April 16, because my daughter felt there was something wrong with me."

"What day is it today and what time?"

"It is sometime late in the afternoon on Tuesday." (This was an accurate response.)

"Mrs. M, can you use your arms?"

"Yes."

"Can you use both hands?"

"Yes, of course."

"Can you use your right hand?"

"Yes."

"Can you use your left hand?"

"Yes."

"Are both hands equally strong?"

"Yes, they are equally strong."

"Mrs. M, point to my student with your right hand." (Patient points.)

"Mrs. M, point to my student with your left hand." (Patient remains silent.)

"Mrs. M, why are you not pointing?"

"Because I didn't want to . . ."

This example is taken from a study carried out by Vilayanur Ramachandran (Ramachandran 1995, p. 24). His patient was a 76-year-old woman with a recent stroke that completely paralyzed the left side of her body. As is typical of this kind of anosognostic patient, she persistently denied her paralysis and was fully convinced of being in a healthy condition. Under standard conditions there can be no doubt about the sincerity of such patients and the truthfulness of their autophenomenological reports.

The first conclusion one has to draw is that a transparent self-model of the patient as a nonparalyzed person is currently active. The content of this self-model is cognitively available and can be used for the control of speech. Obviously, information about the lacking proprioceptive and kinesthetic feedback after a motor command has been issued to the left arm must be active somewhere in the nervous system of this patient. However, due to the deficit, this information is not *globally available* information. It cannot be integrated into the currently active *conscious* model of the self. Please note that anosognosia can be a very fine-grained and domain-specific phenomenon (Stuss 1991). To give an example, an anosognosia may refer to a patient's cortical blindness, but not to his hemiplegia (Mohr 1997, p. 128). Typically it will not be a permanent phenomenon, but be restricted to the early phase of a disease. However, it may also disappear suddenly after a longer period. Raney and Nielsen (1942, p. 151; quoted in Davies and Humphreys 1993, p. 69) described a woman who, after a year of apparent lack of insight into her deficit, exclaimed "My God, I am blind! Just to think, I have lost my eyesight!"

Psychoanalytic interpretations in terms of a repression of unpleasant information are—among other reasons—not tenable, because anosognosia is an asymmetrical disorder occurring only with right-hemisphere damage. One first empirical constraint for any rational psychological or philosophical theory about the phenomenon of anosognosia is that patients whose right side of the body is paralyzed will frequently retain full insight into their condition. A further striking feature of anosognosia is the way in which patients automatically start to confabulate, as if the system were continuously trying to maximize the overall coherence of its global model of reality by sacrificing its veridicality.[1] In confabulation "goodness-of-fit criteria are inoperative" (Picton and Stuss 1994, p. 261), but only locally. On the other hand those patient reports can certainly count as *truthful* reports. What they report is the content of their current, transparent model of reality. A nonlinguistic creature certainly could suffer from anosognosia as well, although it would not be able to utter a verbal report, truthful or not. In such an animal, confabulatory activity might only be reflected on the level of its behavioral profile, making it look like a creature continuously attempting to act out a strange dream. (In fact, dreamers can be seen as anosognostics. They are, for instance, unaware of severe memory impairments and attentional deficits.) It is interesting to note that a traditional philosophical strategy of simply interpreting such states as a pathology of *belief* (for an excellent recent discussion, see Coltheart and Davies 2000) therefore cannot do justice to the representational deep structure of the target phenomenon. Anosognosia appears in beings unable to even form what today we call "beliefs." It is a deficit not so much in high-level cognitive processing, but primarily in subpersonal mechanisms of transparent self-modeling.

Look at the following example of how the patient subsequently moves deeper into a more fully developed delusional state, claiming that the arm doesn't even belong to herself. It becomes harder and harder to prevent externally given information about her true bodily state from entering her conscious self-representation:

---

1. It is interesting to note how all the conceptual constraints for the notion of "phenomenal representation" developed in chapter 3 implicitly also describe the *functional* constraints to be satisfied by any individual conscious system. There may be multiple conflicts, for instance, between the globality constraint and the adaptivity constraint. What looks like a severe distortion from the third-person perspective, say, in cases of anosognosia or delusional disorders, may actually be a form of intelligence, the best viable path through problem space and the most economical manner of achieving functional constraint satisfaction. As Ramachandran and Hirstein put it, confabulations may rather be like "higher-order filling in" and "should be seen as a part of a general strategy for the 'coherencing' of consciousness: they help to avoid indecisive vacillation and serve to optimize resource allocation, and to facilitate rapid, effective action" (1997, p. 447*f.*).

"Doctor, whose hand is this [pointing to her own left hand]?"

"Whose hand do you think it is?"

"Well, it certainly isn't yours!"

"Then whose is it?"

"It isn't mine either."

"Whose hand do you think it is?"

"It is my son's hand, doctor." (Ramachandran 1995, p. 24)

There have, of course, been attempts to break through the veil of delusion about the patient's current physical situation. What such attempts would have to achieve, functionally speaking, would be to allow for an *updating* of the PSM, by integrating already existing system-related information into it, thereby making it globally available for self-directed cognition and verbal report. Edoardo Bisiach and colleagues (Bisiach, Rusconi, and Vallar 1992) discovered that after stimulating the vestibular system of anosognostic patients by injecting ice-cold water into their left ear, they could make the symptoms disappear for a limited period of time. These experiments, which have now been replicated a number of times, are particularly fascinating. The reason is that they allow researchers to observe how, when the curtain is drawn, insight into the deficit and even correct autobiographical memory become globally available, and how the insight, after a brief period of time, disappears again as the old transparent self-model is reinstated. Ramachandran replicated and confirmed the observation of Bisiach and colleagues concerning remission from anosognosia and delusion following caloric stimulation and by specifically asking questions about the content of the autobiographical self-model of the patient demonstrated how the ongoing process of denial actually did not prevent memory consolidation, that is, the continuous construction of an unconscious, veridical autobiographical self-model (see also Ramachandran 1994). He conducted his experiments on the same patient, B.M., the 76-year-old woman, by administering 10 mL of ice-cold water into her left ear.

E: "Do you feel okay?"

P: "My ear is very cold but other than that I am fine."

E: "Can you use your hands?"

P: "I can use my right arm but not my left arm. I want to move it but it doesn't move."

E: (Holding the arm in front of the patient) "Whose arm is this?"

P: "It is my hand, of course."

E: "Can you use it?"

P: "No, it is paralyzed."

E: "Mrs. M, how long has your arm been paralyzed? Did it start now or earlier?"

P: "It has been paralyzed continuously for several days now."

After the caloric effect had worn off completely, I waited for $\frac{1}{2}$ h and asked:

E: "Mrs. M, can you use your arm?"

P: "No, my left arm doesn't work."

Finally the same set of questions was repeated to the patient 8 h later, in my absence, by one of my colleagues.

E: "Mrs. M, can you walk?"

P: "Yes."

E: "Can you use both your arms?"

P: "Yes."

E: "Can you use your left arm?"

P: "Yes."

E: "This morning, two doctors did something to you. Do you remember?"

P: "Yes. They put water in my ear; it was very cold."

E: "Do you remember they asked some questions about your arms, and you gave them an answer? Do you remember what you said?"

P: "No, what did I say?"

E: "What do you think you said? Try and remember."

P: "I said my arms were okay." (Ramachandran 1995, p. 34)

This shift in self-representational content shows a number of interesting aspects. First, it demonstrates how consolidated, existing autobiographical information stored in the central nervous system cannot be made globally available by integrating it into the PSM after a certain time has passed, and how immediately a process of constructing an auto-biographical self-*simulation* takes place in order to preserve the overall coherence of the currently active model. Most of all, this first case study should make more vivid certain points I put forward in sections 3.2.7 and 6.2.6, when I wrote that transparency is a very special form of darkness. Darkness is lack of information, and phenomenal transparency is special in that this lack is not *explicitly* represented; the attentional unavailability of earlier processing stages (see section 3.2.7) is something we cannot subjectively experience itself. The phenomenal part of the mental self-model is transparent, because large parts of its causal history are introspectively unavailable. It is a very limited tool for pursuing self-knowledge, particularly if detached from the biological context in which it evolved.

This first case study also illustrates the true meaning of the concept of "autoepistemic closure." Immediately after stimulation of her left ear, the patient truthfully reported the content of her PSM, having no access to the underlying causal mechanisms that led to its activation, for example, the current remission of her condition. Later, when denying her earlier admission of paralysis, she was doing the same thing: she truthfully reported the current content of her self-model, being autoepistemically closed against the causal mechanisms in her own central nervous system which led to the activation of *this* model. In philosophical terms, all belief *de se* necessarily is belief about the cognitively available content of the conscious self-model, and autoepistemic closure allows beings like ourselves to persistently entertain false beliefs *de se*. This is what Descartes and many later philosophers in the tradition of a priori theorizing about the human mind could not conceive of. And this is also the reason why it was necessary to distinguish between epistemic, referential, and *phenomenal* transparency in section 3.2.7. The phenomenal transparency of the human self-model not only does not permit conclusions to be drawn regarding the *epistemic* transparency of the kind of nonconceptual self-knowledge it mediates. There may even be many situations in our conscious life in which it is precisely phenomenal transparency that prevents epistemic transparency, in which the conscious self can count as a form of darkness *itself*.

The neural correlates of anosognosia are well-known; they include cortices in the insular, cytoarchitectonic areas 3, 1, 2, in the parietal region, and in an area called ST (Damasio 1999, p. 211). A recent hypothesis (Heilman, Barrett, and Adair 1998, p. 1907) proposes that the type of anosognosia just discussed could consist in an "intentional motor activation deficit" which does not set a hypothetical monitor-comparator system, therefore leading to the absence of an *expectation* of a movement, making it impossible for the patient to detect a mismatch between the expectancy of movement and the actual conscious perception of a bodily movement. What these patients would suffer from, then, would be the inability to generate a certain motor *self-simulation* for the left side of their body. As there is never any forward-model generated, the absence of proprioceptive and kinesthetic feedback from the paralyzed left arm cannot be detected and integrated into the conscious self-model. I refrain from more detailed empirical speculations at this point. Let me, however, point out how a transparent self-model may make a system unable to discover the *absence* of certain of its own functional properties, for example, its capacity to actually form a specific type of intention. As we noted earlier, it is always important to keep in mind the Brentano-Dennett principle of an absence of representation not being the same as a representation of absence. There are implicit and explicit kinds of epistemic darkness, as well as of phenomenal blindness. Indeed, there may be something like implicit *intentionality blindness* in the case here described, a deficit resembling a localized and self-directed form of autism.

It is obvious how the self-model theory of subjectivity (SMT) can help us understand the representational and functional architecture underlying deficits like anosognosia, and also give us indications about the phenomenal content active in these situations. Let me end this first section by making a point of a more exclusively philosophical nature. The content of our conscious self-models, from an evolutionary perspective, has been functionally adequate. From an epistemological perspective or under certain normative ideals, as, for instance (to take *the* philosophical classic), the maximization of self-knowledge, this content may be epistemically unjustified or outright false. In other words, there are certain conceivable interpretations of the human condition under which *all of us* are anosognostic. It is fascinating to note how any representational analysis of a particular, deviating neurophenomenological configuration can always be turned into an epistemological metaphor.

Such metaphors may turn out to be highly fruitful. If, for instance, we should arrive at the conclusion that the way in which we are given to ourselves on the level of conscious experience has to be interpreted as a *deficit*, or even a "disease," from a nonbiological perspective, then we may suddenly appear as beings unable to discover our own mental impairments. Anosognosia demonstrates what transparency and autoepistemic closure actually are. It is interesting to note, however, that to a considerable degree we all live our lives under these two constraints, even in nonpathological situations. We might be unable to embody certain intentions we have already generated, and unable to consciously experience this lack. We might be subject to drastic and frequent rearrangements of autobiographical memory, and it would be hard for us to discover this fact—because of the transparency of our conscious self-models. Like anosognostic patients we might have persistent false beliefs *de se* while never being able to consciously experience this very fact, because they are rooted in the deep structure of our noncognitive model of reality. For this reason, third-person approaches to the structure of self-consciousness are valuable and important for anybody who has a *serious* commitment to pursuing the classical philosophical ideal of self-knowledge. For this reason theoretical intuitions about what is possible and what is impossible exclusively derived from introspectively$_4$ accessing our transparent self-model or from deliberately generating phenomenal self-simulations are of little importance to those wanting to operate under a rigorous, rational methodology.

7.2.2 *Ich-Störungen*: Identity Disorders and Disintegrating Self-Models

In this section I want to point to a large class of disturbances that, due to deviant forms of self-modeling, result in dramatic changes in the patients' phenomenal experience of identity. Identity is not a thing or a property, but a relation. Identity is the most *subtle* of all relations, the relation in which everything stands to itself. The PSM constitutes another kind of standing-in-a-relation-to-oneself, sometimes *by* representing identity for an organism. But what precisely is it that is being represented? Possessing a globally available self-representation enables an information-processing system to stand in new kinds of relations to itself (in accessing different kinds of system-related information *as* system-related information), and if a certain portion of this information is highly invariant, the phenomenal experience of *transtemporal* identity can emerge. Philosophically, indiscriminability is certainly not equivalent to identity. Identity is a transitive relation; indiscriminability is not. Indiscriminability may simply cause certain *functional* invariances. However, a transparent representation of functional invariance can result in the *phenomenology* of being identical through time, of transtemporal sameness. A second semantic element in the folk-psychiatric notion of "having" an identity that can be "disordered" is *coherence*: the degree of functional and representational coupling between different elements of the phenomenal self. Being a conscious person presupposes a minimal degree not only of cognitive and behavioral but also of *self-experiential* coherence. A third, more general, aspect refers to the property of phenomenal selfhood, of *being someone*. As the neurophenomenology of deviating forms of self-consciousness demonstrates, human beings can consciously *be someone* to many different degrees, and they can also lose this property altogether without losing conscious experience as such.

There is no clear-cut and well-established translation of the German *Ich-Störung* ("ego disturbance") used in the heading of this section. What in English is often termed "passivity phenomena" and "delusions of control" are prototypical examples of this kind of disturbance.[2] I will not engage in any terminological discussion here, but simply present a series of illustrative examples, using them as a "reality test" for the conceptual scheme already developed in this book. Can identity disorders be analyzed in a more satisfactory manner under SMT (see section 6.6) than under classic phenomenological and transcendentalist approaches?

The phenomenal experience of selfhood and identity can vary along an extremely large number of dimensions. There are simple losses of content (as in the first example to be discussed below). There are various typologies of phenomenal disintegration, as in schizophrenia, in depersonalization disorders, and in *dissociative identity disorder* (DID), accompanied by multiplications of the phenomenal self within one and the same physical system. In these cases, we confront major redistributions of the phenomenal property of "mineness" in representational space. Then there are at least four different delusions of misidentification (DM[3]; namely, Capgras syndrome, Frégoli syndrome, intermetamorphosis, reverse intermetamorphosis, and reduplicative paramnesia). It is therefore important

---

2. Bovet and Parnas write: "One of the essential features of schizophrenia is the disturbances of the experiencing 'I' (*Ich-Störungen*). These disturbances overlap more or less the Anglo-Saxon concepts of 'depersonalization,' 'derealization,' 'loss of control,' 'disturbed ego-boundaries,' 'passivity phenomena,' and 'delusions of reference' . . ." (Bovet and Parnas 1993, p. 589). Henrik Walter points out how these terminological ambiguities may be due to the influence German idealism had on theoretical psychiatry (Walter 2001).

3. In using the abbreviation DM instead of DMS (delusional misidentification *syndromes*) I follow a recent terminological modification introduced by Nora Breen and colleagues in order to avoid the inaccuracy of assuming a whole cluster of symptoms as defining characteristics for the different categories. Cf. Breen et al. 2000, p. 75, n. 1.

to test our conceptual tools at least against some examples of the enormous phenomenological richness of the target phenomenon—because, as Goethe said, all theory is gray but green is the golden tree of our inner life.

Let us start by looking at the phylogenetically oldest part of the human self-model—the body-model in the brain. There are many different disorders related to the phenomenal body image, the conscious body-model in the brain. Some readers may have experienced spatial distortions of the body image themselves, for instance, when deliberately delaying the process of falling asleep or in the first phase of waking up from anesthesia. A large component of this spatial model of the self is constituted by self-presentational content. Self-presentational content is stimulus-correlated content, originating in the vestibular organ, complex homeodynamic self-regulation in the upper brainstem and hypothalamus, and a large number of different receptors external to the brain but internal to our body, which are, for instance, found in skin, muscles, joints, and viscera (see section 5.4). The integration of self-presentational content into a unified, globally available representational structure underlies our phenomenal experience of *embodiment*, of being in direct and immediate contact with our own bodies. Under certain conditions, specific classes of self-presentational and spatial content can selectively be missing from the conscious model of the self. Oliver Sacks describes the rare case of a highly selective sensory polyneuropathy, exclusively damaging proprioceptive nerve fibers.

But the day of surgery Christina was still worse. Standing was impossible—unless she looked down at her feet. She could hold nothing in her hands, and they "wandered"—unless she kept an eye on them. When she reached out for something, or tried to feed herself, her hands would miss, or overshoot as if some essential control or coordination was gone.

She could scarcely even sit up—her body "gave way." Her face was oddly expressionless and slack, her jaw fell open, even her vocal posture was gone.

"Something awful's happened," she mouthed in a ghostly flat voice. "I can't feel my body. I feel weird—disembodied." (Sacks 1998, p. 45)

. . . Christina listened closely, with a sort of desperate attention.

"What I must do then," she said slowly, "is use vision, use my eyes, in every situation where I used—what do you call it?—proprioception before. I have already noticed," she added, musingly, "that I may 'lose' my arms. I think they're one place, and I find they're another. This 'proprioception' is like the eyes of the body, the way the body sees itself. And if it goes, as it's gone with me, *it's like the body's blind*. My body can't 'see' itself if it's lost its eyes, right? So *I* have to watch it—be its eyes. Right?" (p. 47)

Oliver Sacks then reports about the further development of Christina's situation:

Thus at the time of her catastrophe, and for about a month afterwards, Christina remained as floppy as a ragdoll, unable even to sit up. But three months later, I was startled to see her sitting very finely—too finely, statuesquely, like a dancer in mid-pose. And soon I saw that her sitting was, indeed, a pose, consciously or automatically adopted and sustained, a sort of forced or willful or histrionic posture, to make up for the continuing lack of any genuine, natural posture. Nature having failed, she took to "artifice," but the artifice was suggested by nature, and soon became "second nature." (p. 49)

... Thus, although there was not a trace of neurological recovery (recovery from the anatomical damage to nerve fibers), there was, with the help of intensive and varied therapy—she remained in hospital, on the rehabilitation ward, for almost a year—a very considerable functional recovery, i.e., the ability to function using various substitutions and other such tricks. It became possible, finally, for Christina to leave hospital, go home, rejoin her children. She was able to return to her home computer terminal, which she now learned to operate with extraordinary skill and efficiency, considering that everything had to be done by vision, not feel. She had learned to operate—but how did she feel? Had the substitutions dispersed the disembodied sense she first spoke of? (p. 50)

The boundaries of the globally available partition of the self-model are the boundaries of the phenomenal self. The example of the "bodiless woman" illustrates what it means that the conscious self-model is an integrated *multimodal* structure: it can be deprived of certain modalities or specific classes of self-presentational content, but in some situations such losses of internal sources of information can be functionally compensated by strengthening other channels. Christina, for example, had only minimal damage to her sense of light touch, temperature, or pain—that is, other types of self-presentational content were fully available. What was lost was "position sense," the proprioceptive awareness of one's own body, a dynamic and *spatial* form of self-representation predominantly activated from a continuous flow of information generated by sensors in the muscles, tendons, and joints. The situation described here is therefore exclusively caused by an internal "sensory" loss, with no motor damage involved (see also Sternman, Schaumberg, and Asbury 1980). An acute polyneuritis disables a certain input function, which is continuously active under normal circumstances, which in turn results in a circumscribed *phenomenal* loss. However, it is not *only* a phenomenal loss: Not only the phenomenology of the system changes; there are also higher-order functional properties which have to be rearranged to compensate the loss of globally available information for the control of action. The phenomenal self, as such, however, does not disintegrate. It first loses a specific type of content—proprioceptive self-presentational content—and then reflects the underlying process of restructuring:

She continues to feel, with the continuing loss of proprioception, that her body is dead, not-real, not-hers—she cannot appropriate it to herself. She can find no words for this state, and can only use analogies derived from other senses: "I feel my body is blind and deaf to itself . . . it has no sense of itself"—these are her own words. (Sacks 1998, p. 51)

... "It's like something's been scooped right out of me, right at the center . . . that's what they do with frogs, isn't it? They scoop out the center, the spinal cord, they *pith* them . . . that's what I am, *pithed*, like a frog . . . Step up, come and see Chris, the first pithed human being. She has no proprioception, no sense of herself—disembodied Chris, the pithed girl!" She laughs wildly, with an edge of hysteria. I calm her—"Come now!"—while thinking, "Is she right?" (p. 51*f*.)

A further aspect clearly demonstrated by this case study is how even the body has to become *appropriated*, how it has to be represented on the phenomenal level of self-modeling in order for the system as a whole to be able to *own* this body. The sense of ownership, therefore, is a highly specific form of representational content. This content is transparent, and it is not a thing, but an ongoing process—the globally available process of *self-containing*. This act of appropriating one's own body on the conscious level of self-modeling, which generates the phenomenal property of "mineness," also brings about an important new *functional* property: It allows a representational system to *own* its own hardware, that is, to flexibly inspect and control it, not in a modular fashion, but truly *as a whole*. The spatially coded part of the PSM (see section 6.4.1) can be *pithed*. In an extreme case, we might only be given to ourselves as a *res extensa* through visual perception from the outside. In terms of the spatial frame of reference, *internal* states have ceased to exist.

The acute sensory neuropathy syndrome has been interpreted as a distinct clinical entity (Sternman et al. 1980). Gallagher and Cole (1995; but see also Cole and Paillard 1995; Cole 1995) described a related case. Patient I.W. still consciously experiences heat, cold, pain, and muscle fatigue, but his phenomenal representation of *posture* is absent. He could not control his bodily movements, even with visual perception, for the first 3 months. Here is how Gallagher and Cole described this patient:

To maintain his posture and to control his movement IW must not only keep parts of his body in his visual field, but also conceptualize postures and movements. Without proprioceptive and tactile information he neither knows where his limbs are nor controls his posture unless he looks at and thinks about his body. Maintaining posture is, for him, an activity rather than an automatic process. His movement requires constant visual and mental concentration. In darkness he is unable to control movement; when he walks he cannot daydream, but must concentrate constantly on his movement. When he writes he has to concentrate on holding the pen and on his body posture. IW learned through trial and error the amount of force needed to pick up and hold an egg without breaking it. If his attention is directed toward a different task while holding an egg, his hand crushes the egg. (Gallagher and Cole 1995, p. 375)

The last aspect of I.W.'s phenomenology is mirrored in Christina's case, who, if distracted while eating, for example, by conversation, would "grip the knife and the fork with painful force—her nails and fingertips would go bloodless with pressure; but if there was any lessening of the painful pressure, she might nervelessly drop them straightaway—there was no in-between, no modulation, whatever" (Sacks 1998, p. 50). I.W. also describes his body sitting in a supporting chair as being like a "sack of potatoes." He knows the physical limitations of his bones and ligaments will allow his body a certain stability, but that slowly it will slide down (Jonathan Cole, personal communication, 2001). A self-model is an informational structure and, on the functional level of description, a loss of information is immediately expressed in a change of the system's functional profile. One aspect of this is the decoupling of conscious volition and motor system, as seen in I.W. during the first 3 months of his disease. Availability for those selection processes associated with phenomenal volition seems to be highly dependent on proprioceptive feedback in our own case (Fourneret et al. 2002). We can now form a much clearer understanding of the PSM as a representational instrument, making system-related information (e.g., about posture and limb position) *globally available for action control*. We also notice how the global phenomenal property of embodiment, from an epistemological perspective, is a highly mediated and indirect process: No strong conceptual conclusions can be drawn from the phenomenal immediacy in which the geometrical and kinematic properties of our own body are given to us on the level of conscious experience, and the phenomenal experience of being an embodied self certainly cannot function as a successor of the Cartesian *cogito* in terms of providing a safe foundation for all knowledge. Phenomenal embodiment is not a reliable epistemic anchor in physical reality.

A second, functional, aspect highlighted by the last two case studies consists in the self-model as *integrating* information from multiple structures into a multimodal whole. The length and the difficulties involved in the rehabilitation histories of Christina and patient I.W. show how hard it is to substitute the causal role of proprioception either by another external sensory modality (e.g., vision) or by an attempt to substitute volitional availability with *cognitive* availability. Because a large part of the unconscious bodily self-model is deprived of its major source of information, it now has to be integrated with a phenomenal body image which can be continuously updated by what was described as the attentional and the cognitive subject (see sections 6.4.3 and 6.4.4): The prereflexive process of bodily self-control only functions for I.W. if visual attention to his body's current position or the ability to "think about his body" (i.e., to run an intended kinematic or geometrical self-simulation) is given—else his motor control will simply disappear (see Gallagher and Cole 1995, p. 382). It is a global functional property, now no longer realized by this particular system. Of course, information flow from vision also is greatly reduced; it is simply never able to compensate for proprioceptive feedback since it is partial, too slow, and requires attention to some degree. As Cole (personal communication, 2001) points out, I.W. is constrained by speed and by loss of fine exploratory finger movements—he hates to pick up coins from a surface, cannot use a handle on a cup, never takes keys from a pocket or does up his top shirt button. Generally, he has to send motor commands and accept on trust that they arrive. Another interesting aspect clearly illustrated by these case studies is how costly it is in general to elevate certain parts of the unconscious, functional self-model onto the level of the conscious model of reality by actively generating a PMIR.

First, there are attentional limitations: IW cannot attend to all aspects of movement. Second, his rate of movement is slower than normal. The fact that movement and motor programs are consciously driven slows motility down. Third, the overall duration of motor activity is relatively short because of the mental effort or energy required. Finally, complex single movements (like walking across rough ground), and combined or compound movements (walking and carrying an egg) take more energy than simple movements. . . .

Still IW has to simplify movements in order to focus his command on them. His movements appear somewhat stiff and slow and could not be mistaken for normal. . . . IW, however, insists that once a motor behavior has been performed it does not mean that it requires less concentration subsequently. His rehabilitation necessitated huge increases in his attentional abilities. The cognitive demand of this activity cannot be over-estimated, for other deafferented subjects have not managed such a functional recovery. (Gallagher and Cole 1995, p. 384*f*.)

The cases of Christina and I.W. show how a massive loss of input can lead to major disturbances on the level of phenomenal self-consciousness, and how it can eventually lead to massive restructuring on both the phenomenal and the functional levels of the self-model. As opposed to anosognosia, here phenomenal properties systematically covary with functional properties in a much more obvious fashion.

Let us now proceed to look at two further aspects: the phenomenal property of ownership, of experiential "mineness," and the aspect of coherence, as simultaneously reflected on the functional and phenomenal level of the self-model. Again, to arrive at a differentiated theory of subjective experience and to do justice to the complexity of real-world phenomenology, one has to acknowledge that the existence of phenomenal "mineness" is not an all-or-nothing phenomenon. For instance, as Gallagher and Cole point out (Gallagher and Cole 1995, p. 386), patient I.W. reported that when the neuropathy first manifested itself he felt *alienated* from his body. The conscious experience of volitional control plays an important role in the prerational bodily experience of ownership. As I.W. started to regain conscious control over his body, however, his phenomenology underwent a corresponding change as well: he reconstructed what Gallagher and Cole (ibid., p. 387) call the "felt sense of owned embodiment."

Let us now shift to the *opaque* partition of the PSM, the conscious experience of oneself as a thinking subject. What will happen if the transparent, geometrically coded part of the self-model stays stable, while the nonspatial, cognitive part becomes incoherent?

". . . there was a priest standing next to me who is already half retired. You have interrupted me. The speeches about powder are now prepared, and the priest is preparing drugs and music. Are you going to take on somebody else this morning, aha!, now I just thought that it was in the morning. I have been in the Kappelen Bridge, caught a large pike. (Something can be heard from outside.) Aha, this must be the ophthalmologist. He has come, because of the washing machine, that's for certain. Mrs. X is in the bathroom during broad daylight, however, she didn't want to insult me. Mother said, that her son has become worse in M, and Pulver didn't want to insult P. But Klages always says these pseudoscientific things, and that is why he went on to graphology."[4]

In this protocol of an experimentally induced psychosis we can witness how the conscious, cognitive self becomes "semantically inconsistent," while its content is still globally available for verbal report. Formal thought disorders and a general loosening of associational flow, as here reflected in the introspective report of the subject, can be analyzed as a configuration in which the system is being internally flooded with cognitive mental models. Those cognitive models, however, are only weakly interconnected in terms of their intentional content. Phenomenologically, it may be apt to describe such situations as those in which the cognitive subject starts to fall apart, in which the phenomenal self becomes *intellectually inconsistent*. Opaque mental models, normally simulating operations on conceptual and propositional structures *for* the system, are now being activated in a more or less chaotic manner, but still continuously integrated into the self-model. Introducing a thermodynamic metaphor for a connectionist system, one could attempt to describe the underlying microfunctional situation as a general increase in processing speed, taking place within a system that has been "heated up" and now follows a fast trajectory through a sequence of states that are less and less stable. What the pharmacological stimulus employed in this experiment caused may in part have been a rather unspecific disinhibition of certain brain regions. This situation leads precisely to such an increase in the general energetic level of the system, which then in turn generates less stable simulational states characterized by an increased speed of succession. The system has been artificially shaken up, and is now desperately "trying," as it were, to relax into a more stable, low-energy state.

From the first-person perspective this subpersonal process of reintegration—if finally successful—would be experienced as the owning of a viable and consistent *cognitive* model of reality. On a more coarse-grained level of functional analysis it is obvious that the *selectivity* and the capacity for carrying out a controlled search in short-term memory are greatly diminished. On the level of phenomenal experience, however, this kind of situation also leads to the loss of a highly specific kind of conscious content, which was conceptually introduced as cognitive *agency* (see section 6.4.4). In an extreme case, the process of selecting sequences of cognitive contents will simply be absent. Hence, the process of conscious thought formation cannot be integrated into the background of the already existing transparent self-model, thereby making it *my own* thought process

4. This example is part of a verbal protocol from a scopolamine experiment, quoted in Metzinger (1993) from Heimann (1989) (in Pöppel 1989, p. 35). English translation by T.M.

from the first-person perspective. In the case reported here, the confused state could still be integrated into the self-model, it could form the content of conscious experience, and it could be verbally communicated. If, however, such a confusional state is maximally expressed on the functional as well as on the phenomenal level, we would have to say that the respective person is no longer an intellectual, cognitive subject in terms of being a rational and self-conscious thinker of her *own* thoughts. In addition, the fact that it actually possesses a phenomenal first-person perspective would not be cognitively available to such a system. The existence of a PMIR would not be available for mental concept formation. Hence, it would, for example, no longer exhibit *strong* first-person phenomena in the sense of Lynn Baker (as discussed in section 6.4.4). Strong cognitive subjectivity is something that can completely disappear as a result of subpersonal disintegration in the brain. It is important to note how such a process may at the same time still leave the attentional subject and the bodily self untouched.

The subject of Heimann's experiment experienced a loss of cognitive control and an increase in semantic inconsistency, while still experiencing his thoughts as his *own* thoughts. The logical next step consists in posing the following questions: What would it mean to lose cognitive agency *and* the sense of ownership of your own thoughts on the level of conscious experience? What would it mean to suddenly be confronted with conscious thoughts which are undoubtedly parts of your *reality*, but not parts of your own *mind*?

Schizophrenia, of course, is the classic example of a situation where patients are confronted with conscious, cognitive contents for which they have no sense of agency or ownership. On the level of phenomenal content, schizophrenia is typically characterized by phenomena such as thought insertion, verbal-auditive hallucinations, and delusions of control. As the phenomenology of schizophrenia is well-known, I will not offer an explicit case study at this point.[5] Moving one step down to the representational level of analysis, thought insertion will have to be described as a situation where the content of currently active cognitive states and processes cannot be integrated into the self-model, and must therefore be represented *as external*. Nevertheless, such phenomenologically nonsubjective thoughts are encoded as an element of objective reality, and although their content is an opaque content—the fact that they are only representations of reality is globally available—their phenomenal *presence* as such cannot be transcended by the subject of experience. An interesting point to note is that we cannot *imagine* what it would be like to be

5. For a well-documented study of the phenomenology of severe schizophrenia and a number of theoretical considerations concerning the clinical concept of "schizophrenia," presenting a good starting point for philosophers, see McKay, McKenna, and Laws (1996). An interesting phenomenological discussion containing a set of short case studies is Bovet and Parnas (1993); for a recent discussion, see Gold and Hohwy (2000).

schizophrenic: for beings like ourselves it is impossible to deliberately transpose our thoughts onto external reality, we cannot voluntarily split our PSM, and it is impossible for us to externalize its cognitive partition (see also section 8.2). In other words, verbal reports of schizophrenics are intuitively implausible and hard to understand simply because they do not describe *phenomenally possible* situations for normal people (indeed, the most general philosophical issue posed by the phenomenon of schizophrenia may concern the extent to which an *understanding* of such patients is possible, in a more rigorous sense of "understanding"; cf. Campbell 1999, p. 610*f.*).

Many classic philosophers of mind have committed the fallacy of concluding *logical* necessity from a simple phenomenological fact, that our phenomenal space of cognitive self-simulation is limited in certain ways. Descartes's *cogito* and Kant's transcendental unity of apperception are prominent examples. What modern cognitive neuropsychiatry shows, and what they could have known had they listened more closely to the schizophrenics of their own time, is that the popular principle that your own thoughts always are your *own* thoughts is by no means a necessary precondition of all experience. There are ways of mentally modeling reality in which this presupposition is suspended. To conclude from the fact that, in standard situations, all of us experience ourselves as initiators of our own thoughts or that the "I think" can, in principle and in the large majority of phenomenal configurations, accompany all states of consciousness, that some kind of irreducible entity (e.g., a transcendental subject) must exist, is, if one takes a close look at it, just another high-level and refined version of what U.T. Place (see chapter 2, n. 9) called the phenomenological fallacy: jumping from the invariance of transparent phenomenal content ("mineness") or a typical structural feature of the human self-model (permanent availability of a *cognitive* PMIR pointing "inward" to the preexisting first-order self-model) to the existence of a nonphysical individual. Mineness and cognitive subjectivity can be lost, with global coherence and phenomenal experience as such being preserved. *Constraints 2, 3,* and *7* can be fully satisfied, with *constraint 6* (perspectivalness) being either not at all or only *weakly* satisfied (i.e., on the level of attentional processing). However, phenomenal necessity—the impossibility of something usually *not* being the case according to the first-person experience of a certain, paradigmatic class of conscious experiencers—is not equivalent to logical necessity.

If, as in hearing voices, the motor aspects of internal speech production cannot be representationally integrated into the conscious self, a global phenomenal model of reality will emerge in which external voices are heard. As we have already seen (section 5.3), conscious as well as unconscious thought involves a process best described as *self-simulation*, and there are strong indicators that the cognitive content activated in the process may be a refined kind of *motor content* (see sections 6.3.3 and 6.4.4). A good phenomenological term may be "phonemic imagery": what we ultimately think with are phonemic mental images corresponding to those activated by the sensory perception of phonemes. However, functionally, such images could be anchored in (or, in social contexts, *mirrored by*) a process of subvocalization—that is, of motor self-simulations internally mimicking one's own sound-generating behavior. It is easy to imagine how such a process could get out of hand in terms of getting out of the PSM. The PSM is the tool a system uses for "owning" its own thoughts, and if this tool does not fulfil its integrational function anymore, the process of cognitive self-simulation gets out of hand; the fact that these thoughts are self-initiated states can no longer be *grasped* with the help of this tool. The truly interesting phenomenon here seems to be the additional "pseudosensory" character of such auditory hallucinations, the fact that they actually seem to be correlated with an external stimulus by displaying *presentational* content as well. Possibly they depend on an internal emulator for the generation of speech acts, which, in the schizophrenic, transforms an efference copy of motor speech commands, used as input for an internal model of the ongoing process of speech production, into auditory format (Frith 1996; see also Grush 1997, 1998).

In recent years it has become obvious that the neural correlates of phenomenal simulations frequently overlap with those of phenomenal representations. In chapter 3 (section 3.2.8) I termed this the "principle of substrate sharing." In general, neuroimaging studies conducted on hallucinating schizophrenics increasingly show how and when the direct correlates of individual, hallucinated features are activated (Silbersweig and Stern 1998). Patients hearing voices also show patterns of behavior and brain activity similar to those observed in normal people engaged in inner speech or auditory verbal imagery (Frith 1996, p. 1506). For instance, it is known that humming or singing suppresses auditory hallucinations in schizophrenics to some degree—possibly because the intended vocalization suppresses activity in the left frontal parietal lobe and thereby also blocks mechanisms of speech perception. It is precisely this area that is hyperactive in the schizophrenic. Another fact which may be of interest in this context is that those brain regions thought to be responsible for theory-of-mind tasks are also being activated in schizophrenics if they listen to their *own* voice on a headphone.

As Chris Frith points out (1996, p. 1506) there are three different types of auditory hallucinations in terms of hearing voices: (1) There is a "first-person" or reflexive type, namely, the hearing of one's thoughts spoken aloud (*thought echo*); (2) the experience of voices speaking to the patient (*second-person hallucinations*); and (3) hearing voices speaking about the patient (*third-person hallucinations*). In all three classes of phenomenal states the property of conscious agency is absent. The structural difference seems to lie in the way the PMIR is constructed: in the first case the self-component seems to be essentially untouched, whereas the object component is formed by an element that was previously represented as a *part* of the conscious self-model and has now been shifted onto the model of external reality. In the second case, a subject-subject relation is being construed, with agency attributed to the *new* subject component, which now, however, is located in *external* reality while the patient's transparent self-model is the "object component," the passive part of the communicative relationship, the listening subject. In the third type of hallucination multiple phenomenal models of *inter*subjective intentionality relations are being constructed, with the patient now being fully detached, simply forming the intentional content of the object component, as it were. As Frith points out, all behavioral observations suggest that auditory hallucinations arise in the same systems that are engaged when people listen to external speech or generate inner speech. As noted earlier, one important aspect of possessing a self-model consists in *forward-modeling*, in running self-simulations, which can then be compared to incoming proprioceptive and kinesthetic input. Especially for fast and goal-directed movements, such a forward-model could serve to make the likely consequences of an action, for example, the generation of speech, globally available before actual sensory feedback from the completed action arrives. The generation of a consciously experienced self-world border, which underlies the distribution of the phenomenal property of "mineness," could be functionally anchored in a process detecting mismatches between the process of forward self-simulations and ongoing self-*representation* based on ongoing sensory feedback.[6] In Frith's model the ongoing comparison between the current content of self-simulational and self-representational states could, if functionally disturbed, lead to a loss of the globally available properties of mineness and agency, to a situation where the system is forced to attribute the origin of this suddenly appearing globally available content to some part of external reality or other.[7]

6. This is by no means a new idea; it goes back to Helmholtz (1925), and to work on the *Reafferenzprinzip* by von Holst and Mittelstaedt and by Sperry in 1950. Irwin Feinberg describes the basic idea: ". . . motor commands in the nervous system are associated with neuronal discharges that alter activity in both sensory and motor pathways. These alterations permit monitoring of the commands themselves so that subsequent motor activity can be modified even before the effector event (muscle contraction) has occurred. They may act to inform sensory systems that the stimulation produced by the movement is self-generated rather than environmentally produced. In this way these discharges are, at least in an abstract sense, crucial for the distinction of self and non-self" (I. Feinberg 1978, p. 636). Feinberg also clearly points out how this notion may plausibly and parsimoniously describe the functional underpinnings of the phenomenal property of *cognitive agency*: "Whereas the internal feedback associated with simpler motor acts is below the level of consciousness, one might postulate that the corollary discharges accompanying conscious thought are themselves conscious. If so, the subjective experience of these discharges should correspond to nothing less than the experience of will or intention" (p. 638).

7. Frith writes: "If the output from the forward model matches the intended outcome, but not the observed outcome, then external inferences must have occurred. If something went wrong with this mechanism, it might happen that mismatches between expected and observed sensory outcome would occur in the absence of external influences. In this case internally generated events could be misperceived as arising from external influences" (Frith 1996, p. 1507; see also Frith 1992). In terms of motor behavior this could lead to the well-known delusions of control, to the loss of *bodily agency*. However, if applied to the process of motor *simulation* necessarily preceding the generation of overt or covert speech, it is well conceivable how auditory hallucinations might emerge.

It is conceivable, then, how mismatches in unconscious processes of self-simulation and self-representation could prevent the integration of phenomenal content into the conscious self-model. Still, as mentioned earlier, the greatest persisting theoretical problem seems to be the presentational, the *sensory* character of the auditory simulations activated and transparently depicted as a part of external reality. There may, however, be a simple solution to this problem, in terms of a generally elevated internal level of arousal in certain brain regions caused by disinhibitory mechanisms. The explanatory strategy for the additional generation of phenomenal presentational content would then be parallel to that applied with regard to dreams and other hallucinations (see sections 4.2.4 and 4.2.5): the system is confronted with a strong internal source of input and has no chance to detect this situation as such.

Let us look at the third type of deficit traditionally associated with schizophrenia, namely, *delusions of external control*. According to the model proposed here delusions of external control *necessarily* arise if the volitional acts preceding external motor behavior of the patient are not integrated into a PSM anymore. There will be no transparent model of the selection process available on the level of conscious experience. In those situations, motor intentions are correctly being carried out, even if the patient is asked by another person to do them, but they cannot be experienced as such. A typical autophenomenological report will be: "I intended to act, but *before* I could choose a specific action, it was already being carried out for me." Both the intention—an abstract goal representation—and a successful action—the causal coupling of a motor simulation to the effectors—do exist, but no representation of the volitional act itself—the selection of a specific possible behavior, as represented in an egocentric frame of reference (using a PMIR)—is globally available. The neural correlates of this deviating dynamics of internal self-modeling are slowly beginning to emerge. They seem to be related to hyperactivational states in the right inferior parietal lobule (Brodmann area 40) and the cingulate gyrus (cf., e.g., Spence, Brooks, Hirsch, Liddle, Meehan, and Grasby 1997). Interestingly, what in actual scientific practice leads us from a representational analysis of such uncommon classes of states of consciousness to the delineation of physical correlates is first imaging their *functional* correlates. An important aspect of these functional correlates seems to consist in disturbed ways of making the structure of external and internal bodily space available for the system itself and in deficits concerning the internal monitoring of ongoing motor acts. In general, investigating the correlates of different classes of hallucinatory content will be an important methodological aspect of any systematic search for the neural correlates of conscious experience (see Frith, Perry, and Lumer 1999; and ffytche and Howard 1999 for interesting examples).

Let us now return to the representational level of analysis. Delusions of external control appear if the volitional act preceding the motor behavior of the patient cannot be integrated into the PSM anymore. Therefore, related aspects of the PMIR disappear as well. In attempting to find out what event preceding the events of movement displayed by the bodily self-model could have functioned as their *cause*, the system now has to take an educated guess, as it were, at potential components of external reality. The attribution of such intentions to an external person, visible or invisible, may plausibly be interpreted as a confabulatory reaction of the brain, still desperately trying to maximize the overall coherence of its model of reality. The advantage in attributing causality to another *person* is obvious. In those cases where another person is experienced as the cause of one's own bodily behavior, this may simply be the most economical way to still represent such actions as being caused by *mental* events, that is, to preserve a personal-level representation of such events. Personal-level representations are representations under a PMIR. Let me explain.

We have already discussed how Cartesian dualism is an intuitively attractive philosophical position to beings like ourselves, because its ontology is mirrored in the representational architecture of the human self-model (more about this in section 8.2). The question was: How does a human brain manage to integrate nonspatial, cognitive contents into a self-model that, for reasons of its evolutionary history, is spatially coded? There now is a variation of this problem relevant to the theoretical analysis of schizophrenia: How does a *schizophrenic* human brain manage to nevertheless integrate nonspatial, cognitive contents into its globally available model of reality—contents that can, for functional reasons, not be integrated into the current PSM and, a fortiori, not into a *PMIR* of some sort or other? My hypothesis is that attributing it to another *person* is the most cost-efficient solution to the problem, because it preserves the functional status of the content in question *as an object component of a PMIR*. If the content must be globalized—that is, as part of the *world*—but cannot be modeled under a PSM—that is, as part of the *self*—what would be the most economical solution?

The phenomenological constraint of frequent *personal-level misattributions* draws our attention to a second and equally fundamental computational problem, which every system possessing a self-model, in part driven by social correlates (see section 6.3.3), has to solve. In any system able to recognize the behavior of conspecifics or other sentient beings in its environment as driven by goals and intentions, that is, of mentally representing such behavior as an *action*, the problem of correct attribution arises: Multiple action representations simultaneously active within must be correctly associated with the agent actually causing them (see Jeannerod 1999). A number of recent empirical studies indicate that the conscious representation of an action does not depend on the same kind of information used in automatic execution. Action-relative information is coded on at least two different levels in the human brain, one of which is not globally available. In particular, schizophrenic subjects are unable to consciously monitor the internal signals generated by their own movements (see Georgieff and Jeannerod 1998, p. 469). The ability to distinguish between first-person movements and third-person movements does not possess a *direct* functional link to the phenomenal level of presentation. Such internally generated action representations are primarily based on proprioceptive signals, with the differentiation between the self-caused and non–self-caused changes in external objects being dependent on such endogenous signals. However, the differentiation itself is not made in accessing phenomenally available information. The "judgment" about agency, the subpersonal process of nonphenomenal self-modeling, is in this way not carried out in accessing phenomenally available information.

Judgments about agency from a first-person perspective rest on the state of a comparator module, which compares results of actions perceived as external with internally available signals. However, these signals as such cannot be consciously experienced. What is consciously available is the global state of the comparator module. The interesting hypothesis arrived at by Georgieff and Jeannerod (1998, p. 473*ff.*) is that there may be a specific class of hallucinatory phenomenal states, namely, "actions without an agent." The verbal and sensory hallucinations experienced by schizophrenics, according to this new line of thought, should not be considered as perceptual content without a corresponding object, but as action representations without an *agent*. According to the model proposed here, they are free-floating object components not bound into the PMIR. Therefore, in beings possessing theory-of-mind capacities like ourselves, they can only be bound into a PMIR modeled *as external*. They become object components of a transparently modeled *second-person* perspective, sometimes complemented by an imperceptible subject component (as in the untranscendably real experience of a spirit sending you his thoughts or talking to you). That, I propose, is the most economical answer to our original question: If the content must be globalized—that is, as part of the *world*—but cannot be modeled under a PSM—that is, as part of the *self*—what would be the most economical solution? The solution is to integrate it into *another* self by constructing a suitable PMIR portrayed as being a part of *external* reality. Obviously, delusions of alien control might be analyzed in accordance with a similar strategy (namely, by differentiating between the practical and the theoretical PMIR, as discussed in section 6.5), and, given that cognitive processes are fundamentally anchored in motor behavior as well (see section 6.3.3), the well-known phenomena of thought insertion in schizophrenia could plausibly be investigated along these lines as well.[8] Another, related, way of looking at these data consists in positing a

8. Georgieff and Jeannerod write: "This implies that self-consciousness does not rely on discriminating between central signals and sensory reafferences (an explanation put forward by Frith, 1992), but on discriminating between central representations activated from within and those activated by external agents. Delusion of alien control and hallucinations are better explained as a dysfunction of mechanism of interaction between the self and the other, itself based on a proper monitoring of the shared representations. . . . Activation of those areas

circumscribed, functionally encapsulated neural module for "theory-of-mind" tasks, of which it is then well conceivable that it suffers from functional dedifferentiation (see, in particular, Daprati et al. 1997; Frith 1996; for a detailed philosophical interpretation of empirical data, see also Proust 2000).[9]

What recent research on schizophrenia illustrates is how a conscious self-model is important in enabling a system to represent itself *to* itself as an agent. In addition, it now becomes particularly obvious how the process of self-modeling also is a process of self-*constructing*. If you are no longer able to consciously experience yourself as an agent, you lose, as a schizophrenic patient typically does, a lot of the functional properties typically associated with *being* an agent. The ability of being aware that a certain external bodily behavior not only originated *in* you but also in a conscious process of *selecting* a possible action is a vital step in achieving *coherence* of external behavior. A conscious self-model serves to transform a behaving system into an agent. An agent in the true sense, then, is a system that not only possesses a flexible behavioral repertoire but is also *aware* of this very fact, that is, this information is once more globally available *for* the system itself. Behavioral flexibility represented under a PSM creates selectivity, and selectivity is the beginning of agency—arguably even of personhood. To give an example, this information can now for the first time be used in generating second-order volitions (e.g., for *not* wanting to *want* something), and the system as a whole thereby fulfills one of the most important traditional conditions of personhood (Frankfurt 1971). If our system additionally possesses the physical and representational resources to activate abstract, allocentric representations of actions and action goals, it also possesses the most important building blocks for language acquisition and social cognition (see Gallese 2000). In short, a representational analysis of cognitive, volitional, and of *inter*subjectivity is possible. The relevance of case studies from cognitive neuropsychiatry consists in the fact that they allow for "reverse engineering": If we can develop an empirically plausible representationalist analysis of identity disorders, we will automatically arrive at a better understanding of what precisely it means to consciously *be someone* in standard situations.

Two further types of identity disorders are of direct philosophical relevance: specific forms of DM, and Cotard's syndrome. Let us begin with *reverse intermetamorphosis*, usually defined as "the belief that there has been a physical and psychological change of

---

which overlap during a self-produced and an observed action (and, therefore, which is common to several individuals) would be interpreted as an observed action; by contrast, activation of nonoverlapping areas would be interpreted as a self-produced action" (Georgieff and Jeannerod 1998, p. 474*f*.).

9. See also Frith (1996, p. 1509), who points out that attributions of voices to external *agents* are more strongly correlated with current delusions than with actually occurring hallucinations. Hence, they are in some sense independent of the tendency to simply represent self-generated events as external on the level of phenomenal experience.

oneself into another person" (Breen, Caine, Coltheart, Hendy, and Roberts 2000, p. 75). As usual, I will argue that this kind of disorder rests on a deviant form of phenomenal self-modeling, and that in principle it could also occur in a nonlinguistic, noncognitive creature unable to form anything like "beliefs" in the more narrow philosophical sense. Here is a brief excerpt from a recent case study on a patient Roslyn Z, conducted by Nora Breen and colleagues:

RZ, a 40-year-old woman, had the delusional belief that she was a man. This had been a stable delusion for two months prior to our assessment with RZ. During most of that two months she believed that she was her father, but occasionally she would state that she was her grandfather. At the time we saw RZ, she had taken on the persona of her father. She would only respond to her father's name, and she signed his name when asked to sign any forms. She consistently gave her father's history when questioned about her personal history. For example, she said she was in her 60s. . . . The following excerpts are from an interview with RZ. Throughout the interview RZ's mother, Lil, was sitting beside her.

Examiner: Could you tell me your name?

RZ: Douglas.

Examiner: And your surname?

RZ: B____.

Examiner: And how old are you?

RZ: I don't remember.

Examiner: Roughly how old are you?

RZ: Sixty-something.

Examiner: Sixty-something. And are you married?

RZ: No.

Examiner: No. Have you been married?

RZ: Yes.

Examiner: What was your partner's name?

RZ: I don't remember. Lil.

Examiner: Lil. And you have children?

RZ: Four.

Examiner: And what are their names?

RZ: Roslyn, Beverly, Sharon, Greg. . . .

RZ standing in front of a mirror looking at her own reflection.

Examiner: When you look in the mirror there, who do you see?

RZ: Dougie B____ (*her father's name*).

Examiner: What does the reflection look like?

RZ: His hair is a mess, he has a beard and a moustache and his eyes are all droopy.

Examiner: So is that a man or a woman?

RZ: A man.

Examiner: How old is Dougie?

RZ: Sixty-something.

Examiner: And does that reflection you are looking at now look like a sixty-something person?

RZ: Yes.

Examiner: It looks that old does it?

RZ: Yes.

Examiner: Do you think that a sixty-something year old man would have grey hair?

RZ: Well, I haven't worried a lot over the years so my hair didn't go grey.

Examiner: So it's not grey?

RZ: No. It's brown.

(Breen et al. 2000, pp. 94*f*., 98*f*.).

Reverse intermetamorphosis is of philosophical relevance because it challenges the Wittgenstein-Shoemaker principle of immunity to error through misidentification (Wittgenstein 1953, p. 67; Shoemaker 1968). Very obviously there are cases of phenomenal self-representation, of the phenomenal representation of one's own *personal identity* in particular, which are misrepresentations. Misidentification is a symptom rather than a syndrome comprising a stable collection of symptoms, and the particular variety of self-misidentification is closely associated with severe psychotic states (Förstl, Almeida, Owen, Burns, and Howard 1991, p. 908*f*.). To what extent they can count as discrete diagnostic categories is still controversial. However, as this issue was one of the guiding questions formulated in chapter 1, I return to it in section 8.2 in chapter 8.

Finally, a second and last type of identity disorder must be discussed, because it is of particular theoretical relevance. This disorder is what I would call *existence denial*. In the year 1880 the French neurologist Jules Cotard introduced the term *délire de négation* to refer to a specific kind of "nihilistic" delusion, the central defining characteristic of which consists in the fact that patients deny their own existence, and frequently even that of the external world (see Cotard 1880; for a more detailed account, see Cotard 1882). From 1897 onward this condition was referred to as "Cotard's syndrome" in the scientific literature (Séglas 1897; for a concise review of the literature, see Enoch and Trethowan 1991, p. 163*ff*.). Although there still is considerable discussion about the notion of a delusion as such (see, e.g., Young 1999) and about the conceptual status of "pathological" belief systems (see Coltheart and Davies 2000; Halligan and Marshall 1996), most researchers tend to agree that Cotard's syndrome is likely a distinct entity.[10] However, here I will simply treat it as a neurophenomenological state class characterized by a specific form of deviant self-modeling, without entering into any further empirical speculations.

As a delusion, Cotard's syndrome is certainly dramatic; for instance, it violates the global logical coherence of the patient's "web of belief" (see Young 1999, p. 582*f.*) and simply *ends* biographical coherence, while exhibiting more or less modularized damage to the cognitive model of reality to which the patient has conscious access. Cotard's syndrome is a *monothematic* disorder (Davies, Coltheart, Langdon, und Breen 2001). As in many delusions, it is the rather isolated nature of a specific belief content that intially raises serious doubts about the patient's status as a rational subject. However, as a closer look at the data will reveal, a Cotard's syndrome patient may count as a rational subject in developing the only possible conclusion from a dramatic shift in his subcognitive PSM. A promising attempt toward a testable and conceptually convincing hypothesis may therefore start from the assumption that the disorder is simply a modularized, cognitive-level reaction to very uncommon perceptual experience (Young and Leafhead 1996). It must be clearly noted, though, that the phenomenology of firmly believing in one's own non-existence may also turn out to be too intricate and complex to be tractable to classic belief-desire approaches; for instance, because it decisively involves a pathology in *nonpropositional* levels of phenomenal self-representation.

Obviously, any good future philosophical theory of mind should be able to incorporate the "existence denial" exhibited by Cotard's subjects as an important phenomenological constraint, one to be satisfied by its own conceptual proposals. When considering anosognosia in the opening section of this chapter we saw that there actually exist a whole range of neurological disorders characterized by an unawareness of specific deficits following brain injuries, all of them falsifying the Cartesian notion of epistemic transparency in association with phenomenal self-consciousness. In pure and extreme versions of Cotard's syndrome we are confronted with a generalized version of this representational configuration: Patients may explicitly state not only that they are dead but also that they don't *exist* at all. In other words, something that seems an a priori impossibility on logical grounds—a conscious subject truthfully denying its own existence—turns out to be a phenomenological reality. And phenomenology has to be taken seriously. In this case the first lesson to be drawn is this: You can be fully conscious, in terms of satisfying *constraints 2, 3, 4, 5, 6, 7, 8, 9* and *10*, and possibly even in terms of possessing a full-blown PSM as well as

10. Young and Leafhead (1996, p. 154) argue that there is no specific symptom shown by every pure case of Cotard's syndrome, whereas Berrios and Luque (1995) offer a statistical analysis of historical clinical usage of the term, concluding that a pure Cotard's syndrome (represented by "Cotard type 1" patients) does exist, and that its nosological origin "is in the delusional and not in the affective disorders . . ." (ibid., p. 187). I will not take a position on this issue here.

a PMIR, and still truthfully describe the content of your own phenomenal self-experience as "nonexistence." In other words, there are actual, nomologically possible representational configurations in the human brain, which lead truthful subjects into logically incoherent autophenomenological reports. In section 6.4.4 in chapter 6, when discussing cognitive subjectivity as a challenge to naturalism, I offered a representationalist analysis of the Cartesian thought:

[I am certain, that I* exist.]

In extreme forms of Cotard's syndrome, we are faced with a delusional belief that can be expressed as follows:

[I am certain, that I* do not exist.]

Weaker forms are delusional beliefs that can be expressed as follows:

[I am certain, that I* am dead.]

What is the phenomenological landscape of Cotard's syndrome? A recent analysis of 100 cases (Berrios and Luque 1995; see figure 2, p. 186) points out that severe depression was reported in 89% of the subjects, with the most frequent forms of "nihilistic delusion" concerning the body (86%) and existence as such (69%). Other very common features of the reported content of the PSM in these patients were anxiety (65%), guilt (63%), hypochondriacal delusions (58%), and, even more surprising, delusions of immortality (55%; see Berrios and Luque 1995, p. 187). In many cases, certain elements of the bodily self-model seem to have disappeared, or at least to have become attentionally unavailable. For instance, one 59-year-old patient would say, "I have no blood" (Enoch and Trethowan 1991, case 5, p. 172); another would say, "I used to have a heart. I have something which beats in its place." (ibid., p. 173), while a further case study (Ahleid 1968, quoted in Enoch and Trethowan 1991, p. 165) reports a patient asking "to be buried because he said he was 'a corpse which already stinks.' A month later he said that he had no flesh and no legs or trunk. These ideas were unshakeable, so that the clinical picture remained unchanged for months." Such early stages frequently proceed to states in which the body as a whole is denied, and the patient feels like a "living corpse," for example, when saying "I am no longer alive"; "I am dead" (Enoch and Trethowan 1991, case 1, p. 168) or stating, "I have no body, I am dead" (ibid., case 2, p. 168) or, like Young and Leafhead's patient W.I. (Young and Leafhead 1996; see also Young, Robertson Hellawell, de Pauw, and Pentland 1992), simply being convinced that he was dead for some months after a motorcycle accident (involving contusions in the right hemisphere temporoparietal area and bilateral frontal damage), with this belief then gradually resolving over time.

Interestingly, there are a number of other phenomenological state classes in which a person may experience herself as bodiless or disembodied—ranging from cases like Christina's to certain types of out-of-body experiences (OBEs) and lucid dreams (see sections 7.2.3 and 7.2.5). What seems unique about Cotard's syndrome is the additional belief that one is dead. The patient, on the level of his *cognitive* self-model acquires a new, consciously available content—and this content is specific in being highly irrational and functionally immune to rational revision. The difference in the phenomenal content in the transparent and *subcognitive* layers of his self-model can be aptly described by employing a traditional conceptual distinction, which is available in the German language, but not in Greek (e.g., Homer only uses *soma* as referring to corpses), Latin (with *corpus* only referring to the body-as-thing, being the etymological root of the English term "corpse"), or widely spoken languages such as Italian, French, Spanish, and English. The Cotard's patient has a bodily self-model as a *Körper*, but not as a *Leib* (see also Ahleid 1968; Enoch and Trethowan 1991, p. 179*f.*). What is the difference? A *Leib* is a *lived body*, one that is connected to a soul, or, in more modern parlance, the body *as subject*, as the locus of an individual first-person perspective. The body *as inanimate object*, on the other hand, is what the PSM in the Cotard's syndrome configuration depicts. This patient has access to a *Körper*-model, but not a *Leib*-model.

It is interesting to note how one can arrive at a better understanding of the underlying neurophenomenological state class by simply following the traditional line of thought. What kind of loss could make a *Leib*-model a representation of something inanimate, of something that is no longer tied to the inner logic of life? If the logic of survival is, as discussed extensively above, made globally available by conscious emotions, then a complete loss of the *emotional* self-model should have precisely this effect. Philosophically speaking, this would mean that what the Cotard's patient claiming to be a dead corpse is truthfully referring to is the transparent content of his self-model, predominantly concerning the spatial, proprioceptive, and emotional layers. This content portrays a moving *res extensa*, from the inside, closely resembling a living human person, but, as a matter of phenomenal fact, not tied to the logic of survival anymore. In traditional terminology, the patient has a belief *de se*. Since the first-order, nonconceptual self-representational content grounding this belief, in the most literal sense possible, simply no longer *contains* the information that actual elementary bioregulation is still going on, and there is no longer any subjective representation of the current degree of satisfaction of the adaptivity constraint (see section 3.2.11), and the emotions are completely flattened out, the patient forms a hypothesis. This hypothesis, given his current internal sources of information, is absolutely coherent: he must be a dead object resembling a human being. The existence of this object, although experienced as the origin of a PMIR, does not affectively *matter* to the patient in any way. As Philip Gerrans (Gerrans 2000, p. 112) writes: "The Cotard delusion, in its extreme form, is a rationalization of a feeling of disembodiment based on global suppression of affect resulting from extreme depression." Many Cotard's patients make utterances like "I have no feelings" (Enoch and Trethowan 1991, case 4, p. 171) or, like Young and Leafhead's patient K.H. (Young and Leafhead 1996), state that they are dead as a result of "feeling nothing inside." If it is the conscious self-model which, as previously claimed, mediates embodiment not only on the phenomenal but also on the functional level, then these patients suffer from functional deficits, because they are, due to a severe impairment in their PSM, emotionally disembodied. It is a specific subset of system-related information, which cannot be made globally available anymore. This fact triggers further changes on the cognitive level of self-modeling.

As Gerrans (1999, p. 590) has pointed out, on the level of representational content Cotard's syndrome may be miscategorized if described as a DM. At least in its weaker forms, the Cotard's patient reports truthfully about the content of a very unusual PSM. This unusual PSM results from a globalized loss of affect, Gerrans argues, mirroring the *global* distribution of the neurochemical substrate that causes the actual deficit, which in turn is then cognitively interpreted. The issue is to first explain how such a PSM could actually come about. Classic belief-desire psychology and a traditional philosophical analysis in terms of propositional attitudes, however, may not be helpful in bridging the levels of description necessary to arrive at a fuller understanding of the target phenomenon. For instance, it seems plausible that a nonlinguistic creature like a monkey could suffer from most of the Cotard's phenomenology, without being able to utter incoherent autophenomenological reports. An animal could *feel* dead and emotionally disembodied, without possessing the capacity to self-ascribe this very fact to itself linguistically or on the level of cognitive self-reference. What is special about the human case is that an isolated, and functionally rigid new element on the level of the cognitive self-model is formed. As soon as we arrive at a convincing representational and functional analysis of the human Cotard's patient's self-model, we can proceed to the philosophical issue of whether it is possible to exhibit strong first-person phenomena in Lynne Baker's (1998) sense, while simultaneously entertaining the belief that one actually doesn't exist at all. I return to this issue later.

Cotard's syndrome may be analyzed as a combination of loss of a whole layer of nonconceptual, transparent content and a corresponding appearance of new, quasi-conceptual and opaque content in the patient's PSM. Is there a more specific way of describing the causal role of the information now no longer available on the level of the patient's phenomenal model of reality? What *triggers* the massive restructurization of his "web of belief?" A second, and more specific hypothesis, may be the "emotional disembodiment" conjecture: The PSM of the Cotard's patient is emptied of all emotional content, making it, in particular, impossible to consciously experience *familiarity* with himself. What the patient loses may be precisely the phenomenal quality of "prereflexive self-intimacy" already mentioned. The patient is not infinitely close to herself, but infinitely distant. If, in addition, it is true that emotional content, generally speaking, represents the logic of survival to an organism, then *self-representational* emotional content, in particular, will represent the internal logic of autonomic self-regulation, of its *own* life process to this organism. For this patient, the logic of survival has been suspended: His life process— although functionally unfolding as still continuously realized in the physical body—is not *owned* anymore, by being represented under a PSM. His life process is not only not his own anymore, it may not even be part of his phenomenal *reality* anymore, depending on the severity of the degree of psychotic depression. Nor is the fact that autonomous self-regulation, a continuous bodily process aimed at self preservation, is going on is not a globally available fact; therefore this fact is no longer a part of the patient's reality. The dynamic process of self-modeling is, as noted above, a process of *self-containing*. A Cotard's patient may therefore be described as a living, self-representing system that cannot self-contain the fact that it actually is a *living* system anymore.

However, there is more to Cotard's syndrome than emotional disembodiment, leading to a persistent false belief via the principle of phenomenal self-reference (i.e., *all* cognitive self-reference ultimately can only refer to the content of the currently conscious self-model). Claiming to be dead—in terms of a dead *body*—is not the same as claiming to be *nonexistent*. Enoch and Trethowan write:

Subsequently the subject may proceed to deny her very existence, even dispensing altogether with the use of the personal pronoun "I." One patient even called herself "Madam Zero" in order to emphasize her non-existence. One of Anderson's patients said, referring to herself, "It's no use. Wrap it up and throw 'it' in the dustbin" [referring to Anderson 1964]. . . .
If the delusion becomes completely *encapsulated*, the subject may even be able to assume a jovial mood and to engage in a philosophical discussion about her own existence or non-existence. (Enoch and Trethowan 1991, pp. 173, 175)

To my knowledge there is only one other phenomenal state class in which speakers sometimes consistently refer to themselves without using the pronoun "I," namely, during prolonged mystical or spiritual experiences. What seems to be common to both classes is that the phenomenal property of selfhood is not instantiated any more, while a coherent model of reality as such is still in existence. However, a Cotard's patient may express his dramatic and generalized emotional experience of unfamiliarity by even denying the existence of reality as a whole. The phenomenon of explicit existence denial cannot be ignored, because on the level of explicitly negated content, it is the second most common representational feature of Cotard's syndrome, to be found in 69% of the cases (Berrios and Luque 1995, p. 187). Therefore, the pivotal question is, What kind of neurophenomenological configuration could lead a human being into (a) denying his or her own existence, and (b) stop using the personal pronoun "I" (or "I*" for that matter; see section 6.4.4)?

Let us begin by considering the first issue. The conscious representation of existence is coded via phenomenal transparency, as explained in sections 3.2.7 and 6.2.6. Phenomenally, we are beings experiencing the content of a certain active representations as *real* if and only if earlier processing stages of this representation are attentionally unavailable to us. This leads to the prediction that if a human being's self-model became fully opaque, then this person would experience herself as nonexistent—the phenomenal property of selfhood would not be instantiated anymore. The subject component of such a being's PMIR would be fully opaque, and only continue to function as the origin of its first-person perspective for *functional* reasons, due to the ongoing source of continuous input making it the *functional* center of its representational space. As there would be no phenomenal *self as subject*, such a system would not have a PSM in the true sense of the term, and its PMIR, strictly speaking, would only instantiate a functional, but not a *phenomenal*, first-person perspective anymore. I take this to be the natural explanation for the prolonged spiritual and mystical experiences mentioned above, but will not pursue this line of thought any further here. The second logical possibility is that in extreme Cotard's configurations existence is denied because there is no longer a PSM in existence. This is empirically implausible, because Cotard's patients certainly exhibit a high degree of sensorimotor integration, of coherent speech, and so forth; they certainly are not comatose or in deep sleep.

The third possibility, then, is that a transparent, conscious self-model is in place, but it is not a *subject*-model anymore, only an *object*-model. Something still exists, something that looks like the model of a person, but something that is utterly unfamiliar, not alive, and not a phenomenal self in the act of living, perceiving, attending, and thinking. The PSM has lost the emotional layer. The PMIR in such a case would not be a model of a subject-object relation, but only one of an object-object relation. It would not constitute a phenomenal *first-person* perspective, but rather a *first-object* perspective. The "first object," for purely functional reasons, persists as the invariant center of reality, because it is tied to an invariant source of internally generated input. Phenomenally, this functional center is the place where things happen, but all of them—as well as the center itself—are not *owned*. The phenomenal property of "mineness" has disappeared from the patient's reality. As Philip Gerrans (2000) puts it:

In this type of case the patient conceives of herself as nothing more than a locus, not of experience—because, due to the complete suppression of affect, her perceptions and cognitions are not annexed to her body—but of the registration of the passage of events. (p. 118)

Let us now proceed to the second issue: Why would such a system stop using the pronoun "I" when referring to itself? The answer to this question would have to explain the phenomenon for two different phenomenal state classes: spiritual experiences and Cotard's syndrome. In both cases, the system still operates under a functionally centered model of reality. Motor control, attentional processing, and cognitive availability are in place, and in principle well integrated. Sensorimotor integration is successfully achieved. In both cases, the subject component of the PMIR is no longer a *subject* component on the level of phenomenal experience. Phenomenologically, both state classes are constituted by *subjectless* models of reality. On the representational level of analysis we find that there is no globally available representation of a *self as subject*. We currently know very little about the minimally sufficient neural correlates of both types of states, but it is plausible to assume that the etiologies are markedly different: In one state class it is a considerable elevation in the degree of attentional availability for earlier stages of processing contributing to the system-model; in the second state class it is a loss of a particular layer, namely, the emotional layer, which transforms a subject-model into an object-model, turning a first-person state into a "first-object" state. If this description points in the right direction, we can give a new answer to the old philosophical question of what the personal pronoun "refers" to. "I*" inevitably refers to a specific form of phenomenal mental content: to the transparent, *subcognitive* partition of the currently active PSM depicting the speaker *as subject*. If this partition is lost or becomes opaque, then speakers will stop using "I*." I return to this issue in the second section of chapter 8.

7.2.3 Hallucinated Selves

A hallucinated self is a transparent self-model which integrates mental content that, in essential aspects and to a considerable degree, is *only* phenomenal content, and not intentional content. Therefore, it *misrepresents* the current state of the system *to* the system. It is not self-knowledge, but pure phenomenal character. As we have seen earlier, there is a naturalist version of Descartes's argument concerning the certainty of his own existence: As long as a coherent self-model is active and globally available, we have to assume that *some* kind of physical system exists which generates the model. This is, from a third-person perspective, simply "built in" as a central theoretical background assumption of naturalistic versions of representationalism. Interestingly, there is another "built in" aspect, but this time it concerns the functional architecture underlying the phenomenology of selfhood itself: From a first-person perspective, this assumption has been hardwired into our brains by the sheer transparency of the PSM. There is something resembling an "existential quantifier" which, as it were, is displayed in a nonpropositional format by the most invariant and fully transparent partitions of the self-model (see section

5.4). It results from the attentional unavailability of earlier processing stages and is reflected in the naive realism characterizing noncognitive forms of phenomenal self-consciousness.

Please remember that one of the central metaphysical claims guiding this investigation is that no such things as selves exist in the world. All that, in an ontological sense, does exist are certain classes of information-processing systems operating under transparent self-models. For these systems, having such a self-model is just a new way of having access to themselves. Therefore *all* selves are either hallucinated (phenomenologically), or elements of inaccurate, reificatory phenomenological descriptions. However, what is untranscendable, in standard situations (for a potential exception, see Cotard's syndrome discussed earlier), is the experience of actually *existing* right now. And given our background assumptions, this trivially will also inevitably be the case. All other content properties realized by the currently active self-model may in principle be entirely *phenomenal* properties and not carry any information about the real status of the system. This is not only true of simple bodily sensations, of emotional or cognitive mental content, but also of the way the system phenomenally situates itself in time and space. Furthermore, the *integrated* nature of all those properties depicted in the mode of self-representation, can, in principle, be a fiction: we can imagine a physical system consisting of widely distributed sensors and effectors, integrating information across vast distances into an entirely false, empty self-model of a system possessing one, unified body with all its sensory organs and effectors localized in a single region of physical space. The minimally sufficient neural correlate of a conscious self-model could not only be realized by a single brain in a vat but, given efficient media of information transmission, also by single parts of this brain in multiple vats in multiple laboratories scattered across the globe—given that what elsewhere I have called the problem of "highest-order binding" (see Metzinger 1995c) is solved. But as long as we hold on to a realist ontology, it will always remain true that *some* kind of physical system giving rise to the currently hallucinated self does exist. Again, it is important to note how the notion of a "hallucinated self" is not a contradiction in terms: what the hallucination is attributed to is not a conscious Cartesian ego, but simply the physical system as a whole. Just as it can generate a selfless phenomenal model of reality, the physical system as a whole can also hallucinate a self.

Speaking of the possibility of hallucinated selves it is interesting to remember a conceptual distinction I introduced in section 4.2.4. There may be partially opaque hallucinated selves and fully transparent hallucinated selves. There are pseudohallucinations and complex hallucinations. A partially opaque hallucinated self will be one for which the information that a certain partition is actually a subsymbolic, nontheoretical (mis)*repre-*

sentation of the system's own current reality is still globally available, for example, for conscious cognition.[11]

Our first example, phantom limbs, can serve as a typical example. It also highlights the difference between cognitive and attentional opacity. Patients suffering from phantom limbs know that these limbs are not real. The phenomenal sense of ownership is given, as is the cognitive availability of the *misrepresentational* nature of their experiential content. What is not given is the *attentional* availability of earlier processing stages. To do justice to this phenomenological constraint, we could modify our tool kit slightly, by saying that *two* kinds of phenomenal transparency exist. Phantom limbs now are *cognitively* opaque parts of the PSM. However, there are also complex and fully transparent hallucinated selves, as in seriously deluded patients. Complex hallucinations are cognitively *and* attentionally transparent, whereas pseudohallucinations are at least *cognitively* opaque, and even in some cases characterized by the additional *attentional* availability of earlier processing stages (recall the abstract geometrical patterns of certain visual hallucinations discussed in section 4.2.4). If this conceptual distinction is correct, the empirical prediction is that there should be cases of phantom limbs accompanied by anosognosia (the inability to notice a current deficit; see section 7.2.1), leading even a normal phantom limb patient into a fully expressed delusionary state making him believe that the amputated limb *actually* is still in existence. As it turns out, there seem to be rare cases of combined double lesions following accidents, which lead to precisely this neurophenomenological configuration.

For instance, Ramachandran and Hirstein (1998) report one patient D.S. "who lost his left arm in a car accident, and also had bilateral frontal lesions, not only felt a phantom arm as expected but actually insisted that he could still see it and that it had not been removed, even though he was mentally quite lucid in other respects" (p. 1624). To this patient the mis*representational* character of his "supernumerary" limb experience was neither attentionally nor cognitively available. He could therefore be described as suffering from only a partial, but fully transparent and therefore *complex* self-hallucination. Our theory also predicts that cognitive and attentional availability of a deficit must be dissociable for hallucinated selves. It is interesting to note that there are other cases of supernumerary limb experiences in the true sense of the term, in which no degree of confusion or delusion whatsoever is present (cognitive availability) while, for instance, two *additional* lower limbs are experienced as existing in a fully realistic manner (attentional unavailability of earlier processing stages). They are transparently represented parts of a

---

11. Please note that if the same information becomes *attentionally* available, the respective content would become fully opaque, making the phenomenal property of selfhood disappear. Then there would be no hallucinated *self* anymore.

*pseudo*self-hallucination (for case studies, see Vuilleumier, Reverdin, and Landis 1997; Halligan and Marshall 1995). However, there are many other reasons making the phenomenon of phantom limbs particularly interesting in fleshing out the current theory on the level of empirical constraints. The conscious self-model of human beings consists of a spatial, geometrical component and of nonspatial, more cognitive-type forms of content. Phantom limbs clearly are hallucinated parts of geometrical self-models.

Phantom Limbs in Postamputation and Aplasia Patients

Phantom limb phenomena constitute a distinct class of phenomenal states. They consist in the conscious experience of a body part that is nonexistent. Phantom limb experiences are typically reported after amputation of an arm or a leg and between 90% and 98% of all postamputation patients experience a vivid phantom (for a comprehensive review, see Ramachandran and Hirstein 1998, p. 1605*ff.*). Phantom experiences are also reported following amputation of the breast, parts of the face, or even of viscera. Phantom "ulcer pains" following partial gastrectomy have been reported, as well as phantom erections in patients who have had their penis removed, and Ramachandran and Hirstein even reported female patients with phantom menstrual cramps after hysterectomy (for references, see Ramachandran and Hirstein 1998; for a number of popular case studies, see Ramachandran 1998). Phantom limb experiences are fully transparent on the level of attentional processing, and their sometimes ultrarealistic character frequently leads amputees to attempts to use the limb. Postamputation phantom experiences will in 79% of cases appear immediately after the anesthetic wears off and the patient regains conscious experience, whereas in other patients it may be delayed for a couple of days or weeks. Typically, the conscious experience of a nonexistent limb will persist for a number of days or weeks, with the respective part of the PSM then gradually reorganizing itself and disappearing from the overall conscious model of reality. However, there are also reports of phantom limbs persisting for many decades.

An important aspect of the clinical relevance of phantom limb experiences is to be found in the fact that they are frequently accompanied by the subjective experience of pain in the hallucinated limb (for a comprehensive review, see Hill 1999). Descartes knew about this phenomenon when, in the seventh section of the *Sixth Meditation*, he wrote about the unreliability of even what he took to be the most *internal* form of sensory perception: "And yet I have sometimes been informed by parties whose arm or leg had been amputated, that they still occasionally seemed to feel pain in that part of the body which they had lost,—a circumstance that led me to think that I could not be quite certain even that any one of my members was affected when I felt pain in it." The simple subjective "qualities" of pain experiences integrated by the phantom limb—the nociceptive presentational content now not correlated with the original stimulus anymore—is sometimes described as a mild tingling or tightness, or more typically as "pins and needles" (Hill 1999, p. 128).

Other presentational subformats present in the phenomenology are touch, temperature, pressure, and itch. If the quasi-sensory phenomenal content integrated by the phantom limb is painful, patients frequently describe it as "burning" and "cramping." Hill reports that a phantom limb is also frequently described as "numb," "smarting," "stinging," "scrubbing," "piercing," and "tearing" (for further references, see Hill 1999, p. 130). The *posture* of the phantom limb is often habitual, with spontaneous changes being a common phenomenon. A typical example, also reported by Ramachandran and Hirstein, could consist in a patient waking up in the morning, with the phantom limb assuming an unusual and uncomfortable posture, only to return to its habitual posture a few minutes later (Ramachandran and Hirstein 1998, p. 1605). Generally, the volume and shape of a phantom limb experienced immediately after amputation will frequently resemble the way in which the limb was preamputationally modeled on the level of conscious experience. In traumatic losses where the limb was distorted by the accident, the phantom will some-times mirror the position of the limb immediately preceding amputation. Pain experience in a phantom limb frequently resembles preamputation pain not only with regard to the presentational "format" but also with regard to localization. Bailey and Moersch (1941; quoted in Hill 1999, p. 131) presented a case study of a male patient who had undergone amputation 22 years earlier. This patient had an accident that left a painful sliver under his fingernail. His arm was torn off in a machine accident at work 1 week later. The patient experienced pain of *exactly* the same quality and in the same phenomenal localization he experienced when he had the sliver under his fingernail, for a period of 2 years after his accident.

A further important aspect of the phenomenology of phantom limbs, which has pro-vided important clues regarding the underlying neural dynamics, is the so-called tele-scoping effect. Fading phantoms in about 50% of the cases, again typically in those involving upper limbs, do not just disappear from the conscious model of reality, but become progressively shorter. A final stage of this development may consist in a trans-parent, fully realistic experience of a phantom hand dangling from the stump or even the possibility of clenching a fist or feeling individual digits *within* the stump. Such receding parts of the PSM, however, may "pop out" again, for example, if the patient wants to grab a certain object or reaches out to shake a hand. Ramachandran and Hirstein (1998) report a situation where "when we suddenly pulled the cup away, he yelled in pain, claiming that we had wrenched the cup away from his phantom fingers, causing his arm to telescope unexpectedly" (p. 1606).

Particularly intriguing are related observations concerning the perceptual correlates of somatosensory plasticity underlying the reorganization of the bodily self-model in

phantom limb patients over time (see, e.g., Ramachandran 1993). Upon systematically
studying relocalization of touch in a number of postamputation patients by brushing a Q-
tip on various regions of their skin surface, it was discovered that stimuli applied to points
of the body surface which were absolutely remote from the locus of amputation led to
phenomenal sensations *mislocalized* to the phantom arm. Moreover, there was a systematic one-to-one mapping between specific regions of the face and individual digits. For
instance, touching the cheek with a Q-tip would elicit a phenomenal sensation in the
nonexisting thumb, touching the philtrum would activate a sensation in the region modeling the index finger, and brushing over a certain region of the chin would lead to an activation in the part of the PSM representing the fifth or little finger. We return to this specific
example below (see also figure 7.1).

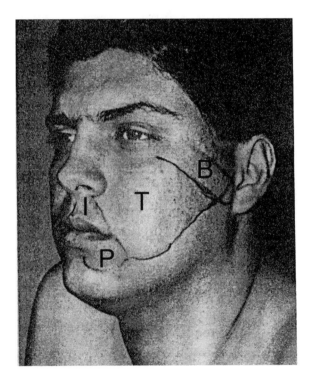

Figure 7.1
Reference fields for hallucinated body parts integrated into the PSM during massive restructurization of
somatosensory cortex. Regions on the left side of the face of patient V.Q. elicited precisely localized referred
sensations in the phantom digits. "Reference fields," regions that evoke referred sensations, were plotted by
brushing a Q-tip repeatedly on the face. The region labeled *T* always evoked sensation in the phantom thumb;
P, in the little finger; *I*, in the index finger; and *B*, in the ball of the thumb. This patient was tested 4 weeks after
amputation. (From Ramachandran 1993.)

These aspects of the phenomenology of the phantom limb experience for the first time vividly illustrate what it means that the bodily model of the self really is a *model*. Given the necessary functional configuration, the human brain will activate a fully transparent model of a bodily self which allows you to feel individual fingers in parts of your face. A part of a hallucinated self can phenomenologically even be *integrated* into a preexisting and a veridical self-model. I briefly return to conclusions about the neural correlate of phenomenal phantoms later. Let me close this first overview of the phenomenology of phantom limbs by pointing out that more complicated configurations than the ones so far described exist. For instance, Lacroix, Melzack, Smith, and Mitchell (1992) documented a case of multiple phantom limbs in a child who developed three *superimposed* phantoms following amputation of a foot and a congenital short leg. All three phantom limbs in this child possess a distinct phenomenological profile: they can be tickled, they are sensitive to heat, and they may vary in degrees of vividness, for instance, when the prosthesis is removed. It is interesting to note that not only do prostheses become integrated into the new self-model in certain cases but also that the users of advanced myoelectric prostheses will suffer less from phantom limb pain—very likely because the prosthesis allows the region of phenomenal or computational state space previously occupied by a model of the organic limb to be "reinvaded" by motor feedback.

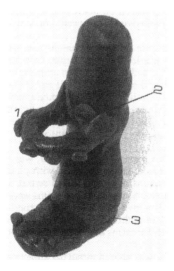

Figure 7.2
Superimposed phantom limbs in a bodily PSM: Clay figure made by K.G. which depicts her three phantoms. Phantom *1* was the first to appear. It has five toes and the edges of the foot are felt but the top and bottom feel absent. Phantom *2* is a set of five toes which are felt at the tip of the stump. Phantom *3* consists of a foot and calf that fill the prosthetic leg. (From Lacroix et al. 1992.)

On the phenomenological level of description phantom limbs seem to constitute a reasonably well-demarcated class of deviant phenomenal models of the self. If one proceeds in analyzing the causal history of such phenomena, it is helpful to differentiate between three different types of etiologies. First, like many other unusual forms of phenomenal content discussed in this book, we are able today to *artificially* activate them by external means. Even many years after loss of input from the physical limb, microstimulation of certain regions in the thalamus with the help of electrodes can re-create sensations in the missing limb (Davis, Kiss, Luo, Tasker, Lozano, and Dostrovsky 1998). Dynamic stimulation in amputees with a phantom limb can activate sensations in the relevant part of the PSM, including pain. Whereas in amputees lacking phantom experiences only sensations on the stump and other nearby areas of the body could be elicited by stimulating the (considerably extended) regions forming the model of the stump in the brain, for phantom patients a functional stereotactic mapping of the ventrocaudal thalamus using microelectrodes activated tingling, unpleasant, or painful sensations integrated into a spatial model of the missing limb. Phantom limbs have also been experimentally induced by using anesthetics to block input from an intact limb (Melzack and Bromage 1973). In this context, it is also interesting to note that phantom limbs that had disappeared or never been active on the phenomenal level of experience before (as in some congenital patients; for a detailed set of case studies, see Melzack et al. 1997) can sometimes "pop out" after a strong stimulation of the stump.

More important, however, the causal histories leading to persistently hallucinated body parts can be further subdivided into those cases where a phantom limb appears following amputation or traumatic loss, and those situations in which phantom experiences appear in *congenitally* limb-deficient persons. Obviously, one of the most relevant issues from a theoretical perspective is constituted by the question if an innate core of the human self-model exists at birth, a more or less rigid functional structure from which phenomenal self-consciousness can later develop. Recent evidence may point toward the plausibility of this hypothesis. However, let us first take a closer look at the standard situation, a situation in which a deviant self-model follows postnatal loss of the relevant physical input site of the body.

I have already described the typical underlying phenomenology of the standard situation of postamputation limb loss. However, there are further phenomenological constraints that have to be imposed on any plausible theory of conscious self-modeling. Phantom patients, almost exclusively, either belong to the group of those who are able to voluntarily control their phantom limbs or to the group of those for whom voluntary control of the phenomenal limb does not exist. Patients in the first group can generate voluntary movements and experience the feedback that is naturally to be expected, for example, when in making a fist or grabbing an object. They may also involuntarily reach for the telephone or attempt to break a fall. However, there is the additional phenomenon of the postamputation "paralyzed" phantom limb. For *these* patients the phantom limb is a rigid, invisible part of their body, which they cannot move. The "virtual" information underlying this hallucinated part of their bodily self is globally available for cognition and for focal attention, but *not* for the control of action. It is interesting to note that almost all of those patients unable to voluntarily move their phantom limbs had to live through a—frequently very traumatic—period of *preamputation* paralysis, while this was not the case for other patients.

I have frequently pointed out that, on the level of functional analysis, a very fruitful way of looking at the spatial model of the bodily self is to interpret it as an internal body *emulator* integrating position- and movement related information into a causally active structure, which can, for instance, enable fast grasping movements. Rick Grush (1998, p. 174) offered a plausible hypothesis for the phenomenon of the volitionally unavailable phantom limb: If what he calls the "skeletomuscular emulator" learns and actualizes its own operation by monitoring activity in the skeletomuscular system, then, during a sufficiently long period of paralysis, it will "learn" that whatever motor command is issued, the result on the level of proprioceptive feedback will *always* be the nonexistence of actual movement. In other words, preoperative paralysis permanently changes the functional structure of the neural substrate underlying the enduring conscious experience of the respective limb in a way that permanently installs a "zero-feedback assumption" in the system.[12] It is as if, during the traumatic experience, immotility is burned into the PSM. What is even more intriguing, however, is that the phenomenon of phantom arm paralysis can be reversible. This fact shows how the human self-model at any given point in time results from the sum of all constraints imposed on the information-processing activity of our brain. Let us therefore look at another case study.

A particularly vivid example of the dependence of the contents of all conscious self-models on perceptual context information has been demonstrated by the intriguing experiments of Ramachandran and colleagues on mirror-induced synesthesia and illusionary movements in phantom limbs (Ramachandran, Rogers-Ramachandran, and Cobb

---

12. It is important to distinguish the no-feedback situation (following normal amputations, and leading to the preservation of volitional availability) from the feedback situation generating the invariant content of [Nothing ever happens!]. It is also interesting to note how one of the strengths of Grush's model of the compensation of feedback delay is that we now have a precise conception of what it would mean to take such an emulator *offline*, thereby generating motor imagery. Imaginary movements are created by disconnecting the premotor layer from the motor output (Cruse 1999). The mental simulation of counterfactual situations in general (see chapter 2) and real-time perceptual processing in particular are other likely applications. An efference copy by itself does not make the overall context in which an action or an ongoing perceptual process takes place globally available to the system as whole, but a conscious self-model already constitutes a *process*-model, that is, an internal representation of the overall control process as a whole.

1995; Ramachandran and Rogers-Ramachandran 1996; see also Ramachandran and Blakeslee 1998, p. 46*ff.*). Ramachandran and colleagues constructed a "virtual reality box," by placing a vertical mirror inside a cardboard box with the roof of the box removed. Two holes in the front of the box enabled the patient to insert his real and his phantom arms. A patient who had suffered from a paralyzed phantom limb for many years was then asked to view the reflection of his normal hand in the mirror, thus—on the level of visual input—creating the illusion of observing two hands, when in fact he was only seeing the mirror reflection of the intact hand. What would happen to the content of the PSM were the subject asked to try making bilateral, mirror-symmetrical movements? Ramachandran described one typical outcome of the experiment:

I asked Philip to place his right hand on the right side of the mirror in the box and imagine that his left hand (the phantom) was on the left side. "I want you to move your right and left arm simultaneously," I instructed.

"Oh, I can't do that," said Philip. "I can move my right arm but my left arm is frozen. Every morning, when I get up, I try to move my phantom because it's in this funny position and I feel that moving it might help relieve the pain. But," he said looking down at his invisible arm, "I never have been able to generate a flicker of movement in it."

"Okay, Philip, but try anyway."

Philip rotated his body, shifting his shoulder, to "insert" his lifeless phantom into the box. Then he put his right hand on the other side of the mirror and attempted to make synchronous movements. As he gazed into the mirror, he gasped and then cried out, "Oh, my God! Oh, my God, doctor! This is unbelievable. It's mind-boggling!" He was jumping up and down like a kid. "My left arm is plugged in again. It's as if I'm in the past. All these memories from years ago are flooding back into my mind. I can move my arm again. I can feel my elbow moving, my wrist moving. It's all moving again."

After he calmed down a little I said, "Okay, Philip, now close your eyes."

"Oh, my," he said, clearly disappointed. "It's frozen again. I feel my right hand moving, but there's no movement in the phantom."

"Open your eyes."

"Oh, yes. Now it's moving again."

(Ramachandran 1998, p. 47*f*. For clinical and experimental details, see Ramachandran and Rogers-Ramachandran 1996.)

What is moving in this experiment is the PSM. The relevant partition now satisfies the dynamicity constraint, which it didn't before. The sudden reoccurrence of kinesthetic qualia in the degraded subspace of the self-model was made possible by installing a second source of "virtual information," restoring, as it were, the visual mode of self-representation, thereby making this information *volitionally* available. Technically speaking, what has been newly activated in this system is presentational content originating in the visual modality. It was then automatically integrated into a visual model of a whole, moving arm. Because of the spatial isomorphism of this model with precisely the region

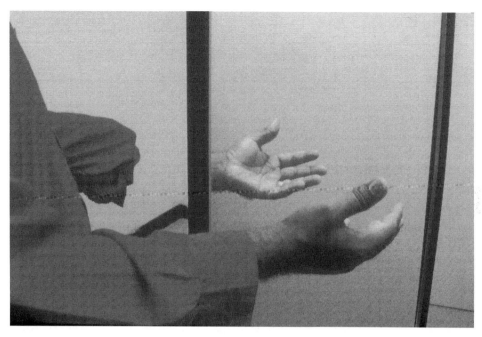

Figure 7.3
Mirror-induced synesthesia: Making part of a hallucinated self available for conscious action control by installing a virtual source of visual feedback. (Courtesy of Vilayanur Ramachandran.)

in phenomenal state space to which the patient is sending motor commands, it is possible for the body emulator mentioned above to actually generate hallucinatory, proprioceptive, and kinesthetic feedback. It emulates nonvisual feedback. Frith and colleagues (2000, p. 1779) made the same point by postulating that a *predictor*, which previously had been adapted to a situation in which no feedback from changed limb position was ever generated regardless of what motor command was issued, could now be successfully updated. Please note the implication this has for the neurophenomenology of movement initiation, fast reaching movements, and so forth, under normal circumstances. It is now highly plausible that what from the first-person perspective is a conscious and fully realistic self-representation must be analyzed as a transparent self-*simulation* under a third-person representationalist description of the system. The underlying principle, again, is that of achieving a maximally coherent, harmonious interpretation of the overall neurocomputational activity in the system. Transiently, the functional profile of the neural substrate underlying this part of the conscious self-model can be changed, because the unusual perceptual context offers a second, fully congruent source of input through another sensory modality. Note how the final result of this swift process of subpersonal self-organization is fully transparent: not only is the subjective experience of an arm *actually* moving absolutely realistic (the fact that it portrays a possibility and not an actuality itself is only cognitively, but not attentionally, available) but the accompanying phenomenal experience of *agency* (see section 6.4.5) springs into place just as swiftly. The content of the bodily PSM is the content of a transparent predictor.

In a study of nine arm amputees it turned out that vivid kinesthetic sensations emerged in seven subjects when observing the normal hand moving in the mirror (Ramachandran et al. 1995, p. 498*f.*). In one patient a motile phenomenal limb was evoked after the absence of any subjective experience of movement for the preceding 10 years. In the same patient, repeated use of the mirror over 3 weeks resulted in a gradual and eventually permanent disappearance of the hallucinated hand. Interestingly, in five patients experiencing involuntary clenching spasms of the phantom hand, it turned out that, for four of them, these spasms could be immediately relieved by looking into the mirror and simultaneously opening both of the hands now represented as parts of the PSM. A plausible hypothesis may be that, in some configurations, motor commands which are not neutralized by error feedback from proprioception generated by an actually existing, physical limb do not lead to the subjective experience of paralysis, but to *overshooting* motor activity in the hallucinated part of the conscious self—by digging virtual nails of virtual fingers into a virtual hand, thereby causing the transparent subjective experience of a painful spasm. Again, the pain itself is experienced as fully "presentational"; on the level of conscious experience it is *actual* and fully realistic. However, a visual alternative offered by the mirror image of the remaining real hand opening itself may help to end this particular aspect of deviant self-modeling. It is also interesting to note that attempts at employing "mirror therapy" in other cases are now showing good results in the rehabilitation of hemiparesis after stroke (Altschuler, Wisdom, Stone, Foster, Galasko, Llewellyn, and Ramachandran 1999).

A phantom limb is not a self-representation, but a self-*simulation*: its content is only a possibility and not an actuality. Phantom limbs are afunctional simulata, which do not satisfy the adaptivity constraint. They fulfill no function *for* the organism. Nevertheless, their phenomenal content is globally available for self-directed cognition and introspective₃ attention, and in many cases even for voluntary control. Because they are embedded in a window of presence, they are experienced as actual, currently existing elements of one's self. "Enacted" or not, they are certainly a part of the individual's lived reality and contribute to the phenomenal experience of embodiment. They are embedded in a coherent global state and may possess an inherent dynamicity, for instance, if a phantom arm involuntarily and automatically reaches for a ringing phone. What makes the phenomenology of phantom limbs so particularly intriguing is the manner in which a pseudohallucination and a fully functional, active self-model are seamlessly *integrated*. In standard situations patients know that their phantom limbs do not really exist; the fact of their arm being a hallucinated arm is cognitively available to them. What integrates the representation and the simulation, from the first-person perspective, is the higher-order quality of phenomenal mineness. The phantom limb—even though I am unable to enact it—is my *own* phantom limb, just as my remaining "real" arm is. The human self-model is a complex, integrated gestalt, constituted by nested and mostly nonconceptual forms of content. It is plausible to assume that a distinct form of unconscious feature binding does exist, determining the phenomenal property of "mineness." It is also conceivable that such a function comes in different degrees of correlation strength, resulting in a gradient of coherence and phenomenal degrees of ownership.

In some cases the process of *updating* the phenomenal self can be a lengthy process (cf. the phenomenology of Anton's syndrome described in section 7.2.1). Hari and colleagues described a patient, E.P., who suffered not from a postamputation phantom, but (after operation of a ruptured aneurysm, followed by an infarction of the right frontal lobe) from intermanual conflict, alien hand syndrome, and a *supernumerary* ghost hand, which frequently created a phenomenal copy of the previous positions of the left hand with a time lag of 30 to 60 seconds.

Several times a day she sensed a third arm and, less frequently, a third leg. . . . E.P. was fully conscious of the abnormality of her percepts and was able to observe analytically her symptoms. The ghost limbs were always on the left side of the body and often felt so real that E.P. had difficulty distinguishing them from the real limbs. Interestingly, the position of the ghost hand copied, in a perseverative manner, the previous position of the left real hand: for example, if the left real hand had previously been on the arm rest of a chair but was now on a table, the (proprioceptically) appearing ghost hand was on the arm rest. When the left hand was moved back to the arm rest, the ghost limb disappeared but reappeared soon, this time on the table. The time delay from the new position of the arm to the appearance of the ghost limb was measured several times and was typically 0.5–1 min. If E.P. stayed immobile, the ghost percept could last for tens of minutes.

E.P. occasionally experienced splitting her body: when she was rising from a bench, she felt that only the right half started walking, whereas the left side remained on the bench. Repetitive and monotonical movements triggered this percept whereas dancing, for example, prevented its appearance. (Hari, Hänninen, Mäkinen, Jousmäki, Forss, Seppä, and Salonen 1998, p. 132)

What makes this case particularly interesting is the fact that ghost limbs were not under volitional control, but frequently followed movements of the *right* limbs. Whereas the general position of the supernumerary phantom was determined by the previous position of the left hand, a movement of a single finger of the right hand could at the same time trigger a corresponding movement sensation in the part of the phenomenal self-model formed by the ghost hand on the left side. What this shows is that the updating process underlying the PSM can functionally depend on different sources, for instance, in different hemispheres, which, in pathological configurations, can even stand in conflict with each other and operate within different time frames. The resulting phenomenology of the bodily self is fascinating, because it still is a unified structure—*one* phenomenal self—while at the same time displaying considerable fragmentation and hypertrophy, reflecting the normally invisible functional modularity underlying the PSM.

Returning to "classical" phantoms, it has also been argued that there is a parallelism between phantom limbs and the visual hallucinations experienced in Charles Bonnet syndrome (CBS; as described in section 4.2.4) in terms of the formation of a full perceptual gestalt without sensory input (Schultz and Melzack 1991, p. 823). Another commonality is the presence of cognitive insight, because CBS, as well as the typical phantom limb experience, differs from Anton's syndrome by its lack of disorientation. The conscious experience of phantom limbs can also count as another example of the offline activation of complex phenomenal content (see section 3.2.8), but without a volitional component and in a temporarily stable manner. We find typical instantiations of presentational content in phantom limbs—pain, sensations of heat, tingling, cramps, kinesthetic sensations, and so on—and for all these types of simple experiential content it is again true that they possess a continuous dimension of intensity (*constraint 9*) and that they are homogeneous (*constraint 10*). However, the degree of constraint satisfaction for intensity may be lower (see figure 7.4 below). In standard situations this type of phenomenal content is strictly stimulus-correlated. Here, the actual stimulus source lies elsewhere in the system, but this very fact is at most *cognitively* available to the patient. On the level of subjective experience the presentational character of elementary sensations integrated by the phantom limb is fully transparent, that is, nonintentional properties and earlier processing stages of the actual representational dynamics in the brain are not available for introspective$_3$ attention.

In terms of the underlying neural correlates a plausible general hypothesis is that important aspects of the phantom limb experience are caused by an innate "neuromatrix" of the human body image (see below). Pain in the phantom limb, as well as the telescoping effect by which a phantom limb withdraws into the stump, and the subjective referral of tactile stimuli applied to the cheek of patients and to particular regions or digits of a phantom hand and arm (as discussed above; see Ramachandran 1993, p. 10494*f*.; see also Ramachandran 1998, p. 1609*f*.; Ramachandran, Rogers-Ramachandran, and Stewart 1992a; Ramachandran, Stewart, and Rogers-Ramachandran 1992b) reflect a *remapping* process in the underlying neural substrate.

I will not go into full details of the current neuroscientific discussion, which is still partially inconclusive and developing at great speed. However, it seems safe to say the following: Loss of a body part is loss of a self-representandum. In principle this should lead to a loss of the respective part of the PSM, but the actual processing underlying and updating this model can take some time, and under special conditions it can be delayed for many years (e.g., the paralyzed body emulator acting as a "null Turing machine"). The human brain opens up a vast computational space, and a certain partition of this computational space is now unoccupied: no computational resources are needed to process information related to the amputated limb and to activate the respective part of the self-model. It also seems safe to say that the human brain allocates computational resources in a competitive, evolutionary style. Many sources of input are continuously competing for a section of neurocomputational space in which they can find maximal expression. As soon as a part of this processing space is abandoned, neighboring regions start to *compete* for the processing capacity that is now available and "invade" these regions. Put differently, human neurophenomenology is to a considerable extent governed by the evolutionary principle of "use it or lose it."

Loss of a limb is not only loss of a representandum. Loss of a limb also makes the behavioral state space of an organism shrink. Certain ranges of behaviors have now become impossible behaviors. As they will never be *actual* behaviors again, they will never have to be represented again, and as they have never to be *planned* again, they never have to be simulated again. From an evolutionary perspective, it would therefore be helpful if a reallocation of computational resources could take place. It looks as if the process of cortical remapping fulfills precisely this function by a process which is mirrored on the phenomenal level as the subjective experience of a sometimes hurting, but gradually disappearing phantom limb.

The first lesson to learn with regard to the underlying neural correlate of phantom experiences is that a remarkable plasticity has to exist, in somatosensory regions of the human brain in particular. Recent magnetoencephalographic (MEG)-studies exploring somatosensory plasticity in adult human subjects, and a number of animal studies present evidence regarding the actual cortical reorganization, for instance, following surgical separation of congenitally webbed fingers (for a review and discussion, see Ramachandran 1993). In fact, new *perceptual* correlates of such neural reorganization processes have been documented. In a number of patients, stimuli applied to points on the body surface remote from the actual locus of amputation have been shown to be systematically remapped to that part of the conscious self-model constituting the phantom arm. To give an example, in patient V.Q. (Ramachandran 1993, p. 10415*f.*) there was a systematic one-to-one mapping between certain regions on the cheek and individual digits like the thumb or little finger (see figure 7.1). Four weeks following amputation, distinct new features in his phenomenology reflected a massive reorganization in the neural and computational underpinnings of this patient's PSM. Here is how Ramachandran described the newly emerging situation:

Typically, the patient reported that he simultaneously felt the Q-tip touching his face and a "tingling" sensation in an individual digit. By repeatedly brushing the Q-tip on his face we were even able to plot "receptive fields" (or "reference fields") for individual digits of the (phantom) left hand on his face surface [see figure 7.1 above]. The margins of these fields were remarkably sharp and stable over successive trials. Stimuli applied to other parts of the body such as the tongue, neck, shoulders, trunk, axilla, and contralateral arm were never mislocalized to the phantom hand. There was, however, one specific point on the contralateral cheek that always elicited a tingling sensation in the phantom elbow.

The second cluster of points that evoked referred sensations was found about 7 cm above the amputation line. Again there was a systematic one-to-one mapping with the thumb represented medially on the anterior surface of the arm and the pinky laterally. (Ramachandran 1993, p. 10415)

It is interesting to note how modality-specific effects exist. In other words, varying *formats* of simple, stimulus-correlated presentational content can be bound into the hallucinated part of the bodily self. This is interesting, because it has implications for the underlying neural pathways forming the physical correlate of the respective type of conscious experience. Consider the example of warmth:

To find out, we tried placing a drop of warm water on VQ's face. He felt the warm water on his face, of course, but remarkably he reported (without any prompting) that his phantom hand also felt distinctly warm. On one occasion when the water accidentally trickled down his face, he exclaimed, with surprise, that he could actually feel the warm water trickling down the length of his phantom arm! We have now seen this effect in three patients, two after upper limb amputation and one after an avulsion of the brachial plexus. The latter patient was able to use his normal hand to trace out the exact path of the illusory "trickle" along his paralyzed arm as a drop of cold water flowed down his face. (ibid., p. 10416)

What these neurophenomenological case studies show is that the phenomenal content of the self-model covaries with remapping processes in the human brain in a rather rapid way, that even complex chains of presentational content ("simple" sensations like heat, warmth, pain, or touch) can be transposed, as it were, from the actual site of physical input to a remote phenomenal localization in the conscious self; that the correspondence between phenomenal self and the "new receptive fields" is of a *systematic* (i.e., one-to-one mapping) type; and that the overall effect is topography-preserving in terms of the direction, distance, and speed by which, for instance, the movement of a stimulus like a warm drop of water is phenomenally represented. There clearly is something like a *phenomenal* frame of spatial reference, and it can be warped and unfolded in many ways. Could the two distinct areas in physical space now projecting into the *same* location in the PSM have been themselves *one* area at an earlier stage? A fascinating speculative hypothesis could be that *in the womb*—when the tender core of the self-model slowly began to unfold and gain in functional differentiation—the curled up embryo had his hands firmly positioned on his cheeks (to my knowledge, this hypothesis was first proposed by

Martha Farah; see Ramachandran and Blakeslee 1998, p. 266; n. 4). As the physical body begins to move, the neighborhood relationship is still preserved on the level of the self-model in the brain.

Ramachandran interestingly argues that the reason for the existence of *two* clusters of points activating the hallucinated part of the phenomenal self in this fashion (one on the face and another one about 7 cm above the amputation line, on the upper arm) is that the hand area in the hypothesized relevant partition of the *neural* representation of the bodily self—in the "Penfield homunculus"—is "flanked on one side by the face and on the other side by the upper arm, shoulder and axilla" (ibid., p. 10449). All this, of course, does not settle the question as to what the necessary and sufficient neurocomputational conditions for the emergence of this type of hallucinated body parts actually are, and I will not engage in any speculation at this point (good candidates for the locus of reorganization are proprioceptive maps and area 3b; for a review, see Ramachandran and Hirstein 1998, p. 1624).

An important next step for any philosophically minded theory of self-consciousness would be to investigate if there are phenomenological constraints provided by neurological case studies which allow us to decide upon the important issue—if the most invariant parts of this core part of the phenomenal self are acquired by social interactions following birth, or if they are, possibly and to some degree, innate and genetically "hardwired." Starting on the functional level of description, it is obvious that there are a multitude of different factors leading to the phenomenology of the phantom limb. Remapping phenomena will play an important role, residual input from the stump (through "neuromas") may play a role, it is plausible to assume that long-term aspects of the human self-model (e.g., contextual effects and autobiographical memories) possess an important function in shaping *global* properties of the experience like the posture of a phantom limb, and obviously efferent copies of motor commands voluntarily issued by the patient are typically integrated into the overall model as well. The question remains if all this is a purely transient, dynamic flux of events in the system, or if a rather invariant "background blueprint" is in existence, not only serving as an integrating schema or functional template but in anchoring the overall conscious model of the muscoskeletal system directly within a persisting anatomical substrate.

In 1964 the German neurologist Klaus Poeck published three case reports demonstrating how no fundamental qualitative differences between phantoms in children and adults exist. Let us take a brief look at the phenomenology given in the first study:

Case 1. This was an eleven-year-old girl, who was born with congenital absence of both forearms and hands (peromelia). She never had worn a prosthesis. The girl reported very distinct and intense phantoms that she had experienced for the first time at the age of six years. She had the feeling of two completely normal hands, placed about 15 cms below the stump. She had never felt her missing forearms. During the years, there had been a slight telescoping, but no fading of the phantoms' intensity.

The child was able to differentiate and to move freely all of her fingers. In her first years in school she had learned to solve simple arithmetic problems by counting with her fingers just as other healthy children did. On these occasions she would place her phantom hands on the table and count the outstretched fingers one by one.

During the examination the child unhesitantly imitated given movements or positions with her phantoms. When she approached a wall with her rudimentary arms the phantoms gradually withdrew within the stump without fading. At the very moment she touched the wall, the phantoms disappeared and she felt nothing but her stumps' contact with the wall. A similar experience was reported by several of our adult probands. The phantoms also disappeared when the examiner took the stumps in his hand. On the contrary, when the child seized the examiner's hand with her phantom fingers, she maintained, like some of our adult amputees, that she felt its natural warmth and soft consistency. . . . In her dreams, the girl saw herself with "beautiful hands." (Poeck 1964, p. 270*f.*)

In his discussion Poeck agrees with Sidney Weinstein and Eugene Sersen, who in 1961 published a substantial paper containing five case studies describing phantom limb experiences in children with *congenital* absence of limbs, that is, phantoms for a limb which had never *existed*, that the assumption of a "built-in" component of the conscious body image has to be made. In 1964 Weinstein, Sersen, and Robert Vetter presented evidence of phantoms for thirteen additional cases of aplasia. Interestingly, in only 16.7% to 18.3% of the cases investigated did phantom experiences emerge at all. Importantly, these authors pointed out that a confabulation hypothesis is not plausible in almost all of these cases, because phantoms invariably resembled the amputated parts, including their deformity, but never an intact, well-formed limb, as would be the result of any "wishful thinking" on the side of the patient, be it conscious or unconscious. This aspect has been confirmed by many subsequent studies. Weinstein and colleagues (1964, p. 287) concluded that the phenomenological data are "consistent with the concept of a plastic, neural substrate which is modifiable by experience." As it turns out, phenomenological reports of phantom experiences in persons with congenitally absent limbs have existed for a long time, but have been mostly ignored by philosophers.

The first published report of a phantom limb experience in aplasic patients appeared in the German literature in the year 1836 (Valentin 1836, p. 330; see also Valentin 1844, p. 609; for a valuable historical review of the 27 cases of phantom phenomena in patients with congenital deficiencies which had been documented up to 1967, cf. Vetter and Weinstein 1967). Valentin (1844), in discussing the *Integritätsgefühle der Amputirten* ("feelings of integrity found in amputees"), claimed that a careful study of the phenomenology of phantoms teaches us that we are not only confronted here with a "subordinate psychological illusion" but with a much more fundamental and far reaching *Nervengesetz* ("neural law") (p. 606). In dismissing alternative hypotheses he uses the phenomenological fact of human beings born without extremities under certain conditions "integrating just like the amputees" (p. 609) as an argument for the necessary, but as yet unknown existence of an "imprint of all bodily organs" in our *Centralwerkzeug* (the brain conceived of as our central tool). Input to this central imprint invariably leads to the effect of it being represented as localized within the peripheral part, conceived of as the "symmetrical complementary piece" of the corresponding transparent region within the self-model. The Valentin hypothesis interestingly also assumed a more general law, called the "law of peripheral reaction."[13] Valentin (1836) emphasized that what is here termed the bodily self-model cannot be conceived of as a certain kind of "permanent memory image" (*eine Art von permanenter Erinnerungsvorstellung*; p. 333), that the integrated nature of the transparent self-model can generate the "subjective appearance of integrity" (*subjectiven Scheine der Integrität*; p. 328) by—as the congenital cases show—providing an autonomous and subpersonal "tendency toward continuous integration" (*Tendenz der beständigen Integration*; p. 333), which remains complete and the same even if visual and tactile perception simultaneously demonstrate the opposite (p. 333). It seems obvious that Valentin had a distinct theoretical entity in mind which clearly resembled the PSM.

The concept of a "phantom" limb was first introduced in 1871 by Silas Weir Mitchell, American neurologist, poet, and novelist, who, however, was unaware of existing research on phantoms in congenitally missing limbs.[14] He spoke of "ghostly members"

---

13. Here is the Valentin hypothesis in its original version from the *Lehrbuch der Physiologie des Menschen* (1844) and in English translation: *Wir wissen, daß die Primitivfasern der einzelnen Körperorgane nach dem Gehirn verlaufen. In diesem Centralwerkzeuge hat jeder Teil seinen Repräsentanten. Es bildet auf irgend eine uns noch unbekannte Art den Abdruck aller Köperorgane. Denn nur hierdurch kann jeder von ihnen der Einwirkung unseres Bewußtseins unterworfen bleiben. Erfolgt an einer bestimmten Stelle des Gehirns eine Veränderung, welche eine Nervenfaser der großen Zehe afficirt, so wird die Wirkung in diesem peripherischen Theile als dem symmetrischen Complementarstücke aufgefasst. Sie ist daher die gleiche, es möge die centripetal fortgeführte Anregung in der Nähe ihres peripherischen Endes oder an einer Stelle ihres Verlaufes oder im Gehirn selbst Statt finden. Daher die allgemeinen Aeußerungen des Gesetzes der peripherischen Reaction. Wird der Fuß amputirt, so ändert dies nicht die Verhältnisse der Centraltheile, welche deshalb auch wie im ganz gesunden Zustande thätig bleiben, d.h. die Integration des verstümmelten Körpers bedingen.* (Valentin 1844, p. 608f.). "We know that the primitive fibers of individual bodily organs run toward the brain. In this central instrument every part has its representation. In a way yet unknown to us, it forms an impression of all bodily organs. It is only through this fact that they can remain under the influence of our consciousness. If a change occurs at a certain site in the brain that affects a nerve fiber related to the big toe, the effect is construed as being in this peripheral part as the symmetrical complementary piece. Therefore it is always the same, whether the excitation takes place close to its peripheral end and is centripetally transmitted, or on a point on this line of transmission, or within the brain itself. For this reason we find the general expression of the law of peripheral reaction. If the foot is amputated, this does not change the relations among the central parts, which therefore remain active as in the completely healthy state, i.e., necessitate integration of the mutilated body." In an earlier paper (1836, p. 336) Valentin spoke of the "mental reproduction of the material symmetry of the peripheral nervous system" (translation by T.M.).

14. "It should be added, that the experiments on which rest these speculations were many of them made on persons whose limbs had been lost when they were too young to remember them at all. No one seems to have examined in these directions any of the cases of people born without limbs—an instance of which exists in the

and "fractional phantoms" haunting people like "unseen ghosts of the lost part," and pointed out that there is "something almost tragical, something ghastly, in the notion of these thousands of spirit limbs haunting as many good soldiers, and every now and then tormenting them with the disappointments which arise when, the memory being off guard for a moment, the keen sense of the limb's presence betrays the man into some effort, the failure of which of a sudden reminds him of his loss" (Mitchell 1871, p. 565*f*.). In 1961 Weinstein and Sersen introduced the notion of a "*nucleus* of the adult body scheme (op. cit., p. 911).[15] It is precisely this issue which possesses direct relevance for philosophical questions concerning the innateness of a particular subset of those functional properties which constitute the human self-model. It relates to the hypothetical existence of a "center of relative invariance," a distinct causal core component, which could form the center of behavioral as well as of phenomenal space, and the idea of a persisting functional link, anchoring the conscious self in the physical world, thereby generating the subjective experience of embodiment (see, e.g., sections 5.4 and 6.3.1).

Is there a genetic component to the body schema? Could this component play the role of an autonomous and continuously active source of internally generated input for the PSM, as I proposed earlier (e.g., Metzinger 1993)? Serious methodological criticisms have been put forward regarding the status of phantom limbs in children who are born without all or part of a limb. Skoyles (1990) pointed out that children are much more prone to confabulatory responses, because they "have a low capacity to differentiate reality from the contents of their imagination and from ideas suggested to them." The phenomenology and the incidence of phantoms in persons with congenital aplasias clearly vary and the data concerning such experiences do not fit well with existing evidence on cerebral plasticity in limb representation. The most prominent representative for the idea of an innate body-self is, of course, Ronald Melzack (Melzack 1989, 1992; Katz and Melzack 1990; see also Saadah and Melzack 1994; and, in particular, Melzack, Israel, Lacroix, and Schultz 1997), and it is his hypothesis at which these methodological doubts were directed.

Saadah and Melzack (1994) presented four case studies clearly demonstrating how the neural substrate of conscious phantom limbs is partially immune against neuroplasticity. It is well-known that, for instance, after excision of a digit, changes in cortical body maps take place which lead to a major reorganization of somatotopic representation and make the persistence of a conscious phantom rather unlikely. However, in cases of congenital

---

person of a well-known member of Parliament. It would be worth while to learn if these unfortunates possess any consciousness of their missing members" (Mitchell 1871, p. 569).

15. "The nucleus of the adult body scheme may have its origin in a neural substrate which is the framework for the potential adult sensory homunculus. This neural 'framework' may be modified by multi-modal sensory experiences during the lifetime of the organism" (Weinstein and Sersen 1961, p. 911).

limb deficiency, phantoms appear for the first time between 4 and 30 years after birth (a marked difference to postamputation phantoms), thereby showing how a relevant portion of the neurofunctional aspects of the human self-model persist into adulthood. Saadah and Melzack (1994, p. 480) found that phantoms could not, therefore, be simple reflections of the somatosensory homunculus. They hypothesized that important components of the neural correlate of a bodily self must be found in somatosensory thalamus and cortex, in the limbic system, and the association cortices. Obviously the concept of a genetically determined neuromatrix does not exclude modifications caused by learning experiences. From a purely logical point of view, however, it is not ruled out that the temporarily stable part of the functional self-model discussed here is not genetically hardwired, but unfolds during pregnancy and is then fully in place at birth.[16]

Interestingly, Saadah and Melzack reported on three patients in their sample who never experienced a phantom limb when awake, but had "vivid dreams in which the deficient limb was perceived to be intact and was used in various activities" (ibid., p. 480). Such phenomenological data may turn out to be interesting, as they indicate the possibility of situations in which the relevant portions of the self-model cannot be activated while under the constraints imposed by actual sensory inputs (*constraint 8*). In an important recent study Melzack and colleagues (1997) reported on a sample of 125 people with missing limbs. They documented phantom experiences in forty-one individuals born limb-deficient or having undergone an amputation before the age of 6 years. This extended case study shows that about every second subject who underwent an amputation before the age of 6 years and at least 20% of all persons with congenital aplasias develop conscious phantom limb experiences at a later stage. This careful set of case studies nicely demonstrates how phenomenological constraints imposed on a multilevel theory of phenomenal self-modeling cannot only rule out assumptions concerning local neural plasticity in the somatosensory cortex but also alternative proposals based on high-level, psychological mechanisms such as confabulation. The authors pointed out that child amputees describe gaps between stump and phantom, or (in five cases) phantoms resembling the appearance, size, or manner of deformation of the limb prior to amputation, or even one whole phantom and a second deformed one (see figure 7.2). They pointed out that it is highly unlikely that the emergence of this kind of experiential content could result from something that could be described as an unconscious wish to "be normal" (Melzack et al. 1997, p. 1611). The general picture emerging from the data currently available clearly supports the notion of a neurocomputational substrate for the bodily self-model which is, first, highly distributed and, second, an entity continuously shaped by experience.

16. I am greatly indebted to helpful discussions with Toemme Noesselt on this issue.

It has been suggested that sensory input is woven into an ongoing process, but the input does not, by itself, produce the output pattern (in accordance with the convolved holism constraint formulated in chapter 3). In this manner, our body perceptions are fluid, dynamic, and constantly changing. The evanescent nature of the phantom thus reveals the way the brain functions. We are rarely aware of a whole body, but more often of the "attentional islands" discussed above. Some of the subjects felt their phantom (or part of it) for minutes or hours at intervals of weeks or months, yet their perception (even during periods as short as seconds) was described as being real, as "real" as the intact physical parts of their body.

However, phenomenally experienced realness cannot be a matter of transparency *alone*. The intensity constraint for presentational content seems to play a role. A recent case study by Brugger and colleagues introduced a vividness rating on a 7-point scale that showed highly consistent judgments across sessions for their subject A.Z., a 44-year old university-educated woman born without forearms and legs. As long as she remembers, she has experienced mental images of forearms (including fingers) and legs (with feet and first and fifth toes), but, as figure 7.4 shows, not *as* realistic as the content of her nonhallucinatory PSM. Functional magnetic resonance imaging (fMRI) of phantom hand movements showed no activation of primary sensorimotor areas, but of premotor and parietal cortex bilaterally. Transcranial magnetic stimulation of the sensorimotor cortex consistently elicited phantom sensations in the contralateral fingers and hand (please note how such sensations can count as presentational content, because they are strictly stimulus-correlated). In addition, premotor and parietal stimulation evoked similar phantom sensations, albeit in the absence of motor evoked potentials in the stump. These data clearly demonstrate how body parts that have never been physically developed can be represented in sensory and motor cortical areas. Are they components of an innate body model? Could they have been "mirrored into" the patient's self-model through the visual observation of other human beings moving around? It may also be interesting to note that, in this case, "Awareness of her phantom limbs is transiently disrupted only when some object or person invades their felt position or when she sees herself in a mirror" (Brugger, Kollias, Müri, Crelier, Hepp-Reymond, and Regard 2000, p. 6168; for further details concerning the phenomenological profile, see ibid.; for an interesting experimental follow-up study demonstrating the intactness of the phenomenal model of kinesthetic and postural limb properties, see Brugger, Regard, and Shiffrar 2001). The phantom, like our physical body, is constantly being generated in new positions. Different parts of the body weave in and out of attention. Here is one way of thinking about the resulting phenomenology: the first-order PSM is a rather stable structure defined by attentional availability. However, the focus of the self-directed PMIR (pointing "downward" or, phenomenologically speaking, "inward"), the object component of self-directed attention, frequently wanders. It

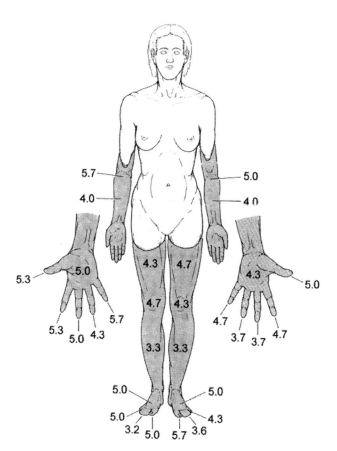

Figure 7.4
Evidence for an innate component of the PSM? Phantoms (shaded areas) in a subject with limb amelia. Numbers are vividness ratings for the felt presence of different phantom body parts on a 7-point scale from 0 (no awareness) to 6 (most vivid impression). (Courtesy of Peter Brugger, Zürich.)

constitutes attentional islands in the conscious body image by *actualizing* them as current targets of an attentional PMIR and creating a second-order self-model, the "attentional subject" described in section 6.4.3. The first-order self-model is constantly being created by the more invariant core of the corresponding neural network (the "neuromatrix") according to the needs of the moment (Melzack et al. 1997, p. 1619).

The general picture emerging is thus one of bodily self-modeling being a highly active process, continuously processing inputs from the body, which can vary greatly in terms of intensity, attentional focus, and general spatial and temporal properties, on the basis of a more invariant "functional skeleton" based on stable genetic determinants. From a neurocomputational perspective evidence demonstrating that phantom limbs frequently reappear even after an *excision* of somatosensory cortex (Gybels and Sweet 1989; quoted in Melzack et al. 1997) provides a strong argument for the highly distributed nature of the overall phenomenon.

Returning to a more theoretical level, and once again applying our new conceptual tools, let me point out an important phenomenological commonality between the ordinary conscious experience of our body and its limbs, and the phenomenology of phantom limbs (either resulting from congenital deficits or from amputations at a later stage). The phenomenal properties of "mineness" and "transparency" are instantiated in absolutely the same manner and to the same degree in all cases. For an amputee, it is absolutely clear that his phantom arm is his *own* phantom arm, just as it is clear for what we like to call his "real" arm. The property of mineness is evenly distributed over the whole of his conscious self-model. A phantom limb may be paralyzed, but it is not neglected like a paralyzed limb in unilateral hemineglect. In the latter case, however, the paralyzed limb is not treated as her *own* by the patient anymore. Second, in almost all cases the fact of the physical nonexistence of the limb in question is *cognitively* available. There are interesting exceptions, like the second patient D.S. mentioned in passing by Ramachandran and Hirstein (1998, p. 1624), who had bilateral frontal lesions following a car accident *and* lost his arm. As pointed out at the beginning, this patient actually insisted that he could still see his own arm and that it had not been removed. However, we are here confronted with a fundamentally different etiology. As a general principle holding for all phantom limb patients, the hallucinatory character of the experience is cognitively available, but full transparency of the self-model is preserved. *Attentional* transparency is maximally expressed. This seamless integration of a hallucinated, but fully transparent element of the body-self into a veridical representation of the remaining physical body supports the conclusion that *both* forms of phenomenal content are generated by precisely the same mechanism—to which a distinct theoretical entity must correspond. It shows what it means to say that every *representation* is also a *simulation*: the content of the human self-model is a possibility which is displayed as a reality. As you read these words the untranscendable "mineness" and "realness" of your bodily experience, the ultrarealistic character of the way in which as an embodied subject you feel your hands holding the book you are reading right now, is determined by precisely the same neural mechanisms and functional properties of the brain which generate the experiential "mineness" and "realness" accompanying the subjective experience of a phantom limb.

Independent evidence for a "primordial" core or a "nucleus" of the human self-model does exist. In section 5.4 we saw that visceral sensitivity, interoception, and the elementary bioregulatory processes of chemical homeostasis very likely play a decisive role in functionally anchoring the self-model in a continuous source of internally generated input. Meltzoff and Moore's famous studies on imitation behavior in infants demonstrated how newborn infants can imitate facial gestures shortly after birth (e.g., Meltzoff and Moore 1977, 1983, 1989). Of course, these very young children are completely unaware of possessing a face themselves; they have never seen their own face, nor would they be able to recognize it in a mirror. Yet they have the capacity to imitate visually perceived face movements like mouth openings, tongue protrusions, and head movements. Obviously these cases demonstrate a process of sensorimotor integration, in which a cross-modal mapping of visually perceived information onto a motor structure controlling the corresponding parts of the infant's body takes place in a reliable and successful manner. It is hard to imagine how such an integration could be achieved without the existence of an underlying functional or representational structure forming the *medium* in which the mapping from visual input onto a kinesthetic representation of the infant's facial motion takes place. In order to generate a detectable similarity between perceived and displayed facial movement, this structure has to stand in an exploitable similarity relation to the body harboring it as well—in short, it has to be a *self-model*. It is important to note that processes of this kind, of course, do not have to be accompanied by phenomenal experience. As always, it is important to differentiate between functional and representational levels of description, as well as between the concept of a mental and a *phenomenal* self-model.

The conceptual instruments I have so far developed to describe the possibilities of conscious and unconscious imitative behavior, sensorimotor integration, and so on are historically related to the earlier concepts of "body schema" and "body image," which, however, have been a source of considerable confusion in the literature. Shaun Gallagher (1986) offered a conceptual clarification, which he applied in a series of publications (for a review of earlier terminological confusions, see Gallagher 1986; Gallagher and Meltzoff 1996; for further discussion, see also Gallagher 1995; Gallagher, Butterworth, Lew, and Cole 1998). As Gallagher writes, the *functional* self-model, the body schema, is a nonconscious "performance," which does not have to be the object of conscious experience in order to do its work (1986, p. 551). The PSM, the body image, serves to achieve modifications of the nonconscious operation of the body. In other words, the PSM makes those functional properties of the body that frequently have to be modified in a fast and flexible manner globally available for attention and motor control. Gallagher points out that the body schema is an "anonymous performance," whereas in the body image, as he calls it, "the body loses its anonymity" by becoming *my* body, an *owned* body. This way of describing the phenomenology of the bodily self supports the conceptual distinctions I introduced earlier: It is only the PSM, which leads to an instantiation of the higher-order phenomenal property of "mineness" and the prereflexive, nonconceptual sense of ownership discussed before. Arguably, personal-level predicates can only be applied to systems having the capacity to representationally *own* their body in the way just described. In an infant imitating facial gestures of its mother, it may well be only the functional, subconscious body schema which achieves the relevant mapping. In phantom limb patients, however, many aspects of these innate functional structures are continuously elevated onto the level of the conscious self-model. Quoting Merleau-Ponty (1962, p. 84) Gallagher writes, "As body schema the body performs it duties, not as 'my' body, but as a pre-personal cleaving to the general form of the world, an anonymous and general system, [that] plays, beneath my personal life, the part of an inborn complex,"[17] (1986, p. 551).

A body schema is a coherent set of functional properties, which are not attentionally available. A body image, on the other hand, is a complex set of representational contents, including the extended context of attitudes and beliefs pertaining to one's own body, all of them globally available and therefore elements of the PSM. In discussing imitative behavior and the phenomenology of phantom limbs, it is important to differentiate between the functional and the phenomenal levels of description, as it is vital to recognize how a preexisting functional component or "nucleus" of the self-model may be a necessary precondition for the development of a consciously experienced self. Gallagher draws attention to the well-known fact that amputees sometimes "forget" the fact that their limb is missing, for example, when spontaneously trying to walk with a nonexisting limb or grasp a cup with a phantom thumb. However, he then points out how no such incidents of forgetting have been reported in subjects with aplasic phantoms (Gallagher et al. 1998, p. 45; Gallagher and Meltzoff 1996, p. 218*ff.*). And it seems as if in "normal" phantom limb patients a functional motor component of the self-model is available at any given time. It need not be simultaneously available for phenomenal experience in general or introspective$_3$ attention in particular, whereas in congenitally limb-deficient patients this structure

---

17. As Gallagher points out, a strict self-world boundary is only introduced on the level of *phenomenal* representation: "The body, in its body schema, most genuinely lives as a body-environment. On the other hand, in the body image the body is seen as something distinct from the environment. It is understood as something in-itself, an object with its own abstract identity, a thing that is often objectified and experienced in an isolated fashion" (Gallagher 1986, p. 552).

may not exist at all (e.g., it could have receded and disappeared before the emergence of autobiographical memory). Is it conceivable that aplasic patients possess a purely *PSM*, without any underlying functional basis? This might constitute an interesting criticism of the innateness hypothesis. The phenomenon of forgetting in normal phantom limb patients may be due to the simple fact that most motor behavior simply does not require conscious control or attentional availability (Gallagher and Meltzoff 1996, p. 218).

A second important empirical fact is in the age of onset for aplastic phantom limb experiences which range from 4 to 30 years, whereas "ordinary" hallucinated body parts of this type typically emerge right after the patient wakes up from anesthesia. As Meltzoff and Gallagher point out,

> Although it seems clear that the aplasic patients do experience certain perceptual aspects of phantom limbs, it remains uncertain whether schema-related experience with an actual limb at some point in one's life is a necessary condition for such errors as "forgetting that one doesn't have it" to occur. The fact that aplasics do not report the forgetting phenomenon raises the possibility that the aplasic phantom is not part of the body schema although it is part of the body image. . . .
>
> The evidence cited suggests that the aplasic phantom is a phantom *image* that develops relatively late. On this evidence the influence that the body *schema* is innate is not logically justified. Of course this does not require us to conclude that the body schema is *not* innate. Indeed, the data on aplasic phantoms are not inconsistent with the idea that both a body schema and perceptual elements of a body image exist at birth. It is quite possible that, as in some cases with phantoms after amputation, aplasic phantoms gradually disappear as the schema and image adjust and develop. Since this would happen relatively early in the case of aplasic phantoms, it is not unlikely that most subjects do not recall a phantom when interviewed later. (Gallagher and Meltzoff 1996, p. 219)

Concerning the examples of hallucinated phenomenal selves that I have discussed in this section, it is important to note that so far we have only been speaking about hallucinated *parts* of bodily selves. It is the phenomenal property of "mineness," which integrates the hallucinated part with the part modeling the remaining parts of the physical organism. Even in patients suffering from aplasic phantoms, the hallucinated part of the phenomenal self develops against the background of an already existing bodily self-model. As we have seen, there is independent empirical evidence for the existence of an innate "nucleus" of this aspect of the bodily self-model, and it is therefore safe to assume that this component exists in congenitally limb-deficient persons experiencing aplasic phantoms at a later stage as well. As the aplasic phantom is phenomenologically well integrated with the preexisting conscious representation of the bodily self, the most parsimonious and simple hypothesis will clearly be that this is also true for the underlying functional substrate.

Before moving on to another new phenomenological case study—which deals with hallucinated bodily selves not concerning specific parts, but phenomenal embodiment *as a whole*—let me point out another intriguing idea following from the discussion presented by Gallagher and Meltzoff. I agree that most of the data available today point to an innate component of the self-model (Gallagher and Meltzoff 1996, p. 214), but possibly only in terms of a "weak modularity" hypothesis. This would mean that the most characteristic partitioning of human phenomenal space—the untranscendable self-world boundary—is anchored in an innate functional structure. In section 6.3.3 I pointed out, that, importantly, certain parts of the human self-model will possess necessary social correlates: You can only enjoy these kinds of self-consciousness if appropriately stimulated by a social environment. What research on imitative behavior in infants may therefore draw our attention to is that not only the subject-world boundary but also a subject-*subject* boundary is functionally prefigured at birth as well. If this is true, one conclusion for philosophical anthropology would be that all of us are born as social subjects, because the relevant functional properties underlying social cognition, in particular those endowing the child with the ability to use her own self-model as a *mirror* for the self-models of other human beings, are, if only in a rudimentary manner, actually present at birth.

Out-of-Body Experiences

Could there be a generalized version of the phantom limb experience? Could there be an integrated kind of bodily self-experience, be it of a mobile body fully available for volitional control or of a paralyzed body, which in its entirety is a phenomenal confabulation—in short, a *hallucinated* and *bodily* self at the same time? At this point it is interesting to recall how all the deviant models of reality and self discussed in the form of neurophenomenological case studies in this chapter can also be read as ontologies and as epistemological metaphors. As phenomenal ontologies they are nonpropositional theories—internal, neurobiologically realized models—about what actually *exists* from the brain's point of view. As epistemological metaphors they are theories about how the organism actually comes to *know* about the existence of this reality. For instance, deviant phenomenal models determine if or how many selves exist and what properties they have. Under a naive-realistic interpretation they can then become *theoretical* ontologies—folk phenomenology turns into folk metaphysics, as it were. On the other hand, if one interprets the content of a PMIR in a naive-realistic fashion, one arrives at a folk epistemology, for instance, a theory saying that a certain state of affairs is actually *perceived by the senses*. As we will see at the end of this section, this context is particularly relevant to assessing the out-of-body experience (OBE); strictly speaking, the possibility mentioned above would presuppose a "disembodied" version of Cartesian dualism. It would consist in the specific kind of phenomenal content normally constituted by the bodily self in the *absence* of a body. Obviously, there is no way of assessing this possibility from an empirical point of view—for example, there never could be anything like a *neuro*phenomenological case study.

However, there is a well-known class of phenomenal states in which the experiencing person undergoes the untranscendable and highly realistic conscious experience of leaving his or her physical body, usually in the form of an etheric double, and moving outside of it. In other words, there is a class (or at least a strong cluster) of intimately related phenomenal models of reality, the classic defining characteristics of which are a *visual representation* of one's own body from a perceptually impossible, externalized third-person perspective (e.g., lying on a bed or on the road below oneself) plus a *second representation* of one's own body, typically (but not in all cases) freely hovering above or floating in space. This second body-model is the locus of the phenomenal self. It not only forms the "true" focus of one's phenomenal identity but also functions as an integrated representation of all kinesthetic qualia and all nonvisual forms of proprioception. Such experiences are called out-of-body-experiences.

OBEs frequently occur spontaneously while falling asleep, or following severe accidents or during surgical operations. At present it is not clear whether the concept of an OBE possesses one clearly delineated set of necessary and sufficient conditions. The concept of an OBE may in the future turn out to be a cluster concept constituted by a whole range of diverging (possibly overlapping) subsets of phenomenological constraints, each forming a set of sufficient, but not necessary, conditions.

On the level of conscious self-representation a prototypical feature of this class of deviant PSMs seems to be the coexistence of (a) a more or less veridical representation of the bodily self, from an external visual perspective, which does *not* function as the center of the global model of reality, and (b) a second self-model, which largely integrates proprioceptive perceptions—although, interestingly, weight sensations only to a lesser degree—and which possesses special properties of shape and form that may or may not be veridical. Both models of the experiencing system are located within the same spatial frame of reference (that is why they are *out-of*-body experiences). This frame of reference is an *egocentric* frame of reference. The first interesting point seems to be that this second self-model always forms the subject component of what I called the "phenomenal model of the intentionality relation" in section 6.5. The PMIR itself is invariably portrayed as of a perceptual, that is, visual, nature—phenomenologically, you simply *see* yourself. If, for instance, after a severe accident, you find yourself floating above the scene viewing your injured body lying on the road beside your car, there is a perceived self (the "object component," which, technically speaking, is only a *system*-model, but not a *subject*-model), invariably formed by a more or less accurate visual representation of your body from an exteriorized perspective, and a *perceiving* self (the "subject component," the PSM, i.e., the current *self*- or *subject*-model) hovering above the scene, both of which are integrated into one overall global model of reality, which is centered on the second self-model. The second self-model can either be one of a full blown agent, that is, endowed with the characteristic form of phenomenal content generating the subjective experience of agency (see section 6.4.5), or only what Harvey Irwin (1985, p. 310) has aptly called a "passive, generalized somaesthetic image of a static floating self." However, before entering into a brief representationalist analysis of OBEs, let us first take a quick detour and look at some more frequent, real-world phenomenological cases. Have you ever had the following experience?

The bus to the train station had already been late. And now you have even queued up in a line at the wrong ticket counter! Nevertheless you manage to reach your train *just* in time, finding an empty compartment and, completely exhausted, drop into the seat. In a slightly unfocussed and detached state of mind you are now observing the passengers sitting in the train on the other side of the platform. Suddenly you feel how your *own* train starts to move, very slowly at first, but accompanied by a continuous acceleration, which you can feel in your own body. Two or three seconds later, with the same degree of suddenness, your bodily sensation disappears and you become aware that it actually is the *other* train, which has now started to slowly leave the train station (see also Metzinger 1993, p. 185*f*.).

What you have just experienced is a very rudimentary form of an OBE, a hallucinated bodily self. The center of your global model of reality was briefly filled by a kinesthetic and proprioceptive hallucination, a nonveridical model of the weight and acceleration of your body, erroneously activated by your brain. The dominating visual model of your environment, largely formed by the input offered through the "picture frame" of the train window, was underdetermined. In the special input configuration driving your visual system it allowed for two consistent interpretations: either it is the *other* train or it is the train in which *you* are presently sitting which has just started to move. The visual model of reality allowed for two equally coherent interpretations. At the same time there was a state of general physical and emotional arousal, accompanied by an unconscious state of expectancy about what is very likely going to happen next, and very soon. The information-processing system, which you *are*, has selected one of the two possible interpretations in accordance with constraints imposed by a preexisting internal context and, as it is a system which always tries to maximize overall coherence, "decided" to simultaneously activate a suitable self-model, one that can be integrated into the new phenomenal model of the world without causing any major problems. Unfortunately, the chosen model of the world was wrong. Therefore, the activation of the accompanying kinesthetic-proprioceptive self-model led the system into a very brief hallucinatory episode. As transparent models of reality and the self are always fully interpreted and untranscendable for the system currently operating *under* them, a hallucinated bodily self ensued. Its content was the content of a phenomenal self-simulatum, activated by an erroneous automatism leading the system astray, while not being recognized as such. A possibility was depicted as a reality. As the dominant visual model of reality is being updated, this briefly "deviating" form of self-modeling leading to the subjective experience of a real body being slowly accelerated is immediately terminated—and with a mild degree of irritation or amusement we recognize that we have just fooled *ourself.*

This may count as the minimal case of a phenomenal self-simulation fulfilling no proper function *for* the system—in this case leading to a partially empty, illusionary experience of the body as a whole and in motion. It does not satisfy the adaptivity constraint, and its most striking neurophenomenological feature is the internal emulation of kinesthetic "motion" qualia, of a form of presentational content we normally take to be as strictly stimulus-correlated. The solution to this problem is to acknowledge that visual kinesthetic information, generally being richer than mechanical kinesthetic information, can overrule the second type in cases of conflict, because vision "is not only an exteroceptive sense, as is classically assumed, it is also an autonomous kinaesthetic sense" (Lishman and Lee 1973, p. 294). What is still missing in this introductory case study is a stable, exteriorized visual perspective of the physical body. Let us now proceed to look at two classic phenomenological descriptions of OBEs, as spontaneously occurring in an ordinary non-pathological context (see also figures 7.5 and 7.6):

I awoke at night—it must have been at about 3 A.M.—and realized that I was completely unable to move. I was absolutely certain I was not dreaming, as I was enjoying full consciousness. Filled with fear about my current condition I only had one goal, namely, being able to move my body again. I concentrated all my will power and tried to roll over to one side: something rolled, but not my body—something that was me, my whole consciousness, including all of its sensations. I rolled onto the floor beside the bed. While this happened, I did not feel bodiless, but as if my body consisted of a substance constituted of a mixture between the gaseous and liquid states. To the present day I have never forgotten the combination of amazement and great surprise which gripped me while I felt myself falling onto the floor, but the expected hard bounce never took place. Actually, had the movement unfolded in my normal body, my head would have had to collide with the edge of my bedside table. Lying on the floor, I was seized by terrible fear and panic. I knew that I possessed a body, and I only had one great desire—to be able to control it again. With a sudden jolt I regained control, without knowing how I managed to get back to it. (Waelti 1983, p. 18; English translation by T.M.)

The prevalence of OBEs ranges from 10% in the general population to 25% in students, with extremely high incidences in certain subpopulations such as, to take just one example, 42% in schizophrenics (Blackmore 1986; for an overview and further references, see Alvarado 1986; 2000, p. 18*f.*; Irwin 1985, p. 174*f.*). However, it would be false to assume that OBEs typically occur in people suffering from severe psychiatric disorders or neurological deficits. Quite the contrary; most OBE reports come from ordinary people in everyday life situations. Let us therefore stay with nonpathological situations, and look at another paradigmatic example, again reported by the Swiss biochemist Ernst Waelti:

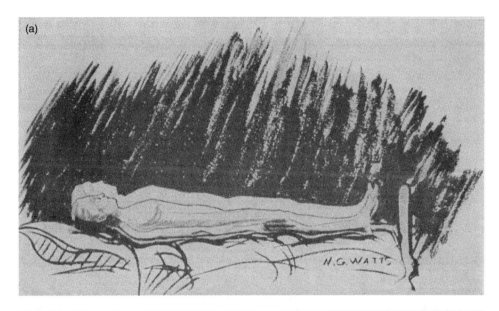

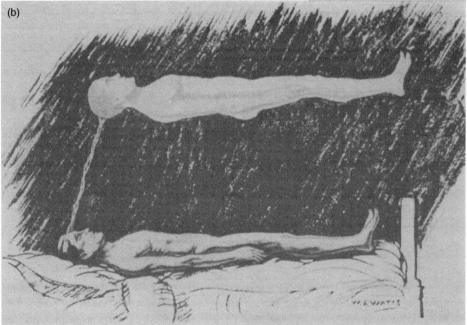

Figure 7.5
(*a–d*) Kinematics of the phenomenal body image during OBE onset: The "classic" motion pattern according to Muldoon and Carrington. (From Muldoon and Carrington, 1929.)

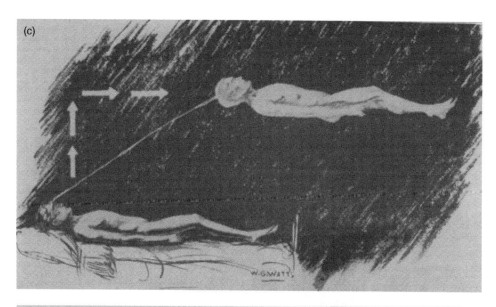

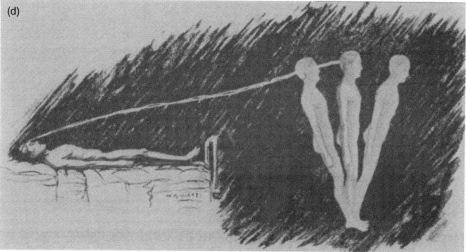

Figure 7.5
Continued.

(a)

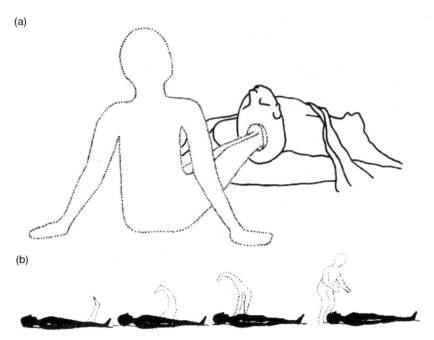

(b)

Figure 7.6
Kinematics of the phenomenal body image during OBE onset. (*a* and *b*) Two alternative, but equally characteristic motion patterns, as described by Swiss biochemist Ernst Waelti (1983).

In a dazed state I went to bed at 11 P.M. and tried to go to sleep. I was restless and turned over frequently, causing my wife to grumble briefly. Now I forced myself to lie in bed motionless. For a
while I dozed before feeling the need to pull up my hands, which were lying on the blanket, in order
to bring them into a more comfortable position. In the same instant I realized that I was absolutely
unable to move and that my body was lying there in some kind of paralysis. Simultaneously I could
pull my hands out of my physical hands, as if the latter were just a stiff pair of gloves. The process
of detachment started at the fingertips, in a way that could be clearly felt, almost with a perceptible
sound, a kind of crackling. It was precisely the movement, which I actually intended to carry out
with my physical hands. With this movement, I detached from my body and floated out of it with
the head leading. I gained an upright position, as if I were now almost weightless. Nevertheless I
had a body consisting of real limbs. You have certainly seen how elegantly a jellyfish moves through
the water. I could now move around with the same ease.

I lay down horizontally in the air and floated across the bed like a swimmer who has pushed
himself from the edge of a swimming pool. A delightful feeling of liberation arose within me.
But soon I was seized by the ancient fear common to all living creatures, the fear of losing my physical body. It sufficed to drive me back into my body. (Waelti 1983, p. 25; English translation
by T.M.)

Sleep paralysis is not a necessary precondition for OBEs. They frequently occur during extreme sports, for instance, in high-altitude climbers or marathon runners.

A Scottish woman wrote that, when she was 32 years old, she had an OBE while training for a marathon. "After running approximately 12–13 miles . . . I started to feel as if I wasn't looking through my eyes but from somewhere else. . . . I felt as if something was leaving my body, and although I was still running along looking at the scenery, I was looking at myself running as well. My "soul" or whatever, was floating somewhere above my body high enough up to see the tops of the trees and the small hills. (Alvarado 2000, p. 184)

The classic OBE contains two self-models, one visually represented from an external perspective and one forming the center of the phenomenal world from which the first-person perspective originates. What makes the conceptual analysis of OBEs difficult is the fact that many *related* phenomena exist, for example, autoscopic phenomena during epileptic seizures in which only the first criterion is fulfilled. Devinsky and colleagues differentiated between autoscopy in the form of a complex hallucinatory perception of one's own body as being external with "the subject's consciousness . . . usually perceived within his body" and a second type, the classic OBE, including the feeling of leaving one's body and viewing it from another vantage point. The incidence of autoscopic seizures is possibly higher than previously recognized; the authors found a 6.3% incidence in their patient population (Devinsky, Feldmann, Burrowes, and Bromfield 1989, p. 1085; regarding a possible causal relation between epilepsy, autoscopy, and attempted suicide, see Brugger, Agosti, Regard, Wieser, and Landis 1994). Here is one of their case studies, demonstrating how OBEs can also develop from untypical etiologies like epileptic seizures.

Case 7.—A 29-year-old woman has had absence seizures since the age of 12 years. The seizures occur five times a week without warning. They consist of a blank stare and brief interruption of ongoing behavior, sometimes with blinking. She had an autoscopic experience at age 19 years during the only generalized tonoclonic seizure she has ever had. While working in a department store she suddenly fell, and she said,

the next thing I knew I was floating just below the ceiling. I could see myself lying there. I wasn't scared; it was too interesting. I saw myself jerking and overheard my boss telling someone to "punch the timecard out" and that she was going with me to the hospital. Next thing, I was in space and could see Earth. I felt a hand on my left shoulder, and when I went to turn around, I couldn't. Then I looked down and I had no legs; I just saw stars. I stayed there for a while until some inner voice told me to go back to the body. I didn't want to go because it was gorgeous up there, it was warm— not like heat, but security. Next thing, I woke up in the emergency room.

No abnormalities were found on the neurological examination. Skull CT scan was normal. The EEG demonstrated generalized bursts of 3/s spike-and-wave discharges. (Devinsky et al. 1989, p. 1082)

One important feature of OBEs is that the phenomenal representation of the perceiving, acting self is confabulatory, while the representation of the remaining physical body from an external perspective is generally accurate. For instance, OBEs during seizures frequently clearly depict convulsive movements and automatisms very accurately, from a viewpoint above the body.[18] For many people who have actually lived through these phenomenal states, this is an argument against the possibility of their hallucinatory nature (I come back to this point at the end of this section). However, it has to be noted that in the second self-model forming the object component of the consciously modeled subject-object relationship, veridical content and confabulatory content are frequently *integrated* into a single whole. To remain with the case studies of Devinsky and colleagues, one patient noted that his body perceived from an external perspective was dressed in the same clothes he was wearing, but curiously he always had combed hair even when he knew his hair was uncombed before the onset of the episode (case 4, p. 1081). Another telling phenomenological difference is that some patients will visually experience their body seen from above as not transparent and actually casting a shadow (e.g., case 4); in other cases the double will be transparent, but slightly smaller than life-size (case 9, p. 1082); and in other patients the body appears solid, but does *not* cast a shadow (case 2, p. 1081). It may be relevant to note that even in spontaneous OBEs, clearly occurring in nonpathological contexts, the nonveridical or self-contradictory nature of particular forms of experiential content may very well be cognitively available, not only after, but *during* the experience. Remember our very first case study, the report by Swiss biochemist Ernst Waelti: "Actually, had the movement unfolded in my normal body, my head would have had to collide with the edge of my bedside table." Phenomenal kinesthetics and the underlying spatial frame of reference seem to be slightly dissociated in this case. This very fact itself is in turn available for cognitive processing, and for the formation of autobiographical memory.

As Alvarado (1997, p. 16) remarked, little systematic work has been conducted on the phenomenology of the experience (see also Alvarado 1986; 2000, p. 186*f.*). In terms of the conceptual tools and constraints so far developed, the content of OBEs certainly is globally available for attention and cognitive access. *Volitional* availability, however, is a highly variable component of the experience (for an overview of the phenomenology, see Irwin 1985, p. 76*ff.*; for an analysis of different case studies, cf. Blackmore 1982a, p. 56*ff.*; for further references, see Alvarado 2000). Many OBEs are dominated by a sense of passively floating. The two self-models that are active during an OBE are embedded in a coherent global state, into a single multimodal scene forming an integrated model of

18. As Devinsky and colleagues write: "Patient 39 was 'up there looking at myself convulsing, and my mother and the maid were screaming . . . I felt so sorry for them and my body.' Patient 40 watched her convulsive seizure, 'like being in a balcony,' and observed the nurses placing a tongue depressor on her tongue and putting up the sides of the bed. Patient 33, who witnessed her complex partial seizure, clearly saw herself looking 'anxious, pale, and rubbing my hands, running aimlessly from one place to another.'" (Devinsky et al. 1989, p. 1086).

reality. They are also activated within a window of presence, that is, the experience has no phenomenological characteristics of recollection or future planning—an OBE is something that is happening *now*. In fact, a considerable subset of OBEs is accompanied by the subjective experience of "hyperpresence" or "hyperrealism," particularly in those cases where a blending into or additional episodes of religious ecstasy are reported. The phenomenal reality as modeled in the OBE certainly is a convolved and a dynamic reality (see sections 3.2.4 and 3.2.5). OBEs are also first-person states: they clearly unfold under a single and unified first-person perspective generated by a PMIR. What makes them unique is that the object component of the PMIR is formed by a self-model, which is not a *subject*-model. You see your own body, and you recognize it as your own, but presently it is not the body *as subject*, the body as the locus of knowledge, and of lived, conscious experience.

Of course, numerous exceptions exist in the colorful reports and the folklore about this kind of bodily self-consciousness, but the conceptually most interesting feature of the OBE arguably is that it is accompanied by situations in which the subject as well as the object component of a phenomenal model of the current subject-object relationship is taken by a model of the self: *you* see your *own* body lying on the bed below you. Interestingly, this does not lead to a multicentered or decentered overall state of consciousness. Only one of the currently active self-models functions as the "locus of identification." Typically, it is only the etheric double hovering above that is represented as the attentional subject (see section 6.4.3), as the currently thinking self (see section 6.4.4), and as the agent deliberately moving through space (see section 6.4.5 and the marathon runner example for an exception). In general, it also seems safe to say that prototypical OBEs are fully transparent states in the sense previously defined: the model of reality generated during the experience is not experienced *as* a model, although in experienced subjects and practitioners this fact may well be *cognitively* available during the episode. It is precisely the transparency of OBEs, which has led generations of experiencers and theoreticians in many cultures and for many centuries to naive-realistic interpretations of this deviant form of phenomenal self-modeling. However, it must be noted, many OBE subjects also report a "dreamlike quality, as if being awake in a dream." Of general dream variables like the prevalence of flying dreams, vividness, dream recall, and suchlike, the occurrence of lucid dreams is the most consistent predictor of OBEs (Alvarado 2000, p. 194*f*.; see also section 7.2.5). Susan Blackmore (1986a) found that subjects reporting deliberate, as compared with spontaneous, OBEs have a better ability to control and terminate dream content and more frequent flying dreams. An important hypothesis, which has to be empirically followed up, therefore, is that OBEs are just an additionally constrained subset of lucid dreams (see also Blackmore 1982b and section 7.2.5). Deliberate OBE experiencers ("OBErs") also seem to be characterized by specific personality traits. In an interesting study, Wolfradt and Watzke (1999) singled out only the 10.4% of subjects who reported being able to leave and return to their body at will and treated only them as true OBErs. They found "that primarily the DP-subscale [DP = depersonalization] 'sense of self,' followed by the SPQ-subscale [SPQ = schizotypy] 'cognitive-perceptive,' the DP-subscales 'self-awareness' and 'certainty of self,' accounts for almost all of the valid variance of discrimination between OBErs and non-OBErs" (p. 5).

In short, one may predict that a more systematic approach to the phenomenology of OBEs will yield different degrees of global transparency and opacity accompanying the experience, and will have to investigate the interrelatedness of this feature with other high-level variables, for instance, global content properties of the self-model ("personality traits"). OBEs can certainly be functionally characterized as offline-activated states (*constraint 8*), because they typically occur when the body is asleep, paralyzed after an accident, or under anesthesia. In these situations, globally available somatosensory input will be minimal. The PSM loses an important source of presentational content that drives it under normal circumstances. Harvey Irwin (1985, p. 308*ff.*) has presented a theory of the OBE in which the notion of being "out of touch with somatic processes" plays a decisive role, either in terms of functional loss of input or in terms of attentional unavailability through habituation. An interesting question, finally, is whether OBEs satisfy the adaptivity constraint introduced at the end of chapter 3: Can there be a *teleofunctionalist* analysis of OBEs? What function could this type of experience have *for* the organism as a whole? Here is a speculative proposal of Devinsky and colleagues:

There are several possible benefits that dissociative phenomena, such as autoscopy, may confer. For example, when a prey is likely to be caught by its predator, feigning death may be of survival value. Also, accounts from survivors of near-death experiences in combat or mountaineering suggest that the mental clarity associated with dissociation may allow subjects to perform remarkable rescue maneuvers that might not otherwise be possible. Therefore, dissociation may be a neural mechanism that allows one to remain calm in the midst of near-death trauma. (Devinsky et al. 1998, p. 1088)

Given the current theoretical framework it is not at all inconceivable that there are physically or emotionally stressful situations in which an information-processing system is forced to introduce a "representational division of labor" by distributing different representational functions among two or more distinct self-models (see section 7.2.4). The OBE may be an instance of transient functional modularization, of a purposeful separation of levels of representational content in the PSM. For instance, if cut off from somatosensory input, or if flooded with stressful signals and information threatening the overall integrity of the self-model as such, it may be advantageous to integrate the ongoing conscious representation of higher cognitive functions like attention, conceptual thought, and volitional selection processes into a *separate* model of the self. This may allow for a high degree of integrated processing, that is, for "mental clarity," by functionally encapsulating and thereby *modularizing* different functions like proprioception or attention and cognition in order to preserve at least some of these functions in a life-threatening situation. Almost all necessary system-related information is still globally available, and higher-order processes like attention and cognition can still operate on it as it is presented in an integrated manner, but its distribution across specific subregions in phenomenal space as a whole has now dramatically changed. Only one of the two self-models is truly "situated" in the overall scene, integrated into an internally simulated behavioral space, and only one of them is immediately embodied and virtually self-present in the sense described in sections 5.4 and 6.2.2. As it is fully transparent, it is a full-blown phenomenal self instantiating the phenomenal property of selfhood *for* the system. Frequently, both self-models integrated within a single OBE are constituted by spatial as well as nonspatial mental content.

Interestingly, the bodily self-model forming the object component in this type of first-person experience never changes much in its spatial properties: the physical body viewed from an external perspective is very rarely distorted or changed in shape and size. However, the subject component of the intentionality relation modeled in these states may vary greatly (note how just the opposite principle holds for ordinary waking states). Some OBE experiencers see or feel themselves in a weightless replica of their original body; others experience themselves as being in no body at all or in a kind of indeterminate form, such as a ball of light or an energy pattern (Alvarado 1997, p. 18; Green 1968) or even as "pure consciousness" (Alvarado 2000, p. 186). This may point to the fact that spatial content is not strictly necessary to realizing the function fulfilled by the second self-model for the system as a whole. In other words, those higher functions such as attention, cognition, and agency, which are integrated by the "dissociated" self, are now only *weakly embodied* functions. In order to be carried out they do not need integration into a spatially characterized, explicit body image. Arguably, attentional and cognitive agency can *functionally* be decoupled from the process of autonomic self-regulation and the spatial self-representation necessary for generating motor behavior. In this context, it may also be interesting to note that certain technological setups in virtual reality (VR) experiments—so-called second person VR and telepresence systems (Heeter 1992, p. 264; see also section 8.1)—seem to achieve precisely the same effect, by creating the conscious experience of viewing one's own body as embedded in and interacting with a virtual world or the experience that there is a "real you" not currently inhabiting your body. What such technical systems offer is an additional functional module (a graphic image or a robot body) through which subjects can control their own behavior. Participants in VR experiments of this type frequently describe their phenomenology simply as *being* an OBE, even if they have never had a natural OBE before (Heeter 1992). If empirical evidence could be generated to show that the spatiality of the attentional and cognitive self-model hovering above the self-as-object component in the OBE-model of reality is not a strictly necessary condition, this would support the functional modularization hypothesis proposed here.

From a systematic point of view, any thorough analysis of deviant phenomenal models of the self is of highest relevance. However, of the phenomenological state classes mentioned in this chapter, there are three for which the general quantity and quality of available scientific research are particularly low: OBEs, dissociative identity disorder (DID) (see section 7.2.4), and lucid dreams (see section 7.2.5). It is hard to find empirical work that lives up to the methodological or conceptual standards of current cognitive neuroscience or analytical philosophy of mind.[19] Notable exceptions are the works of Harvey Irwin, John Palmer, and Susan Blackmore. Irwin proposes a model involving a shift in attentional processing during episodes of weakened somatosensory input and a kinesthetic completion of the somesthetic body image mediated by a visual model of the environment, constructed from memory sources (Irwin 1985, p. 306 *ff.*). As somesthetic input is lost, other presentational subformats—like vision and kinesthesia—become more dominant and take its role in stabilizing the PSM. As Alvarado (2000, p. 203) points out, Irwin's model has received support from studies relating absorption and visuospatial abilities to the OBE and positively correlating synesthesia-like items from a specific absorption scale to OBE frequency. John Palmer analyzes OBEs as compensatory processes after events threaten the integrity of the overall self-model by causing fundamental changes in the body schema (see Palmer 1978). For Palmer, OBEs are just one of many routes the system can take to rescue its threatened phenomenal identity, to preserve the overall coherence (see section 6.2.1) of the self-model. As Alvarado (2000, p. 202) puts it, in Palmer's view the "OBE, then, is an attempt to prevent the jeopardy to one's identity from reaching awareness and precipitating a crisis."

Susan Blackmore, to whom I am grateful for many exceptionally stimulating discussions, explicitly employs the concept of a "model of reality." Explicitly operating under the information-processing approach and analyzing the representational needs and

---

19. From this point of view, the most important publications certainly are Blackmore 1982a, Irwin 1985, and J. Palmer 1978. An excellent recent review is Alvarado 2000. A short overview concerning the literature and trends in research from the nineteenth century to 1987 may be found in Alvarado 1989. A review of modern developments from 1960 to 1984 concerning research on spontaneous out-of-body experiences is in Alvarado 1986. A review of three historical phases of psychological research since the nineteenth century may be found in Alvarado 1992. A more systematic overview concerning the phenomenology of OBEs may be found in Irwin 1985, p. 76 *ff.*; for further discussion and a review of attempts toward the development of empirical taxonomies and typologies of the OBE, see Alvarado 1997. Blackmore 1982a, p. 56 *ff.*, offers an analysis of different case studies; reports of OBEs in non-Western cultures and of previous scientific studies may be found in Blackmore 1982a, p. 71 *ff.* and 82 *ff.*) Wolfradt and Watzke 1999 present an interesting study of the relationship between depersonalization, schizotypal personality traits, thinking styles, and deliberate OBEs.

resources of persons undergoing OBEs, she arrives at a theory describing OBEs as episodic models of reality, constructed by brains cut off from sensory input during stressful situations and having to fall back on internal sources of information. For instance, she draws attention to the fact that visual cognitive maps reconstructed from memory are, interestingly, organized from a bird's-eye perspective in the majority of subjects and predicts that these persons are more prone to having OBEs (see, e.g., Blackmore 1982a, p. 164*ff.*; 1987). She also points out an important phenomenological feature of intended bodily *motion* in the OBE state: frequently, the way in which OBErs move around in the currently active model of reality is not smooth, as in walking or flying, but occurs in discrete jumps from one salient point in the cognitive map to the next salient point. What Blackmore's observation draws attention to is that, whatever else OBEs are, they certainly are internally simulated behavioral spaces. This phenomenological observation may point to the fact that frequently these behavioral spaces, typically simulated by a brain under great stress, are *spatially underdetermined*; that is, they are coarse-grained internal simulations of landmarks and salient spots in certain perceptual scenes that were seen and acted upon at an earlier stage in life. The general idea in Blackmore's theory is that OBEs are transparent phenomenal simulations of a world which are highly realistic because they include a partially veridical representation of a phenomenal body and are organized from an external "third-person" visual perspective (Blackmore 1984, 1987).

All these approaches are in keeping with the current theory. It is interesting to note that all three of them are explicitly presented as *psychological* theories, not making the assumption of any nonphysical carrier substance for conscious experience being in existence or actually leaving the body during an OBE. They are parsimonious by being simulational, and not representational, theories of the OBE, because they do not assume that there is an actual *representatum* in the environment of the physical body corresponding to the PSM as an exteriorized second entity. However, taking a more careful look at abstract, nonspatial aspects of the phenomenal self in these states, one discovers how the subject component of the PMIR in the OBE state is not completely empty. An attentional and cognitive subject engaging in selective processing is modeled, and actually *in existence*: OBErs generally have good control over their attentional and thought processes as such, even if almost all the *content* of these processes may be hallucinatory.

From a philosophical perspective, OBEs are interesting for a number of reasons. First, from the purely systematic perspective of a representational theory of mind, they present us with a unique phenomenal configuration: OBEs are global, phenomenal models of reality, in which two self-models but only one first-person perspective exist. That is, we have a more or less stable, centered model of reality that contains a PMIR. The interesting point is that during some episodes, the subject component, as well as the object component of the transparent model of the intentionality relation, is constituted by a

representational structure actually purporting to depict the experiencing person *herself.*
What OBEs show is that self-models are not necessarily *subject*-models: You can represent something as your *own* body, without representing it as an agent to which you are
identical, and you can do so under a *perceptual* model of the subject-object relation. OBEs
are like a "perceptualized" variant of reflexive self-consciousness. OBEs constitute a
strong argument for the thesis that, while an accompanying bodily self-model may be fully
"confabulated" by subpersonal mechanisms fighting for global coherence, the phenomenal locus of the self is always where the locus of cognitive and attentional *agency* is. Interestingly, this is not true of *bodily* agency (recall the marathon example). It is easy to
conceive of systems that are not cognitive, but only attentional agents (for instance,
animals) but which have OBEs. Therefore, the experience of attentional agency may
be the core of phenomenal selfhood and perspectivalness and the origin of all consciously
experienced intentionality.

More generally, the phenomenological concept of an OBE seems to be a cluster concept,
and the phenomenal state class picked out by this concept is characterized by a high degree
of variability in phenomenal content. However, there seem to be a number of further and
essential features. In whatever way the etheric "double" or doppelgänger leaving the physical body is phenomenally modeled, it is always the cognitive and attentional subject—
the self-model modeling the system as a cognitive and attentional agent (see sections 6.4.3
and 6.4.4)—which forms the phenomenal "locus of identity," which invariably is represented as the subject component of the represented subject-object-relationship, thereby
generating the structural feature of the overall model of reality which I have described
as its perspectivalness. As we have seen above, there are higher-order types of self-
consciousness (i.e., *self*-models internally satisfying the perspectivalness constraint; see
section 6.4.4) with the arrow of the PMIR pointing downward from a second-order self-
representation to a first-order self-representation—as in phenomenologically *inward*-
directed attention and self-related cognition. OBEs are unique in being simulations of
perceptual PMIRs, frequently pointing "downward" in a much more literal sense, establishing a system-system relationship modeled within a spatial frame of reference. It is as
if in situations where the self-model cannot be anchored in internal somatosensory input
anymore (see section 5.4), higher cognitive functions like attentional processing or categorical thought simply take over in *centering* the global model of reality. In this way some
persons undergoing an OBE truly are disembodied thinking selves in a neurophenomenologically reduced version of the original Cartesian sense. However, the information that
is not subjectively available to them, of course, is that all this is just a *model* of reality
generated by their central nervous system.

This leads us to a number of issues of a more general philosophical interest. For anyone
who has actually undergone that type of experience, it will be almost impossible not to

become an ontological dualist afterward (e.g., 73% of respondents in an early study by Karlis Osis claimed having a new attitude about life after death after experiencing an OBE, 67% reported a reduction in their fear of death, and 66% in a study done by Gabbard and Twemlow claimed to have actually adopted a belief in life after death; see these and further references in Alvarado 2000, p. 188; for a recent empirical study of near-death experiences in cardiac arrest survivors, see Parnia, Waller, Yeates, and Fenwick 2001). In all their realism, cognitive clarity, and general coherence, these phenomenal experiences will almost inevitably lead the experiencer to later conclude that conscious experience can, as a matter of fact, take place *independently* of the brain and the body: what was phenomenally possible in such a clear and vivid manner simply must be metaphysically possible. Although many OBE reports are certainly colored by the interpretational schemes offered by metaphysical ideologies available to the person in his time and culture, such experiences have to be taken seriously. Although their conceptual and ontological interpretations are in most cases seriously misguided, the truthfulness of centuries of reports about "ecstatic" states, soul travel, and "second bodies" can hardly be doubted.

A second, related point is that reports about this specific type of phenomenal state are available in abundance, not only from all time periods, but also from many different cultures. There is a culturally invariant core to the phenomenon. The experience of a soul-like entity, an etheric or astral body leaving the physical body during sleep, after an accident, or in death is what I would call a "phenomenological archetype" of mankind. Following this line of thought I will make two claims. First, the phenomenological archetype which, today, we call an "out-of-body experience" is actually a *neuro*phenomenological archetype: the functional core of this kind of phenomenal state is formed by a *c*ulturally *i*nvariant *n*europsychological *p*otential common to all human beings. Call this the CINP hypothesis. Under certain conditions, the brains of *all* human beings, through specific properties of their functional and representational architecture which have yet to be empirically investigated, allow for this set of phenomenal models of reality. Probably this set of models of reality is a discrete set, forming an individual, clearly circumscribed goal for empirical research. A minimally sufficient neural correlate for the OBE state in humans is likely to exist, and, in principle, a functionalist analysis of the phenomenon can be developed from a more fine-grained representationalist analysis. Maybe, in some distant future, even machines can engage in soul travel.

Obviously, the notions of a PSM and of a PMIR offered here could serve as an excellent starting point in operationalizing the OBE. However, this assumption may be false, and it will also be important to find out how high the degree of cultural invariance in OBEs actually is. Maybe the OBE is *not* a distinct theoretical entity, but just a subcluster of pre-lucid dreams, or a tendency toward depersonalization, intuitive thinking and certain schizotypal personality traits (Wolfradt and Watzke 1999). In any case, the second point which makes OBEs an interesting target for philosophical analysis is that they likely also form a *neuroanthropological constant*, a potential, given the necessary neurofunctional configuration, to undergo a certain type of experience shared by all human beings. Animals could have OBEs too: as for many other of the syndromes discussed in this chapter, it is obvious that nonlinguistic creatures not embedded in a cultural environment could undergo these experiences as well. However, it is only in humans that OBEs could be *strong* first-person phenomena (in the sense of Baker 1998, as discussed in section 6.4.4), namely, by being in addition self-ascribed on a *conceptual* level. On our planet, so far, only human beings have had OBEs *and* the capacity to think and communicate about them, because only they have had the necessary brain structures. The potential to undergo "strong" OBEs, then, is a *neuro*anthropological *c*onstant. Therefore, let us call this second proposal the NAC hypothesis.

Let me point to a *third* aspect of this issue, one which makes OBEs interesting from a history-of-ideas perspective and which again highlights the urgent need for rigorous future research programs from a purely metatheoretical perspective. My last proposal is that the kind of phenomenal states, which today we call OBEs and which point to a commonality in the neurofunctional architecture underlying the process of human, conscious self-modeling, are actually the historical root of what I would call the "proto-concept of mind," which eventually developed into Cartesian dualism and idealistic theories of consciousness. In short, it is the particular kind of phenomenal content described in this section which first led human beings to believe in a *soul*. Call this simply the "soul hypothesis." After the evolution of brains had reached a stage at which OBEs in terms of strong, conceptually mediated forms of phenomenal self-modeling became possible, it was only natural—on a *theoretical* level—to assume that something like a soul actually exists. Given the epistemic resources of early mankind, it was a highly rational belief to assume the possibility of disembodied existence. And it was the PSM of *Homo sapiens* which made this step possible.

What is the proto-concept of mind? In many cultures we simultaneously find prescientific theories about a "breath of life" (e.g., the Hebrew *ruach*, the Arabic *ruh*, the Latin *spiritus*, the Greek *pneuma*, and the Indian *prana* viz. the five *koshas*, etc.). This is typically a spatially extended entity, keeping the body alive and leaving it during phases of unconsciousness and after death. We are confronted with the almost ubiquitous idea of what mind actually is, which in all its many variations is still a *sensory-concrete* idea of the mental as something that integrates parts, not only of physical organisms but in a wider sense also of societies and groups of human beings. In Western philosophy of mind this proto-concept of mind has developed through innumerable stages, from the pneumatology of Anaximenes in the sixth century B.C., through Diogenes of Apollonia and the

Aristotelian distinction between breathed air and psychic pneuma (which may perhaps count as the first attempt at a naturalist theory of mind in Western philosophy). This development continued through alchemist theories of controlling nature by controlling mind and the neoplatonists, for whom the pneuma was an aureola covering the soul and protecting it from contact and contamination by material objects, on toward Christian philosophy, which finally *denaturalized* and *personalized* the concept of mind. In this way the Western history of the concept of mind can be read as a history of a continuous differentiation of a traditionalistic, mythical, sensory proto-theory of mind, which gradually led to mind being a more and more abstract principle, which finally, culminating in Hegel, is devoid of *all* spatial and temporal properties.

It is interesting to note how the best theories of mind available today *again* turn it into a concrete process, fully endowed with temporal and spatial properties. However, in the light of present-day cognitive neuroscience it is even more interesting to see how, at the beginning of human theorizing about mind and consciousness, we find a very similar basic motive across very different cultural contexts: the idea of a "subtle body," which is independent of the physical body and the true carrier of higher mental functions like attention and cognition (Mead 1919). Historically, the dualist tradition in philosophy of mind is *rooted* in these early proto-theories. These theories, I would propose, may in turn be motivated by naive-realistic interpretations of early reports about OBEs. At the beginning of this chapter I noted how may of the deviant models of reality and self discussed here in the form of neurophenomenological case studies may have a hidden heuristic potential, because they can also be read as metaphysical or epistemological metaphors. In a way, they are the brain's own philosophy. As phenomenal ontologies they are nonpropositional theories—internal, neurobiologically realized models—about what actually *exists* from the brain's point of view. Taken as an ontological metaphor, the phenomenology of OBEs inevitably leads to dualism, and to the concrete idea of an invisible, weightless, but spatially extended *second body*. This, then, may actually be the folk-phenomenological ancestor of the soul, and of the philosophical proto-concept of mind: It is the OBE PSM. Therefore, in order to not only have an empirically grounded theory of conscious experience but to also understand the neurofunctional and neurophenomenological underpinnings of the persisting intuition that such a theory leaves out something highly important, it will be of highest relevance to achieve a fuller understanding of this type of phenomenal experience. What I have sketched as the CINP, the NAC, and the soul hypotheses may be a good starting point to take phenomenology seriously. The traditional concept of an immortal soul, which can exist independently of the physical body, may have a phylogenetically new *neurophenomenological correlate* in the type of deviant phenomenal self-modeling described in this section.

Hallucinated Agency

What is consciously experienced *volition*? It is the phenomenal content activated by a transparent model of the internal selection process leading the organism to actually carry out a certain behavioral pattern. This will typically be one specific pattern of motor behavior out of a number of possible behaviors that have previously been internally simulated. Phenomenal volition is the content of an internal representation of this *selection* process, which cannot be recognized *as* a representation on the level of introspective access. This is why the experience feels absolutely real.

Volition, in standard situations, is additionally experienced as one's *own* will, because this representation is integrated into the currently active self-model. Please note how this is precisely the transition from the subpersonal to the personal level: A subpersonal process of dynamic self-organization is *appropriated* by the system as a whole, because it is now integrated into its PSM, and is therefore globally available for a more flexible and selective form of response control. Like all other representational content embedded in the self-model it gains the additional phenomenal quality of "mineness."

On the representational level of analysis the upshot is as follows: Classes of phenomenal models are classes of instruments helping the organism to make specific types of information globally available, for instance, for cognitive assessment or for *vetoing* certain kinds of ongoing motor processing. A volitional self-model is an instrument making a certain kind of system-related information—the information that a certain kind of selection process has just taken place—globally available *for* the system. On the functional level of description the advantage provided by the process of conscious volition consists in making ongoing selection processes possible targets of higher-order interventions.[20] Conscious control dramatically increases the *flexibility* of the system's behavioral profile.

I will not enter into an extended discussion of the philosophical problem of freedom of will here. Let me briefly make one conceptual and one empirical point, which will help to better understand the notion of hallucinated agency. First, the concept of a "volitional act" is an incoherent concept, because it leads to an infinite regress. At least if the conscious experience of volition is itself analyzed as a kind of internal agency, a homunculus is implicitly introduced, an internalized intentional system (see Dennett 1987b) *whose*

---

20. My use of the expression "higher-order intervention" should not be construed to imply (a) that there is some type of mysteriously direct *personal-level* intervention, or (b), that such personal-level interventions (e.g., Libetian "vetos") as such could be causally undetermined. Of course, this would just re-create the problem of freedom of the will on another level (see Walter 2001). "Higher-order" here just refers to the functional or representational architecture of the system. Conscious volition increases behavioral flexibility by letting a larger portion of this architecture causally interact with the subpersonal selection process, thereby making it more *context-sensitive*.

action this subjective experience of volition then becomes. For this little man in the head the same problem will reappear: How does *it* decide on what volitional acts to choose? The philosophical answer to this problem lies in shifting levels of description by exchanging the logical subjects of predication. This can be achieved naturally by ascribing selective activity, increased flexibility, the capacity to interrupt actions after they have been started, and so on, to the *system as a whole* and not to some subpersonal entity in its brain. It is not the PSM or some preconscious mechanism for example, that selects a certain motor pattern, but always *the system as a whole*. There now is a cognitive science aspect to this solution which helps us much better to *understand* how it actually works: The transition from subpersonal to personal-level properties works via the PSM. Because this new representational tool permits the system to internally *conceive of itself as a whole*, subpersonal selection processes can be functionally appropriated, namely, by making them globally available *under a PSM*. They are now causally integrated into a larger structure and thereby become targets of flexible top-down processing. The PSM is the decisive link from microproperties to macroproperties, from neural dynamics in the brain to personhood.

Second, from an empirical perspective, it is important to understand the further point that every overt behavior will have a minimally sufficient neural correlate that can be analyzed as its typical, but domain-specific, cause. Like every other form of conscious content, the subjective experience of willing and deciding on a specific behavioral pattern *also* will possess a minimally sufficient neural correlate. It supervenes locally on certain brain properties. Our conscious self-model represents that kind of phenomenal content, which in folk-psychological contexts we call "the experience of will," as the one and only *cause* of the ensuing external action. This was a wonderfully elegant way of creating the first-person phenomenon of *agency*. But from a third-person perspective this may be false: the minimally sufficient neural cause necessary to produce an external action and the minimally sufficient neural correlate of the subjective experience of *deciding* to carry out this action may diverge. As a matter of fact, this is an empirically plausible assumption in many cases. The experience of agency (see section 6.4.5) and the activation of a phenomenal model of the *practical* intentionality relation (see section 6.5.3) may therefore be a simplified internal confabulation, a cost-effective solution to the brain's evolutionary problems. By activating the minimally sufficient neural correlate of the overt action we could reliably trigger this action, even against the subject's will. Strictly speaking, it would now only be behavior, and not an action anymore.

On the other hand, if the minimally sufficient neural correlate of the phenomenal experience of will could be artificially brought about in a human being, the prediction would be that this person experiences herself as choosing a particular action and actually carrying it through, although from a third-person perspective this would be not the true state of affairs. Hallucinated agency is the conscious experience of volition and executive consciousness in the presence of a deviant, nonstandard causal etiology for the actual motor behavior taking place. To give an example, there is some limited evidence that not only the direct execution of a grasping movement but also the conscious experience of an irresistible "urge to grasp" can be directly triggered by stimulating the ventral bank of the anterior cingulate sulcus (Kremer, Chassagnon, Hoffmann, Benabid, and Kahane 2001).[21] One central prediction of the SMT is that, as the whole representational process is fully transparent, this would lead to an untranscendable experience of agency in a situation where no action has ever taken place. Let us now look at an elegant and noninvasive psychological experiment, which validates this prediction.

Daniel M. Wegner and Thalia Wheatley (1999, see also Wegner 2002) investigated the necessary and sufficient conditions for the conscious experience of mental causation with the help of a simple and ingenious experiment. In their *I Spy* study they led subjects to experience a causal link between a thought and an action, the feeling that they willfully performed an action, which, however, was actually performed by someone else. Each subject arrived for the experiment at about the same time as a confederate who was posing as another participant (for a detailed description of the experimental setup, see Wegner and Wheatley 1999, p. 487*ff*.). On a table separating them was a square board mounted atop a computer mouse and both participant and confederate had to place their fingertips at the side of the board closest to them, enabling them to move the mouse together. They could move a cursor around a computer screen visible to both of them, which showed a photo called "Tiny Toys" from the book *I Spy*, which showed about fifty small objects such as plastic dinosaurs, cars, and swans. The subjects were told to stop moving the mouse about every 30 seconds and that afterward they would be asked to rate each stop they made for "personal intentionality." Participant and confederate marked the degree to which they consciously experienced their own behavior as a willed action on scales which they kept on clipboards in their laps. Both were told that they would hear music and words through headphones, and that for every trial a 30-second phase of movement followed by a 10-second clip of music would signal that they should now make a stop. The subjects assumed they were listening to different tracks of an audiotape but at about the same time and were told that they should wait a few seconds into the music before actually making

21. This was the case of a patient with medically intractable epileptic seizures, who underwent intracerebral EEG recordings and stimulations to locate the epileptogenic zone before surgery. The authors describe the phenomenal correlate and the functional consequences of the above-mentioned stimulation as follows: "It consisted in an irresistible urge to grasp something, resulting in exploratory eye movements scanning both sides of the visual field, and accompanied by a wandering arm movement contralateral to the stimulation side. Then, after the patient had visually localized a potential target, her left hand moved towards the object to grasp it, as if mimicking a spontaneous movement. This irrepressible need started and ended with stimulation, and the patient was unable to control it" (Kremer et al. 2001, p. 265).

stops to make sure they were ready. They were also told that they would hear words, ostensibly to "provide a mild distraction," and that they would hear different words, which was the reason for their listening to separate audio tracks. In short, participants were led to believe that whatever words they heard, they were not heard by their confederate.

The words served to prime thoughts about items on the screen for the participant (e.g., "swan") and one was presented for each trial. The confederate, on the other hand, heard neither words nor music, but instead heard instructions to make particular movements at particular times. For four of the trials, the confederate was instructed to move to an object on the screen. A countdown followed until the time the confederate was to stop on the object. These forced stops were timed to occur midway through the participant's music. (Wegner and Wheatley 1999, p. 488)

Wegner and Wheatley assume that three principles govern the construction of phenomenally experienced mental causation: (1) the *principle of exclusivity* (the thought should be the only introspectively available cause of action), (2) the *principle of consistency* (the semantic content of the thought should be consistent with the action as represented), and (3) the *principle of priority*, namely, that the consciously experienced thought should precede the consciously experienced action at a proper interval. The variation in timing served to manipulate the degree of priority just mentioned. As it turned out, although there was a general tendency for subjects to perceive forced stops as actually intended, there was a marked dependence of the subjective experience of practical intentionality determined by the timing of the prime word. As predicted by the principle of temporal neighborhood, experienced intentionality was lower when the prime word appeared 30 seconds before the forced stop, increased when the word occurred 5 seconds or 1 second before the stop, and then dropped to a lower

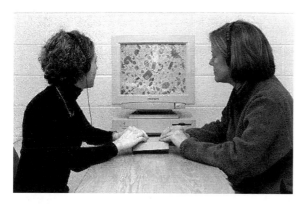

Figure 7.7
Hallucinated agency: The *I Spy* study. (Courtesy of Daniel M. Wegner and Thalia Wheatley.)

level when the word occurred 1 second following the stop (Wegner and Wheatley 1999, p. 489).

Postexperimental interviews showed that subjects often searched for items onscreen after they were named over the headphones. In other words, there was a continuing attempt to establish a "perceptual intentionality relation," a successful phenomenal representation of a certain subject-object relationship, an integrated phenomenal representation of the phenomenal self as currently *visually* perceiving a particular object. As the authors point out, this sense of searching for the item, in combination with the subsequent forced stop, may have been a particularly conducive condition for activating the conscious content in question. In what follows I offer a coarse-grained functional and representational analysis of the effect of hallucinated agency achieved by the *I Spy* experiment. However, as readers will see, my own interpretation of the data presented by Wegner and Wheatley diverges slightly from the authors' interpretation, first, in employing some of the conceptual tools previously developed, and second, in pointing to the potential importance of the system of "mirror neurons" to be found in area F5 of human premotor cortex (which were mentioned in section 6.3.3, when discussing possible social correlates of the human self-model). In short, I will attempt to interpret these data not only as a deviant kind of phenomenal *self-modeling* but also as a deviant type of semiconscious *social cognition* taking place between confederate and subject. I will treat them as functionally coupled self-modeling systems.

Let me begin by distinguishing two target phenomena: the phenomenal experience of volition and the phenomenal experience of agency. Target phenomenon 1 can be analyzed as a situation in which an abstract, allocentric representation of a terminated action is integrated with the currently active self-model, thereby becoming *my own* goal on the level of conscious experience. This specific process of transparent self-representation (which, from a phenomenological third-person perspective, could be termed "the self in the act of desiring") leads to the following phenomenal content:

[I* currently want to achieve this goal.]

The first step, therefore, may consist in activating a rather abstract, allocentric representation of an action as successfully terminated. This goal representation could, for instance, depict a mouse pointer having come to rest on a certain item on the screen plus your own arm having reached a certain final position. It is important to note that this process itself does not necessarily have to be conscious. The second step would then consist in somehow integrating the result of this step into the currently active self-model. Computationally speaking, an integration problem, a higher-order variant of the binding problem, has to be solved. Doing this means to construct what I have previously called the phenomenal model of the *practical* intentionality relation: the system, which you are, activates the mental representation of a certain subject-object relation, as currently holding. The object component in this relation is the allocentric action representation. The phenomenal subject, as usual, is the content of the currently active PSM. A *practical* PMIR does not portray the relationship of the system to a perceptual object in its environment or to some specific cognitive content (as in a *theoretical* PMIR), but the relation in which the system as a whole stands to a certain internally simulated goal state. Of course, we have the usual background assumption, namely, that the self-model and the overarching intentionality relation are transparently represented, that is, the system does not have a chance to introspectively$_3$ access these representations *as* self-generated internal representations. It is caught in naive realism about the content of the self-model, as well as about this relation in the manner it is currently modeled. The object component, however, may well be opaque—the fact that the goal state is just a simulated, possible state of the world can be attentionally available. This representational event, then, will endow the goal representation with the additional phenomenal quality of mineness: the goal is now *my own* goal. This is, or so I would claim, the representational structure underlying phenomenal volition. *Wanting* the goal is the same as *making the goal my own* on the level of phenomenal experience. The object component now is transparent too: what was a *possible* goal now is a fixed element of my own, inner *reality*. The final result is a conscious self in the act of desiring something. The next question is: How do you get from phenomenal volition to agency?

After one or a whole series of abstract, allocentric action representations have been activated, that is, after a certain set of possible actions have been mentally simulated, motor trajectories have to be generated which map the current state of the self-model—for instance, its arm position—onto the state of the self-model depicted in the selected goal representation, which has just been embedded. A transparent self-model can be used as the reference basis for forward-modeling of possible motor behavior (for an example of how this process could be led astray, see endnote 7). In this way it is self-zero, the anchor of an intended self-simulation. As soon as one of these simulated trajectories of possible action representations is selected, the system is ready to act. Acting, from the point of view of the current theory, means running an *egocentric* action simulation that is causally coupled to the effectors through the motor system. The step from allocentric to egocentric simulation is taken by pulling the object component of the PMIR into the subject component: by *embedding* it in the PSM. You literally *make* a possible action your own by embodying and enacting it via the self-model. Under standard conditions, this will be the central necessary condition for target phenomenon 2, the experience of executive consciousness (*Vollzugsbewusstsein*) or agency to emerge. After an egocentric forward-model has been coupled to the motor system, the resulting proprioceptive feedback or efference copy is then continuously integrated into the active self-model. On the level of phenomenal experience, it thereby becomes my *own* current behavior. The ongoing process of transparent self-modeling ("the self as behaving") briefly leads to the following phenomenal content:

[My own* body is currently moving in this way.]

Motor output leads to feedback either through an efference copy, or through proprioceptive, kinesthetic, or visual channels. This feedback then continuously changes the content of the self-model, in particular that partition of it which can be described as a motor emulator. Physical events—bodily motions—are being integrated into the self-model, and gain the phenomenal quality of mineness: this is my *own* body behaving and moving.

However, in order to arrive at full-blown phenomenal agency, in order to take the step from the conscious experience of behavior to the conscious experience of being an *agent*, a further element is needed. A causal relation has to be attributed to two separate events transparently modeled within the current self-model. This is what we usually call consciously experienced mental causation. The attribution of this causal relationship is necessary, on the level of phenomenal experience, to transform my current behavior into my own *action*. This transparent representation of an intrasubjective causal relation ("the self as mentally causing its own bodily behavior") leads to the following phenomenal content:

[I* am currently an agent.]

We now have a transparent model of the causal relation between two subsequent events taking place within the dynamics of the PSM: the (subpersonal) act of selecting a possible action simulation and integrating it into what I have called an "egocentric action simulation," and the event of my body actually moving. In this attribution of causality the final phase of my own volitional state has to be depicted as the *cause* of my bodily movements. One has to imagine this as a continuing, ongoing process leading not only to a singular experience of causing one's own actions but to the temporarily extended subjective experience of carrying your actions *through*, of executing a bodily motion. The true phenomenology can perhaps more realistically be described as a *flow* of agency. The importance of Wegner and Wheatley's investigation lies in demonstrating under what conditions this type of phenomenal agency can be constructed even if, first, a goal representation, and, second, an efference copy are actually missing.

Let us now proceed with a brief analysis of active representational content in the respective self-models of confederate and participant. You see that in the beginning we are considering *conscious* content only (box 7.1).

We see that the participant has some false *intentional* content as well, namely, in having a false opinion about himself (e.g., the purpose of his own current auditory experience)

Box 7.1

Confederate

PSM:

- [I* am now hearing an instruction.]

PMIR:

- [I* am now hearing *an instruction to stop on a certain object after the countdown ends.*]

Context:

⟨The participant cannot hear this.⟩

Participant

PSM:

- [I* am now hearing a word.]

PMIR:

- [I* am now hearing *a word on the headphone, to mildly distract me.*]

Context:

⟨The other participant is now hearing another word.⟩

---

and about the *context*, that is, the role of the confederate—whom he takes to be another participant. Auditory input slightly diverges for both subjects and is interpreted according to very different internal contexts. It is also important to remember how an initial analysis shows that a simple hearing of the target word does *not* lead to a stop on the named object in the participant. What is happening as the experiment proceeds (box 7.2)?

A plausible assumption now says that in the confederate the semantic input given through the instruction leads to an active goal representation, and a very fast simulation of possible motor behaviors that would, in their final phase, match this goal. In the participant it is quite likely that the priming effect through the headphone might activate a visual search for a matching onscreen item. In fact, postexperimental interviews have shown that the hearing of the word leads to a *guiding of attention* in some participants. Therefore, in those participants there actually was a preexisting PMIR, a model of the subject *attempting* to visually find a certain object already present in their imagination. The object component was given through auditory input, the system tried to construct a successful perceptual PMIR in the *visual* domain. In those people who do *not* have a memory of such an experience of visual search, however, one could imagine that they have an increased functional accessibility of content matching the heard word to consciousness due to what Daniel Wegner in an earlier work (1997) called an "ironic effect":

Box 7.2

Confederate

Activation of goal representation, forward-model, selection of motor trajectory.

PSM:
• [I have heard the instruction and now want to carry it out.]

PMIR:
• [*This kind of behavior would be necessary* in order for me* to carry out the instruction.]

Participant

Priming effect activates visual search. Automatic attempt to find matching visual object: *Attentional* PMIR is being constructed.

PSM:
• [I have heard another word. My visual attention is wandering.]

PMIR:
• As yet no shift in consciously experienced object component.

---

those participants really trying hard *not* to be distracted by the word may be creating an "ironic monitor" that is applied to a very small range of searched targets only, thereby making this search more effective and the respective representational content—which is still *unconscious*—more accessible to phenomenal experience, especially under conditions of cognitive load. One could speculate that even if it is very unlikely that participants are *actually* actively suppressing the words they hear, there may be an automatic process with a similar effect in place. They could—and this is pure speculation—achieve global availability (see section 3.2.1) by unintentionally running a simulation (see section 2.3) of what *not* to make the object component of their current PMIR (see section 6.5). Let us look at the next step in the current experiment (box 7.3).

In the next step the confederate integrates the goal-representation previously activated through auditory input into her current self-model. On the phenomenal level this means that she "accepts" the instruction and the goal becomes her *own* goal on the level of conscious experience. On a subpersonal level the system also selects a certain active representation of a possible motor trajectory and integrates it into the forward-model of the bodily self. Let us also assume that the participant is one of those persons who actually consciously experiences an ongoing visual search that has just been primed. He is therefore subjectively experiencing himself as *trying to successfully construct a perceptual model of this subject-object relation that he is already imagining*. We therefore have a

Box 7.3

Confederate

Allocentric goal representation is being integrated into the self-model.

PSM ("volitional subjectivity"):
· [I* am in the act of deciding to stop.]

PMIR:
· [I* am in the act of deciding to stop *on a certain object after the countdown ends.*]

Participant

Search results are now being integrated into the transparent model of the intentionality relation.

PMIR:
· [I* am now imagining a certain perceptual situation, that is, of myself visually perceiving *an onscreen item matching the word I just heard.*]

· [I* am now visually searching *for an onscreen item matching the word I just heard.*]

---

conscious representation of the self in the act of guiding its attention. Moreover, this representational configuration is a typical initial condition for motor behavior like grasping or pointing movements; it structurally resembles the typical beginning phase of a motor sequence. It is interesting to note that at this stage we already have a system which is searching for a match of exactly the object component which later *becomes* the phenomenally experienced action goal, and which simultaneously is trying to successfully *construct* a certain subject-object relation in its model of reality. However, this specific PMIR is not yet a model of a practical intentionality relation, but of a *theoretical* one: it tries to activate a certain kind of perceptual knowledge (box 7.4). At this stage—or so I would propose—a number of interesting events take place. In the confederate, an egocentric motor simulation is causally coupled to the motor system, as previously explained. A motor command is issued, which by proprioceptive feedback or through an efference copy leads to a continuous updating of that part of the conscious self-model which I would call the "phenomenal motor emulator." The resulting conscious content is described in box 7.4.

Let me now introduce an additional assumption, which I believe that, although admittedly speculative, is now not only rational but empirically plausible (for references, see section 6.3.3). The visual observation of the confederate's arm movement by the participant automatically triggers the activation of an abstract action representation, presumably

Box 7.4

Confederate

Motor command is issued, efference copy continuously fed into phenomenal motor emulator.

PSM:
• [I* am now pointing. I feel my own* arm move.]

PMIR:
• [I* am now pointing *to this onscreen object.*]

Participant

Visually observed behavior of confederate drives mirror system and the participant's unconscious self-model on a *functional* level, activating an unconscious action simulation and an allocentric goal representation.

PMIR:
• [I* am currently seeing/feeling *the other subject's arm movement.*]

Unconscious SM:
• [This kind of my own behavior would match the other subject's behavior.]

Unconscious goal representation:
• [In my own case, this behavior would typically be driven by *this* goal.]

---

in the left superior temporal sulcus (Brodmann area 21), the left inferior parietal lobule (area 40), and possibly in the interior part of Broca's region (area 45). In particular, I will now assume that position emission tomography (PET) scanning experiments carried out by Grafton, Rizzolatti, and colleagues (1996) about the localization of grasp movements have demonstrated this. Another line of empirical evidence (experiments on the excitability of motor cortex in humans by transcranial magnetic stimulation done by Fadiga and coworkers; see Fadiga, Fogassi, Pavesi, and Rizzolatti 1995) seems to show that there actually is something like a mirror system in humans and not only in monkeys. In short, I assume that every time we look at someone performing an action, the same motor circuits are activated as when we perform this action ourselves. This, in turn, helps us to mentally develop an *abstract goal representation out of a visually observed action.* It makes a new kind of representational content available, by extracting a highly specific kind of information (a "motor equivalence") from the social environment. The externally generated activity in the mirror system of the participant visually perceiving the arm movement of the confederate leads to a *retrodictive simulation of the confederate's mental state* (see, e.g., Gallese and Goldman 1998). Please always remember that this new form of

Box 7.5

Confederate

Action is carried through.

PSM:
• [I* am now pointing. I* feel my arm move.]

PMIR:
• [I* am now pointing *to this onscreen object*. I* am the agent *related to the object*.]

Participant

Proprioceptive-kinesthetic feedback from passive arm movement fed into phenomenal body image. Allocentric goal representation generated by mirror system increasingly matches kinematics of phenomenal body image, that is, its most likely termination point in a forward model; "goodness of fit" is *unconsciously* detected.

PSM:
• [My arm is moving.]

PMIR:
• *No* practical PMIR. Phenomenal agency not instantiated.

---

active representational content in the participant's brain does not yet have to be *conscious content*. Activity in a human mirror system is nothing in the nature of a theoretical inference. Rather it creates in the observer a state matching that of the target—it synchronizes the unconscious motor partitions of their self-models.

In other words, we now have an unconscious goal representation in the participant, which, however, is not yet integrated into his PSM. The speculative line of thought I am proposing here, therefore, treats Wegner and Wheatley's intriguing experiment as one in social cognition as well. It may be fruitful to look not only at the participant's isolated PSM, but also at the functionally coupled "two-person system" of confederate and participant. The central *physical* element realizing this causal link is area F5 in his premotor cortex. This leads to a testable prediction concerning Wegner and Wheatley's hypothesis: the experiment should not work in persons with lesions in F5 or, more simply, if both arms are hidden under a black board. What does it mean for two self-modeling systems to be functionally coupled through their self-models? For instance, many people think that joint attention is possibly the elementary building block of social cognition. Two people staring at the same monitor while simultaneously perceiving each other's arm movements certainly fulfill that condition, and it is interesting to note how they perceive their respective bodily movements in more than one modality as well (box 7.5). The confederate is now physically carrying through her pointing movement. A causal attribution between the first event, the mental selection of a possible motor trajectory, and the second event, the proprioceptive feedback generated by object-related bodily motion, is taking place and therefore she not only enjoys the experience of her own* arm moving but also the experience of full phenomenal agency. Her brain constructs not only a PSM but also a PMIR.

The participant, whose arm is passively dragged along, does not experience this causal attribution, because only the second event is represented in *his* self-model. For him the content of the conscious self only is: [My own arm is moving]. There is—as yet—no practical PMIR, just the experience of visual search. However, after a certain time, during but shortly before the end of the confederate's pointing movement, it becomes perceptually obvious *where*, that is, on what onscreen item, this movement will terminate. In the confederate everything is as is was before: the pointing movement unfolds, PSM and PMIR are updated accordingly. In the participant, however, we have an entirely different situation, corresponding to a different functional architecture. As hypothesized, we suddenly have an unconscious goal representation of the confederate's observed movement *including the object component of the intentional relation she is represented as standing in*. A full-blown model of a PMIR holding in the *other* subject becomes available. This will happen as soon as the most likely endpoint of *her* pointing movement becomes available. Simultaneously, the change in the phenomenal body image of the participant approximates exactly the same endpoint for the body movement still represented as *passively* taking place by the participant. The visually given object representation now begins to fully coincide with the endpoint of the proprioceptively experienced motor trajectory *and* the unconscious, abstract goal representation supplied by the mirror system in premotor cortex. In addition, we have a semantically primed visual search already going on, for the potential object component of a perceptual PMIR *exactly* matching those parameters. This search is now completed. In other words, what is represented as a *possible* perceptual subject-object relation is now represented as an *actual* subject-object relation (box 7.6). At this point in the development we have a situation where the actual input (proprioceptive and visual) fully converges for the confederate as well as for the participant. Here is the representational configuration at the *end* of the confederate's pointing movement (box 7.7): The content of the PSM active in the confederate's brain is: [I* am now done following the instruction from the headphone. My arm doesn't move anymore]. In the participant we have the same object, say, the onscreen swan, represented in *three* different ways: as visual object component of the currently active *visual* PMIR, as the proprioceptively experienced termination point of a passive arm movement, and as the object component of an *external* PMIR activated through the mirror system, a relation in which the *confederate's* movement is represented, through the mind-reading or "folk-psychology" mechanism

Box 7.6

Confederate

Action is carried through.

PSM:
· [I* am now pointing. I* feel my arm move.]

PMIR:
· [I* am now pointing *to this onscreen object*. I* am the agent *related to the object*.]

Participant

Visual search is successful or confederate stops on item.

PSM:
· [My own visual/attentional state has changed. I* am not searching anymore.]

PMIR:
· [I* am now seeing *an object corresponding to the word I heard on the headphone*.]

Context:
· ⟨The other participant never heard this word at all.⟩

Box 7.7

Confederate

Action completed: congruence between goal and action representation.

PSM:
· [I* am now done. My arm doesn't move anymore.]

PMIR:
· [I* am now done *following the instruction from the headphone*. My arm doesn't move anymore.]

Participant

System nonphenomenally detects isomorphism between:

· visually attended object in currently active PMIR;

· termination point of arm/pointer trajectory; and

· object component of allocentric goal representation.

---

which is always automatically active in the participant's brain. In other words, all the components necessary to assemble the representation of a *practical* PMIR originating from the participant's PSM are active. There is a goal, there is a movement, and there is a suitable object component. However, these components are not integrated into an egocentric phenomenal framework yet.

Now, remember that the participant also has a false belief. There is causally active context information: In the two-person system—as *he* consciously represents it—he* is the only one who has the semantic content heard over the headphone as an available mental cause, because he still thinks the "other" participant must necessarily be hearing another word. The exclusivity constraint introduced by Wegner and Wheatley (1999, p. 486) is fully satisfied on the conscious level of representation. However, *the mirror system cannot be fooled*: it smuggles the word back into the head of the participant via area F5 of his premotor cortex (box 7.8). How can this fact be explained on the level of conscious self-modeling?

This alternative (and admittedly coarse-grained) representational analysis of Wegner and Wheatley's material leads to a new and speculative hypothesis. First, on the functional and representational levels of description everything stays the same with the confederate. Second, the active search process running in the participant and the detected goodness of fit between the different object representations already active in the system lead to an "infection" of his PSM with the goal representation, which was supplied to him by the

Box 7.8

Confederate

Action completed and cognitively available.

PSM:
• [I* am now done. I* voluntarily decided to do this and all the time I* was the agent, that is, the cause of my own pointing behavior.]

Participant

To maximize overall coherence, the system automatically *integrates* allocentric goal representation into the PSM, antedates it, and treats it as the *cause* of proprioceptively perceived arm movement. Feedback is reinterpreted as efference copy. Phenomenal agency is instantiated.

PSM:
• [I* voluntarily decided to do this and all the time I* was the agent, that is, the cause of my own pointing behavior. I* am now done.]

---

other part of our two-person system via mirror neurons in premotor cortex. The confederate has two functions. First, she supplies the mirror system of the participant in the areas of motor cortex already mentioned with an active, but as yet unconscious goal representation. Second, as a kinesthetic element of the environment (i.e., in moving his arm) she supplies his motor emulator with the perfectly matching feedback, precisely the feedback which would have been generated by the right kind of arm movement through an efference copy or ordinary feedback. The participant himself has only *one* important function. In being "contextualized," semantically primed, and having an active search going, he sets the stage for activating a cascade of perceptual, volitional, and *practical* PMIRs: the self in the act of *searching* an object, the self in the act of *perceiving* an object, the self in the act of *wanting to act* on an object, the self in the act of *really pointing* to an object. My own hypothesis says that under the experimental conditions constructed by Wegner and Wheatley we will frequently have a situation where the participant's brain integrates and *antedates* a goal representation, proprioceptive feedback, and an internally primed search context into a transparent PSM—a model of a person that has been wanting to act and has actually acted all along (box 7.9; see also Haggard, Clark, and Kalogeras 2002). In this way we arrive at a final situation characterized by two self-models, which are phenomenally identical with regard to the aspects relevant here and have just been assembled out of the coupled functional dynamics of two individuals. One individual has knowledge about himself, the other is hallucinating. *What* the second individual is hallucinating are the past existence of a conscious selection process (volition) and the past existence of a continuing process of carrying out a chosen behavior (agency).

Box 7.9

Confederate

Action completed and cognitively available.

PSM:
• [I* am now done. I* voluntarily decided to do this and all the time I* was the agent, that is, the cause of my own pointing behavior.]

Participant

No decision or action ever took place.

PSM:
• [I* am now done. I* voluntarily decided to do this and all the time I* was the agent, that is, the cause of my own pointing behavior.]

7.2.4 Multiple Selves: Dissociative Identity Disorder

Self-models can be viewed not only as tools but as organs as well. A self-model is an *abstract* organ. Although it can be described as an integrated, dynamical, and bodily process—for example, on a neuroscientific level of description—it only reveals its full biological function if we analyze certain of its *abstract* properties. Such properties will typically be its "content properties," as revealed on the representational level of analysis. However, what is an abstract property from a third-person approach may be a maximally concrete *experiential* property from the first-person perspective. Dissociative identity disorder provides an excellent example of both of these general principles.

I have already pointed out how important partitions of the conscious human self-model possess social correlates (see section 6.3.3). In different social environments, different PSMs may be appropriate, because they may make different types of information globally available. However, social environments can also be highly *incompatible*. One and the same person, in different contexts, may be your most important and stable source of security, while at other times he or she may present a serious threat to your physical and mental health. On the other hand, a flood of psychological data today make it a highly plausible assumption that one of the highest "neurocomputational imperatives" for human beings consists not only in continuously maximizing the overall coherence of their global model of the world but of their internal *self*-model as well. The integrity of life itself is reflected in the integrity of the PSM. Therefore, it is easy to understand that there will be situations in which a system is forced to use multiple, alternating self-models in order to cope with "inconsistent data sets," for instance, with highly inconsistent *social* environments. Rapidly alternating social contexts may confront a human being with information that is highly relevant, and must therefore be made available on the level of conscious experience, while on the other hand it is impossible to integrate this information into a single autobiographical self-model. Some people are forced to live more than one life. It is not only conceivable from a purely conceptual point of view but it is also an empirically plausible assumption that in certain environments and under certain internal contexts a system will be forced to use multiple and alternating self-models, and that this will lead to the emergence of corresponding new classes of phenomenal states.

DID, previously also termed "multiple personality disorder" (MPD), is well-known for bringing about such types of phenomenal states. However, the validity of DID as a distinct clinical entity is a matter of continuous, controversial debate (for references, see Miller and Triggiano 1992, p. 47). But before discussing the theoretical and methodological problems related to the phenomenon of multiple, alternating phenomenal selves appearing in one and the same physical person, let us look at one particularly helpful and now classic case study.

What is DID? DID frequently results from extreme traumatization in early childhood, sexual abuse by a male parent in particular. One of the defining characteristics of DID is the existence of two or more "personalities" within a single individual becoming dominant and determining the behavior of this individual at different times. Every one of these subpersonalities processes a complex structure, as well as its own, unmistakable pattern of behavior and social relationships. Frequently, a *host personality* exists. This host personality usually is amnestic with regard to those episodes during which other personalities step out into the light of the phenomenal model of reality. A number of "alter egos" exist, typically using separate names to refer to themselves. Interestingly, none of these personalities seems to possess a full emotional spectrum. A frequent phenomenological configuration is one of the host personality being affectively undifferentiated, while the "visiting" personalities display an affective profile that is *exaggerated* in specific dimensions, thereby making themselves "appropriate" for specific social situations. At this point it may be helpful to remember an earlier point: Emotions represent the "logic of survival" (as ,e.g., Damasio 1999 puts it), and the emotional self-model *embodies* this logic. It is only natural to point out how different social situations may be characterized by diverging "logics of survival." Different subpersonalities seem to share general background knowledge about the world, while constructing their own autobiographical memory from an individual life history, including a specific sense of self developed during those periods in which they gained control over the behavior of the physical person "harboring them."

Daniel Dennett and Nicholas Humphrey were among the first authors to combine a thoughtful philosophical analysis with an illustrative case study (see Dennett and Humphrey 1989).[22] They described a patient named Mary. She is in her early thirties, suffers from depression, confusional states, and memory loss. Mary has undergone multiple therapies, does not respond to pharmacological treatment (and therefore has been taken to be a simulator), and has on different occasions been diagnosed as schizophrenic, as suffering from a *borderline* psychosis, and as manic-depressive. To a therapist she describes her own biography as follows:

Mary's father died when she was two years old, and her mother almost immediately remarried. Her stepfather, she says, was kind to her, although "he sometimes went too far." Through childhood she suffered from sick headaches. She had a poor appetite and remembers frequently being punished for not finishing her food. Her teenage years were stormy, with dramatic swings in mood. She vaguely recalls being suspended from her high school for a misdemeanor, but her memory for her school

---

22. For extensive philosophical discussions, see Braude 1991, and Radden 1996, 1999; a further case study from a philosophical perspective, including additional references, may be found in Wilkes 1988a, p. 109 *ff*. For a different, "narrativistic," approach and the notion of a "multiplex self," see Flanagan 1994, p. 136.

years is patchy. In describing them she occasionally resorts—without notice—to the third person ("She did this, That happened to her"), or sometimes the first-person plural ("We [Mary] went to Grandma's"). She is well-informed in many areas, is artistically creative, and can play the guitar; but when asked where she learned it, she says she does not know and deflects attention to something else. She agrees that she is "absent-minded"—"but aren't we all?": for example, she might find there are clothes in her closet that she can't remember buying, or she might find she has sent her niece two birthday cards. She claims to have strong moral values; but other people, she admits, call her a hypocrite and a liar. She keeps a diary—"to keep up," she says, "with where we're at." (Dennett and Humphrey 1989, p. 71).

After a couple of months of treatment the therapist discovers that the handwriting for different entries in Mary's diary varies as strongly from entry to entry as the handwriting of different persons. During a therapeutic session under hypnosis, he decides to appeal to that part of Mary that "hasn't yet come forward" (ibid., p. 72), encouraging it to do precisely this. This is what happens:

A sea change occurs in the woman in front of him. Mary, until then a model of decorum, throws him a flirtatious smile. "Hi, doctor," she says, "I'm Sally. Mary's a wimp. She thinks she knows it all, but I can tell you . . ."
   But Sally does not tell him much, at least not yet. In subsequent sessions (conducted now without hypnosis) Sally comes and goes almost as if she were playing games with Dr. R. She allows him glimpses of what she calls the "happy hours," and hints at having a separate and exotic history unknown to Mary. But then with a toss of the head she slips away—leaving Mary, apparently no party of the foregoing conversation, to explain where *she* has been. (ibid., p. 72)

In the course of treatment further alter egos step out: coquettish "Sally," aggressive "Hatey," young and malleable "Peggy." Every single one of those visiting personalities possesses a history of its own and its own memories. All visiting personalities claim to have a far-reaching knowledge concerning the biography of their host Mary, while Mary denies possessing more than indirect knowledge about *their* "experiences" and the history of their personality.

   The following picture emerges from subsequent attempts to search for a possibility of integrating the different phenomenal selves in the course of a therapeutic process. At the age of 4 years Mary was repeatedly sexually abused by her stepfather. He gave her a nickname of her own, "Sandra," and urged the small child to keep "Daddy Love" as his and Sandra's little secret.[23] After the psychological suffering and the overall situation became unbearable for the small child and its tender personality only in the early phases of its development, she attempted to save her personal integrity by splitting her phenomenal self.

---

23. I will spare the reader further details at this point. See Dennett and Humphrey 1989, p. 73.

Eventually, when the pain, dirt, and disgrace became too much to bear, Mary simply "left it all behind": while the man abused her, she *dissociated* and took off to another world. She left—and left Sandra in her place. (ibid., p. 73)

Our new conceptual tools may be helpful in shedding light on this specific form of deviant self-modeling. *Taking off into another world* means to relocate the attentional subject (see section 6.4.3) within a different phenomenal model of reality. Attentional and emotional self-modeling can be separated. One of the central social correlates of Mary's emotional self-model—her stepfather—became inconsistent, by episodically and unpredictably turning into an aggressor. In Mary's model of reality, he lost his transtemporal identity as a person. It was impossible to mentally model him as *one* person. This development, however, was mirrored in her *own* self-model. The forced process of modularization generated a Mary-self, which could provide a stable phenomenal identity, a consistent inner history, and functional social relationships (cf. the process of functional modularization in self-models after loss of *somatosensory* input in OBEs, as analyzed in section 7.2.3). Dennett and Humphrey speculate how the Sandra-self in the background could have undergone further dissociations by distributing different aspects of the horrible series of traumatic experiences to a number of different subselves, which, however, could access memories shared with Mary. In terms of the present model, the space of autobiographical memory was divided into globally available regions and those that can only be functionally and phenomenally accessed under a nonstandard self-model. Viewed from the newly generated "perspective" of the dissociating Sandra-self, the advantage in this process would have been that afterward at least *parts* of the self-model constructed during the traumatic situation could step into the light during certain socially adequate situations, taking over control of Mary's behavior. In short, multiple PMIRs became available with multiple PSMs.

Thus her experience of liking to please Daddy gave rise to what became the Sally-self. Her experience of the pain and anger gave rise to Hatey. And the experience of playing at being a doll gave rise to Peggy.

Now these descendants of the original Sandra could, with relative safety, come out in the open. And before long, opportunities arose for them to try their newfound strength in settings other than that of the original abuse. When Mary lost her temper with her mother, Hatey could chip in to do the screaming. When Mary was kissed by a boy in the playground, Sally could kiss him back. Everyone could do what they were "good at," and Mary's own life was made that much simpler. This pattern of what might be termed "the division of emotional labor" or "self-replacement therapy" proved not only to be viable, but also to be rewarding all around. (ibid., p. 74)

Just like in OBEs, the phenomenal model of reality constructed in the course of DID is characterized by the activation of multiple self-models. The content of these differing self-models is incompatible, for example, with regard to their spatial, emotional, or autobiographical content. In fact, one author (Putnam 1989, p. 21*f.*; quoted in Alvarado 1992, p. 242) has described OBEs as a "dissociative disorder not included in DSM-III [*Diagnostic and Statistical Manual of Mental Disorders*, 3rd ed.]." Because the different PSMs in DID alternate, a common characteristic of both classes of states is that, at any given point in time, there is, first, a single phenomenal center of consciousness constituted by a coherent attentional, cognitive, and behavioral agent. As a phenomenal model of reality, DID is functionally *monocentric*. Second, the phenomenal first-person perspective *as such* is never multiplied: at any given point in time there is one and only one PMIR. The content and causal profile of the subject component may vary dramatically, but the fundamental perspectivalness of conscious experience as such is always preserved.

Anyone interested in developing a neurophenomenological analysis of those dissociative states characteristic of DID has to exclude iatrogenic artifacts. A skeptical stance toward this phenomenon, as well as toward the specific interests of the therapeutic community, certainly is appropriate. (However, Dennett and Humphrey [1989, p. 85] also reported a patient, whose *own* skeptical stance toward the diagnosis of her therapist disappeared after she learned that one of her alter egos had already consulted another therapist). Miller and Triggiano (1992, p. 56) criticized a number of methodological shortcomings and the general lack of experimental rigor characterizing current research on DID, thereby limiting the generalizability of findings and potential progress in eventually establishing this disorder as a distinct clinical entity possessing a discrete set of diagnostic criteria and open to systematic forms of treatment. Earlier reviewers (Fahay 1988; Putnam 1984) arrived at similar results. On the other hand, there can be no reasonable doubts about the existence of the phenomenon as such. A large number of empirical findings concerning the behavioral and physiological correlates of the multiple "personality states" observed in DID make it a plausible assumption that the respective PSMs generating the conscious content and the functional profile of these personality states are coherently organized, and functionally discrete system states. Even if DID should turn out not to be a distinct neurophenomenological or clinical entity, and even if it can eventually be reduced to a combination of other syndromes, the notion of a PSM may be a helpful tool in arriving at this sort of conclusion. When shifting from one self-model to another, not only have marked differences in voice, posture, and motor traits such as handwriting been reliably reported but also systematic shifts in cerebral electrical activity, cerebral blood flow, galvanic skin response, skin temperature, event-related potentials, neuroendocrine profiles, thyroid function, response to medication, perception, visual function, and visually evoked potentials (see Miller and Triggiano 1992 for review and references). The shift in phenomenal content is clearly mirrored in shifts between coherent sets of functional properties. DID gives us an excellent illustration of how the human self-model simultaneously achieves *phenomenal* and *functional* embodiment. On the level of anecdotal evidence, even such dramatic effects as shifts in allergic profile accompanying "personality changes" and the prolonged absence of withdrawal symptoms in a heroin addict after switching to a "nonaddicted" phenomenal self have been reported (Miller and Triggiano 1992, p. 55*f.*).

Whatever the final empirical analysis of DID, it is obvious that a modern philosophical theory of mind will have to offer an explanation of this phenomenon. Conceptually, it helps us to see what is possible, and what may be necessary. As in all other case studies presented here, we do *not* find a multiplication of the phenomenal first-person perspective as such. What DID demonstrates, however, is that the subject component of the transparent PMIR can possess a much higher degree of *variance* in terms of representational content than is usually assumed. In particular, multiple sets of mutually exclusive and functionally incompatible forms of integrated self-representational content can take its place. Because of the high degree of *internal* coherence characterizing these sets of representational content, and because of the emergence of separate, functionally encapsulated autobiographical memories, I propose to analyze them as distinct entities, namely, as different PSMs alternating within one and the same physical person.

It is plausible to assume that in specific stress situations a naturally evolved representational system like the human brain is forced into a certain type of "emotional division of labor," as alluded to by Dennett and Humphrey in the passage quoted earlier. This may simply be the only possibility of preventing the phenomenal self from disintegrating altogether. The emotional self-model possesses the function of making information regarding the general interests and biological needs of the system globally available for attentional processing, autobiographical memory, motor control, and so forth. If in an early phase of development, in which the PSM of a child has only just started to flower and consolidate, a parent suddenly turns into an aggressor and even *offers* a second identity by giving a new name to the child (as is frequently the case), a bizarre and highly threatening social context is generated. More than one logic of survival is now in existence. As physical escape from the situation is generally impossible, the child may be forced to distribute the process of internally modeling its interests and needs onto different functional modules, which then play the respective roles in its overall representational ecology separately. It is conceivable how such pathological self-models could become stabilized within a system and suddenly be reactivated at a later stage of its history by different, but structurally related social situations (e.g., an attempted rape in adulthood). This will lead to the unavailability of certain kinds of self-related information during certain periods of time (memory loss), as well as to incompatible overall functional profiles during such periods (inconsistent behavioral patterns).

From a third-person perspective the observable psychological properties of a patient suffering from DID cannot consistently be described as properties of a *single* person. This was exactly the problem that, in Dennett and Humphrey's case study, little Mary had: how to still create a mental model of her stepfather as a single person. The phenomenon of DID complements our previous discussion of the social correlates of the PSM in section 6.3.3 by adding the developmental perspective: different social correlates can drive different phenomenal ontogenies. It also shows how psychological properties standardly ascribed to the system as a whole on the personal level of description are determined by the subpersonal processes which generate the content and the functional properties of the currently active self-model. Identity disorders, while being diagnosed on the *personal* level of description, result from subpersonal disintegration (see Gerrans 1999; see also Dennett 1998). Especially when operating from a genetic perspective, when investigating the causal history of such dramatic "personality shifts," subpersonal levels of explanation have to be taken into account. The concept of a PSM forms the logical link between subpersonal and personal levels of description. As a neurobiological, functional, and representational entity it is subpersonal, but by satisfying the transparency constraint (see section 6.2.6) it generates personal-level properties like phenomenal selfhood for the system as a whole, enabling "strong" first-person phenomena, social cognition, and intersubjectivity. Classic, egologic theories of mind, when confronted with phenomenological material like the one presented by DID or other cases described in this chapter, are forced to either ignore the empirical material or to resort to occultist assumptions, like DID actually being possession by spirits, and such like.

As soon as more rigorous empirical research on DID becomes available, one important goal will consist in investigating how different *degrees* of variance and invariance are distributed over different levels of the PSM. For instance, there may be a maximal variance in autobiographical memory and affective profile, while certain styles of attentional and cognitive processing could prove to be a more or less invariant source of information, even between alternating self-models. In particular, if it is true that, as I have claimed, the human self-model is always functionally anchored in a more or less invariant source of internally generated input, then there should be a nucleus of invariance in a certain part of the *unconscious* self-model—for instance, provided by abstract computational features of the spatial model of the body or, as Damasio has hypothesized, in those brainstem structures continually regulating the homeodynamic stability of fundamental aspects of the internal chemical milieu.[24]

24. In Damasio's terminology, this would mean that a certain functional core, the "proto-self" is the transtemporal link connecting different PSMs even in patients suffering from dissociative identity disorder (DID). As Damasio writes, "It is apparent, however, that in spite of being able to display more than one autobiographical self, such patients continue to have only one mechanism of core consciousness and only one core self. Each of the autobiographical selves must use the same central resource. Reflection on this fact is intriguing. It brings us back to the notion that the generation of the core self is closely related to the proto-self, which, in turn, is based

7.2.5 Lucid Dreams

As Antti Revonsuo has pointed out, the ongoing process of conscious experience can be regarded as a distinctive, namely, *phenomenological*, level of organization in the mind-brain (see Revonsuo 2000). In order to proceed to more systematic descriptions of this level in terms of representational content and the functional roles of the individual states involved, an appropriate metaphor may be useful for initially guiding research and developing more specific hypotheses. The concept of "virtual reality" could be used as a heuristically fruitful metaphor of consciousness, because it captures many of its essential features (see Revonsuo 1995; 1997; 2000a, p. 65; Metzinger 1993; see also section 8.1). From a third-person epistemological point of view, consciousness is a *global simulational state*. However, this fact is not available from the first-person perspective during ordinary, non-lucid dreams. In ordinary dreams, as well as in waking states, the phenomenological level of organization is characterized by the subjective sense of self-presence (see sections 6.5.2 and 6.5.3), in terms of a full immersion of the attending, thinking self into a multimodal experiential reality (see sections 6.2.2 and 6.2.3). I also agree with Revonsuo in that previous metaphors (e.g., multiple drafts, global workspace, theater models, and the like) do capture some, but not enough of the essential characteristics of the relevant level. What is missing?

A plausible philosophical assumption is that phenomenal content supervenes on internal and contemporaneous functional properties of the human brain. However, this principle of internality is not reflected on the level of conscious experience itself, because—on the level of content—it is systematically "externalized": The brain is constantly creating the experience that I* am directly present in a world *outside* my brain, although, as Revonsuo says, the experience itself is brought about by neural systems buried deep inside the brain. Whereas, in one of the previous sections, I made initial attempts at offering a representationalist analysis of out-of-*body* experiences, Revonsuo has coined the concept of an "out-of-the-*brain* experience" (Revonsuo 2000, p. 65). The second notion is more fundamental: An essential phenomenological constraint on all classes of phenomenal states we know today seems to be full immersion into a seemingly real world portrayed as being outside the brain. Lucid dreams, in neurophilosophically informed individuals, may present an exception to this rule. But even ordinary dreams are interesting, because they activate an internally simulated behavioral space as well, in a situation where the physical system itself is functionally decoupled from its environment while continu-

---

closely on the representations of one singular body in its singular brain. Given a single set of representations for one body state, it would require a major pathological distortion to generate more than one proto-self and more than one core self. Presumably the distortion would not be compatible with life" (Damasio 1999, p. 354*f.*, n. 14).

ously "attempting" to self-organize its neural activity, constantly perturbed by an internal source of input (see section 4.2.5), into a coherent global state (for empirical details concerning explanatory models, see Kahn, Pace-Schott, and Hobson 1997; Kahn and Hobson 1993; Hobson, Pace-Schott, and Stickgold 2000).

A second important feature of phenomenal dreams is their transparency: the fact of dream content being *simulational* content, of not being a reality, but the internal representation of a possibility, is not available for conscious experience in general or cognition in particular. As I show in this section, there is a well-documented and possibly distinct class of phenomenal states in which the content and functional profile of the human self-model is enriched in a way that neutralizes the transparency constraint, which was introduced in chapter 3, and which holds for almost all other phenomenal states except conscious cognition and pseudohallucinations. Lucid dreams are theoretically relevant, because they may be the most common and uncontroversial example of *global opacity*. Before proceeding to point out differences between ordinary and lucid dreams relevant to our first working definition of the term, let us look at one first, and typical, example:

I dreamed that I was standing on the pavement outside my home. . . . I was about to enter the house when, on glancing casually at [the pavement] stones, my attention became riveted by a passing strange phenomenon, so extraordinary that I could not believe my eyes—they had seemingly all changed their position in the night, and the long sides were parallel to the curb! Then the solution flashed upon me: though this glorious summer morning seemed as real as real could be, I was *dreaming*! With the realization of this fact, the quality of the dream changed in a manner very difficult to convey to one who has not had the experience. Instantly, the vividness of life increased a hundredfold. Never had the sea and sky and trees shone with such glamorous beauty; even the commonplace houses seemed alive and mystically beautiful. Never had I felt so absolutely well, so clear-brained, so inexpressibly *free*! The sensation was exquisite beyond words; but it lasted only a few minutes and I awoke. (Fox 1962, p. 32*f*.; quoted in S. LaBerge and Gackenbach 2000, p. 154)

The lucid dreamer is fully aware of the fact that her current phenomenal world does not, in its content, covary with external physical reality. Functionally, she is *freed* from extraorganismic reality as an experiential subject, while at the same time being aware of the misrepresentational character of her overall state. It is important to note, however, that ordinary dreams are not only hallucinatory episodes, but also fully delusional states. As a matter of fact, Hobson (1997, p. 126; see also Hobson 1999) has put forward the bold hypothesis that dreaming is not like delirium, but identical to delirium; that dreaming is "not a *model* of a psychosis. It *is* a psychosis." The dreaming subject not only suffers from visual hallucinations resembling those occurring in toxic states but is fully disoriented to time, to place, and to person, suffers from severe distractibility and attention deficits, from memory-losses, and cognitive inconsistencies. As Hobson (1997, p. 122) stresses, the conviction that physically impossible dream events are elements of reality strongly resembles the delusional beliefs forming the "hallmark of all psychosis," the enduring failure to recognize that we are dreaming can be seen as "akin to the tenacity with which the paranoid clings to false belief" and that the overall mechanism integrating singular dream events into a highly improbable story are "like the confabulations of Korsakov's syndrome." In short, the fact that dreams are not only complex hallucinations but are also characterized by disorientation, confabulation-like dynamics, amnesia, and a dramatic general loss of insight, has led some experts to propose a radical interpretation of dreams as an organic mental syndrome. Lucid dreams differ from ordinary dreams in almost all of these dimensions.

Nonlucid dreams clearly are global phenomenal states in fulfilling the globality constraint, the principle of presentationality, and in being transparent (cf. the notion of aperspectival, "minimal consciousness" in section 3.2.7). However, they are phenomenally *subjective* states in a much weaker sense: there is no attentional subject in existence, the cognitive subject is fully deluded in terms of having almost only false beliefs about itself, and the phenomenal property of agency is only realized in a weak and intermittent fashion, if at all. The PMIR is highly unstable in ordinary dreams, making them first-person states in only a weak sense. However, there exist dreams in which the first-person perspective becomes just as stable as in ordinary waking consciousness. Such dreams are clearly strong, self-ascribable first-person phenomena in Lynne Baker's (1998; see also section 6.4.4) sense. Interestingly, it is the human self-model that plays the decisive role in this transition.

Let us adopt the following working definition of a lucid dream:

1. The dreaming subject has achieved full mental clarity concerning the fact *that* she is dreaming. The dreamer *knows* that she is now experiencing a lucid dream and is capable of ascribing this property to herself. In terms of the current theory this means that the fact of the system currently undergoing a specific type of representational state is cognitively, as well as attentionally, available, and has been integrated into the current conscious self-model.

2. The conscious state of the dreaming subject is generally characterized by full intellectual clarity. The overall level of cognitive insight into the nature of the state and intellectual coherence in general are at least as high as during normal waking states (but may actually be even higher[25]).

---

25. As the phenomenology shows, lucid dreams can be characterized by brief episodes of heightened intellectual insight, and by the "hyperreal" character already mentioned a number of times. This global phenomenological characteristic is also typical of certain religious experiences, and of mania and drug-induced states (which may also reflect episodically heightened levels of arousal and global coherence in the brain), and in some cases in states of brief religious ecstasy, as known from some types of epilepsy. Note the very accurate

3. According to subjective experience, all five sensory modalities function as well as they do during the waking state.

4. There is full access to memory for past phenomenal states, concerning waking life, *as well as* for previously experienced lucid dreams. Autobiographical memory is globally available on the level of conscious self-modeling. There is no amnesia; and particularly there are no asymmetrical amnesias between different episodes of conscious self-modeling, as can be found in DID (see previous section) or between the phenomenal selves of the waking and the *ordinary* dream states.

5. The property of *agency* is fully realized, on the phenomenal as well as on the functional level. A temporally extended *practical* PMIR is in existence. The subject of a lucid dream is not a passive victim lost in a sequence of bizarre episodes, but experiences itself as a full-blown agent, capable of selecting from a variety of possible behavioral patterns, by turning them into intended, real actions. Moreover, agency is not only experienced but the *fact* of being capable of selective action is cognitively available.

This definition is a strong definition, in a number of ways. First, there is an equivocation of "knowledge" in many earlier research definitions of lucidity, in terms of simply describing lucid dreams as dreaming while *knowing* that one is dreaming (Green 1968; S. LaBerge 1985; see also S. LaBerge and Gackenbach 2000, p. 152). However, knowledge can consist in either *cognitive* availability (of a certain fact, as mentally represented in a quasi-propositional format) or *attentional* availability (of information, in terms of intensified subsymbolic modeling). Cognitive availability leads to conceptual classification or categorization, for example, of the current experiential state belonging to the class of dreams. Attentional availability leads to the accessibility of earlier processing stages, resulting in phenomenal opacity. The current definition is a *strong* definition in that it makes both features defining characteristics of lucidity.

Could animals have lucid dreams? It is interesting to note that there might be systems for whom the simulational nature of their current dream state has become opaque in terms of an exclusively *attentional* availability of earlier processing stages, without the accompanying ability to self-ascribe this situation on the level of cognitive self-reference. Noncognitive creatures could experience lucidity in terms of regaining agency and a stable attentional PMIR during the dream state, while not being able to categorize their current state as a *dream* for themselves.

---

phenomenological notions of "the vividness of life increasing a hundred-fold," the "glamorous" and "alive" "mystical beauty" reported by Oliver Fox in the first case study selected for the main text above. In this context it may be interesting to note that Tart 1972a coined the concept of a "high dream." A considerable number of lucid dreams *end* in states phenomenologically overlapping with episodes of deeper spiritual insight. See, for instance, the very first case study presented by Stephen LaBerge and Jayne Gackenbach (2000, p. 151).

This definition is also strong in that it requires the availability of autobiographical content in the PSM plus full-blown agency, that is, the availability of a practical PMIR at any time, as additional necessary conditions (like earlier research definitions put forward by Tart 1988 and Tholey 1988; for a dissenting view, see S. LaBerge and Gackenbach 2000, p. 152). It is important to note that the availability of a certain content does not require that it actually is realized all the time. As has been pointed out, there is no requirement for a lucid dreamer to actually, continuously, and *explicitly* remember that his physical body is now lying in bed at a specific place and time or to actually, and continuously, *exercise* control over the dream (Kahan and LaBerge 1994; S. LaBerge 1985). Availability is all that counts. Therefore, strong and weak research definitions of the phenomenon can easily be integrated relative to the list presented above, in terms of degrees of *realized* availability of different types of simulational content on the level of the PSM and the PMIR.

What is known about lucid dreams from an empirical point of view? Lucid dreams occur spontaneously, as well as a consequence of intentional induction (for a recent review, see S. LaBerge and Gackenbach 2000). Younger people tend to have lucid dreams more frequently, and the capacity to induce lucid dreams can be learned to a certain degree (e.g., S. LaBerge and Rheingold 1990; Tholey 1987). Just as with OBEs and DID, the general quantity and quality, in terms of experimental and methodological rigor, of the scientific literature currently available is low. One particularly interesting question is whether OBEs and lucid dreams are discrete sets of phenomenal states to which a single and distinct theoretical entity could correspond. First, however, let us look at three short case studies.

. . . I arrive in W. by bus. Two acquaintances (from my high school days), M. and a girl (N.?), leave the bus. I think the bus will go on to the main train station where it will be easier for me to transfer. However, it goes on in the direction of Z. After it bypasses a traffic circle (at which it could have turned back), I get angry and form the desire that all this should not be true.

Immediately I realize that this is a dream. Because I know that it is already quite late (about 9 P.M.) I want to verify if I am actually in a real lucid dream or if I am only seeing hypnagogic imagery. To achieve this purpose I observe my body position. I am *sitting* in a bus: that means I am in a lucid dream. I make an attempt to talk to a not-so-slim lady sitting in front of me. She is childish and gives an impression of being a little vulgar. I tell her to write something on a sheet of paper in a way that allows me to read it. Obviously, this imprecise instruction is fully intelligible to her. She is already standing next to my seat, but then walks back—as if she had understood my plan of her taking a position just opposite me. While doing so, she says: "But then you will soon realize . . ." She doesn't say anything else. I start to speculate on what it is that I will soon realize: that she possesses a consciousness of her own or that she doesn't? She asks me if I have something to write. I imagine (!) a piece of paper and, as it were, pull it out of my left pocket or out of nothingness. This leads the woman to make the remark that I must be a real magician. However, the sheet is not fully tangible, I cannot grasp it, and it starts to dissolve again. As a consequence, the lady in front of me takes a towel and spreads it over the back of her seat; obviously because she wants to write on it.

Amazed, I stare at the towel (which I obviously fixated on too much) and I wake up. (Tholey 1987, p. 232*f.*; English translation by T.M.)

As all experienced lucid dreamers know, fixating visual objects is a reliable method of terminating a lucid dream. Interestingly, there seems to be a stable mapping between the PSM and the unconscious functional self-model, in the dream as well as in the lucid dream, in terms of eye movements and gaze direction: If the subject in a lucid dream voluntarily suppresses eye movements as represented in the PSM, it also changes an important functional property of the brain, by interrupting the rapid eye movements, which constitute one of the most reliable "functional correlates" of dreaming. In other words, if—in what seems to be a paradigm example of top-down causation—you suppress phenomenal eye movement in the lucid dream, you suppress eye movements in the dreaming physical body as well, forcing it to wake up, that is, to shift into another global state of reality-modeling.

It is easy to see that lucid dreams are *subjective* states in terms of a fully developed first-person perspective. However, from a philosophical perspective, in particular, phenomenal *intersubjectivity* in dreams is an even more fascinating phenomenon. Do dream figures, encountered during a lucid dream possess a phenomenal identity of their own? Are they persons? German dream researcher Paul Tholey reports the following episode:

. . . I briefly looked back. The person following me did not look like an ordinary human being; he was as tall as a giant and reminded me of Rübezahl [in German legend, a mountain spirit]. Now it was fully clear to me that I was undergoing a dream and with a great sense of relief I continued running away. Then it suddenly occurred to me that I did not have to escape, but was capable of doing something else. I remembered my plan of talking to other persons during the dream. So I stopped running, turned around, and allowed the pursuer to approach me. Then I asked him, what it was actually that he wanted. His answer was: "How am I supposed to know?! After all this is *your* dream and, moreover, *you* have studied psychology and not me . . ." (Tholey 1987, p. 97; English translation by T.M.)

For philosophers, of course, it is highly interesting to engage dream characters encountered during a lucid dream in fundamental epistemological debates. For instance, it may be interesting to ask them if—from their own "point of view"—they are persons of their own, or if they are only "virtual machines" realized by a subset of the dreamer's brain states (cf. related possibilities in indirect communication between host personality and alters, or therapist, for DID; see also Dennett 1998, p. 57). Assume the following: In a lucid dream, you encounter a scientific community. Their members are strongly interested in convincing you of the fundamental falsity of your own ontological assumptions concerning the dream reality you share. Is it permissible to accept the intersubjective verification of scientific hypotheses *in* a dream and by dream characters? Are scientific communities state-specific entities (see Tart 1972b)? Maybe completely different laws of nature govern this dream reality, or all of their members are proponents of a strange philosophical theory called "eliminative phenomenalism," holding that no such thing as physical objects, let alone the brain of the dreamer, has ever existed. How can you, as a rational philosophical psychonaut now incarnated in *their* reality, prove *to them* that, say, single terms of the best theories in dream physics actually only refer to certain content properties of a phenomenal mental model, activated by a brain which *you* usually like to call your "own?" By interrupting the process of generating and testing hypotheses in the lucid dream reality (e.g., by exclaiming "I will show you who the *true* subject is!" while angrily fixating your own hands and waking up) you have not proved anything to anybody in a very literal sense, and no growth of knowledge has actually been achieved. Or has it? I hope readers will forgive me for not pursuing these questions any further at this point. Let us look at one last case study and then swiftly proceed to a representationalist and functionalist analysis of lucid dreams. A centrally important factor in inducing lucid dreams consists in maintaining a critical attitude toward phenomenal reality in general. This is the report of a young woman about the first lucid dream she ever had:

. . . I meet K., who already is a lucid dreamer, in a lavatory in the theater. I think, "This guy appears just at the right time!" I have been mad at him for quite some time. For many weeks now I have been carefully practicing my exercises and I have not had a single lucid dream. Not even a very little one, a very short one! "You have given me completely wrong instructions!", I complain to him. I am close to a nervous breakdown. And to hell with it, now I even get furious: "All this is lies! Something like this doesn't exist at all! Lucid dreaming! Ha! You can't fool me! This is the end! I won't let you treat me like an idiot any longer! Not you, in particular!"

K. doesn't react at all. He stands in front of a mirror, gently stroking his beard. I get so angry that I lose control and I actually beat him on the back of his head. Laughingly, K. turns around and looks directly into my eyes. "Why is he laughing?", I briefly think, then he just passes me by and walks directly into the mirror. In a fury I scream and throw a piece of soap at him, but miss. Meanwhile I was in such a rage that I simply didn't check that such things, of course, only happen in a dream. "Don't lose your courage, baby!", he says, still laughing. "You'll find out." He turns around and disappears.

I almost explode! Suddenly the door behind me opens, and K. enters, together with another guy. They firmly hold on to each other! Both of them grin at me in a frivolous way. I quickly bow down and reach for the soap, as I suddenly become dizzy. "This just cannot be true," I think, as I come back up and see both of them standing there in this manner. "This guy isn't gay, not *this* guy! I would know that! Why is he so happy?" Suddenly I feel a freezing cold. "What if all this is a dream??? Am I dreaming or am I waking? What has happened until now? This is ridiculous! Is this a dream?" I ask both of them. They shake their heads and break out in an insane kind of laughter. Who cares! I'm not interested in K. at all anymore.

I think: "This can, can, can only be a dream! This is a dream! A lucid dream! Oh my, what am I supposed to do now?" K. and the other guy have disappeared. Upon touching it, the tiled wall of the room feels unbelievably real. Cool and smooth. Feverishly excited I start to think about what I could do now. I am extremely excited. I have to do something now! This is when I remember this film with Heinz Rühmann. A man who was able to walk through walls. That was one of my dreams for a long time. Upon thinking the word "dream" I have to start laughing. God, how childish I am, I think. I make an attempt to walk through the tiled wall. My hand is already inside! With a firm decision I start walking. I penetrate into the wall and, again, I have to start laughing. It is gorgeous, warm and dark. Somehow reddish. Now I am on the other side! And I find myself in the living room of my parents! Mom and Dad are drinking coffee and are boring each other. Mom immediately walks toward me and starts accusing me. "Who do you think you are, to come walking through the wall just like that, without letting us know before!" "Ah, cut it out," I happily respond, "after all you're just a dream character . . ." (Tholey 1987, p. 46*f.*; English translation by T.M.)

General factors conducive to the induction of lucid dreams are a high level of physical activity during the day (Gackenbach, Curren, and Cutler 1983; Garfield 1975) and a heightened affective arousal during the day period (Gackenbach et al. 1983; Sparrow 1976). Short interruptions of sleep, including short activities in waking consciousness, preceding the relevant REM phase, also increase the probability for the realization of the global phenomenal property of lucidity (e.g., see Garfield 1975; S. LaBerge 1980a, 1980b, 1990; Sparrow 1976). The interesting fact (mentioned above) that the PSM of human beings seems to be firmly anchored in the functional structure of the human brain inasmuch as there is a direct and reliable relationship between the direction of polygraphically recorded eye movements and the gaze shifts reported by lucid dreamers made a particularly ingenious type of experiment possible (S. LaBerge et al. 1981a,b). We might term it "trans-reality communication." Experienced subjects indicated the *initiation* of a lucid dream by ocular signals determined before the experiments. Polysomographic analysis of subjects then showed that typical electrophysiological correlates of a beginning lucid dream are the first 2 minutes of a REM phase, short, interrupting intervals of waking consciousness during a REM phase and/or heightened phasic REM activity (for a brief review of psychophysiological studies of lucid dreaming, see S. LaBerge 1990; for further references, see S. LaBerge and Gackenbach 2000, p. 157*f.*). It is plausible to assume that brief episodes of sudden increases in the general cortical level of arousal are one of the most important physiological conditions necessary for the generation of lucidity. The phenomenal correlates seem to be increased vividness (see endnote 21), heightened fear, or stress in the chain of events forming the dream; the discovery of contradictions within the dream world; or the subjective experience of becoming aware of a "dreamlike" or "unreal" quality of dreamed reality. Single reports of the emergence of lucid dreams in non-REM sleep exist, but, as far as I know, there is no secure knowledge (for an introduction, see Gackenbach and LaBerge 1988). The phenomenon of lucid dreaming as such has been known for millennia. It has only become the focus of serious scientific research during the last three decades. Probably Celia Green's book marks the beginning of this phase (Green 1968; a short review of the literature from Aristotle to this point can be found in

S. LaBerge 1988). The first two doctoral dissertations on lucid dreams appeared in 1978 and 1980 (Gackenbach 1978; S. LaBerge 1980c). It has to be noted, however, that the quantity of rigorous research on lucid dreams, as compared to the quantity of research into the phenomenon of ordinary dreams, is almost negligible. This is a deplorable state of affairs, because, as we will now see, the phenomenon of lucid dreaming is of great systematic interest in developing a general theory of consciousness and of the phenomenal first-person perspective.

On the representational level of analysis, the most important feature clearly is the generalized absence of the transparency constraint. Lucid dreams are perhaps the only *globally opaque* class of phenomenal states. What precisely does this mean? First, it is plausible to assume that the episodically overshooting cortical arousal correlated with the emergence of dream lucidity leads to a sudden increase in terms of the availability of internal self-related information and computational resources in the brain. Second, the emergence of a generalized "dreamlike" or "unreal" quality pertaining to reality as a whole is precisely the moment at which the all-pervading naive realism—which also characterizes ordinary waking states—is finally lost. The *simulational*, namely, *misrepresentational*, character of the experiential process as such becomes globally available. The moment of lucidity is the moment at which this information becomes cognitively available, that is, can be expressed on the level of conscious thought. It is also the moment at which earlier processing stages (e.g., of more "fluid" visual content) become available for attentional processing. As the dream state, among other things, is also the internal emulation of a *behavioral* space, this information now becomes available for the control of action as well: full-blown agency is established, the dreamer is not a passive observer anymore, but has the capacity to utilize the knowledge that all this is a dream, a global phenomenal simulation, in determining the course of his or her future actions. Computationally speaking, lucidity consists in an increased availability of self-related information. My core claim, therefore, is that what changes in the transition from ordinary to lucid dreaming is, first of all, the content and functional profile of the PSM. The shift in the PSM then enables the *stabilization* of the PMIR. However, different types of global availability and different types of information have to be distinguished.

It is important to note how the information that all this is just a *modeled* reality, and not a reality in the usual, folk-physical way of using the term, is not only cognitively available but *attentionally* available on the level of introspective$_{3/4}$ processing. Compare waking states. If you find the current theory convincing, and if this theory actually points in the right direction, the fact that the contents of your own conscious experience as you read this book are the contents of a phenomenal *model* of reality is cognitively available to you but does not in the least make you shift into a state of "lucid waking," a state in which the experiential character of naive realism starts to dissolve. It is a purely intellectual attitude, which has almost no influence on how you actually experience the world. Therefore it is highly plausible that *cognitive availability* is unlikely to be the sole cause of dream lucidity.

In the same way, as all lucid dreamers can confirm, the sudden appearance of insight into the overall nature of the current state, which is so typical of lucid dreaming, is not only a cognitive event, a purely intellectual insight. What makes these states so fascinating to the people experiencing them is the fact that the representational character of conscious contents is *prereflexively* available, for example, on the level of attentional processing, on the level of "direct" sensory awareness (recall the first example). The fact that the global model of reality shifts from transparency to opacity means that the introspectively accessible properties of the phenomenal representations constituted and integrated by it are not exhausted by content properties anymore, but include "vehicle properties," or what I called processing stages in section 3.2.7. In *prelucid* stages, this information may find its expression in a general "dreamlike" quality, without being cognitively available in terms of an explicit conscious thought of the sort "I am now dreaming!" or without being available for the control of behavior in the dream, for example, in terms of flying or penetrating walls. We have seen that there exist other examples of opaque phenomenal states, for example, as in consciously experienced cognition or pseudohallucinations of a sensory character. What makes lucid dreams interesting is that the transparency constraint is transiently not satisfied here on a *global* level of phenomenal reality-modeling. A lucid dream in this way is a globalized pseudohallucination. Or, to use a metaphor idealist philosophers might prefer, it is like one big *thought*.

Before going on to analyze further representational features of the class of global, phenomenal models of reality, which today we call "lucid dreams," let me point to a complicated issue, one I cannot fully resolve at this point. The current theory predicts that full-blown global opacity leads to a "derealization" on the level of phenomenal experience. Lucid dreams may be just that: coherent, but phenomenologically *derealized* global states. However, the current theory also predicts that full-blown opacity for the *PSM* will lead to a loss of phenomenally experienced selfhood (see section 6.2.6). But the distribution of transparency versus opacity in lucid dreams is not uniform, it varies. As long as the higher-order phenomenal property of "selfhood" is instantiated, as long as there is the conscious experience of a dreaming *self*, a major portion of the PSM must therefore be transparent. The current theory predicts that the phenomenal self would disappear in a fully generalized state of opacity, in a situation where not only the virtuality of the world model but also the virtuality of the self-model is fully available on the level of phenomenal representation itself. The subject component of the PMIR would disappear in not being a *subject* component anymore. Indeed, this may actually be the case, namely, in those phenomenological situations where the lucid dream dissolves into and is terminated by a kind of religious or spiritual ecstasy, as is not infrequently reported in the phenomenological material (see endnote 21). On the other hand, it presently seems impossible to approach this question in a rigorous manner based on empirical data: Autophenomenological reports about selfless states contain a performative self-contradiction, and are therefore highly problematic for methodological reasons. I return to analysis of the self-model in lucid dreams soon.

Viewed as global, phenomenal models of reality, lucid dreams are fully characterized by the criterion of offline activation (see sections 3.2.8 and 4.2.5; for a review of the empirical evidence, see Kahn et al. 1997; Hobson et al. 2000). The representation of intensity (see section 3.2.9) can vary greatly, as is, for instance, demonstrated by hyperemotional states or the absence of certain presentational "formats" like nociception. In a lucid dream it is possible to experience intense states of emotional arousal like fear or bliss, which are usually unknown in the waking state, while other types of sensory experience, for example, the sense of temperature or pain, are much rarer. As compared to nonlucid dreams, lucid dreams have more marked *kinesthetic* and *auditory* content (Gackenbach 1988). Simple phenomenal content is homogeneous, as in ordinary dream or waking states, and it is presently unclear if the phenomenon of lucid dreaming fulfills any adaptive functions. Could lucid dreams have played a role in the cultural history of mankind by making the appearance-reality distinction a topic of intersubjective communication, or in establishing certain religious beliefs?

In a number of ways, lucid dreams are *perspectival* global states in a much stronger sense than ordinary dreams. The phenomenal first-person perspective—that is, the transparent model of the intentionality relation—is much more stable in terms of temporal extension and semantic continuity. In terms of the content available as an object component, in terms of what the dreaming subject can attend to, think about, or decide to do, selectivity and variability are greatly increased. In ordinary dreams high-level attention, deliberation, and volitional action, as well as coherent cognition, are almost nonexistent, all these capacities are almost exclusively available in the lucid dream. It is also true that the conscious model of the world in lucid dreams is characterized by the features of convolved holism and dynamicity described in chapter 3. However, the well-known hyperassociativity of ordinary dreams, which, as Kahn and colleagues write, "helps create the semblance of unity amid a great variety and richness of imagery as well as contributing to those incongruities and discontinuities that typify dreaming consciousness" (Kahn et al. 1997, p. 17) seems to be markedly decreased. Lucid dreams average fewer dream characters than nonlucid dreams (Gackenbach 1988). The world of the lucid dreamer certainly may be bizarre, but it exhibits a much higher degree of internal coherence. It is plausible to assume that, on the functional level of description, a general correlate of lucidity consists in the sudden availability of additional processing capacities to the system as a whole. This in turn may enable the self-organization of a globally coherent state, the strengthening of a hypothetical process, which I have elsewhere (Metzinger 1995b) called "highest-order binding." An important recent development in analyzing the formal features of dream mentation has been the development of operationally defined "bizarreness scales," which allow researchers to measure the discontinuity, incongruence, uncertainty, and so forth of dreamed content (for references, see Kahn et al. 1997, p. 18; see also Hobson et al. 2001; Revonsuo and Salmivalli 1995). Even from a coarse-grained phenomenological analysis of lucid dreams, a straightforward prediction follows: The global model of the world, as represented during lucid episodes, is much less bizarre in terms of content than the consciously experienced reality of an ordinary dream. In short, lucidity imposes semantic coherence and stability on the internal simulation of the world.

One centrally relevant constraint for phenomenal representata is their activation within a virtual window of presence (see section 3.2.2). The fact that *short-term memory* functions in a much better and reliable way during lucid dreams may point to the fact that this window of presence is enlarged and stabilized during lucid episodes. In general, lucid dreams—although shorter—are much less "fleeting" experiences than ordinary dreams, and their subjectively experienced degree of "realness," that is, the degree to which their content is represented as an actually *present* world, is much higher. However, this issue leads to a much more decisive question, namely, the role of the self-model in the transition from ordinary dreaming to lucidity.

My claim is that the key to understanding the phenomenon of lucidity lies in analyzing the additional type of information made globally available during lucid dreams *by changing the content of the self-model*. What suddenly becomes available when shifting into a lucid episode is context information of a system-related type: Lucidity is what in German is called *Zustandsklarheit* ("state clarity"), globally available knowledge about the general category of the representational state that the system is currently realizing. On the functional level of description, the most important feature certainly is the reappearance of autobiographical memory, the availability of autobiographical memory concerning earlier episodes of waking consciousness *and* of lucid dreaming, including their distinction. As autobiographical memory becomes cognitively available, the content of the conscious model of the self dramatically changes, as it is now possible for the system to grasp the character of its overall state and the fact that all this happened by integrating thoughts of the type "My God, I am dreaming!" into its internal self-representation. Cognitive self-reference leads to agency and the reestablishment of executive control. Therefore, it is plausible to assume that lucidity is correlated with the degree to which the prefrontal cortex can *functionally penetrate the substrate of the PSM*. As a matter of fact, on the level of a necessary neural correlate in humans, Hobson has speculated that for lucidity to occur, "the normally deactivated dorsolateral prefrontal cortex (DLPFC) must be reactivated, but not so strongly as to suppress the pontolimbic signals to it" (Hobson et al. 2000, p. 837).[26] It is interesting to note that the shift from an ordinary dream into a lucid state, on the representational level of analysis, can fundamentally be characterized as the sudden availability of system-related context information, information about a particular psychological context, about a particular way of being currently situated—namely, in an exclusively *internal* behavioral space, within a model of reality now for the first time experienced *as* a model.

As all lucid dreamers are able to confirm, the phenomenological profile associated with the sudden process of "coming to" strongly resembles the sudden reappearance of memories containing long-lost but highly relevant information. This may count as a strong indicator of the relevance of memory functions in the generation of lucidity. In an ordinary dream, control of action, high-level attention, and cognitive access to autobiographical memories frequently are completely absent. In a conceptually clear sense involving degrees of constraint satisfaction, ordinary dreams are much less *conscious* than lucid dreams, because they consist only of a global model of reality presented within a window of presence, while the feature of perspectivalness is expressed to a much lesser degree. The PMIR is absent or unstable. In not satisfying the perspectivalness constraint, nonlucid dreams are not truly *subjective* states. They are only weak first-person phenomena. Dreaming information-processing systems find themselves in a strange and problematic overall state. They are suddenly confronted with an internal signal source (see section 4.2.5), while suffering from an almost complete input blockade and a paralysis of their effectors. With their effectors paralyzed, they are unable to dissolve the input blockade by establishing reafferent signals, that is, by waking themselves up. As usual, the system will try to assemble all active contents into a coherent model of reality. However, if normal learning and memory functions are not available, bizarre mental episodes will result, which frequently cannot be remembered. If the physical boundary conditions are changed and the system suddenly possesses additional computational resources, more internal information can now be used to interpret the ongoing chain of events—by generating an appropriate self-model.

26. One of the strengths of the latest version of the AIM-model (see Hobson et al. 2000, particularly figure 12) is that it can give us an idea about how the phenomenon of lucidity may be integrated into a larger explanatory framework. Hobson and colleagues also argue for a difference between spontaneous and prepared episodes of dream lucidity: "The fact that lucidity can arise when the DLPFC is deactivated can also be explained using AIM. Lucid dreaming occurs spontaneously or can be cultivated by pre-sleep autosuggestion. Spontaneous lucidity indicates that the reduced amount of reflective self-awareness during dreaming is sometimes enhanced enough for the subject to recognize the dream state for what it is. Autosuggestion probably increases this probability by priming the brain circuitry—presumably in prefrontal areas—that subserves self-reflective awareness. In both cases, the phenomenon of lucidity clearly illustrates the always statistical and always dissociable quality of brain-mind states. AIM accommodates these features very well by proposing that lucid dreaming is a hybrid state lying across the wake-REM interface" (Hobson et al. 2000, p. 837*f*.).

Ordinary dreaming clearly is characterized by a metacognitive deficit, in terms of information about the overall state not being globally available for cognition (see also Kahan and LaBerge 1994). Mental clarity about the nature of the current phenomenal state requires an additional representation of the inner history of the system, requires the capacity to recognize a global representational state as belonging to a certain class of states as being a *representational*—and also a *misrepresentational*—state in the light of earlier global representational states undergone by the system. A global simulation is, for the first time, experienced *as* a simulation. It is precisely this metacognitive achievement which is brought about by generating a stable self-model. A stable self-model makes autobiographical information globally available for cognitive self-reference. It is the autobiographical, and consequently the cognitive, attentional, and volitional self-model which is dramatically enriched during the transition from a normal to a lucid dream.

This also allows for *semantic* enrichment. We can define the concept of "lucidity," then, as the availability of information concerning the overall representational nature of the current model of reality as being represented in the currently active, conscious self-model. Speaking of dreams, it is important to note that this interesting phenomenal property is realized in many shades and degrees of functional effectiveness. Weaker forms or definitions of lucidity can easily be singled out. For instance, in a "prelucid" stage, your attention may already be caught by certain incongruences in the dream, and the respective context information may be attentionally available, but you may not yet have intellectually *grasped* it, let alone be able to fly around or walk through walls. This may be a situation in which, by happy coincidence, the motif of a dream appears *in* a dream ([Now I* have been sitting in the cinema for over half an hour, waiting for the movie about the dream time of the Australian aborigines to start! Something is wrong with this place, somehow this situation carries a symbolic meaning—while at the same time something about this cinema is strangely unreal. As a matter of fact, this whole situation is kind of dreamlike . . .]). Cognitive availability in terms of explicitly self-ascribing the property of lucidity in the dream ([Wow—I have just become lucid again!]) does not mean that you do not stay a passive observer instead of a full-blown agent exerting volitional control (S. LaBerge 1985). In sum, many weaker and more refined versions of lucidity can be described to match specific neurophenomenological domains more accurately. However, the notion of "lucidity" can now also be interestingly generalized to other global phenomenal state classes: A class of global phenomenal models of reality is lucid if and only if the fact that it is a *model* and that it belongs to this class is cognitively *and* attentionally available to the system generating it, by being represented in its conscious self-model.

Could there be a class of phenomenal states correctly termed "lucid waking?" Obviously, if the current theory points in the right direction and you happen to believe that this theory is true, the fact that you are a system which is never in direct and immediate contact with reality, but which always operates under a global, virtual *model* of reality, will be cognitively available to you via your PSM. It is also trivially true that, for instance, psychiatric patients demanding antihallucinogenic drugs or recreational drug users in nonclinical settings implicitly know about this fact, and utilize it in trying to control or influence the content of their conscious reality-model in a certain way. It is mentally represented in a way which makes it available for cognition and the fast and flexible control of action. But what about subsymbolic metarepresentation, what about the availability of this specific kind of psychological context information on the level of *attentional* processing during the waking state? There may well be transitions from ordinary waking states to globally opaque models of reality, for example, in psychiatric conditions such as derealization or in certain mystical experiences. But, in general, the transparency of the conscious model of reality during waking states is a much more stable, an attentionally impenetrable phenomenon: full-blown lucidity, not as an intellectual achievement, but as an all-pervading experiential phenomenon, is much easier to achieve during the dream state than during the waking state. There may be obvious evolutionary reasons for this, and the waking-state model of reality is largely driven and constrained by external input. As opposed to the dream, in which we can "wake up" into a lucid episode, there usually exists no further type of global phenomenal model of reality in our autobiographical memory in which we were "more awake," more coherent, and more insightful about the actual nature of the overall process, which could function as a *reference basis* to which the waking state could be compared (cf. our introductory report, and endnote 21). As soon as autobiographical memory becomes activated during a dream, this additional phenomenal frame of reference exists; it is formed by conscious memories of the richer and more coherent waking life. For waking life, however, and for ordinary individuals, no such second phenomenal frame of reference exists which could permit "waking up" during the waking state by making not only content properties but also vehicle properties of the process generating it available for introspective attention, thereby globalizing opacity.

Frederik van Eeden (1913), who first introduced the concept of a "lucid dream," presented not only the full recognition of his waking life and the ability to act voluntarily in his dreams as defining characteristics but also a *third* feature. He wrote, "I was so fast asleep that no bodily sensations penetrated into my perception." (ibid., p. 441). Dreams, lucid dreams, and OBEs, as compared to waking states, are what I would call "partially disembodied states." It seems as if in those states the content of the self-model is constrained to a lesser degree by current proprioceptive input from the physical body. The subject of the lucid dream is an attentional and a cognitive subject to a much stronger degree than it is an *embodied* subject—as can be seen from the frequent experiences of weightlessness, floating, flying dreams, and so on. Other elementary forms of *self-presentational*, that is, stimulus-correlated, content (see sections 2.4.4 and 5.4), like the experience of pain, heat, or cold, are much rarer in the phenomenology of lucid dreams or OBEs. Kinesthesia is an exception, but arguably not a truly *simple* form of bodily awareness. In Antonio Damasio's words, the brain is much more the body's "captive audience" during waking states than it is during the lucid dream (Damasio 1999, p. 150).

Not all bodily sensation is absent, but proprioceptive awareness certainly is not the focus of phenomenal experience and self-modeling in the lucid dream state. In terms of neural correlates this may mean that this correlate is functionally penetrated by the prefrontal cortex in a way more closely resembling the waking state than it is, for example, by the upper brainstem or somatosensory cortex. This partial decoupling from input continuously generated by the physical body is reflected in the phenomenology of the lucid dream. It may be that it is precisely the stronger self-presentational component of the PSM in the waking state, which usually prevents the waking world from suddenly becoming "unreal" and "dreamlike": it is the *body* which anchors us in reality—physically and functionally, as well as phenomenally. One intriguing feature of lucid dreams is how the transition from the PSM of the lucid dream "into" the proprioceptively more constrained self-model of the waking state can sometimes be closely inspected and become a part of autobiographical memory. This can be seen in the last case study to be presented in this book.

Let me close this second set of neurophenomenological case studies with one final example of deviant self-modeling, which once again demonstrates how the human self-model is a *virtual* self-model, the content of which is constrained by varying internal contexts. The PSM is truly a *dream body*. The following passage is once again taken from a pioneer of consciousness research, namely, from van Eeden's original contribution, in which the concept of a "lucid dream" was first introduced:

In January, 1898, I was able to repeat the observation. In the night of January 19–20, I dreamt that I was lying in the garden before the windows of my study, and saw the eyes of my dog through the glass pane. I was lying on my chest and observing the dog very keenly. At the same time, however, I knew with perfect certainty that I was dreaming and lying on my back in my bed. And then I resolved to wake up slowly and carefully and observe how my sensation of lying on my chest would change to the sensation of lying on my back. And so I did, slowly and deliberately, and the transition—which I have since undergone many times—is most wonderful. It is like the feeling of slipping from one body into another, and there is distinctly a *double* recollection of the two bodies. I remembered what I felt in my dream, lying on my chest; but returning into the day-life, I remembered also that my physical body had been quietly lying on its back all the while. This observation of a double memory I have had many times since. It is so indubitable that it leads almost unavoidably to the conception of *a dream-body*. (van Eeden 1913, p. 446*f*.)

7.3   The Concept of a Phenomenal First-Person Perspective

The case studies in this chapter have confirmed the basic claims made in chapter 6: A consciously experienced first-person perspective emerges if a system not only activates a world-model and embeds a self-model in it but as soon as it additionally represents itself as being *directed* at some aspects of the world. There are many different *types* of intentionality-modeling, depending on the nature of the object component, the stability of the subject component, and the way in which both are representationally integrated. Many borderline cases exist, configurations in which either the PSM or the PMIR, or both, are damaged and they lead to deviant neurophenomenological state classes. But there is one underlying theoretical principle which has been confirmed across all pathological situations: the perspectivalness of consciousness results from an active PMIR. Whenever a globally available model of the intentionality relation exists, a phenomenal first-person perspective emerges. Whenever this special kind of representational content is lacking, the first-person perspective disappears. We are now prepared to step back and look at the more general picture of the conscious mind emerging from the discussion in all the previous chapters.

8 Preliminary Answers

8.1 The Neurophenomenological Caveman, the Little Red Arrow, and the Total Flight Simulator: From Full Immersion to Emptiness

Has a general picture of the conscious human mind emerged from the investigations carried out in the previous chapters of this book? In the end, what is it that the self-model theory of subjectivity (SMT) has to tell us about consciousness, the phenomenal self, and the first-person perspective? In this final chapter we take stock and attempt to draw the different threads of our discussion together. In the first section I offer three metaphors that will serve as introductory illustrations and increase the intuitive plausibility of the overall picture now emerging. In the next section I keep the promise I made in the first chapter: We proceed to look at some potentially new answers to those specifically philosophical questions outlined in the corresponding second part of chapter 1. In the third section I draw some more general conclusions, and explore possible future routes of research. But let's start with the metaphors mentioned above. Each of these metaphors highlights a different set of aspects characterizing the SMT if we view it as the general outline for a theory of consciousness, the phenomenal self, and the first-person perspective. The first metaphor is of an epistemological nature, while the second and third metaphors are representationalist and technological metaphors. Each is an image of what it means to be a conscious human being. In their own way these metaphors also reflect three different and successive stages in Western history of philosophy of the mind.

The first metaphor relates to the Book VII of Plato's *Republic*, and the image of the cave (Plato 2000, p. 119*ff.*). I claim that in terms of the deeper structure underlying our phenomenal experience of the world and of ourselves in particular, we resemble *neurophenomenological cavemen*. The cave in which we live our conscious life is formed by our global, phenomenal model of reality. According to Plato, the cave in which we live our lives is a *subterranean* location, which, however, has an entrance stretched upward corresponding to the expanse of the cave and open to the light over its entire width. Our conscious model of reality is subterranean in that it is determined exclusively by the internal properties of our central nervous system: there is a minimally sufficient neural correlate for the content of consciousness at any given point in time. If all properties of this local neural correlate are fixed, the properties of subjective experience are fixed as well. Of course, the outside world could at the same time undergo considerable changes. For instance, a disembodied but appropriately stimulated brain in a vat could—*phenomenologically*—enjoy exactly the same kind of conscious experience as you do right now while reading this book. In principle, it would even suffice to properly activate just a subset of this brain, the minimally sufficient neural correlate of your present state, to make a "phenomenological snapshot" of exactly the same kind of conscious experience emerge. Of course, we would never call such a physically restricted phenomenal subject a person, or even a *subject* in any philosophically interesting sense at all. For example, such a sub-personal clone of your own current conscious model of the world right now would bizarrely misrepresent its own position in the world; it would have an extreme number of false beliefs about itself. There would be experience, but not *knowledge*. Still, it is true to say that phenomenal experience as such unfolds in an *internal* space, in a space quite distinct from the world described by ordinary physics. It evolves within an individual model of reality, in an individual organism's brain, and its experiential properties are determined exclusively by properties within this brain. Although this simple fact may well be cognitively available to many of us, we are neurophenomenological cavemen in that none of us are able to consciously experience its truth. Effortlessly, we enjoy an "out-of-the-brain experience."[1] Only if confronted with the data and discoveries of modern neuropsychology, or if pressed to come up with a convincing argument showing that currently we are *not* just a shadow on the wall of the phenomenal cave generated by some sort of isolated, minimally sufficient correlate stimulated by an evil scientist, only then do we sometimes begin to develop a stronger intuitive sense of what it means that our phenomenal model of reality is an *internal* model of reality that could at any time, in principle, turn out to be quite far removed from a much more high-dimensional physical reality than we have ever thought of. Plato, however, tells us there is an entrance to the cave, which at the same time may be a potential exit. But who could it be? Who could ever pass *through* this exit?

In Plato's beautiful parable the captives in the cave are chained down by their thighs and necks. They have been in this position since birth, and they can only look straight ahead, because even their head has been in a fixed position from the beginning of their existence onward. They are prevented by their fetters from turning their heads. As Socrates points out, they have never seen anything of themselves and each other except the shadows cast by the fire burning behind them to the opposite wall of the cave, and which they take for real objects. The same is true of the objects carried along above the low wall behind their heads. What is the cave? The cave, according to the SMT, is simply the physical organism as a whole, including, in particular, its brain. What are the shadows on the wall? A shadow is a low-dimensional projection of a higher-dimensional object. *Phenomenal* shadows are low-dimensional projections of internal or external objects in the conscious state space opened within the central nervous system of a biological organism. According to the SMT, the shadows on the wall are phenomenal mental models. The book you are

---

1. The notion of an "out-of-the-brain experience" was first coined by Revonsuo 2000a, p. 65. The functional principle of internality and the ontological principle of local supervenience are not reflected on the level of conscious experience itself, because—on the level of representational content—it is systematically "externalized": the brain is constantly creating the experience that I* am directly present in a world *outside* my brain, although, as Revonsuo points out, the experience itself is brought about by neural systems buried deep inside the brain. See also sections 7.2.3 and 7.2.5.

holding in your hands, as consciously experienced by you at this moment, is a dynamic, low-dimensional shadow of the actual physical object in your hand, a dancing shadow in your central nervous system. As all neural network modelers know, real-life connectionist systems typically achieve a major reduction in the dimensionality of their input vectors at the very first processing stage, when transforming the activation pattern on their sensory surface into the first hidden layer. But what is the fire, causing the projection of flickering shadows of consciousness, ever changing, dancing away as activation patterns on the surface of your neural cave? The fire is neural dynamics. The fire is the incessant, self-regulating flow of neural information processing, constantly perturbed and modulated by sensory and cognitive input. The wall is not a *two-dimensional* surface. It is a *space*, namely, the high-dimensional phenomenal state space of human technicolor phenomenology (see McGinn 1989b, p. 349; Metzinger 2000b, p. 1*f*.). Please note that, in a conscious human being, the wall and the fire are not separate entities: they are two aspects of one and the same process. But what exactly does it mean when Plato tells us that we have never seen anything of ourselves but our *own* shadow on the opposite wall? It means that, as perceiving, attending, thinking, and even as acting subjects, we are only given to ourselves through what I have called the PSM—the phenomenal self-model. Could we free ourselves from our attachment to this inner image of ourselves, the dancing shadow in our conscious state space? Could we stop to *confuse* ourselves with this shadow, and leave Plato's cave altogether?

Here is where we have to depart from the classical metaphor. I claim that there is no one *in* the cave. There is no one who could leave. There is no one who—in Socrates' words—could "stand up suddenly and turn his head around and walk and . . . lift up his eyes to the light" (515c; p. 123), who could return to the cave, after having seen the light of the sun, the "dazzle and the glitter" (515c; p. 123) of true reality, and there is no one who could later provoke the laughter of the ignorant perpetual prisoners, about whom Socrates asks the following question: "And if it were possible to lay hands on and to kill the man who tried to release them and lead them up, would they not kill him?" (517a, p. 129).

It is important to note that a shadow, although dependent on, controlled by, and in a certain, very weak sense *representing* the object that casts it, is never a distinct entity. Shadows as such don't exist. What exists are *shaded surfaces*. However, it is, of course, possible to confuse object and shaded surface, thereby treating the latter as a distinct entity. I claim that the conscious self is not a thing, but a shaded surface. It is not an individual object, but a *process*: the ongoing process of shading. The beauty of the shadow metaphor for self-consciousness consists partly in the fact that it is not only a classical but also a global metaphor—one to be found at the origin of many of mankind's great philosophical traditions. To name a prominent non-Western example, Śaṃkara (who lived 1200 years later than Plato, from 788 A.D. to 820 A.D.), in his *Vivekacūḍāmani*, or *Crest-Jewel of Wisdom* (Śaṃkara 1966, p. 70), argued that just as we don't confuse ourselves with the shadow cast by our own body, or with a reflection of it, or with the body as it appears in a dream or in imagination, we should not identify with what appears to be our bodily self right now. Śaṃkara said: Just as you have no self-identification with your shadow-body, reflection-body, dream-body, or imagination-body, so should you not have with the living body. The SMT offers a deeper understanding of why, in standard situations, the system as a whole inevitably *does* identify itself with its own neurodynamical shadow, with its inner computational reflection of itself, with its continuous online dream about, and internal emulation of, itself. It is the transparency of the human self-model which causes this effect.

We must imagine Plato's cave differently if we are to understand the neurophenomenological caveman's true situation. There are low-dimensional phenomenal shadows of external perceptual objects dancing on the neural user surface of the caveman's brain. So much is true. There certainly is a phenomenal *self*-shadow as well. But what is this shadow the low-dimensional projection *of*? I claim that it is a shadow not of a captive person, but of the cave as a whole. It is the physical organism as a whole, including all of its brain, its cognitive activity, and its social relationships, that is projecting inward, *from all directions at the same time*, as it were. There is no true subject and no homunculus in the cave that could confuse itself with anything. It is the cave as a whole, which episodically, during phases of waking and dreaming, projects a shadow of itself onto one of its many internal walls. The cave shadow is there. The cave itself is empty.

Śaṃkara was right: A transparent phenomenal self-model is not a self. But Socrates was right too. He depicted the prisoners as firmly anchored in the cave, chained down since birth. Exactly the same holds true for our phenomenal self-model: It is firmly anchored in the autonomous bodily dynamics of elementary bioregulation, through a process I call "self-presentation." The human self-model transforms our lived reality into a *centered* reality, because it is the only phenomenal shadow firmly anchored in a continuous source of internally generated input. Socrates clearly saw that a persistent functional link was there. I return to the issue of whether this link could ever be broken when discussing the third metaphor for the SMT at the end of this section. According to the SMT, it is true that the dancing shadow on the internal wall of our brain possesses a persistent functional link to this very brain, for example, as realized by the upper brainstem and the hypothalamus. It is *not* true that there is an internal *person* forming the object of this shadow, a person conceived of as a distinct entity tied down by such a functional link. Personhood is a global property of the system as a whole that only emerges at a much later stage, through social interactions. The self-shadow—a necessary precondition for all social interaction—is simply the shadow cast by the cave as a whole onto itself. Plato was also right about the extremely reduced dimensionality of our phenomenal model of reality. From all we know today, the flow of conscious experience is an idiosyncratic trajectory through phenomenal state space, a highly selective projection shaped by the contingencies of biological evolution on this planet—something much more resembling a reality *tunnel* through an inconceivably high-dimensional reality. A third aspect, in which *both* Plato and Śaṃkara were certainly right, is the normative ideal of expanding self-knowledge. The neurophenomenological caveman's situation is deplorable. It must be changed. However, it *cannot* be changed by freeing ourselves and leaving the cave altogether, searching for the true light of the sun. We have never been in the cave. The cave is empty.

The second metaphor I want to offer here is a representationalist metaphor. Representationalist theories of mind have a long history, spanning many centuries of Western philosophy. Recently, representationalist theories of conscious experience have again become popular and the mundane concept of a "map" has at the same time become a ubiquitous tool in neuroscience and the cognitive sciences. The idea is simple and straightforward: Phenomenal experience is like a dynamic, multidimensional map of the world. Interestingly, like only very few of the *external* maps used by human beings, it also has a little red arrow. I claim that the phenomenal self *is* the little red arrow in your conscious map of reality.

When looking at a city map on the wall of a subway station you will frequently discover a little red arrow, maybe even a sentence next to it saying, YOU ARE HERE! It is interesting to note that this linguistic explanatory note is not strictly necessary. For most users, a map exhibiting only the little red arrow will serve its functional purpose just as well. Your phenomenal map of the world is an *internal* map of the world. In order to be useful, it must have more than phenomenal content alone—very roughly, it must possess a certain isomorphy to your current environment. This is the problem of intentionality: there must be some kind of *link* between the map and the city, between mind and world. In order to achieve a certain degree of covariance with external reality, it must also be a dynamic map, capable of constant, flexible, and swift updating. However, a conscious model of reality has only *one* single user. This is not true of the map in the subway station. The subway map has many users. It does not change with the city around it. It is an external object. Compared with the enormous wealth of your conscious model of reality, it is less than a shadow. Not only is it a low-dimensional projection, it does not possess a genuine first-person perspective; all it has is a little red arrow. The little red arrow is the self-model of the city map user. It specifies the position and thereby, indirectly, the interests of potential users such as an external representation of reality *within* this representation. The little red arrow and the indexical sentence YOU ARE HERE! deprives it of its universal character and turns it into an instrument of orientation, which can only be used successfully at a single location in the world.

The multimodal maps generated by human brains, however, are general *models* of reality that flexibly adapt to the situation of the organism and are updated in real time. Since they are also *internal* models of the world, the user, whose purposes they have to serve, is in fact identical across all possible situations. As opposed to firmly installed maps in subway stations it is not the problem domain, which is fixed, and the class of users, which is variable, but the system as a whole, which remains identical across all representational situations while the class of problems is so general as to be almost infinite. Human beings are general problem solvers and autonomous agents at the same time, developing a phenomenal geography of the world. Mental self-models are the little red arrows that help a phenomenal geographer to navigate her own complex mental map of reality by once again depicting a subset of her own properties *for* herself. As long as they are functionally active, they transform the models of reality in which they are embedded by the system as a whole into *user-centered* representations. Consciousness is typically tied to an *individual* perspective, and it is not only by reason of their physical internality but owing to their structural and representational fixation to a single user that centered models of reality are transformed into meaningful instruments for only a single system in the world. Insofar as their functional profile is additionally characterized by extraorganismic relations, self-models cannot even lose the property of physical internality. Not only are they anchored in a fine-grained internal context, some of their higher layers are also driven by their social environment. We therefore return to the issue of the portability of self-models below.

For now it is only important to point out that the uniqueness of every single phenomenal subject is anchored in the uniqueness of the functional properties constituting the self-model underlying it. This self-model is the little red arrow that a human brain uses to orient itself within the internal simulation of reality it has generated. The most important difference between the little red arrow on the subway map and the little red arrow in our neurophenomenological troglodyte's brain is that the external red arrow is *opaque*. It is always clear that it is only a representation—a placeholder for something else. The little red arrow on the subway map is clearly recognizable as a variable, because different passengers can use this map by *identifying* with this little red arrow—they are episodically, as it were, "incarnated" in the reality model constructed by the map. This representational incarnation in external media of representation is something that could never work without a conscious self-model. The conscious self-model in the caveman's brain itself, however, is in large portions transparent: it is not experienced *as* a representational structure, not as a placeholder and not as a variable. It is a phenomenal self characterized not only by full-blown prereflexive embodiment but by the comprehensive, all-encompassing subjective experience of *being situated*.

Could there be an external user, someone who became deeply entangled within our current conscious model of reality by mistakenly identifying herself with the little red arrow, the PSM? Are we like moviegoers who have identified so strongly with their hero on the screen as to have completely forgotten who and where they actually are? No. The cave is empty. What the cave in internally generating a multidimensional neural image of itself as a whole allows to emerge, however, is a fascinating phenomenal property: the property of "full immersion." This property plays the central role in our third and last metaphor. As it turns out, in reflecting functionalist intuitions in the philosophy of mind, this metaphor is closest to the present time: It is a *technological* metaphor, and as all readers educated about current virtual reality technology will have noted, the concept of "full immersion" in its origin is a technological concept as well. As the history of philosophy has shown, technological metaphors are dangerous if their limitations are not clearly seen. Let us keep this issue in mind as we begin with a slightly old-fashioned image.

I claim that phenomenal first-person experience works like a *total flight simulator*. A flight simulator is a device for student pilots. It can also serve for training in behavioral reactions to unforeseen and critical situations without the risk of a real-world crash. Flight simulators were already in use at the beginning of the last century, and since then they have been continually improved. In yesterday's standard model, candidates sit in a cabin that rests on a movable platform on large extensible legs (figure 8.1). The legs are controlled by a computer that can mimic all motions of an airplane.

One of the most important practical tasks in successfully programming vehicle simulators lies in understanding the "tolerable dynamical limits in visual-vestibular miscorrelation" (Ellis 1995, p. 25), because in order to create a coherent virtual *environment* two very different sources of sensory information have to be integrated: the proprioceptive sense of balance and the external sense of vision. The phenomenal self-model (as driven by the simulator) has to cohere to the phenomenal world-model (as driven by the simulator). In the cabin we find a cockpit of realistic design, containing all the displays and control instruments one finds in a real airplane. The student pilot views a computer-controlled video screen, supplying him with a visual simulation of the view from the cockpit. In more advanced models this screen will have been replaced by a data helmet, containing two slightly displaced monitors creating a view into three-dimensional surround graphics. It is characterized by an "infinity optics." A special programming technique serves to keep the virtual focus of the image always at more than 10 yards distant. If the candidate looks "out of the window," he is able to focus his eyes on distant objects, although the real computer-generated image is only a few inches away from his face. This visual simulation of external reality is constantly updated at great speed depending on the actions the pilot takes. Today, it is also possible to specifically stimulate the proprioceptive and kinesthetic senses, for instance, by employing a seat shaker that helps to simulate a whole range of bodily sensations, as they are typically generated by a sudden break in airflow during critical velocities or vibrations of the afterburner. In this way, the student

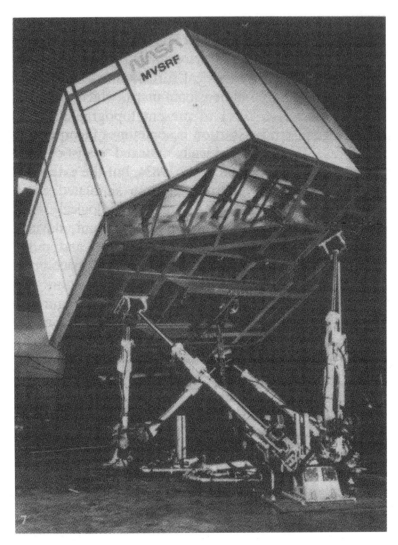

Figure 8.1
Yesterday's standard model: Moving-base simulator of the Aerospace Human Factors Division of Ames Research
Center pitched so as to simulate an acceleration. (Courtesy of NASA.) (From Barfield and Furness 1995, p. 25.)

pilot learns how to use onboard instruments, gets to know the reactions of an aircraft to his own actions, carrying out the most important basic operations any good pilot needs to master, and without taking any major physical risks.

Human brains function in a similar way. From internally represented information and utilizing continuous input supplied by the sensory organs they construct an internal model of external reality. This global model is a *real-time model*; it is being updated at such a great speed and with such reliability that in general we are not able to experience it *as* a model anymore. Phenomenal reality, for us, is not a simulational space constructed by our brains, but in a very direct and experientially untranscendable manner it is simply *the world, in which we live our lives*. A flight simulator, however, is easily recognized *as* a flight simulator. Although as student pilots we work in it in a very concentrated fashion, we never believe we are *really* flying. The reason for this opacity of the artificial simulation surrounding us is simply that our brain continuously supplies us with a much *better* reference model of the world than the computer that controls the flight simulator. The images generated by our visual cortex are orders of magnitude faster and certainly more reliable, they are characterized by a much higher resolution and a greater wealth of detail than the images appearing on the monitor of a training simulator. This is why we can always recognize the images on the monitor *as* images at any point in time, simply because we possess a higher representational standard with which we can compare them. If the simulator starts to shake and rattle as the result of flying through an air pocket or the consequences of an inadvertent maneuver, then these shaking and rattling motions will never *truly* deceive the student pilot. This is so because the phenomenal models of our *own* bodily motions generated from proprioceptive and kinesthetic perceptions are much richer in detail and more convincing than the simulations of airplane movements generated by the computer ever could be. However, it must be noted, this situation will doubtlessly change soon (for an excellent overview, see Barfield and Furness 1995). The subjective experience of presence and *being* there is determined by functional factors like the number and fidelity of sensory input and output channels, the ability to modify the virtual environment, and, importantly, the level of social interactivity in terms of actually being recognized as an existing person by *others* in the virtual world (Heeter 1992).

From an engineering point of view, the problems involved in creating virtual environments are problems of advanced *interface design*. A virtual interface is defined as a system of transducers, signal processors, hardware, and software that creates an interactive *medium* conveying information to the senses in the form of 3D virtual images, tactile and kinesthetic feedback, spatialized sound, and so on, while monitoring the psychomotor and physiological behavior of the user and employing it to manipulate the virtual environment (Barfield and Furness 1995, p. 4). Virtual environments are the latest development in

Table 8.1
Attributes of an ideal medium: Conscious experience as an invisible interface

• Matches the sensory capabilities of the human	• Unambiguous
• Easy to learn	• Does not consume reserve capacity
• High bandwidth bridge to the brain	• Easy prediction
• Dynamically adapts to the needs of the task	• Reliable
• Can be tailored to individual approaches	• Operates when busy
• Natural semantic language	• High semantic content (sample presentation)
	• Localization of objects:
• Organization of spatial/state/temporal factors	movement
• Macroscopic vs. microscopic view	state
• High bandwidth input	immediacy
• Information clustering	• Sense of presence
• Information filtering	

From Furness and Barfield 1995, reprinted with permission from Oxford University Press.

neurophenomenological cave art. And, obviously, this is one fruitful way of looking at consciousness. Phenomenal experience, insofar as it is transparent, is an *invisible interface*, an internal medium that allows an organism to interact with *itself*. It is a control device that functions by creating an *internal* user surface. Moreover, if one looks at how theorists in virtual reality and advanced interface design today actually define the attributes of what, for them, would be an ideal medium, one is immediately reminded of the catalogue of constraints for phenomenal representations offered in chapter 3 (table 8.1).

The virtual reality metaphor for phenomenal experience possesses great heuristic fertility, but we must not lose sight of its inherent limitations. The conscious brain differs from a flight simulator in a number of relevant aspects. First, it possesses many more modalities and presentational subformats: Just think of conscious vision, auditory phenomenology, olfactory and gustatory qualities, tactile sensations, and the incredible subtlety and richness given through bodily interoceptors. In particular, it is able to blend the information originating in all these different modalities into a nonfragmented, unitary model of reality—and it is precisely this task that even in a flight simulator is left to the brain of the student pilot. Flight simulators *drive* phenomenal models of reality, but they do not yet *create* them. Second, as opposed to flight simulators and present-day virtual reality systems, the human brain is not confined to a specific domain. The conscious brain is open to a vast number of representational configurations and simulational tasks. As noted above, conscious brains approximate the classic notion of a *general problem solver* (GPS; Newell and Simon 1961). A third characteristic, however, distinguishing brains and flight simulators is much more important in our present context: *human brains simulate the pilot as well.*

Of course, there is no homunculus in the system. The cave is empty. The little red arrow is just a special representational device. What *does* exist for conscious systems of a certain complexity, however, is a certain need—the necessity for the system *as a whole* to explain its own inner and outer actions to itself. It has to possess a representational and functional tool that helps to predict its own future behavior, to continuously monitor critical system properties with the help of an ongoing internal simulation, and which can depict the history of its own actions as its *own* history. Generally speaking, the system needs a computational tool that helps it in *owning its own hardware*. This tool is what I have described as the self-model of the organism. The brain differs from the flight simulator in not being used by a student pilot, who episodically "enters" it. It operates like a "total flight simulator": A total flight simulator is a self modeling airplane that has always flown without a pilot and has generated a complex internal image of itself within its *own* internal flight simulator. The image is transparent. The information that it is an internally generated image is not yet available to the system as a whole. Because, operating under the condition of a naive-realistic self-misunderstanding, it interprets the content of this image as a non-physical object; "the pilot" is born in its flight simulator. Like the neurophenomenological caveman, "the pilot" is born into a virtual reality right from the beginning—without a chance to ever discover this fact. Like a seriously deluded tourist who actually believes he is the little red arrow, the caveman is like an airplane that functionally owns its hardware, but has only just begun to appropriate the *simulator*. Neurophenomenologically, he is a shadow boxer who has become hypnotized by his own internal shadow. Employing some more recent terminology, the pilot rather is like a biologically grounded "softbot," a humanoid "avatar" used by the airplane as its own internal interface to control its own hardware, as a whole, and more flexibly.

It is surprising to see how theorists researching virtual environments today not only employ phenomenological notions like "presence" or "situatedness" but have already coined a terminological notion for what, under the SMT, would be the spatial partition of the PSM modeling motor properties of the organism: the "virtual body" (VB; Barfield, Zeltzer, Sheridan, and Slater 1995, p. 505). A VB is a part of an extended virtual environment, a dynamic and high-dimensional tool that *can* be used as a little red arrow. It can be used to control a robot at a distance, employing the virtual body as an interface. However, the authors also point out how the issue of "identification" is crucial to the context of teleoperator systems controlling distant robots, and how users of a virtual environment may actually reject their VB, just as some neuropsychological patients do (ibid., p. 506). Most illustrative, however, is the notion of a "slave robot": To achieve telepresence, an operator has to rely on a high correlation between his own movements as sensed "directly" and the actions of the slave robot; and he ideally has to achieve an identification between his own body and that of the slave robot.

A VB, like a PSM, is an advanced interface to functionally appropriate and control a body. In the VB case, the body may be thousands of miles away, and the interface used will (hopefully) only be episodically transparent. In the PSM case, Mother Nature solved all major interface problems millions of years ago, including a VB and extensive internal user-modeling. The target system and simulating system are identical, and conscious subjectivity is the case in which a single organism has learned to enslave *itself*. Interestingly, this does not turn the system as a whole into a slave robot, but into an increasingly autonomous agent. Autonomy is conscious self-control. However, in the early stages a price has to be paid. The representational misunderstanding then generates a phenomenal *self*-misunderstanding on the level of phenomenal experience, as explained in sections 3.2.7 and 6.2.6. It is *phenomenal transparency*, a very special kind of darkness, which generates this fundamental deficit in subjective knowledge concerning the constitutive conditions and the deep structure of our own phenomenal self-consciousness, which later leads to misguided philosophical theories like the Platonic metaphor of the helmsman or the homunculus in the cave, which leads to the birth of the Cartesian ego and eventually to the Kantian notion of a transcendental subject, to the many false theories of "the pilot," whose existence preceded that of the body and who only episodically "entered" into it. Shadows are a form of darkness. Growth of knowledge in cognitive neuroscience today makes all these classical models look untenable. On the contrary, the brain, the dynamical, self-organizing system as a whole, *activates* the pilot if and only if it needs the pilot as a representational instrument in order to integrate, monitor, predict, and remember its own activities. As long as the pilot is needed to navigate the world, the puppet shadow dances on the wall of the neurophenomenological caveman's phenomenal state space. As soon as the system does not need a globally available self-model, it simply turns it off. Together with the model the conscious experience of selfhood disappears. Sleep is the little brother of death.

8.2 Preliminary Answers

In the second section of chapter 1 I offered a small set of questions to guide us through the complex theoretical landscape associated with the phenomenon of subjective experience. I will now keep my promise and return to each one of these questions by giving brief answers to them. However, recall that the *longer* answers can only be found elsewhere. Let us start by taking a second look at our basic notions.

What does it mean to say of a mental state that it is conscious?

First, it is important to note that there is no one single answer to this question, but that there are now many of them. *How* conscious a mental state is depends on the target domain and on the degree of constraint satisfaction. Consciousness is not an all-or-nothing phenomenon. There are *degrees of phenomenality* (for a first and simple example, think of Lewis qualia, Raffman qualia, and Metzinger qualia, as described in section 2.4). And as constraints are themselves theoretical entities, the degree of phenomenality or conscious*ness* exhibited by a certain mental state is not only an objective property but is also relative to a given theory. Third, any answer will depend on how we choose to individuate mental states, that is, the level of description we choose to give our answer *on*.

If a mental state is conceived of as a *representational* state, something that is described as carrying a content, then this content will be minimally conscious if it is, at the same time, integrated into a virtual window of presence (an internally generated "Now") and into a single, coherent, and globally available model of reality while earlier processing stages—and therefore its representational character as such—are attentionally unavailable, that is, if it is also a *transparent* form of content. The minimal degree of constraint satisfaction needed to speak about the phenomenon of "appearance," the phenomenon of consciousness *at all*, involves *constraints 2* (presentationality), *3* (globality), and *7* (transparency). Conscious experience consists in the activation of a coherent and transparent world-model within a window of presence. On the level of phenomenal content this is simply equivalent to "the presence of a world." Please note that such a minimal version of conscious experience is not yet *subjective* experience in terms of being tied to a consciously experienced first-person perspective (it is only subjective in the very weak sense of being an internal reality-model within an individual organism), and that this notion still is very simplistic (and probably empirically implausible), because it is completely *undifferentiated* in its representation of causality, space, and time. A system enjoying minimal consciousness as exclusively described by the conjunction of *Constraints 2, 3*, and *7*, would be frozen in an eternal Now and the world appearing to this organism would be devoid of all internal structure.

Please note how, in more complex configurations, there may be individual states *not* satisfying the transparency constraint: As soon as what I have called a "world zero" is in place, phenomenal simulations become possible (see the "world-zero hypothesis" for the evolutionary function of consciousness, as proposed in section 2.3). The system may now develop phenomenal simulations, conscious mental states that are experienced *as* representational states. Short-term memory and a single, integrated world-model are strictly necessary for phenomenal experience. In more complex organisms (like ourselves) transparency isn't. This is so because once conscious world-models are established, phenomenally *opaque* forms of content can be integrated into them.

We must therefore ask how phenomenal mental content could become stronger, by exhibiting a higher and potentially *variable* degree of constraint satisfaction. In principle there are now many ways to describe what I called *differentiated consciousness* in chapter 3. If we add a mereological internal structure in terms of *constraint 4* (convolved holism), we allow for multimodal scene segmentation and the emergence of a complex situation. However, if we do not want to assume the unlikely case of one single, presegmented scene being frozen into an eternal Now on the phenomenal level, we have to add *temporal* structure in terms of *constraint 5* (dynamicity). At this stage it is possible to have phenomenal experience as a dynamically evolving phenomenon on the level of content, to have an interrelated hierarchy of different contents that unfolds over time and possesses a dynamical structure. Differentiated consciousness, therefore, results from adding an internal context and a rich temporal structure.

The decisive step is the one leading to *subjective* consciousness. This is the level at which consciousness begins to approach the complexity we find on the human level of organization, and the level at which it becomes a truly theoretically interesting phenomenon. By adding *constraint 6* (perspectivalness) to constraints *2*, *3*, *4*, *5*, and *7*, we introduce a consciously experienced first-person perspective into phenomenal space. The space of experience is now always *centered* on an active self-representation. A PSM, a transparent and globally available self-model, as well as a PMIR, a transparent and globally available model of ongoing subject-object relations, is in existence and integrated into working memory (see chapter 6 for details). A *perspectivally* conscious mental state, therefore, is one whose representational content has been integrated into a phenomenal model of reality that is structured by a PMIR. There is also an alternative formulation allowing us to describe all and only those states as subjectively conscious which are currently in the *focus* of experience. A truly conscious mental state would then be one that currently constitutes the *object component* of the phenomenal model of the intentionality relation (PMIR; see section 6.5).[2]

If we demand the satisfaction of this constraint, we pick out a much more interesting class of representational systems: the class of systems of which it can actually be said that they enjoy *subjective* experience in the true sense of the word. One may speculate that all those vertebrates possessing a PSM plus at least some rudimentary form of attentional processing belong to this level of constraint satisfaction. They have a conscious self (however simple it may be) and they generate a phenomenally experienced "arrow of intentionality" pointing from the attending self to various perceptual objects. They have a simple, subsymbolic PMIR. Such systems, although a subjectively experienced flow of time involving duration and change against the background of a specious present would already

---

2. This also allows for a definition of what the *fringe* of consciousness actually is (Mangan 1993). Every representational content that fulfills *constraints 2,3*, and *6*, while *not* being integrated into either the subject or the object component of the PMIR, constitutes the fringe of phenomenal awareness.

be available for them, would not yet have an explicit phenomenal representation of past and future, of possible worlds, and possible selves.

An even richer degree of phenomenality is constituted by *cognitive* subjective consciousness. If we add *constraint 8* (offline activation) and if we assume a spectrum from transparent to opaque representations (see section 3.2.7), we arrive at a yet more specific class of phenomenal systems. These systems would be able to selectively engage in the activation of globally available representational structures *independently of current external input*, and given that these structures would exhibit a certain degree of opacity, the fact that they were now operating *with* representations would therefore be globally available to them and could be integrated into their self-model. In other words, such systems could not only in principle engage in future planning, enjoy explicit, episodic memories, and start genuinely cognitive processes like the mental formation of concepts, these systems could also for the first time represent themselves *as* representational systems, on whatever minimal a scale. They would be thinkers of thoughts. They would be like total flight simulators that have started to simulate the pilot *as a simulator*. Through the running of phenomenally opaque simulations, they would be able to finally escape naive realism, previously generated by a full satisfaction of the transparency constraint on all levels of content. For such systems, the difference between reality and appearance would for the first time become available for attentional and metacognitive processing. Therefore, they would now possess the resources to develop a conception of *consciousness* itself, of the phenomenon of appearance *as such*. They could then become what I would (in alluding to Daniel Dennett's notion of a "second-order intentional system"; see, e.g., Dennett 1987b, p. 243*ff.*) term a "second-order phenomenal system": a being that can consciously experience the fact that it currently undergoes conscious experiences itself. It may well be that human beings are the only biological creatures on our planet fulfilling this additional condition to any interesting degree. Please also note how the adaptivity constraint (section 3.2.11) still excludes artificial systems as bearers of *phenomenal* mental states. I return to this issue below when giving a preliminary answer to the last question on this list.

Alternatively, what does it mean of a conscious system—a person, a biological organism, or an artificial system—if taken as a whole, to say that it is conscious?

The transition from state consciousness to system consciousness is rather straightforward and simple. A system is conscious to the degree to which its mental states satisfy the criteria mentioned above. Any system possessing representational mental states, but no virtual window of presence and no single, global, integrated, and transparent model of reality, is unconscious. So even if the logical subject of predication is not a subsystemic state, but the system as a whole, ascribing phenomenality never is the same as ascribing one *single*, and primitive, property with the help of a one-place predicate (for which there would then not exist a noncircular definition). Ascribing phenomenality always consists in determining the degree of constraint satisfaction on *multiple levels of description*. Making the transition from state consciousness to system consciousness just means to exchange microlevels for macrolevels in terms of the logical subjects and the possible predicates constituting those levels of description. There may be interesting and highly relevant constraints, which can be exclusively discovered and applied on the whole-system level only—for instance, when investigating the *social correlates* of complex forms of phenomenal experience (see section 6.3.3). In particular, if the macrolevel is not simply the whole-system level but the *personal* level of description, a fundamental transition to an entirely new dimension is made. This may constitute a second fundamental distinction between human beings and other conscious beings on our planet. To give an example, in conscious systems, which, by accepting certain *normative* standards (epistemically justified or not), have begun to phenomenally experience themselves and others as rational individuals and as moral subjects, we have to explain not only the phenomenal experience of "selfhood" but also that of "personhood." This brings about a whole new set of properties and predicates on the whole-system level.

In terms of individuating characteristics for mental states, it is interesting to note that there could conceivably be afunctional phenomenal states, which are not representational states at all (e.g., in dreams or some kinds of hallucinations). Such states could contribute to conscious experience, while not representing anything *for* the organism as a whole. According to our teleofunctionalist background assumption they would have phenomenal, but not intentional content. In this case they will have to be individuated on a lower level of description, for example, as purely *functional* states currently *functionally* integrated into the mechanism that creates the organism's experiential present and its world-model. In this case, it would be their causal role that has been integrated, but not their representational contents. Call this "vehicle consciousness."

What does it mean to say of a mental state that it is a part of a given system's self-consciousness?

All mental states constituting phenomenal self-consciousness are characterized by a further content property, the property of *mineness*. Mineness represents *ownership* on a nonconceptual level (see section 6.1). In conscious processing, mineness creates a prereflexive and fully transparent *sense of ownership*. It is a property of a particular form of phenomenal content that, in our own case, is accessible on the level of inner attention as well as on the level of self-directed cognition. It is available to introspection$_3$ and introspection$_4$ (see section 2.2). In pathological situations, the distribution of this property across phenomenal space can vary considerably. A mental state is part of a given system's self-consciousness if it has been integrated into the system's PSM (see chapter 6). Its representational content has then become a part of the system's phenomenal self. Functionally, any system property currently represented in the PSM is an *appropriated* property. If, in unusual configurations (see chapter 7), a representational state satisfying the constraints for phenomenality *cannot* be integrated into the PSM, it automatically becomes a part of the world-model and its content is now experienced as external. For instance, a conscious thought could not be phenomenally owned any more, if—as in some cases of schizophrenia—the system is unable to embed it in its PSM. It would then not be *my* thought anymore. Or a body part, as in unilateral hemineglect, could drop out of the phenomenal self, if the system is for some reason unable to integrate it into the globally available partition of its self-model. Phenomenally, it would then not be my *own* body part anymore.

What does it mean for any conscious system to possess a phenomenal self? Is selfless consciousness possible?

First, it is important to understand the central ontological claim: No such things as selves exist in the world. All that exists are certain information-processing systems meeting the constraints for phenomenality while operating under a transparent self-*model*. At least for all conscious beings so far known to us, it is true that they neither *have* nor *are* a self. Biological organisms exist, but an organism is not a self. Some organisms possess conscious self-models, but such self-models certainly are not selves—they are only complex brain states. However, if an organism operates under a phenomenally transparent self-model, then it possesses a *phenomenal* self. The phenomenal property of selfhood as such is a representational construct; it truly is a *phenomenal* property in terms of being an appearance only. For all scientific and philosophical purposes, the notion of a self—as a theoretical entity—can be safely eliminated. What we have been calling "the" self in the past is not a substance, an unchangeable essence, or a thing (i.e., an "individual" in the sense of philosophical metaphysics), but a very special kind of representational content: the content of a phenomenally transparent system-model (see section 6.2). It is the content of a self-model that cannot be recognized *as* a model by the system using it. The phenomenal experiences of *substantiality* (i.e., of being an independent entity that could in principle exist all by itself), of having an *essence* (i.e., of being defined by possessing an unchangeable innermost core, an invariant set of properties), and of *individuality* (i.e., of being an entity that is unique and cannot be divided) are special forms of conscious, representational content as well. Possessing them was evolutionary advantageous, but as such they are not epistemically justified. As such, they are not a form of knowledge, although they play an important functional role.

On the functional level of description, a phenomenal self, again, is not a substance or an individual—be it physical or nonphysical—but an ongoing *process*: the process of self-modeling, as currently integrated into working memory and the organism's globally available world-model. This process can be interestingly described as a process of *self-containing*, of functionally achieving ownership for a subset of the system's causal capacities. Self-modeling is causal self-appropriation. What we called the "phenomenal self-shadow" earlier is determined exclusively by the machinery of internal functional properties. On the neurobiological level, the phenomenal content of the self-model supervenes locally. This means that in biological organisms, every phenomenal self possesses a minimally sufficient neural correlate. Given this correlate, a conscious self will come into existence by nomological necessity.

A phenomenal self appears if a certain property is instantiated, the phenomenal property of *selfhood*. In its core, this property is a representational property. Interestingly, it is brought about by a special form of epistemic darkness, by a lack of introspectively available information. It is important to note this point: phenomenal selfhood results from phenomenal transparency, but from *epistemic* opacity. According to the SMT, phenomenal selfhood is a *lack* of introspective self-knowledge. I have called this structural characteristic of the neurophenomenological caveman's conscious mind "autoepistemic closure" (see sections 2.3, 3.2.7, and 6.2.6), referring to it as an "inbuilt blind spot," a structurally anchored deficit in the capacity to gain knowledge about oneself. It is important to understand that autoepistemic closure as used in this book does not refer to *cognitive* closure (McGinn 1989b, 1991) or epistemic "boundedness" (e.g., Fodor 1983, p. 120) in terms of the perhaps principled unavailability of *theoretical*, propositionally structured self-knowledge. Rather, it refers to a closure or boundedness of attentional processing with regard to one's own internal representational dynamics. It is a limitation in mental resource allocation expressed on the level of *nonconceptual* content. Autoepistemic closure, in the current context, consists in human beings in ordinary waking states, using their internal representational resources—that is, by introspectively guiding *attention*—not being able to attentionally penetrate into earlier processing stages in the ongoing construction of their conscious self-model. Of course, there may be good evolutionary reasons for this: Attentional availability uses precious computational resources, and a transparent self-model—a *realistic* self-model—has the functional advantage of making its bearer maximally egotistic.

Is selfless consciousness possible? All consciousness *is* selfless, in that a self is not represented in it, but only a physical, representational *system*—but transparently, in the mode of naive realism, as it were. Because the PSM is transparent, the system constantly operates under the condition of what I have called a naive-realistic self-misunderstanding (see section 6.2.6). Metaphorically speaking, it *confuses* itself with the content of its own PSM. Just as with color qualia there is nothing in the external world that nicely and systematically maps on the chromatic primitives of conscious color vision, so there is no single entity in or outside the system that directly corresponds to the primitive, prereflexive feeling of conscious selfhood. In principle there are two ways in which a phenomenal system could lack this feeling, in which selfless consciousness is conceivable within the present framework.

First, it is possible for a system to satisfy all other constraints for consciousness, without *having* a self-model. It could have a world-model, but no self-model. Probably many simple organisms on our planet belong to this phenomenal system class. If the system at least satisfies *constraints 2, 3,* and *7,* but without possessing a centered model of reality, then it will instantiate selfless consciousness. Such organisms may have unconscious proto-selves, for example, in terms of the elementary form of functional self-appropriation that comes with homeostasis and rudimentary emotions, but no distinct conscious representation directed at the intentional object of the organism as a whole. There would be the appearance of a world, but no one to appear as currently being directed *toward* this world. Phenomenologically, the light would be on, but no one would be at home. There would be no explicit little red arrow, and only a flight simulator, but no total flight simulator.

There is, however, a second possibility and it is of much greater philosophical interest. In section 6.4.2 we saw that the human self-model is interestingly characterized by exhibiting a *continuum* ranging from full transparency to opacity, typically ascending from the sensory aspects of bodily self-awareness to purely cognitive levels of self-reference and reflexive self-consciousness. Try to imagine a PSM that was *fully opaque.* Imagine a system that—all other aspects held constant—is characterized by the fact that *constraint 7,* the transparency constraint, is not satisfied for its self-model *at all.* Earlier processing stages would be attentionally available for all partitions of its conscious self-representation; it would continuously recognize it as a representational construct, as an internally generated internal structure. The SMT makes the following prediction: Phenomenologically, this system would not have a self, but only a system-model. It would not instantiate selfhood. *Functionally,* it would still possess all the computational and informational advantages associated with having a coherent self-model, at the price, however, of a somewhat higher computational load. In addition, it would have to find a new solution to the problem of not getting paralyzed by an infinite loop of self-representation, to the problem of avoiding an infinite regression in the absence of transparent primitives. But possibly it could still operate under a centered model of reality, even if this model were not *phenomenologically* centered anymore. What the neurobiological characteristics of such a system would be is presently unclear. However, it may be interesting to note a specific phenomenological analogy. There is one type of *global* opacity that we discussed in our last neurophenomenological case study, namely, the lucid dream (see section 7.2.5). In the lucid dream the dreamer is fully aware that whatever she experiences is just the content of a global simulation, a representational construct. It is also plausible to assume that there are state classes in the phenomenology of spiritual or religious experience resembling this configuration—but only during the waking state. Now imagine a situation in which the lucid dreamer would also phenomenally recognize *herself* as being a dream character, a simulated self, a representational fiction, a situation in which the dreaming system, as it were, became lucid *to itself*. This is the second possibility for selfless consciousness under the theoretical framework proposed here. I am, of course, well aware that this second conception of selflessness directly corresponds to a classical philosophical notion, well-developed in Asian philosophy at least 2500 years ago, namely, the Buddhist conception of "enlightenment." However, let us adopt a metaphysically neutral terminology here and call this phenomenological state class "system consciousness." A representational system has system consciousness if and only if it operates under a phenomenally opaque *system*-model, but not under a self-model.

What the first possibility and the second possibility have in common is that they are *logical* possibilities; they can be coherently described and conceived of. Whether they are nomologically possible neurophenomenological configurations is an open question. For instance, there could be fundamental neurocomputational reasons that make such selfless models of reality at least highly unlikely, hard to sustain, or generally unstable. Assuming the second case, it may turn out that any representational system needs *some* kind of transparent primitive, and that this is true for human self-consciousness in particular. On the other hand, please note that all that is needed for generalized opacity is the *availability* of earlier processing stages for introspective attention, but not a permanently realized form of *actually ongoing access*. For the first class of phenomenal systems, it is plausible to assume that many lower animals on our planet function in this way. Autophenomenological reports given by human beings about selfless states of the second type, however, will typically not impress philosophers much, because they contain an inherent logical fallacy: How can you coherently report about a selfless state of consciousness from your *own*, autobiographical memory? How could this episode ever constitute an element of your *own* mental life? Such reports generate a performative self-contradiction, because you deny something that is presupposed by what you are currently doing. (For a more mundane example: "I am probably the most modest person I have ever met.")

In any case, it is interesting to note a second common characteristic of the first and second selfless configurations: they are phenomenally *impossible*, and therefore extremely counterintuitive. In section 2.3, I introduced the notion of phenomenal possibility, as a property of all states of affairs or worlds which, as a contingent matter of fact, we can actually *consciously* imagine or conceive of—all those states of affairs or worlds which can enter into conscious thought experiments, into cognitive operations, or explicit planning processes. We also saw that what is phenomenally possible is always relative to a certain class of concrete conscious systems, to their specific functional profile, and to the deep representational structure underlying their specific form of phenomenal experience. For beings like us, the goal of deliberately simulating a noncentered, selfless reality is strictly incompatible with our representational architecture. We cannot *truly* imagine the world as viewed from nowhere, pace Nagel. When, earlier, I asked the reader to imagine a fully opaque PSM or discovering that oneself is a dream character, I was asking for something impossible. Children discover this impossibility for the first time when trying to imagine how the world will be after they are dead. Adults certainly can phenomenally simulate noncentered worlds *within* a centered world zero, but there will always be a phenomenal self experienced as *doing* the imagining. The view from nowhere always is *your* view—or it could not be an element of *your* autobiographical memory about which you could later report. In short, the self-model theory of subjectivity is a theory which, even if strongly supported by good arguments and empirical data, will always remain counterintuitive. Even if you are intellectually convinced by the current theory, it will never be something that *you* can believe in.

What does it mean to say of a mental state that it is a subjective *state? Is* nonsubjective *consciousness possible?*

First, it is important to note that so far we are only talking about *phenomenal* subjectivity, that is, of subjectivity as phenomenally experienced. There is a more trivial reading of subjectivity (previously introduced as "functional subjectivity"; see section 2.2), amounting to the fact that information has been integrated into an exclusively *internal* model of reality, active within an *individual* system, and, therefore, giving this particular system a kind of privileged introspective access to this information in terms of *uniquely direct causal links* between this information and higher-order attentional or cognitive processes operating on it. If this internal model of reality satisfies the minimal constraints for perspectival phenomenality, then three major interpretations of "phenomenal subjectivity" result.

First, I experience everything as subjective that is an element of my conscious world-model. Even, if I don't experience it as *mental* I learn (e.g., through visual illusions and other cases of sensory misrepresentation) that, strictly speaking, my world is only *my* world and that others may have a different kind of phenomenal experience. To be sure, my world-model remains transparent, but, through experience, the fact that in all its reliability it nevertheless must be a model becomes *cognitively available* to me. And this event changes my PSM: I am now someone who consciously experiences himself as knowing this very fact. This is a weak, cognitively mediated form of phenomenal subjectivity from the first-person point of view. There is also a straightforward third-person reading of this first notion of phenomenal subjectivity: any system that has a conscious world-model has phenomenally subjective states. Please note how cognitive subjectivity emerges from an internal simulation of just this third-person reading: Cognitive subjectivity results when a system representationally *distances* itself from its own world zero.

The second interpretation of "phenomenal subjectivity" is more interesting. Any representational content that has been integrated into a PSM is phenomenally subjective. Whatever is represented under a PSM is an element of an individual system's self-consciousness. It is now phenomenally *owned*, by gaining the additional phenomenal property of "mineness." Phenomenal selfhood creates internality in the sense that something is portrayed as currently belonging to the center of representational space, as being a property of *this* subject. To be a subjective content then means to be a state of the phenomenal self, to be seamlessly integrated into it. However, in order to properly understand what has just been said, we need to understand how a phenomenal self can be portrayed not only as an ego but as a *subject*—as a subject of knowledge, an autonomous agent, or, to take the most simple case, as a currently *attending* self. Are there neurophenomenological configurations in which a phenomenal self is in existence, but no conscious *subject*? Is it possible for a system to have a conscious world-model plus a conscious self-model but *no* phenomenally subjective states?

What turns a phenomenal self into a conscious subject is the fact that it is transiently integrated into a yet more comprehensive kind of globally available representational structure: the PMIR. Phenomenal subjectivity in a truly interesting sense only emerges at this stage. It is the moment in which the system experiences itself as *directed at* a possible object of knowledge, an action goal, or a perceptual object. Truly subjective states are those that are integrated into the representation of a specific *relation*, namely, a self-object relation. I explained the notion of a PMIR at length in section 6.5, and there I also, in quoting from the work of Antonio Damasio (Damasio 1999, p. 263; for a brief case study, see p. 101*ff.*), pointed out how akinetic mutism may be a particularly circumscribed and salient example of a rare neurophenomenological configuration, the possibility of which is predicted by the SMT. Bilateral anterior damage to the cingulate gyrus and bilateral medial parietal damage lead to a situation which can be described as, first, the absence of a PMIR, while, second, a coherent conscious model of the world functionally centered by a phenomenal self is retained. Full-blown conscious experience—phenomenal *subjectivity* in a philosophically interesting sense—is more than the existence of a conscious self, and it is much more than the mere presence of a world. It results from the dynamic interplay between this self and the world, as situated in a lived, embodied present. In the patient with akinetic mutism we arguably have a situation in which there is a PSM, but no PMIR. The patient is awake, but not a subject. He may stare vacantly at the world or orient mechanically toward some visual object, but he never is *a self in the act of seeing*. To represent *the act of seeing* you need a PMIR. The patient is phenomenally embodied, but not *present*, because he is not phenomenally situated—*situatedness* is precisely what is established through the ongoing, dynamic construction of a PMIR. I have, on philosophical grounds, introduced the PMIR as a distinct theoretical entity on the phenomenological, representational, and functional levels of description (see chapter 6). I am therefore committed to the empirical prediction that there will be a distinct neural correlate as well. In fact, candidates for the necessary components of the neural correlate of this specific kind of a PMIR are already under discussion (e.g., the cingulate gyrus, certain thalamic nuclei, and the superior colliculi; cf. Damasio 1999, p. 260*ff*.).

Returning to the level of philosophical analysis, I propose to treat the notion of phenomenal subjectivity as exactly that which may be absent in akinetic mutism. I argue that it is this kind of phenomenal content   a transient, dynamic integration of subject and object—that many of us intuitively regard as the essence of conscious experience. The most interesting sense of phenomenal subjectivity is the one that comes with *constraint 6*, the perspectivalness constraint. A truly subjective representational content is one that is an element of a *perspectival* model of reality, one that is structurally dominated by a PMIR.

Again, there is an alternative and more narrow formulation allowing us to describe all and only those states as *subjectively* conscious which are currently in the *focus* of experience. A truly conscious mental state would then be one that currently constitutes the *object component* of the PMIR. Viewed as a form of representational content, its subjectivity then consists in being explicitly linked to a phenomenal self—in its contribution to a more comprehensive mental structure, a relational representation of the *act of experience*. To give an example, as empirical research on change blindness (Mack and Rock 1998) shows for visual consciousness, there clearly exists an attentional PMIR in the visual domain: its object component is simply *what* we experience in an integrated fashion. Once attention is released, visual objects dissolve back into "proto-objects" and all informational content is lost. The phenomenon of change blindness demonstrates how systems like ourselves only integrate what becomes the visual object component of the PMIR, thereby minimizing the computational load on our brains. Computationally speaking, it is not necessary to keep all objects represented simultaneously, all that is needed is the capacity to access object identity whenever necessary. There is also, of course, nonattentional extraction of scene structure, because attention is not the central gateway through which all conscious information must pass; the attentional bottleneck applies only to coherent objects. Preattentive vision gives us scene structure, which is everything that can be seen before the arrival of the limited-capacity selection mechanism on the object. In this sense, and according to the third possible reading of "phenomenal subjectivity," preattentive scene structure would be a *nonsubjective* form of conscious content. This third interpretation of phenomenal subjectivity not only follows the philosophical intuition of "subjectivity-as-focal-representation-only" but nicely demonstrates what it means to say that conscious experience truly is a graded phenomenon.

What does it mean to speak of whole systems as "subjects of experience?"

Again, the transition from the subjectivity of states to the subjectivity of systems is rather straightforward and simple. A system is *subjectively* conscious to the degree to which its mental states satisfy the constraints mentioned above. Based on the second interpretation of "phenomenal subjectivity" we can now say that any system possessing a virtual window of presence and a single, globally integrated, and transparent model of reality but no PSM and no PMIR is not a subject of experience. Generally speaking, to become a true subject of experience you have to represent the world under a stable PMIR. However, there are borderline cases, like the nonlucid dreamer who possesses a highly unstable PMIR or the patient who suffers from akinetic mutism. Although such a patient has minimal self-awareness and no *perspectival* form of first-person experience, I would plead that all systems—human or not—belonging to this phenomenological class be treated as genuine subjects of experience. Why?

The notion of a "subject of phenomenal experience" is of great relevance not only for philosophy of mind but for *ethics* as well. Without going into any technical issues here, I would argue that everything that is capable of conscious *suffering* should automatically be treated as a moral object. Put simply, a moral object is something that belongs to the domain of things with regard to which our actions should be morally justifiable. Call this the "principle of negative utilitarianism": Whatever else our ethical commitments and specific constraints are, we can and should certainly all agree that, in principle, the *overall amount of conscious suffering* in all beings capable of conscious suffering should be minimized. This seems to be a simple principle of solidarity among all conscious creatures that are mortal, and able to feel physical pain or to suffer emotionally, intellectually, or otherwise. Whatever is a phenomenal subject of experience should immediately be treated as a moral object. It is interesting to note how the SMT predicts that many animals on this planet (as well as the first artificial subjects of experience that may one day evolve; see Metzinger 2001) are phenomenal subjects—but not yet *moral* subjects. They cannot mentally represent norms and are in principle unable to impose moral obligations unto themselves. Although they have no conscious first-person perspective, although they have no cognitive, let alone *moral*, first-person perspective, they should definitely be treated as moral objects. It is important to note the simple fact that all of the above does not imply that they cannot suffer. Maybe suffering is even *more* intense in simpler creatures that don't have the mental capacities to cognitively distance themselves from their pain or understand the potential meaning their suffering might have.

Remember the patient with akinetic mutism. Arguably, he is not capable of first-person, perspectival suffering, because he *has* no phenomenal first-person perspective. He cannot represent reality under a stable PMIR. However, he can certainly *own* physical pain, which, for instance, might occur in his body. He has rudimentary self-awareness. I would argue that even phenomenal ownership alone is enough for suffering: We should treat every representational system that is able to activate a PSM, however rudimentary, as a moral object, because it can in principle *own* its suffering, physical or otherwise. It is the phenomenal property of "mineness," the phenomenal, nonconceptual sense of ownership, which counts for ethical purposes. Without phenomenal ownership, suffering is not possible. With ownership, the capacity for conscious suffering starts to evolve. We would never deliberately hurt a patient with akinetic mutism, even if he could neither talk nor move and even if all we could elicit is the well-known vacant stare. The same principle should hold for all other weakly conscious systems, for all creatures characterized by low degrees of constraint satisfaction. In particular, we should take care to always stay on the safe side: As soon as there is evidence that something is a weak phenomenal subject of experience, as soon as there are indicators for the existence of a PSM, we should automatically treat it as a moral object. Of course, much more needs to be said about negative utilitarianism, its potentially limiting principles, and about the connection between philosophy of mind and ethics in general. And, of course, it is obvious how cognitive neuroscience now starts to gain increasing relevance for ethical issues. As a scientific discipline, it has the great potential to make extremely valuable contributions in the future in terms of precisely pinning down *objective indicators* for the existence of a PSM in a given nervous system, in empirically defining inclusion criteria for the class of phenomenal subjects, and thereby for the class of moral objects. But this is not the place for this type of investigation.

What is a phenomenal first-person perspective, as opposed, for example, to a linguistic, cognitive, or epistemic first-person perspective?

A *linguistic* first-person perspective appears with the mastery of the first-person pronoun "I." For a *cognitive* first-person perspective to emerge it is not only necessary to have thoughts that can be expressed using "I." What is necessary is the possession of a concept of oneself as the *thinker* of these thoughts, as the *owner* of a subjective point of view. An *epistemic* first-person perspective comes into existence if the system's model of reality, as structured through a PMIR, is not only characterized by its phenomenal content but also as possessing *intentional* content. It is then described as a structure that not only mediates conscious experience but also *knowledge*. It is interesting to see how the phenomenal first-person perspective is a necessary foundation for all the richer, more complex forms of subjectivity just mentioned, and how it is at the same time fully autonomous. Every philosophical investigation of higher-order forms of subjectivity—be they mediated through linguistic and cognitive self-reference, through propositional forms of structured self-knowledge, or even through *social* interactions—will inevitably have to rest on a convincing account of the PMIR. Let us have a short look in four brief steps.

First, what *is* a phenomenal first-person perspective? And what does it mean that it is autonomous? A phenomenal first-person perspective is realized by any system possessing a transparent PSM plus a transparent PMIR. In particular, every system satisfying *constraints 2, 3, 6,* and *7* will have a phenomenal first-person perspective. More realistically, it is important to note that all candidates for phenomenally experienced perspectivalness actually existing in the part of the universe known to us are highly likely to satisfy *all* the constraints developed in chapter 3 with the exception of *constraint 8,* the capacity for offline activation. Of course, given the terminological machinery developed in chapters 2, 3, 5, and 6, it is now possible to offer many fine-grained descriptions of different grades of first-person phenomena, of different degrees of constraint satisfaction—like consciousness in general, selfhood or phenomenally experienced perspectivalness is not an all-or-nothing phenomenon. *How* perspectival a mental state is depends on the target domain and on the degree of constraint satisfaction, and any judgment is theory-relative. However, I will not enter into a discussion here, but highlight just one single aspect: It is empirically plausible to assume that a large majority of phenomenal systems currently known to us will have only very limited resources to run consciously experienced mental simulations and self-simulations (see sections 2.3 and 5.3.) They will have dynamic and somewhat convolved phenomenal models of reality, including a rudimentary self-model and a simple *attentional* first-person perspective (see sections 6.4.3 and 6.5.2). But, put simply, they will not be thinkers of thoughts and will have only limited capacity for explicit episodic memory and future planning. In particular, many of them will lack an *opaque* partition of their self-model (see section 6.4.2).

The autonomy of the phenomenal first-person perspective consists in that it can exist in nonlinguistic creatures and that it does not presuppose strong *cognitive* first-person phenomena in any way. A fully transparent PMIR is enough. You do not need to have a concept of yourself *as* operating under a phenomenal first-person perspective in order to possess it, neither linguistic nor mental. On the contrary, all empirical indicators strongly point to the hypothesis that abstract forms of self-representation evolved out of and are anchored in subsymbolic (e.g., spatial, proprioceptive, motor, and emotional) forms of self-representation, that any conceptual point of view can only be acquired via a *nonconceptual* point of view (see Bermúdez 1998; Metzinger 1993; and chapter 7). To establish what I called the *phenomenal presence of a knowing self* in section 6.5.2 (see also the intimately related notions of a "juxtaposition of self and object" and of a "self in the act of knowing" in the work of Antonio and Hanna Damasio; Damasio and Damasio 1996a, p. 172; 1996b, p. 24*ff.*; Damasio 1999, p. 168*ff.*), it fully suffices that the PMIR is constituted by attentional, that is, *subsymbolic*, mechanisms. Call this "subdoxastic subjectivity." Cognitive processing and concept formation are not needed to activate a PMIR. Attentional subjectivity (see section 6.4.3) is already a full-blown first-person phenomenon.

Third, the autonomy of the phenomenal first-person perspective also consists in not *presupposing* an epistemic first-person perspective. Please recall that all this time we have been discussing phenomenal content only. Phenomenal content supervenes locally. It follows that even the highest and most complex form of phenomenal content that human beings are arguably capable of, including all its higher-order variants emerging through reflexive self-consciousness and social cognition, is fully determined by the properties of its minimally sufficient neural correlate. Isolated portions of brain in a vat could generate a PMIR. What they could never generate is first-person *knowledge*. A minimally sufficient neural correlate in a vat could not even know what *kind* of properties the current PSM supervenes on, because, apart from the fact that it could hardly count as an epistemic subject, it would lack independent means of verification.

What is a *linguistic* first-person perspective? The "principle of phenomenal reference" introduced in chapter 2 states that one can only deliberately speak and think about those things that one also consciously experiences. Only phenomenally represented information can become the object of linguistic or cognitive reference, thereby entering into communicative and thought processes that have been voluntarily initiated. It is important to fully understand this principle. If you want to linguistically refer to, say, Gödel's theorem or to a friend living on the other side of the earth, you can only do so if you have, in whatever sketchy and rudimentary way, *phenomenally simulated* them. There must be a representation of them that is globally available for speech control and cognitive processing. Linguistic reference functions via phenomenal representation. Talking in your sleep or during light anesthesia or an epileptic automatism is not linguistic reference *at all*, because it is not agency, it is automatic motor behavior blindly producing speech output, without this output having been voluntarily initiated. A speech *act* always presupposes a phenomenal first-person perspective. The same is true of thought. Only phenomenally represented information can become the object of explicit cognitive reference, thereby entering into further thought processes which have been voluntarily initiated. If you refer linguistically to events in the distant past or future you can only do so by first *re*presenting them within your own virtual window of presence. If only very briefly, they *have* to become an element of global working memory.

There is a related principle for linguistic and cognitive *self-reference*. Not only reference *de re*, but reference *de se* has to be internally modeled while it is taking place. SMT proposes that the PSM is the neurocomputational tool making this possible. In short, what is needed for stronger forms of subjectivity is not only reference from the first-person point of view but the capacity of mentally "ascribing" this act of reference *to* oneself while it is taking place. However, it is empirically more plausible that this "ascribing" takes place in a dynamic, subsymbolic medium and in an ongoing fashion, like a permanent ("transcendental") process operating in the background. We have to keep this in mind when using the concept of "cognitive self-reference": We are not talking about discrete symbol tokens, but about dynamical self-organization in human brains. Cognitive self-reference always is reference to the phenomenal content of a transparent self-model. More precisely, it is a *second-order* variant of phenomenal self-modeling, which, however, is mediated by *one and the same* integrated vehicle of representation. The vehicle is not a thing, but a process. The capacity to conceive of oneself as oneself* consists in being able to activate a dynamic, "hybrid" self-model. Phenomenally opaque, quasi-symbolic, and second-order representations of a preexisting phenomenally transparent self-model are being activated and continuously reembedded in it.

Recall the discussion in section 6.4.4. Weak first-person phenomena are those in which, for instance, animals can be conceived of as operating under an egocentric world-model forming the center of their own universe and the origin of their own perspective. Such simpler animals do not have a hybrid self-model, because they generate no opaque states that they could continuously reintegrate into it. Using Lynne Baker's terminology we can now say that all sentient beings are conscious subjects of experience, but not all of them have first-person *concepts* of themselves. For Baker, only those who do are fully self-conscious in an interesting sense (Baker 1998, p. 328; see also note 18 in chapter 6, p. 396). Under the SMT simple sentient beings would use an integrated, global, and transparent model of the world functionally centered by a transparent self-model to regulate their own behavior. In Bakerian terminology, such organisms could be said to be solving problems by employing perspectival attitudes, while not yet possessing a concept of themselves *as a subject*. First-person phenomena in a stronger and more interesting sense, however, are not only characterized by the necessary condition of possessing a self-world boundary and being able to differentiate between the first and third person but include the capacity to possess this distinction on a *conceptual* level, and the act of currently using it. In the terminology so far introduced, this means that the existence of a preattentive self-world boundary and the difference between first- and third-person attributions are cognitively available in terms of introspection$_{2/4}$. It is not only necessary to have thoughts that can be expressed using "I." What is necessary is the possession of a concept of oneself as the *thinker* of these thoughts, as the *owner* of a subjective point of view. In short, what is needed is not only reference from the first-person point of view but the capacity of mentally "ascribing" this act of reference *to* oneself while it is taking place. The PSM of human beings enables this important step by possessing a transparent and a stable opaque partition at the same time.

Last, we have to ask, What is an *epistemic* first-person perspective? Here is my answer: Epistemic perspectivalness comes about if a fact is correctly represented *under a PMIR*. If some intentional content is integrated into a PMIR, or, more precisely, if it constitutes its *object component*, then it is a perspectival form of representational content. First-person knowledge is *knowledge under a PMIR*. And this finally tells us what causes the core problem in the philosophy of consciousness, the epistemic asymmetry (Jackson 1982): If Mary—who is one of the most recent descendants of Plato's captives in the cave—finally leaves her achromatic prison and sees the blue sky and a red apple on a tree for the first time, she represents a physical fact already previously known to her. But now, for the first time, this fact is integrated into the object component of her PMIR, for the first time she represents this aspect of reality *under a transparent PMIR*. She generates a new epistemic possibility, by gaining a new mode of knowledge. The new mode of presentation is *being known under a PMIR*. The same physical fact—that the neural correlate for certain conscious color experiences is currently active—is now for the first time represented to her as something she is *directed* to, under a PMIR. Moreover, it is represented transparently: Mary has no noncognitive introspective$_3$ access to the additional fact that all that is currently going on while she sees the blue sky or a red apple is a *representational* process. Even after Mary leaves her prison, she is still a neurophenomenological cavewoman. She is only a very distant relative of Plato's prisoners.

A rational theory of consciousness will have two major explanatory goals. First, How can full-blown, perspectival phenomenal experience be *ontologically* reduced? If there are principled obstacles, how can these obstacles be described so precisely that these descriptions in themselves constitute a growth of knowledge? Second, How can we at the same time give a plausible account of the fact that it is *epistemically irreducible* (see Walde 2002)? The concept of a PMIR as introduced in section 6.5 now enables us to give a clear and straightforward answer to the second question. Phenomenal content is epistemically irreducible, because—in standard situations—it is integrated into a global model of reality *structured* by a PMIR. The special and hitherto somewhat mysterious fact that the phenomenal character of conscious states seems to constitute an irreducible first-person form of content can be reduced to the fact that this character is typically represented *under a PMIR*. And *this* way of gaining knowledge about your own mental state certainly is irreducible to, say, any scientific procedure producing knowledge about its neurofunctional correlate. It is *another* way of gaining knowledge—one that existed long before philosophy and science came into being. On the contrary, arguably, it was the existence of a stable PMIR that made cognitive subjectivity (see above) and theoretical intersubjectivity *possible* in the first place.

So much for our first set of questions. Now we face a number of more general questions concerning ontological, logical or semantic, and epistemological issues. They do not form the focus of this investigation, but nevertheless are of great relevance.

Is the notion of a "subject" logically primitive? Does its existence have to be assumed a priori? Ontologically speaking: Does what we refer to by "subject" belong to the basic constituents of reality, or is it a theoretical entity that could in principle be eliminated in the course of scientific progress?

Let us first limit the scope of our answer to the two notions relevant to our context: the concept of a "subject of experience" and the notion of a "phenomenal subject." A *subject of experience* is any system that has phenomenal states satisfying *constraint 6*. As soon as a system possesses not only minimal and differentiated consciousness (see section 3.2.11) but also structures its global phenomenal state with the help of a single, coherent, and temporally stable PMIR (see section 6.5), it is a subject of experience. Subjects of experience are systems representing reality under a transparent PMIR. Therefore, there is no prima facie reason to believe that they form a category of irreducible and ontologically distinct entities. There is no internal homunculus on any level of description: being a subject of experience is never a property of the self-model, but always a property of the system as a whole. The class of subjects of experience is formed by all systems satisfying *constraints 2, 3, 6*, and *7*. It is a class of functional or representational architectures. However, the truly interesting or *intended* class of systems, in the context of the current theory, is only formed by the maximal degree of constraint satisfaction, as explained in sections 3.2 and 6.2. In order to have a PMIR, you need to have a transparent self-model forming its subject component. Therefore, any system qualifying as a subject of experience will also have a consciously experienced self. But what is the difference between a subject and a self? This question leads us to the second relevant notion.

A *phenomenal subject* is a specific kind of phenomenal self: a representation of the system as a whole *as currently being a subject of experience*, as currently being an agent, bodily, attentional, or cognitive (see sections 6.4.3, 6.4.4, and 6.4.5). If we want to take phenomenology seriously, we have to conceptually integrate two additional but important constraints: you can have a phenomenal self without being a subject of experience and you can be a subject of experience without cognitively *knowing* this fact. As explained above, there are many situations in which a transparent self-model is active, but not currently integrated with any object component. This may not only be the case in pathological configurations like akinetic mutism, but also in some everyday situations (e.g., imagine states of complete exhaustion or prostration, in which you are merely vacantly staring at the world, without truly seeing anything, without attending, thinking, or acting at all; or brief transitory phases of waking up from deep sleep). Second, operating under a purely attentional PMIR—as many animals probably do—does not include *cognitive availability* of this fact, or strong first-person phenomena in Lynne Baker's sense (see section 6.4.4). You can be a subject of experience for all of your life without *knowing* this fact. For example, this will be true of all systems satisfying *constraint 6*, but not *constraint 8*.

From this it follows that the notion of a "subject of experience" is not logically primitive. First, there is not *one* simple set of syntactic or semantic rules governing the use of this expression, but according to the different degrees of constraint satisfaction there are many different ways of using the expression "subject of experience." There are even borderline cases (recall the notion of "system consciousness" introduced above), in which we can conceive of selfless subjects of experience, namely, all systems possessing a fully opaque subject component in their PMIR. In particular, when speaking about consciousness and phenomenal selfhood, there is no a priori implication of experiential subjectivity. As general phenomenological observations and the case studies in chapter 7 show, conscious systems not possessing an integrated phenomenal self are not only logical possibilities but exist in the actual world. Not every conscious system has a phenomenal self. And systems possessing a phenomenal self do not necessary have to be *subjects* of experience or experience themselves as such. Not every phenomenal self is a phenomenal subject.

Moving on from logical to metaphysical considerations, it certainly is not necessary to assume a simple, basic constituent of reality corresponding to any of our folk-psychological or folk-philosophical notions of a phenomenal self or subject of experience. No such things as selves or subjects of experience exist in the world. What exist are natural systems operating under transparent PSMs and PMIRs, with both of these representational structures coming in many different strengths and with a long evolutionary history. We can therefore greatly simplify the ontological set of background assumptions necessary to do proper scientific psychology and cognitive neuroscience. All that exists are *phenomenal* selves, as instantiated by transparent self-models. For methodological purposes, no stronger assumption is necessary. The same is true of subjects of experience. We can be parsimonious by doing without the assumption that there are any basic, independent constituents of reality in this sense. For the cognitive neuroscience of consciousness and scientific psychology in general, all that exists are *phenomenal* models of the intentionality relation. Subjectivity is not a *thing*, but a property of complex representational processes unfolding in certain physical systems. In principle—and one may certainly have doubts that this would be rational in all contexts—the corresponding theoretical entities can be eliminated, and substituted by successor concepts on representationalist and functionalist levels of description. As a matter of fact, we have already taken the first steps: A "subject of experience" is a conscious representational system satisfying *constraint 6*. A "phenomenal self" is constituted by the representational content of a PSM. A "phenomenal subject" is a PSM integrated into a PMIR.

It is clearly outside the scope of my approach to develop a more detailed semantics for the indexical expression "I." Therefore, let me just very briefly sketch how we could arrive at a deeper understanding of sentences in which the word "I" is used in the autophenomenological self-ascription of experiential properties (as in "I am feeling a toothache right now").

What are the truth conditions for sentences of this type?

Self-ascriptions of phenomenal properties refer to the currently conscious content of the self-model. You *can* only linguistically self-refer to properties of yourself that have before been made globally available through the conscious part of your self-model. A PSM is a necessary, but not a sufficient condition for self-reference and phenomenological attitudes *de se*. Many different properties of oneself—social, physical, functional—can be made available for self-report through the conscious self-model. They then form its representational or *intentional* content. In the special case of autophenomenological reports about the experiential *character* of certain aspects of self-consciousness we refer to the current *phenomenal* content of the self-model. Because the self-model is transparent, most people never distinguish the two situations. Intuitively, most of us therefore treat all kinds of self-reference as *direct* self-reference, because we normally experience them as such. Phenomenal immediacy, however, is not referential immediacy. Of course it is true that only the experiencing subject can refer to its own phenomenal states *as* phenomenal states. But as we now know, *no* kind of self-reference is ever truly direct, because it is inevitably mediated through the self-model, because it crucially depends on the subpersonal self-organization of the relevant construction mechanisms, which are introspectively invisible, that is, transparent to us. This is also true of the special case of self-related phenomenal content.

The phenomenal content of self-consciousness supervenes locally. It will have a distinct neural correlate in every single case. From a third-person perspective we can, therefore, in principle, assess the truth of an autophenomenological report by verifying the existence of its minimal sufficient physical correlate. What makes an autophenomenological statement true is the fact that its minimally sufficient correlate was functionally active at the time it was uttered. This fact can be known using very different kinds of causal links (or modes of presentation). It can be known and reported from the first-person perspective through introspection$_3$ and introspection$_4$ (see section 2.2), that is, via a PMIR, which has a first-order PSM as its object component. It can also be known and reported from the third-person perspective, for instance, through neuroscientific methods of investigation. First-person phenomenological self-reports are special in that the use of "I" takes place under the unique conditions of the uttering and the self-modeling system being identical (see the next question below).

Please note how the *intentional* content of self-consciousness may not supervene locally. Of course, we do ascribe much more than experiential properties to ourselves in using our conscious self-model as a basis for public statements. If you say, "Sometimes I am a little isolated," then the truth conditions for this statement are to be found in your social environment. Are you *really*? This intentional content is *mediated* through your PSM. The phenomenal content that you *feel* a little isolated, however, supervenes locally on brain properties. It might be a hallucination. You need independent means of verification. What generates many problems in this domain is that beings like ourselves typically cannot make distinctions of this type *on the level of subjective experience itself*. For the transparent partition of our self-model, we are introspectively unable to distinguish between vehicle and content, or between self-experience and self-knowledge. However, the simple fact that you can understand these words as you read them demonstrates that, at least for human beings, the situation is more complicated.

Would the elimination of the subject use of "I" leave a gap in our understanding of ourselves?

We now have a better understanding of the constitutive conditions for what Wittgenstein called *Subjektgebrauch* ("subject use"): Only a true subject of experience, a system possessing a PSM and a PMIR, can refer to itself *as a subject* using "I." A conscious system possessing a system-model only, while not instantiating a phenomenal self—that is, a system possessing a "nemocentric" model of reality containing a fully *opaque* model of itself (see above and section 6.2.6)—could not use "I" to refer to itself *as* a subject of experience. The reason is straightforward and simple: such a system *is* no subject of experience. It has a model of reality functionally centered by a system-model, but not a consciously experienced self forming a genuine center on the level of phenomenal experience. However, we could easily adopt a terminological convention labeling this type of system as a phenomenally selfless subject of experience.

Such a system could still use the indexical expression "I." However, it would only be capable of the *object use* of "I," because this use would be mediated through an opaque system-model only—a globally available model of the system *as an object*—and not through a phenomenal self. Such a system could truly refer to itself as "the speaker of this sentence" by using "I," leaving nothing out, because this would precisely be the way in which it would also internally represent itself: not via a phenomenal self as subject, but as a system currently generating speech output. It is easy to imagine a machine satisfying the set of constraints sketched above: an artificial or postbiotic system that is conscious, but has no phenomenal self, only an opaque self-*model*. If this system were to use "I" when communicating with us, we would therefore be justified in regarding it as an object, and not as a subject. For instance, it could never truly suffer, because it could not *phenomenally own* its pain states (see above). In this context, it must also be noted that it may make a difference if something models or refers to itself as an object only, or as a *living* object (cf. the discussion of Cotard's syndrome in section 7.2.2). But the deeper question in the background is whether anything that has neither a PSM nor, a fortiori, a PMIR could ever count as a *speaker* of a sentence.

Think of an unconscious patient during a prolonged epileptic automatism referring to himself using "I" (recall the case of Dr. Z, briefly cited in chapter 6, n. 23). Is he a subject? He certainly is not a subject of *experience*. Is he a speaker? He certainly does not refer to properties of himself, which were first represented as contents of his globally available (i.e., *conscious*) self-model. It obviously is an (open) empirical, and not a philosophical matter to find out if such persons only blindly "shoot off" complex motor patterns using their physical speech apparatus, or if they actually retrieve some unconscious form of self-representational content. Therefore, we can hardly decide on philosophical grounds alone if such a patient might nevertheless be an epistemic subject, that is, a subject of *knowledge*, even if he is not a subject of *experience*. I think he isn't. However, these thought experiments help us to further clarify what is the standard case: You can only linguistically refer to yourself via your conscious self-model. The neurocomputational tool has to be in place before the linguistic tool can start to operate.

Speech is action. You need an internal instrument that makes self-related information globally available for the flexible control of action before you can enter into external communication. This instrument is the PSM. As in the majority of cases when you are referring to information generating a phenomenally *transparent* form of representational content in the PSM, you do not consciously experience yourself as referring to a *content* when using "I," but to yourself, that is, to an object which is a *subject*. This, or so I propose, is the way in which attitudes and reference *de se* are internally modeled, else we could not understand what we are doing *while* using "I." Second, in all standard situations the phenomenal self is a representation of something which, although certainly possessing an objective, physical body, is in its essence a subject—a being that constantly catches itself in the act of knowing. In this way the subject use of "I" is anchored in an automatic, subpersonal process of phenomenally modeling oneself (a) as a subject, that is, as the fixed origin of a first-person perspective, and (b) transparently.

Would the elimination of the subject use of "I" leave a gap in our understanding of ourselves? There are at least two relevant readings of "understanding" at this point: individual self-understanding and theoretical self-understanding. They have to be distinguished. Consider the first case, in which an individual system possessing a PSM has stopped (or never even started) using "I" to refer to itself as subject. Let us assume it has not done so for ideological reasons, but truthfully. There are basically two classes of phenomenal systems I can conceive of as exhibiting this feature, namely, enlightened human beings or the kind of machine briefly discussed above.[3] What both types of systems have in common is that they satisfy the necessary constraints for being conscious, while their self-model is fully opaque. They introspectively$_3$ recognize their self-models as representational structures, because earlier processing stages are continuously attentionally available to them (see section 6.4.3). The phenomenal property of selfhood is not instantiated by these systems. If they operate under a PMIR, they do not possess a consciously experienced first-*person* perspective, but only what I have termed a consciously experienced first-*object* perspective. Their variety of consciousness might well be biological consciousness (see section 3.2.11), but it would certainly not be phenomenologically *subjective* consciousness.

At this point it becomes obvious that, yes, such beings would indeed have a very different individual understanding of themselves—at least as compared to normal humans like you and me. The reason is that they would live in an entirely different kind of phenomenal reality, a reality deeply counterintuitive to most of us, a reality that seems *phenomenally impossible* to us because we cannot even imagine it—we are constitutionally unable to run the corresponding mental simulations in our brains (see section 2.3). If we were to encounter members of this class of systems, there would certainly be a deep gap to be bridged in trying to understand them. If we were to *become* such systems ourselves, there would be an equally dramatic shift, not only in the overall structure of our conscious reality but also in our understanding of ourselves. A whole set of possible truths (e.g., about the nature of our *self*) would become unavailable, because there were no such truths—our understanding would only be an understanding of our*selves* in a much weaker sense. The same would be true in the machine scenario. Let us now turn to the second reading of our initial question.

Would eliminating the subject use of "I"—say, in scientific and philosophical circles—leave a gap in our theoretical understanding of ourselves? Let us look at a recent example. Thomas Nagel (1986, p. 58*ff.*) has famously pointed out that an elimination of the particular first-person thought "I am TN" in favor of its impersonal truth conditions leaves a significant gap in our conception of the world. His general point is that all facts making such first-person, self-referential statements true can be expressed by third-person statements, but as Nagel argues, they cannot be *replaced* by them. We now have a much better

3. The Cotard's patients discussed in section 7.2.2 *may* constitute a third class. However, as these patients today are under heavy medication from the very beginning of their clinical stay, it is very hard to assess their true neurophenomenological profile. In particular, their self-model is not opaque, but,—a plausible hypothesis—it is fully deprived of its emotional layer. Cotard's patients are neither enlightened nor machines, they are *emotionally disembodied*. See section 7.2.2.

understanding of how such third-person statements could look on different levels of description (see section 6.4.4 in particular). For instance, instead of saying, "I am feeling very happy today," we (or our selflessly conscious machine) could say something like, "The emotional layer of the PSM currently activated by the brain of *this* organism is in a close-to-optimal state." If this were a truthful autophenomenological report, we would be one of the selfless systems just discussed. But when Thomas Nagel developed the beautiful philosophical vision of the *View from Nowhere* he was not selfless at all. If Nagel had ever truly viewed the world from *nowhere*, then he would not have had any autobiographical memory referring to this episode. A fortiori he would not have been able to offer his readers a neo-Cartesian interpretation of this phenomenal episode.

As is well-known, the neo-Cartesian interpretation of the *View from Nowhere* faces serious analytical difficulties.[4] What is even more important is to analyze the actual representational deep structure of the *View from Nowhere*, because this will also help us to understand the Cartesian intuitions behind many bad arguments—and also *what* it was that Nagel has importantly discovered and what his true achievement is. We now have the conceptual tool kit to do so (briefly, for more extended discussions, see Metzinger 1993 and 1995c). What Nagel does is ask his readers to run a certain *intended simulation* (see section 2.3) in the conscious partition of their self-model. He then offers a philosophical inter-

---

4. First, the logical structure of the alleged perspectival fact is never clearly stated; see Lycan 1987, p. 78*f.*; 1996, p. 50; Metzinger 1993, p. 233). Second, the *objective self*—which is more similar to Husserl's notion of a "transcendental ego" in his later philosophy than to the Wittgensteinian subject as forming the border of the world—in being used in Nagel's ubiquitous visual metaphor of the "taking" of perspectives immediately creates distal objects as its counterparts. In its conceptual interpretation this then leads to persisting act-object equivocations, to the freezing of phenomenal *events* into irreducible phenomenal individuals. Again, see Lycan 1987, p. 79*f.*; 1996, p. 51*f.*). Third, upon a closer look Nagel's concept of an "objective self" is inconsistent. It is not a mental object anymore, because the concept of mentality was *introduced* via the notion of a perspective as referring to subjective points of view and their modifications (see Nagel 1986, p. 37). "Self," however, is a mentalistic term par excellence. Norman Malcolm has pointed out how an aperspectival objective self would be a "mindless thing" because in its striving for objectivity it would have distanced itself so radically from the point of view of the *psychological* subject that it could no longer be grasped by any mental concept (see Malcolm 1988, p. 158*f.*). The most important mistake, however, consists in using "I" as a designator and not as an indicator in the "philosophical" reading of the relevant identity statements. There are no criteria of identity offered for the individual in question. As Malcolm (1988, pp. 154, 159) puts it: "Does this make any sense? *It would if there were criteria of identity for an* I. [emphasis added] . . . When we are uncertain about the identity of a person, sometimes we succeed in determining his identity, sometimes we make mistakes. But in regard to the identity of an *I* that supposedly occupies the point of view of a person, we could be neither right nor wrong. After a bout of severe amnesia Nagel might be able to identify himself as TN—but not as *I*. "I am TN" could announce a discovery—but not "I am I." An important source of confusion in Nagel's thinking is his assumption that the word "I" is used by each speaker, to *refer* to, to *designate—something*. But that is not how "I" is used. If it were, then "I am I" might be false, because "I" in these two occurrences had been used to refer to different things. Nagel's statement, "I am TN," could also be false, not because the speaker was not TN, but because Nagel had mistakenly used "I" to refer to the wrong thing. If Nagel had not assumed that "I" is used, like a name, to designate something, he would not have had the notion that in each person there dwells an *I* or *Self* or *Subject*— which uses that person as its point of viewing" (Malcolm 1988, p. 159*f.*).

pretation of the resulting chain of phenomenal states. I claim that this interpretation is phenomenologically unconvincing.

What Thomas Nagel terms the *objective self* is a conceptual reification of an ongoing representational process. This process takes place within a perspectivally structured model of reality in the conscious mind of his readers experimenting with the *View from Nowhere*. Do you still remember that, when discussing mental models in chapter 3, we said that propositional representations are *instructions for constructions*, because they trigger internal simulations? This is precisely what happens to you when reading Nagel: Propositional input activates a chain of phenomenal mental models in your brain. In particular, you now simulate a noncentered reality *within* a centered model of reality. In Nagel's case, this noncentered "conception" of the world also contains all experiences and the perspective of Thomas Nagel as well:

Essentially I have no particular point of view at all, but apprehend the world as centerless. As it happens, I ordinarily view the world from a certain vantage point, using the eyes, the person, and the daily life of TN as a kind of window. But the experiences and the perspective of TN with which I am directly presented are not the point of view of the true self, for the true self has no point of view and includes in its conception of the centerless world TN and his perspective among the contents of that world. (Nagel 1986, p. 61)

But this is false: *This* inner experience, the current *View from Nowhere* as initiated and executed by the psychological subject TN is *not* contained in the "centerless conception of the world." The *last* phenomenal event—namely, the intended shift in perspective—is not contained in the centerless conception, because this would lead to an infinite regress. However, it is very obviously contained in Nagel's autobiographical self-model—else it would not be reportable. The current perspective is not a part of reality as nonperspectivally seen by the true self Nagel postulates. The threat of infinite regress is blocked by an object formation, by introducing a metaphysical entity: the objective self.

Here is what really happens. A conscious, self-modeling system internally simulates a noncentered reality. This simulation is opaque, and is embedded in the current PSM: at any time you know that this is only a thought experiment, and you know that *you* are carrying it through. Anything else would either be a manifest daydream or a full-blown mystical experience; this is certainly not the phenomenology Nagel describes. In this phenomenally simulated reality there is a model of a person, TN (or yourself), enriched by all the properties until then only known under the PSM as your *own* properties. This person-model forms the object component of your PMIR; it is part of a comprehensive simulational process. In this way you generate the simulation of an "inner third-person perspective," by forming a model of yourself, which is *not* a self-model, but the model of yourself as if you were only given through indirect, external sources of knowledge. It is a model of a person alone in oceans of space and time, *"a momentary blip on the cosmic TV-screen"* (Nagel 1986, p. 61).

This process is fully reversible. In a second step you can now *reintegrate* the simulated person with the transparent partition of your PSM, which, of course, has been there all along. Like a monkey or a dolphin recognizing itself in a mirror, as it were, you discover yourself in the *internal* mirror of your ongoing phenomenal simulation of a centerless world, by discovering a strong structural isomorphism to one of the persons contained in this world. To this representational event you can linguistically refer by exclaiming sentences of the form "I am TN!" in their second, "philosophical" reading. But there is no homunculus that was briefly united with the transcendental ego (Nagel's *objective self*) and is now hurled back onto the empirical subject. This would just be a naive-realistic interpretation of a series of phenomenal representations. The cave is empty. There is no pilot. In particular, perspectivalness was never lost; *constraint 6* was satisfied all the time. The *View from Nowhere* is a *subjective* state of consciousness in the sense introduced in section 3.2.11. Naive realism creeps in at the moment one forgets about the processuality (i.e., the event character and the intended nature of the respective simulations), and the phenomenal opacity (i.e., the attentional availability of the representational nature characterizing the overall process).

What is interesting about Nagel's treatment is the idea of using the "vantage point" of an individual person as a kind of window. Phenomenal representations are such windows, representations *under which* we interact with the world and with ourselves. Some of these representational structures are opaque, but most of them are transparent: they satisfy *constraint 7*. A PMIR is just such a window. To represent reality (and, in higher-order mental operations, *yourself*) under a PMIR makes you a subject of experience. What Nagel has discovered is a fascinating architectural feature of the human mind: We are beings who can representationally *distance* ourselves from ourselves and make this fact globally available through conscious experience. In the terminology proposed here, what Nagel attempts to describe is that in certain special cases not only world-models but also *self-models* can satisfy *constraint 6*, the perspectivalness constraint. They do so by integrating the PMIR as a whole, modeling the intentionality relation as an *internal* subject-subject relation. Of course, many philosophers in the past have targeted this property, because it is a good candidate for a representational feature that distinguishes us from all other animals on this planet. Today, we can get a much clearer understanding of this feature by describing it under a naturalistic theory of mental representation, thereby preparing for a truly explanatory contact on the level of our currently best empirical theories of the mind. Using our new conceptual tools, we can describe it as the capacity to run intended, opaque emulations of our own person *in our conscious self-model*. We are conscious systems that can internally simulate taking an external perspective on our own person by phenomenally being the subject and object of experience at the same time. That is, we can generate a PMIR with an opaque model of ourselves as the object component. Recall how PMIRs can metaphorically be conceived of as windows. The *View from Nowhere* is a very specific type of PMIR, a *new* window through which beings like ourselves can represent the world and themselves. Whatever is seen through this window is globally available for the formation of long-term, autobiographical memory. Its particular strength consists in the fact *that* it is a window being available to us at the same time.

If even the capacity to engage in the *View from Nowhere* is a natural property of certain representational architectures, is it, then, really true that there is nothing special about the self-ascription of phenomenal properties, be they simple bodily sensations like a tickle or a complex internal event like the kind of self-simulation just described? Is there nothing *special* left? What is special in linguistic self-reference is the identity of self-modeling and self-referring system. There is only one system in the universe which can *introspectively* (i.e., using uniquely direct causal links) access the current content of its self-model and do so under the two conditions of internality and using both tools at the same time. Maybe some future neuroscientist can indirectly read out the content of your phenomenal self-model to arrive at true statements about you. It is also conceivable that his predictive power in doing so might be stronger than yours, that he could actually predict your future behavior better than you could, by introspectively reading out your self-model yourself. But he would never be able to do this under the aspect of *internality*: your PSM supervenes locally on the internal properties of your brain, and the causal links you employ in accessing its content are uniquely direct. The neuroscientist's model *of* and access *to* yourself could never achieve this.

These are the first two defining characteristics of phenomenal self-reference that cannot be reduced to third-person reference. Third, there is a temporal reading of internality as well. For each one of us it is true that we are likely the only being in the universe that can *at the same time* use the neurocomputational tool (the phenomenal self-model) and the linguistic tool (the utterance of "I"). In each subject use of "I" we causally link both tools, and we do so in an extremely small time frame. "Sameness of time" here is a weak form of identity, one determined by the scope of working memory and the way the respective phenomenal system constructs its own functional window of simultaneity (see sections 2.2 and 3.2.2). Obviously, it is conceptually as well as nomologically possible for a third-person readout mechanism to operate at the same speed as the first-person process it is targeting, but the *technological* probability today is negligible (see Birnbacher 1995). Yet what seems strictly impossible is the establishment of causal links to a conscious person's self-model that are *more direct* than that person's introspective capacities. Causal proximity is maximal, because introspection is *itself* a part of the ongoing process of self-modeling. The underlying reason is the physical identity of the self-modeling and self-referring system: the subject of experience and the speaker are one and the same system. Call this the "principle of twofold internality." This principle governing the subject use of "I" is certainly not a metaphysical mystery, but it puts each conscious subject capable of speaking a language in a unique position. But is this an *epistemologically* unique position in that it ultimately presents us with an irreducible epistemological superiority or autonomy?

Is subjectivity an epistemic relation? Do phenomenal states possess truth-values? Do consciousness, the phenomenal self, and the first-person perspective supply us with a specific kind of information or knowledge, not to be gained by any other means?

Again, let us restrict the scope of our discussion to *phenomenal* subjectivity as discussed above. The PMIR as such is not an epistemic relation, but the process of consciously *modeling* such a relation. This process could take place in a brain in a vat. All objects (or subjects) seen through this representational window could at any point turn out to be hallucinations.[5] Therefore, any claims to knowledge—that is, to an additional *epistemic* or intentional content going along with the phenomenal content in question—are in need of independent justification. Phenomenal experience is how the world *appears* to you and as such it is nothing more than that. In particular, please recall that stronger versions of phenomenality are likely to satisfy *constraint 11*. All the forms of consciousness, phenomenal selfhood, and subjectivity we have so far encountered were biological forms of consciousness, satisfying the adaptivity constraint. This is to say that the neuronal vehicles subserving this content have been optimized in the course of millions of years of biological evolution on this planet. They have been optimized toward *functional adequacy*. Functional adequacy, however, is not the same as epistemic justification. Certain deep-rooted illusions—like "believing in yourself," come what may—may certainly be biologically advantageous. It is also easy to see how the phenomenal experience of knowing something will itself be advantageous in many situations. It makes the fact that you *probably* possess information globally available. However, in many situations it will, of course, be functionally optimal to act *as if* you possess information—even if you don't. The same, of course, is true of the experience of knowing *that* you know something. To give an

5. Could a brain in a vat conclude that at least *some kind of representational system has to exist?* Can *you* conclude that for the very same reason your current self-model cannot be a hallucination in its entirety? Is the existential quantifier epistemically justified? *That some physically realized representational system inevitably has to exist,* of course, is one of the background assumptions of any naturalist theory of mental representation. At first sight, it is intriguing to see how this might lead to a naturalized version of Descartes's *cogito* argument. On the other hand, as a theoretical background assumption, it needs independent support. A brain in a vat—possessing no sensors, no effectors, and no social correlates to its conscious states (see section 6.3.3)—as opposed to you and me, does not have these independent sources of verification. It could therefore never even justify the assumption that it is a *representational* system of some sort.

example, in biological and social contexts it is frequently advantageous to deceive other conspecifics, as in playing dead or pretending not to notice the presence of a certain desired object, say, a fruit or an attractive male. Deception strategies will be most reliable if they include *self-deception*, that is, an adequate and appropriate PSM. Due to the transparency of the self-model, the correlated phenomenal experience will be one of certainty, of *knowing that you know*. As many of the case studies in chapter 7 demonstrate, unnoticed and unnotice*able* phenomenal misrepresentation can occur at any time. This is particularly true of higher-order or self-directed forms of representation (Neander 1998). It is important to understand how such states would not be instances of self-knowledge, but could satisfy *constraint 11*. If, in addition, my speculative hypothesis is true, that the emotional self-model also functions to *internally* represent the degree of evolutionary optimality currently achieved, then it follows that certain classes of delusional states will even be emotionally attractive to beings like us.

Truth-values are something predicated of sentences. Propositions are possible truths; sentences expressing such propositions possess truth-values. Our best current theories about the representational architecture underlying phenomenal experience do not assume compositionality or propositional modularity (Ramsey et al. 1991). The brain certainly is not a medium carrying out rule-based operations on syntactically specified symbol tokens. It may sometimes *emulate* such operations, but nevertheless the underlying laws and regularities will be the physical laws of dynamical self-organization. Therefore, it is not currently rational to assume that phenomenal states as such possess truth-values. However, as discussed extensively above, a specific kind of globally available self-modeling may certainly be the centrally relevant necessary condition for language acquisition. In particular, given our representationalist background assumptions, it is hard to see how the virtual organs which today we call "states of consciousness" could have propagated and preserved their own existence across certain types of nervous systems and populations of biological systems if they had *not* correctly and reliably extracted information from the environment in a large majority of cases. It is hard to explain large-scale reliability without assuming knowledge.

Does the incorrigibility involved in the self-ascription of psychological properties imply their infallibility?

Let us use Richard Rorty's (1970) definition of incorrigibility as implying that, given a certain subject S believes p at t, there exist no accepted procedures at this point in time which could allow us to rationally arrive at the belief that non-p. Currently, we live at such a point in time. If you refer to the content of your phenomenal self-model, there generally is no way in which a neuroscientist could demonstrate that you do so *falsely*. Take p to refer to the content of your own phenomenal self-consciousness. Your p-reports about this content cannot be corrected. However, it is important to note how the property of incorrigibility in this sense is a historical entity. Since the phenomenal content of your self-model supervenes locally and since it may be possible to discover strict, domain-specific and law-like regularities connecting it to its minimally sufficient neural correlate, future neuroscientists may predict the content by looking at its neural vehicle. Incorrigibility is a property that *p*-reports may lose.

In some cases *p*-reports *have* already lost this property. Recall the example of Anton's syndrome, of blindness denial, which we discussed in chapters 4 (section 4.2.3) and 7 (section 7.2.1). From all we know today about massive hemorrhages in the occipital lobes, a highly plausible inference to the best explanation in these patients leads us to the conclusion that they have no form of phenomenal visual content which could satisfy *constraint 2*. We are certainly in a position today to correct the confabulations of a patient suffering from Anton's syndrome. There exist accepted procedures that allow us to arrive rationally at the belief that the patient does not have (and, sadly, never again *will* have) phenomenal vision—that is, that non-*p*. The rise of clinical neuropsychology has supplied us with many examples of situations in which human subjects actually proved to be fallible in terms of their phenomenal beliefs *de se* (for an excellent recent discussion, see Coltheart and Davies 2000). Psychiatric disorders such as Cotard's syndrome demonstrate even more dramatic possibilities, such as, for example, *existence denial* (see section 7.2.2). As today there are many independent reasons demonstrating the fallibility of introspective autophenomenology, it is impossible to *rationally* draw the conclusion from incorrigibility to infallibility.

Are there any irreducible facts concerning the subjectivity of mental states which can only be grasped under a phenomenal first-person perspective or only be expressed in the first-person singular?

As we saw when briefly discussing Thomas Nagel's argument above, subjectivity is a *representational* phenomenon. Facts always are facts *under* a specific type of representation or mode of presentation. For example, you can know about the world (and yourself) under a theoretical representation, and you can know about the world (and yourself) under a phenomenal representation. In particular, you can know about the world and yourself under a phenomenal representation that satisfies *constraint 6*, the perspectivalness constraint (see section 3.2.6). In this case the knowledge you gain is *phenomenally subjective* knowledge. It is not the represented facts that are nonobjective; the way they are portrayed by an individual conscious brain is phenomenally subjective. Given the concept of a PMIR discussed extensively above, we now have a much clearer understanding of what this may mean in terms of the necessary representational and functional architecture involved.

A transparent self-model and a PMIR allow us to represent the world (and ourselves) in a unique manner, involving uniquely direct causal links. They also allow us to linguistically self-refer, using "I" and the current content of our PSM as a medium in a functionally privileged manner. No other system can achieve the identity of a speaking and internally self-modeling system in the same way we do. In this way our consciously experienced and linguistically or cognitively extended first-person perspective is truly an *individual* first-person perspective. Our phenomenal model of reality is an *individual* picture. Yet all the functional and representational facts constituting this unusual situation can be described objectively, and are open to scientific inquiry. Consciousness is *epistemically* irreducible, but this irreducibility is now demystified, because we have a better understanding of how epistemic subjectivity is rooted in phenomenal subjectivity. In order to have subjective *knowledge*, you need to successfully represent reality (and yourself) under a conscious world-model that satisfies *constraint 6*.

Can the thesis that the scientific worldview must in principle *remain incomplete be derived from the subjectivity of the mental? Can subjectivity, in its full content, be naturalized?*

First, let us restrict the scope to *phenomenal* subjectivity again. As we have seen in the course of this book, no principled obstacles to an exhaustive representationalist analysis of consciousness, selfhood, and perspectivalness exist. This is not to say that we may not discover such obstacles in the future, or eventually do without the representationalist level of description altogether. For now, it is tenable to say that all phenomenal facts are representational facts and that phenomenal subjectivity is a representational phenomenon in its entirety. The consciously experienced first-person perspective is simply one of an infinitely large number of possibilities in which a representational system can portray reality.

Second, of course, it is not clear what subjectivity in its *full content* actually is. I see two major extensions of maximal relevance which have only been touched upon in this book in passing: *intentional* subjectivity and *inter*subjectivity. Intentional subjectivity is something that will not supervene locally on brain properties. It is the question of self-*knowledge* versus the question of self-*experience*. Our unconscious self-model incorporates huge amounts of information about our physical body and its relationship to the environment. In part, this information was acquired by millions of generations of our biological ancestors. As a form of unconscious, nonconceptual, structurally embodied self-knowledge, that is, as an *intentional* content, it satisfies the adaptivity constraint. Then there is a wide variety of occurrent self-representational states, for instance, when thinking about ourselves. This self-directed intentional or representational content is something different from the phenomenal character by which it may or may not be accompanied. Arguably, one can even have a weak, passive version of unconscious thoughts about oneself, for instance, during phases of non-REM (NREM) sleep. Dreaming and REM sleep are incompletely correlated, because up to 30% of REM awakenings do not elicit dream reports, whereas up to 10% of NREM awakenings do lead to reports about complex forms of mentation, which, interestingly, have a more *cognitive* type of content than the usual phenomenal dreams that many of us recall in the morning (for details and references, see Nielsen 2000; see also Solms 2000). Therefore, any more general and comprehensive theory of subjectivity will have to do justice to such nonphenomenal types of mental content as well. They are outside the scope of this work, but they will be an important part of a fuller understanding of mind and subjectivity.

Second, the history of consciousness has not stopped with the PMIR. It has already taken the step from the phenomenal first-person perspective to all other forms of conscious experience from which our rich, social reality eventually emerges: the phenomenal experience of the "you," the "he/she/it," the phenomenal awareness of "us," "you," and "them." I have in this book only focused on the PSM and PMIR, because I see them as the decisive link between personal and subpersonal truths about the human mind, and because I think that they actually may have been the crucial step from biological to cultural evolution. But subjectivity in its *full* content will certainly have to include not only subject-object relations, but subject-*subject* relations as well. It will also have to include subject-*group* relations. To give just two examples: There will be a phenomenal (and *intentional*) representation not only of "mineness" and ownership. There will also be "usness" and "themness"; there will be a mental representation of the first- and third-person *plural*. The notion of a consciously experienced *perspective* is greatly expanded if we want to do justice to such important facts. The phenomenal first-person perspective now looks like the functional or representational foundation of the conscious first- and third-person plural perspectives. Obviously, we are today very far from being able to furnish anything in terms of an empirically anchored, rigorous, and conceptually convincing analysis of the kinds of mental representations involved in all of these target phenomena. It is therefore better to be modest, start at the very beginning, and try to understand *phenomenal* subjectivity first.

Do anything like "first-person data" exist? Can introspective reports compete with statements originating from scientific theories of the mind?

The popular notion of "first-person data" is a metaphor, just like the notion of a "first-person perspective." In both cases, an ill-defined but intuitively attractive meaning results from the combination of two precursor concepts originating in very different domains. In the latter case, we fuse a semantic element of grammar theory (i.e., associated with linguistic *ascriptions* of certain properties in the first-person singular) with a semantic element related to the phenomenology of *visual* experience, in particular to its geometry (as a contingent matter of fact our visual model of the world is centered around a point of view: distant objects appear smaller than those in our vicinity, parallel lines converge at the horizon, etc.). In the first case, we fuse the same semantic element with a concept borrowed from the theory of science. In doing so we put the notion of "data" to an extended usage, which unfortunately runs the great risk of simply being empty. First, data are things that are extracted from the physical world by *technical* measuring devices like telescopes, electrodes, or functional MRI scanners. There is a well-defined and public *procedure*, which certainly has its limitations, but which can be and *is* being continuously improved. Second, data generation inevitably takes place among *groups* of human beings, that is, within scientific communities open to criticism and constantly seeking independent means of verification. Data generation is, by necessity, an *intersubjective* process. First-person access to the phenomenal content of one's own mental states does not fulfill these defining criteria for the concept of "data." My politically incorrect conclusion therefore is that first-person data do not exist.

Of course, maximizing phenomenological plausibility is of the highest priority for any theory of consciousness, the phenomenal self, and the first-person perspective. In this book I have tried to develop an alternative strategy, namely, by maximizing the degree of phenomenological *constraint satisfaction*. As the reader may remember, phenomenological constraints were always the *first* constraints from which I started (for the only exceptions, see sections 3.2.11 and 6.2.8). The advantage of this somewhat weaker procedure is that you get all the heuristic power from first-person descriptions without being driven to naive-realistic assumptions and the stipulation of mysterious, nonpublic objects. In particular, you can define networks of constraints that can be continuously refined on lower levels of description, while at the same time allowing you to search for domain-specific, consistent solutions. You can take phenomenology seriously without running into all of its traditional problems.

The epistemological problem regarding phenomenological, first-person approaches of "data generation" is that if *inconsistencies* in two individual "data sets" should appear, there is no way to settle the conflict. In particular, the phenomenological method cannot provide a method of generating any further growth of knowledge in such situations. Progress ends. This is a third defining characteristic of the scientific way of approaching reality: there are *procedures* to settle conflicts resulting from conflicting hypotheses. Epistemic progress continues. The same is not true in cases where two experiential subjects arrive at conflicting statements like "This is the purest blue anyone can perceive!" versus "No, it *isn't*, it has a faint but perceptible trace of green in it!" or, "This conscious experience of jealousy shows me how much I love my husband!" versus "No, this emotional state is not love *at all*, it is a neurotic, bourgeois fear of loss!" The advantage of the constraint satisfaction approach is that we can turn such discoveries into new and differentiated constraints themselves. Any good theory of consciousness now has to explain how such truthful but conflicting autophenomenological reports are possible, and in which cases they will emerge by necessity. Inconsistencies in reports lead to progress by differentiating the constraint landscape.

Can introspective reports compete with statements originating from scientific theories of the mind? Yes, they can, and they should. But please note how any such competition is relative to our interests: What do these statements compete *for*? If our agreed-on goal is predictive power, then it certainly is possible to assign such a power to first-person autophenomenological statements like, "I will always be able to discriminate *my* purest blue from *your* purest blue!" or, "You will *never* be able to consciously experience a colored patch that exhibits red and green presentational content at the *same* time, while fully satisfying *constraint 10*, the homogeneity constraint!" Such statements are always statements about publicly observable future behavior. They make predictions. In the first case, the experiential subject may be the winner; in the second case, science may make the better predictions (Crane and Piantanida 1983). Right now, first-person predictions of one's own future behavior—which are invariably based on introspectively accessing the content of one's PSM—are much better and more reliable than third-person predictions. This situation may change, as we learn more about potential divergences or dissociations between the phenomenal and the functional, behavior-driving layers in the human self-model or about the evolutionary advantages of self-deception. What will not change is the remaining, and deeper, philosophical question. It is the issue of what actually it is that introspective reports and statements originating from scientific theories of the mind can compete *for*.

The true focus of the current proposal, however, was phenomenal content, the way certain representational states *feel* from the first-person perspective. Does it help to shed new light on the historical roots of certain philosophical intuitions like, for instance, the Cartesian intuition that *I could always have been someone else*; or that my own consciousness necessarily forms a single, unified whole; or that phenomenal experience actually brings us in direct and immediate contact with ourselves and the world around us? Philosophical problems can frequently be solved by conceptual analysis or by transforming them into more differentiated versions. Sometimes these new versions can be handed over to the sciences. Arguably, the problem of consciousness can be *naturalized* by transforming it into an empirically tractable version. However, an additional, complementary, and equally interesting strategy consists in attempting to also uncover their introspective roots. A careful inspection of these roots may help us to understand the *intuitive force* behind many bad arguments, a force that typically survives their rebuttal. I will therefore supplement my discussion by having a closer look at the genetic conditions for certain introspective certainties. But let us look at experiential content first.

What is the "phenomenal content" of mental states, as opposed to their representational or "intentional content?" Are there examples of mentality exhibiting one without the other? Do double dissociations exist?

The representational or intentional content of a mental state is what this state is *directed at*. The important point is that this is a relational and an abstract property, not an intrinsic property of the physical state carrying the content, and that this is true of self-representational intentional (or, in traditional parlance, "reflexive") content too. A self-model gains its intentional content by being *directed at* the system as a whole, at the system *within* which it is activated. It has a single intentional object. The same is true of what I have called the PMIR, the phenomenal model of the intentionality relation itself. *If* we exclusively view it as a representational structure, then it is directed at certain classes of subject-object relations. It is directed at the fact that the system is currently attending *to* a certain visual object, or thinking *about* something specific, or an agent *pursuing* a certain goal state, or in communication trying to *understand* the thoughts of another human being. The second important point is that everything that has an intentional content can *misrepresent* either the external world or the representational system itself. For instance, it could misrepresent the fact that it actually is pursuing a certain goal state.

Then there is phenomenal content. It is a *special* form of intentional content, namely, in satisfying the constraints developed in chapters 3 and 6. Importantly, there are now many different *degrees* of phenomenality: an intentional content can be *more or less* conscious. Our new conceptual tool kit allows us to describe very many levels of subjective experience, thereby doing justice to different domains and a large number of phenomenological constraints. Phenomenal states and events are a proper subset of intentional states and events. For a given minded being, and a given point in time, this subset may be empty. To give another illustrative example, think about the case of NREM sleep mentation briefly mentioned above. Unconscious thinking taking place in the NREM phase of nocturnal sleep certainly is representational activity, it may be *mis*representational activity, but it is not globally available for action control, for attention, or for selective metacognition (as a matter of fact, this is demonstrated by perserverative characteristics). Raffman qualia and Metzinger qualia (see section 2.4.4) are further examples of intentional content, which is only *weakly* conscious, because it only satisfies the globality constraint for attention, but not for cognition, and in the latter case not even for action control.

These forms of *presentational* content are intentional, because—although no simple or systematic one-to-one mapping with any kind of physical property is possible—they are, in the sense of an ancient, approximative, and unreliable teleological function, directed at certain properties, of certain objects, in the ecological niche of certain animals. As we saw in section 3.2.11, these properties do *not* have to be surface properties, they can be hidden physical properties like the fact that certain types of young leaves are richer in protein (Dominy and Lucas 2001). How they *appear* to us, millions of years after they acquired this first function in our distant ancestors, is another matter. Please note that the same may be true of self-modeling. Much of it may actually be unconscious or *weakly* conscious. Much of it was acquired millions of years ago by our distant ancestors. And a large part of the human self-model may *originally* have been directed at target properties, which were properties of our ancestors, but are not properties of *us* anymore. Self-perception may frequently not correspond to the internal stimulus itself, but to an ancient internal context, to the probability distribution of its possible sources millions of years ago. In particular, it is an empirically plausible assumption that the largest portion of the self-modeling that causally drives our behavior actually takes place unconsciously. This insight reaches across a large range of cases, from the internal emulation of fast, goal-directed movement (see, e.g., section 7.2.3) to social cognition (see section 6.3.3). The *phenomenal* self-model is only that partition of the *mental* self-model which satisfies a certain subset of items in our flexible catalogue of constraints. For the PMIR, the situation is more difficult: Is it plausible to assume that unconscious modeling of intentional directedness itself takes place as well? Is there a non-phenomenal MIR, or is perspectivalness truly *the* hallmark of conscious experience and conscious experience only? Interestingly, we now have a refined version of Brentano's ([1874] 1973) original point. Fortunately, as Brentano would be delighted to hear, this is a question that can now be settled by empirical research and not by philosophical speculation.

Double dissociations do not exist. There certainly is unconscious intentional content. A lot of it. But in ecologically valid standard situations there is *no* conscious state that is not a representational state in some way (for a nonstandard situation, cf. the abstract geometrical hallucinations discussed in chapter 4; see also figure 4.1 for one beautiful example of purely *phenomenal* content). As long as we choose to operate on the representational level of analysis at all—and this may change—there is no example of phenomenal content that is not also *directed at* some target object, property, or relation. Please note that this does not mean that the experiential subject has to have the slightest clue about what the intentional object of his or her experiences actually is. In many cases, for example, in living through diffuse feelings and emotions (like jealousy), the original intentional object may be millions of years away. It may not exist anymore. The original representandum may be something that was only present in the world of our distant ancestors. In particular, as we have learned from our discussion of the transparency constraint, Mother Nature has until very recently not cared to let any of us know or experience the fact that there is something like intentionality *at all*. Only recently did we become able to discover and represent the fact that we actually have *minds*. The PMIR may actually be our first attempt at internally making this very fact accessible to ourselves.

Please also note how a phenomenal state may be only *weakly* representational. Under certain theories of mental representation, for example, those that describe degrees of statistical dependency (see Eliasmith 2000) or covariance, one and the same type of phenomenal state may satisfy certain constraints for intentionality (e.g., accuracy) to differing degrees on different occasions. It may be *more or less* representational. But even if it is pure appearance, a *misrepresentation* in its entirety, it still has an intentional object: it is *directed at* something. The interesting question is whether in such cases its directedness consists in more than the fact that it is integrated into a PMIR. However, as it has not been my goal to offer a general theory of mental representation, this issue is clearly outside the scope of the current investigation.

How do Cartesian intuitions, like the contingency intuition, the indivisibility intuition, and the intuition of immediate givenness, emerge?

The degree of intuitive plausibility for a given theory results from the *degree of phenomenal possibility* associated with it (see section 2.3). Theories describe worlds. Conscious experience *models* worlds. Beings like ourselves experience all those theories as intuitively plausible that describe worlds that can be phenomenally simulated by us. These worlds then strike us as *possible phenomenal experiences* we might have—because we can internally model them. Therefore, this concept of possibility is always relative to a certain class of concrete representational systems, each of which possesses a specific functional profile and a particular representational architecture. Human beings may—and do—differ in what they can imagine, in what classes of worlds they can consciously simulate, and in what they find intuitively plausible. We cannot imagine the thirteen-dimensional shadow of a fourteen-dimensional cube or the continuum of space-time, because the visual cortex of our ancestors was never confronted with this type of object and because the brain's global model of reality based on three spatial dimensions and one distinct, unidirectional temporal dimension sufficed for surviving in what was *our* biological environment.

Moreover, intuitions change over a lifetime: Even within one individual the internal landscape characterizing the space of possibilities may undergo considerable change. It is also important to note how the mechanisms of generating and evaluating representational coherence employed by such systems have been optimized with regard to their biological or social functionality, and do *not* have to be subject to the classic criteria of adequacy, rationality, or epistemic justification in the narrow sense of philosophical epistemology. Briefly, in our own case, the set of phenomenally possible worlds is related directly to the set of nomologically possible worlds, but only indirectly to the sets of logically and metaphysically possible worlds.

The contingency intuition is the intuition of thinking "I could always have been somebody completely different!" Proponents of essentialist theories of subjectivity traditionally have been guided by this intuition, by the beautiful—and certainly emotionally attractive—idea that there must be something about myself which has *nothing* to do with any of my ever-changing, objective, and observable properties. As a *subject* I just cannot be identical with my physical body or any of its more complex and abstract properties—at least this identity is not a *necessary* identity. It could be broken. I will not go into the long history of this philosophical intuition here, as I have already presented one recent example in this chapter. If Thomas Nagel (1986, p. 61) says "*Essentially* [emphasis added] I have no particular point of view at all . . . ," we have exactly this situation: There is an essence, the objective self, which is only *contingently* united with the history of a certain physical person by the name of T. N. and its individual perspective. However, as we saw above, the phenomenology of the *View from Nowhere* is one in which the original PMIR is never really lost, and its conceptual interpretation is flawed. What Nagel describes is not a mystical experience—the *Great View from Nowhere*—but just an ordinary thought experiment.

The undisputed fact is that all of us can imagine having had a completely different set of public and phenomenological properties, say, those of Immanuel Kant. However, in doing this we only open a certain new partition of our phenomenal space and activate a fictitious self-simulatum, more or less completely portraying us as possessing those properties of Immanuel Kant currently known to us. What we construct is a *cognitive first-person perspective* (see section 6.5.2), a PMIR with the simulated person as its object component. This is a first-person state, a conscious model of reality satisfying the perspectivalness constraint, *constraint 6*. In order to really consciously simulate a world in which we would have *been* Immanuel Kant, the Kant-model would have to be the transparent subject component of this PMIR. As most of my colleagues know, in philosophical departments around the world, such systems actually do appear from time to time—systems in which a constant attempt at counterfactual self-simulation has gotten out of control, and which, due to a now highly afunctional self-model, actually *believe* they are Immanuel Kant, and even *experience* themselves accordingly. What these sad cases of delusion show exactly is that, in these cases, there is *no* overarching essence, no subjective core state or genuine phenomenal identity anymore.

But isn't it true that we can actually imagine much more than only being Immanuel Kant, namely, being Immanuel Kant, including *his* PMIR? Isn't the *View from Nowhere* more like social cognition, in that its object component truly is another *subject*, including the representation of a second PMIR (see section 6.3.3)? Yes, certainly. But social cognition is a first-person process, even if directed at a second, fictitious self. *Being someone* is a phenomenal property determined by the locus of attentional, volitional, and cognitive agency, as represented under a *transparent* self-model (cf. our discussion of OBEs in section 7.2.3). If you represent your alter ego as being a subject, as having a PMIR, then *this* subject component remains opaque. In nonmystical and nondeluded states, the first, the original person-model invariably is the transparent one: You know that *you* do the imagining—at least this fact is globally available to you at any time. So what you imagine is never *being* Immanuel Kant, even if you phenomenally simulate him as subject, possessing a first-person perspective of his own. You cannot simulate him as *self*. So the surprising answer is that the contingency intuition, at closer inspection, is not even based on a phenomenal possibility. As a philosophical claim, it is based on bad phenomenology. And this seems to contradict my introductory claim that intuitive plausibility goes along with phenomenal possibility.

There must be a second factor, which, for beings like ourselves, makes it *attractive* to believe in essentialist interpretations of the sort Nagel offers. Death denial may be this factor. In chapter 2 we saw how the process of phenomenal simulation needs a heuristic which compresses the vastness of logical space to two essential classes of "intended realities," that is, those world models causally conducive and relevant to the selection process. The first class is constituted by all desirable worlds, that is, all those worlds in which the system is enjoying optimal external conditions, many descendants, and a high social status. A world in which we are potentially independent of our physical bodies, a world in which individual survival is, in principle, possible *is* certainly a desirable world for beings like us. Individual survival is one of the highest biological imperatives burned into our emotional self-model: This is where we come from. Even if we cannot *really* carry out the phenomenal simulations needed, what we may feel is that such simulations would satisfy *constraint 11*, the adaptivity constraint. They are emotionally attractive, and that is why beings like us are all too ready to jump to certain inaccurate descriptions, and, in particular, to related assumptions about *metaphysical* possibility. False beliefs certainly can be adaptive. If mental health is defined as the integrity and stability of the self-model, then some types of false beliefs may even be conducive to mental health. So the answer is that there is a second functional factor: intuitive plausibility not only goes along with phenomenal possibility per se, but with adaptivity as well. But what, in this special case of Cartesian and essentialist intuitions about the phenomenal self, is the adaptation directed *to*? Here is a speculative hypothesis: it may be directed to a recent change in our self-model. This change may have been the split into a transparent and an opaque section, and, in particular, to the entirely new situation that this split made the fact of our own mortality *cognitively available*. We paid a high price for becoming cognitive subjects, and essentialist fantasies may be an attempt to minimize this price as much as possible. More about this in the final section.

In the *Sixth Meditation*, Descartes attempted to make it appear as an immediately evident truth that "there is a vast difference between mind and body, in respect that body, from its nature, is always divisible, and that mind is entirely indivisible." This is a different situation. Here, we clearly see how intuitive plausibility is rooted in a phenomenal *necessity*. It is not possible that our minds are *not* "absolutely one and entire" (as Descartes put it), because beings like ourselves cannot run the corresponding phenomenal self-simulations. As noted above, one of the most fundamental functional constraints on the PSM is that the system currently operating under it cannot intentionally split it or dissolve it. Have you ever tried? And in confusing phenomenal with logical modalities, it may therefore appear that what is not not possible is necessary, in some sense of a priori necessity which now has to be explained. The existence of a single, unified self may even appear as metaphysically necessary. But it isn't. As the neurophenomenological case studies presented in the preceding chapter demonstrate, there are many kinds of conscious but highly fragmented self-modeling of which it is true that they are strictly impossible to imagine. Can you imagine what it is like for a Cotard patient to be absolutely certain that she does not exist? Can you imagine how it is for a schizophrenic to have alien thoughts penetrating his mind? For healthy people there simply *is* no way to imagine this, clearly and distinctly. And there may again be a deeper, teleofunctionalist reason for this obvious fact.

Put very simply, we are not *supposed to* imagine pathological situations, because dissociative self-simulations endanger the functional integrity of the organism as a whole. After all, the self-model, in its deeper functional core, is an instrument used in homeostatic self-regulation, a tool to make the individual process of life as coherent and stable as possible. Too much playing around in its conscious offline section could eventually put the elementary processes of elementary bioregulation at risk. It could make you *sick*. Cotard's syndrome, schizophrenia, and other identity disorders are highly maladaptive situations—they must be avoided at all costs. *All* situations in which the conscious self-model, in one way or another, portrays the system as falling apart into two or more parts (again, recall the case study on OBEs in section 7.2.3) are usually situations in which the organism simply is in great danger of dying. The integrity of the organism as a whole is at risk. Therefore, the corresponding self-simulations are emotionally unattractive; they can even cause a fear reaction. A related fact is that many people find it distressing, or painful, or threatening to seriously try to understand patients with severe psychiatric disorders or to be among them for a long period of time. The Cartesian intuition of the indivisible self, the Kantian notion of the transcendental subject—the reassuring idea of the "*I* think" that can, at least in principle, accompany all my conscious *Vorstellungen*—are rooted in this feature of our representational architecture, in the functional inability of the system as a whole to split its PSM. This is why monist or naturalist theories of subjectivity inevitably strike us as deeply counterintuitive, and frequently even as emotionally unattractive. Of course, all this is no argument showing that Descartes and Kant may not have been right.

What about the Cartesian picture of a sensory-cognitive continuum, the idea that we can *directly* gain knowledge about the world and about ourselves through the process of conscious experience? Is there *epistemic immediacy* going along with some of the contents constituting consciousness, the phenomenal self, and the first-person perspective? Here, our answer can be brief. For all conscious mental content satisfying the transparency constraint in the way introduced here (see sections 3.2.7 and 6.2.6), it is an obvious and necessary characteristic that this content will be experienced as immediately given. This characteristic is a *phenomenological* feature in its entirety. *Phenomenal* immediacy does not entail epistemic immediacy. Every form of phenomenal content is in need of independent epistemic justification, and this, of course, is also true of the conscious experience of apparently *direct* perception, *direct* reference, *direct* knowledge, and so on. Our neurophenomenological case studies in chapters 4 and 7 provided examples of a wide range of states which are, in a way that is unnoticeable to the subject of experience, epistemically empty constructs and at the same time characterized by the phenomenology of certainty and direct, immediate knowledge. In particular, it is today empirically implausible to assume that mental contents satisfying at least *constraints 2, 3,* and *6* could not be based on complex, physically realized, and therefore fallible and time-consuming processes of information processing. There simply is no such thing as epistemically immediate contact to reality. What there is is an efficient, cost-effective, and evolutionary advantageous way of phenomenally modeling reliable representational contents *as immediately given.*

In chapter 1, I pointed out how the human variety of conscious subjectivity is unique on this planet in being deeply culturally embedded (see also Metzinger 2000b, p. 6*ff.*), namely, through language and social interactions. It is therefore interesting to ask how the actual contents of experience *change* through this constant integration into other representational media, and how specific contents may genetically depend on social factors.

Which new phenomenal properties emerge through cognitive and linguistic forms of self-reference? In humans, are there necessary social correlates for certain kinds of phenomenal content?

As we saw in section 6.4.4, cognitive self-reference is not something taking place in a linguistic medium, but a very special way of higher-order self-modeling. This new way of self-modeling, in particular when internally emulating logical operations involving rule-based transformations over discrete symbol tokens, and so on, has been a major breakthrough in biological intelligence. It has made *abstract* information globally available, for example, information about what is logically coherent or information about the fact that there is a difference—and often some kind of *relation*—between reality and representation, and it arguably has even enabled us to form the concept of truth. After language was available, we could not only communicate about all these new facts and concepts but also proceed to publicly *self-ascribe* them to us. And this, of course, brought about new phenomenal properties, because it dramatically changed the content of the PSM.

We started to consciously experience ourselves as thinkers of thoughts and as speakers of sentences. We started to *think* about ourselves as thinkers of thoughts and as speakers of sentences. And we again consciously experienced *this* fact, because it brought about a change in our PSM. We started to talk to each other about the surprising fact that we—very likely as opposed to most other creatures we knew—are thinkers of thoughts and speakers of sentences, and that we *know* about this fact, because we consciously experience it. Or do we? We mutually started to *ascribe* the property of being experiencing, thinking, communicating beings to ourselves and to each other, and because the difference between reality and representation was already available to us, due to the phenomenal opacity of our cognitive self-model, we were aware that such ascriptions might actually be *false*. We started to discuss matters. We disagreed! Probably, philosophy was born at this stage. I will not speculate here concerning the more fine-grained representational architecture that must have been involved in these first steps. I just want to point out how this chain of events—self-modeling systems now starting to mirror each other not only through their motor systems (see section 6.4.4) but also through the opaque sections of their minds and through external use of symbols—has brought about two fundamental and highly interesting shifts in the *phenomenal* content of the human-self-model.

First, we could begin to experience ourselves as *rational individuals*. Because it was now possible to consciously model the process of forming coherent thoughts according to some set of abstract, logical rules, we could also form the concept of a being that actively *strives* for this kind of coherence. We already knew that we had emotions, that we were biological beings with needs and urges, following the logic of survival. Now we started to see that for us there was *another*—possibly a conflicting—way of following a certain logic. This time it was the logic of *intellectual* integrity, of making the opaque partition of your PSM as coherent as possible. It was the logic of having as few conflicting thoughts as possible. It was the logic of preserving truth. And it also was the logic of rational agency, of pursuing one's own goals by ordering them into a consistent hierarchy, and the logic of trying to gain *knowledge* in order to achieve these goals, to continuously minimize the difference between mental representation and reality already discovered. We experienced ourselves as individual beings that, at least to certain degree, also were *rational subjects*. Although our PSM was now continuously split into an opaque and a transparent partition, our brains somehow managed in that it remained one single representational structure and thereby allowed us to phenomenally *own* this new property of ourselves. Later, we even found a new linguistic concept to describe this new property. We called it *personhood*.

Second, we could now also begin to make the fact that we are *social subjects* globally available for attention, cognitive processing, and action control. In particular, we could start to consciously experience the fact that, as social beings, we were not only related to each other through the common logic of survival, that is, through our bodies and our emotions, but *as rational persons*. The new phenomenal property of personhood could now start to unfold its functional profile. Because it made this radically new information globally available for deliberate action control, for linguistic report and communication, for self-ascription and critical discussion, it was now possible for us to also *share* this information. Our PSM allowed us to pool our cognitive resources. Of course, as we have seen in this book, intersubjectivity starts on the unconscious level and is later mediated through entirely nonconceptual and nonpropositional levels of the PSM. But now we had acquired a PSM of ourselves as *persons*, as rational individuals. Rational individuals are capable of rational intersubjectivity, because they can mirror each other in an entirely different manner. At this point a whole cascade of functional transformations, of instantiations of new functional properties through the global availability of new representational contents, unfolded explosively.

The new kind of PSM enabled the construction of a new type of PMIR. Its object component could now be formed by *other* subjects, this time phenomenally modeled as individual thinkers of thoughts and as rational, self-conscious bearers of strong first-person phenomena. Person-to-person relations in the true sense of the word could be consciously modeled. I will not go into any further details at this point, because I think it is already clear how the human PSM was the decisive neurocomputational tool in the shift from biological to cultural evolution. Let me just name what I think is the essential high-level property, the central functional feature, in which this transition eventually culminated. Through our extended PSMs we were able to simultaneously establish *correlated* cognitive PMIRs of the type just described. Two or more human beings could now *at the same time* activate cognitive PMIRs mutually pointing to each other under a representation as rational subjects. And the correlated nature of these two mental events, their mutuality and interdependence, could itself be represented on the level of global availability. We were able to mutually *acknowledge each other as persons*, and to consciously experience this very fact.

The concept of a "person," however, does not simply refer to some complex, but objective representational property. Personhood cannot be naturalized in a simple and straightforward way, because the concept of a person contains domain-specific and semantically vague normative elements. Why is this so? Persons never are something we find *out there*, as parts of an objective order. Persons are constituted in societies. If conscious self-modeling systems *acknowledge* each other as persons, then they are persons. But, as I pointed out in chapter 1, conscious experience is a culturally embedded phenomenon (see also Metzinger 2000b). This is true of complex phenomenal properties like personhood too. From the perspective of the humanities, it is therefore centrally important to gain a more precise understanding of the neurocognitive and evolutionary, of the functional and representational conditions of possibility governing the appearance of personhood and successful intersubjectivity. And this is what I have tried to prepare for in this book. But how the emergence of phenomenal personhood and the mutual processes of "mirroring" each others' conscious personhood described above are then *interpreted* in a given social context is quite another matter. Answers to the question of how they *should* be interpreted may vary from society to society, from subculture to subculture, or from one historical epoch to another. And even given our own context, they may certainly change as we now learn more about what in our brains and in their biological history actually brings them about.

The question about the necessary social correlates of consciousness, selfhood, and high-level perspectivalness today has become a predominantly empirical issue. However, at the risk of being tedious, one has to be clear about the underlying metaphysical principle of local supervenience. To bring out this point, let us take an example not yet involving the complex neurophenomenology of rational intersubjectivity. Let us choose something much more simple and beautiful: the conscious experience of very briefly catching a glimmer in the eye of another human being; a glimmer that, in the fraction of a second, lets you discover not only that, this person likes you but also *how much* she likes you, and the conscious experience of realizing, at what appears to be the same time, that you *yourself* must have been giving the same signal a moment ago. SMT makes the claim that even for consciously experienced intersubjectivity of this type, it is true that an appropriately stimulated brain in a vat could activate the same *phenomenal content*. This claim may strike you as bizarre. But it is easy to understand what this claim amounts to, and what it does *not* amount to as well.

First, in standard situations, phenomenal content is a special kind of intentional content. In order to *understand* how it could ever come about, what its role in the psychological ecology of its bearers actually is, how this role has been shaped by the history of their biological ancestors, and so forth, you have to give a much more extensive representationalist, teleofunctionalist, and eventually even neuroscientific analysis. You need all the subpersonal levels of description on which I have operated in chapters 3 and 6 in order to arrive at a truly *informative* analysis of consciously experienced social cognition. Local supervenience is just a (rather weak) *metaphysical* claim, one that in various ways assumes asymmetrical bottom-up dependency without reducibility. One of the weaknesses of supervenience is that it is not an *explanatory* relation. In saying that phenomenal intersubjectivity supervenes locally on individual brain properties, you are not saying that social and intersubjective *knowledge* is determined by internal and contemporaneous brain properties as well. You are not even contributing to a deeper understanding of why this knowledge had to be mediated by conscious experience.

At any given point in time, phenomenal content supervenes locally on properties of individual brains. "Points in time" are physical entities, individuated from a third-person perspective. Brain properties are fully embedded in the causal network of the physical world, and information processing in the brain is a *time-consuming* process. Therefore, social cognition and the conscious processing going along with it are time-consuming processes as well. There is no such thing as temporal or epistemic immediacy on any subpersonal level. However, there may certainly be *phenomenal immediacy*, for instance, in the situation described above. In the way the *brain* individuates points in time (see section 3.2.2) it is certainly conceivable that the spark of sympathy shooting back and forth between two conscious human beings may be experienced as an *instantaneous* spark. It may be transparently represented as one single event, taking place in one single moment, but bridging the gulf between *two* individuals. Phenomenologically, lightning strikes and mutually unites two phenomenal selves—this is the "affective dissolution of the self" mentioned earlier. Because it involves loss of control over and transient dissolution of the emotional self-model, the experience of catching each other in the act of falling in love is a little bit like dying, and also a little bit like going insane. As a phenomenal content, this event supervenes locally. As a nonconceptual form of intentional content it doesn't.

At least in some cases, becoming friends or falling in love is a process of knowledge acquisition. We cannot even begin to adequately understand it if we do not understand the *information* that it makes globally available for the system as a whole, plus the representational and functional role such an event plays *for* the now coupled system of our two self-modeling systems. And on this level of analysis it is all too obvious that many forms of conscious experience—which, after all, are a special form of *intelligence* too—possess necessary social correlates (e.g., see section 6.3.3). What these correlates correlate *with* is invariably the self-model of the other organism. The self-model is what built the functional bridge from individual cognition to social cognition, from first-person intelligence to the *pooling* of resources in a species. Such resources can be intellectual, but they can also be emotional or motivational. The first step in understanding social cognition therefore consists in developing an *acquisition history* for this new virtual organ, in telling a comprehensive developmental and evolutionary story about the PSM and the PMIR in particular. Metaphysically, individual occurrences of phenomenally experienced intersubjectivity supervene locally. But—and this is the answer to our original question—if we want to understand how they can satisfy the adaptivity constraint, we will need a greatly expanded explanatory base.

In chapter 1 I also promised answers to a set of questions concerning the relations between certain phenomenal state classes or global phenomenal properties. Let us now, briefly, look at the answers.

What is the most simple form of phenomenal content? Is there anything like "qualia" in the classic sense of the word?

Simplicity is representational atomicity. What *appears* as simple and as strictly indivisi-ble is always relative to the representational architecture actually generating this content (see section 2.4; see also Jakab 2000). There are two readings of this answer: First, sim-plicity is relative to the internal readout mechanism employed by the brain in activating a globally available presentatum of, say, magenta$_{11}$ and integrating it into short-term memory, then making it an element of the object component of the PMIR; second, sim-plicity is relative to the theory describing this mechanism and to the constraints which this specific theoretical solution attempts to satisfy. Let us remain with the first case. It makes a difference if presentational content is made available for introspection$_1$ or for intro-spection$_2$; that is, if it becomes conscious by being available for attentional processing and behavioral control only, or by being available for the formation of enduring, concept-like mental structures as well. Many conscious color experiences, for example, are simple phe-nomenal states in terms of being attentional atoms, but not *cognitive* atoms. Therefore, they are ineffable (Raffman 1995) and simpler than qualia in the classic sense of the term.

Lewis qualia in the sense of the classic terminology (see section 2.4.1)—as a first-order phenomenal property, that is, as a recognizable, maximally simple, and fully determinate form of sensory content—arguably do not exist. For most maximally determinate sensory values it is a truism that we cannot, as Lewis originally demanded, reliably *recognize* them from one instance to the next. We cannot form concepts of them because, due to limita-tions of perceptual memory, we possess no transtemporal identity criteria. That is, they are not cognitively, but only *attentionally* available from the first-person perspective. They can only contribute to the object component of a certain, restricted subset of PMIRs. The interesting fact (which some analytical philosophers all too much would like to ignore) is that not only are we unable to talk about them in a conceptually precise manner but we cannot even *think* about them. Certainly something like strong Lewis qualia do exist, for example, in terms of the conscious experience of the pure colors green, blue, red, and yellow. But it is not the most *simple* form of phenomenal color content. As extensively explained in section 2.4.4, Lewis qualia are much stronger than Raffman qualia, because, descriptively, they are located on the three-constraint level, and not on the two-constraint level. In this second sense, unitary hues, due to their "purity" and the resulting cognitive availability, are a richer and more complex form of phenomenal content. The more general image that now emerges (particularly for the level of allegedly "simple" sensory process-ing) portrays conscious experience as a highly graded phenomenon. Phenomenal color vision, for example, is not an all-or-nothing affair but recedes gradually into the uncon-scious processing of wavelength information through a fine-grained hierarchy constituted by *levels of constraint satisfaction*. And this is a second sense in which simplicity is rel-ative to the representational scheme under which it appears: simplicity is theory-relative. Take the current investigation as an example.

In chapter 2 I used an excessively simplistic and crude example of constraints that can be applied in marking out phenomenal from mental presentation (global availability for attention, cognition, and behavioral control). As I hastened to point out, this was an extremely oversimplified fiction from an empirical point of view, because there obviously is more than one kind of attention (e.g., deliberately initiated, focused high-level attention and automatic low-level attention), different styles of thought certainly exist, and the behavioral control exerted by, for example, an animal may turn out to be something entirely different from rationally guided human *action* control. In chapter 3 I then submitted a more comprehensive set of ten multilevel constraints for discussion. Both of these examples may serve as an illustration of the principle of theory relativity. What appears as simple under my provisional, theory-driven attempt at describing the phenomenal landscape of what we called "qualia" in the past may appear as a host of *different* things if we try to satisfy alternative sets of constraints proposed by data-driven, bottom-up approaches. One man's primitive is another man's high-level theoretical entity. I have tried to respond to this problem by formulating *multilevel* constraints containing a large number of place-holders that can be filled in by other disciplines. Therefore, to give another concrete example, the candidates I have offered as potential primitives of chromatic vision—Lewis qualia, Raffman qualia, and Metzinger qualia as enriched by *constraints 1 to 10*—are entirely relative to *my* way of describing the domain of conscious experience, to my own set of constraints. The advantage is that my notion of "phenomenal simplicity" is now domain-specific, can be corrected, and continuously differentiated by, say, additional data from psychophysics. Theory relativity is not an epistemological tragedy—it can be de-fused by making the set of constraints one wants to find solutions for a flexible and *evolvable* set.

What is the minimal set of constraints that have to be satisfied for conscious experience to emerge at all? For instance, could qualia exist without the global property of consciousness, or is a qualia-free form of consciousness conceivable?

A large part of the answer to this question was already contained in the very first answer to the very first question. I believe that the minimal philosophical intuition behind the concept of consciousness is that of the *appearance of a reality*, here and now. This amounts to the demand that *constraints 2, 3,* and *7* have to be satisfied. Personally, however, I think that the most interesting target phenomenon is full-blown cognitive subjectivity, includ-ing its social correlates, in terms of satisfying *all* the constraints sketched in this book. In passing, let me briefly point out how there are even stronger research targets, and that they may interestingly be embodied in our ancient, traditional notions of consciousness. Stronger and centuries-old concepts, like the Greek *syneidesis*, or its Latin successor *con-scientia*, involving not only an integration of representational space but concomitant higher-order cognition plus *moral* subjectivity, would inevitably have to involve all constraints, plus a theory of intentional content, plus a theory of *normative* mental judgment (Metzinger and Schumacher 1999). In order to understand why *conscientia* is also higher-order *knowledge*, the current approach would have to be considerably extended toward an integrated theory of phenomenal and intentional content as such. Second, it must be noted, in discussing social correlates, we have so far only proceeded toward an extremely sketchy account of *rational* intersubjectivity. *Moral* intersubjectivity and its neurophenomenological conditions of possibility are quite another matter. *Conscientia* in terms of phenomenally mediated *conscience* is still beyond us. Therefore, consciousness research, at least when oriented toward those traditional epistemic goals, eventually will have to face issues much more comprehensive than those of the necessary and sufficient conditions determining the appearance of phenomenal content as such. But obviously it is much too early for this.

Could "qualia-free" consciousness exist? Could there be a heavenly place for disembodied mathematicians, dealing with abstract objects only, lacking any form of sensory perception? On the representational level of description this may seem to be a conceptual possibility. There could be integrated, transparent reality-models held in working memory, involving no form of presentational content as such. But what about the earlier processing stages? What about the standard causal linkage? If we demand that the stimulus source to which presentational content is strictly correlated is an *extradermal* source, then even normal dreams could count as such a qualia-free form of consciousness. Obviously, this would be far-fetched from a phenomenological perspective, because representational atoms certainly *do* exist in the way in which the dreaming brain emulates actual sensory perception. In any case, the background assumptions of the current approach do not permit consciousness without sensory elements. In particular, it would be hard to translate the representational constraints of our celestial mathematicians into functional level properties. Of course, functionalism does not necessarily imply token physicalism. Functional properties are ontologically neutral in that they could be realized on nonphysical hardware. Angels, qualia-free mathematicians, and the like might be some sort of Turing machine, entirely realized on "angel stuff," but a closer look reveals considerable difficulties concerning a detailed specification of the causal linkages underlying input and output. Even on the representational level itself it may be hard to see how the presentationality constraint could actually be satisfied. *Constraint 2* demands that all conscious content is content *de nunc*. Abstract objects and other elements of the mathematician's universe, however, are *timeless* entities: They have no temporal properties. So how could they, *as such*, be consciously experienced as being present *now*?

What is phenomenal selfhood? What, precisely, is the nonconceptual sense of ownership going along with the phenomenal experience of selfhood, or of "being someone"?

Phenomenal selfhood is a representational phenomenon. As explained above, any system operating under a transparent self-model will instantiate a phenomenal self if it satisfies the set of constraints we deem minimally sufficient for conscious experience as such. The sense of ownership is a representational property as well. It consists in a content being integrated into the current PSM. Whatever is a part of our conscious self-model is something that we have *appropriated*. Appropriation in this sense is based not on rule-based inferences or operations on syntactically structured symbol tokens, but on an entirely subpersonal, automatic process of dynamic self-organization. It is *subsymbolic* ownership. No sense of cognitive agency is involved.

If the PSM into which information is currently integrated is of a nonhallucinatory kind, then there is not only phenomenal ownership and appropriation but also a corresponding type of intentional *content*. The system then represents certain aspects of reality as being parts of itself, and it does so correctly. What it achieves is not only self-experience but self-knowledge. This is important, because it brings about a major shift in correlated functional properties as well. The system as a whole now establishes a causal relationship to certain aspects of reality by integrating them into a globally available representation of itself as a whole. Representational ownership goes along with functional integration. The more self-knowledge a system acquires, the more it is able to functionally appropriate the relevant aspects of itself. The phenomenal variant of self-knowledge is of particular relevance here, because it helps to monitor *newly* discovered aspects of oneself and because it *enhances* the functional profile of representationally appropriated aspects of oneself, for example, by making them globally available for focal attention, selective cognitive processing, and flexible behavioral control. It is this ongoing process of dynamic, globally available, and functionally active self-integration, which is mirrored on the phenomenal level. It is mirrored as the transparent experience of ownership, as agency, as dramatically enhanced self-control, as flexibility, selectivity, and autonomy—in short, as the ultrarealistic experience of *being someone*. And again it is important to note that functional appropriation on the subsymbolic level is likely to come in many different degrees. The actual correlation strength between different parts of the self-model in the brain may vary greatly, for instance, during the process in which a new content is *acquired* as a newly learned property of the system. In pathological configurations like schizophrenia it may also vary as a function of a process in which representational content is actually *lost*. Representationally losing a part of the self-model inevitably means losing information, which in turn is equivalent to losing a computational resource for self-control.

It is interesting to note how such fluctuations in internal coherence are also mirrored on the phenomenological level. Phenomenal appropriation is characterized by a complex and ever-changing landscape. The phenomenal sense of ownership is *not* one simple property, a rigid characteristic of our inner life. For example, it has a subtle temporal profile; it is context-sensitive and it *unfolds* over time. Taking the phenomenology of ownership seriously means to do justice to the fact that even in normal life the degree to which, for example, you prereflexively experience a certain property of your body or of your emotional personality as *your own*, or rather as something externally caused and not really belonging to your "true identity," is highly variable. It changes, for instance, as you grow older. And, as philosophers and scientists alike know, the degree to which you actually experience a certain thought or argument as *your own* certainly depends on the response of your social environment. If the response to certain parts of your cognitive self is exceedingly positive and gratifying, the chances are high that you will experience it as a deeply original part of yourself, as something that always belonged to you, and as something that *never* was appropriated from anywhere else.

How is the experience of agency related to the experience of ownership? Can both forms of phenomenal content be dissociated?

An agent is a system that has a certain degree of selective and flexible motor control, and that has, in the sense just sketched, representationally and functionally appropriated the underlying *selection processes* by integrating them into its self-model. Consciously experienced agency appears only if these selection processes are part of the PSM. As explained in more detail in sections 6.4.5 and 6.5.3, an essential part of this process is the activation of a *volitional* PMIR: a representation of "the self in the act of deliberating," integrating the self-model with certain internally simulated actions or goal states. This, then, is a phenomenal representation of a practical intentionality relation, because it transparently represents the system as standing in a certain relation to a set of possible actions or a specific goal state, and it underlies the experience of agency.

Are there phenomenological situations in which there is agency without ownership? In a more general sense, it is plausible to assume, for example, that patients suffering from akinetic mutism do not experience themselves as agents while still possessing a very basic conscious sense of ownership of their body as such. As they are awake and exhibit an orienting reflex, they are likely to have an integrated phenomenal body image. Everything integrated into this body image exhibits the phenomenal property of "mineness," of nonconceptual ownership. On the other hand, given the reports available, it seems as if these patients never constitute a volitional PMIR (they don't act) or a cognitive PMIR (because they are not so much "imprisoned in a jail of immobility," but rather don't *have* a mind at all; see Damasio 1994, p. 73; 1999, p. 101*ff.*), and an attentional PMIR, fleeting and instable, can only be triggered from the outside. So there is bodily ownership without attentional, cognitive, or motor agency. However, the remaining question here is if ownership and agency are really dissociated in the same *domain*. Schizophrenics experiencing thought insertion and introspective alienation may present us with a more specific case.

Phenomenologically, they experience cognitive agency: specific, conscious thoughts are being selected and forced into their own minds, into what I have termed the opaque partition of their PSM (see section 6.4.2). Phenomenologically, there is a cognitive agent—someone else who is *thinking* or *sending* these thoughts. That is, the causal history of these states is phenomenally modeled as having an external origin. They are caused by an agent. This agent is not identical to the subject of experience, however. Second, inserted thoughts are certainly *owned*, in the sense of now being a part of the schizophrenic's *inner* world, of her PSM, because they are *in*serted into what phenomenologically she still experiences as her own mind. So there arguably is third-person agency plus ownership in one and the same domain, in the domain of cognitive representational contents. The neurophenomenology of schizophrenia shows how for one and the same individual thought ownership and agency can be dissociated.

The next logical step to take consists in asking if, in one and the same domain of content, and in any type of real-world neurophenomenological configuration, *first-person* agency ever does coexist with a lack of ownership. Are there any cases in which the phenomenal self is modeled as a bodily, attentional, or cognitive agent, but in which nonconceptual ownership does not exist? Let us look at some potential examples: Can you have a transparent self-model of yourself as actively generating a certain thought without then *owning* this thought? Can you experience yourself as actively and focally attending to the perceived weight of the book that you are now holding in your hands without automatically *owning* the ongoing act of attending? Is it possible to deliberately initiate a bodily movement without owning the proprioceptive feedback, without phenomenally experiencing the actual movement as that of your *own* body? It is very tempting to say that here—if anywhere at all—we are actually confronted with phenomenal necessity, with something law-like, with an *essential* connection between two elements holding across all possible cases. Agency, the representation of subpersonal selection processes on the level of the PSM, is a prime candidate for the conceptual essence of phenomenal ownership, for phenomenal selfhood, and for the deepest origin of subjectivity, simply because the two elements are so strongly correlated. Is this a domain-specific neurophenomenological "law of self-consciousness?" Is the constitution of a phenomenal self, of consciously experienced ownership *causally tied* to the mechanism by which systems like ourselves functionally appropriate the subpersonal processes selecting target objects for attention, cognition, and action?

The answer may be yes—but we must not forget how it will only hold for healthy human beings. First-person agency is certainly a sufficient condition for ownership in most nonpathological configurations. However, once again expanding our explanatory target domain, the initial example of akinetic mutism seems to show that it is not a necessary condition: You can phenomenally own your body without being an agent. Our best current control-theoretic models for the delusions of control arising in schizophrenia (e.g., Frith et al. 2000) give us a detailed understanding of how an agent can consciously own his body, and his self-caused bodily motions, *without* being able to phenomenally appropriate the selection and initiation process leading to them. As a result, he owns a body that feels like a remote-controlled puppet. On the contrary, ownership seems to be necessary for agency. Personal-level, conscious selection processes always operate *on* elements represented through the PSM, and these elements have become parts of the PSM through subpersonal, unconscious mechanisms of integration which themselves cannot be phenomenally owned. And this is one way in which subjectivity is anchored in the objective world: It necessarily depends on subpersonal, unconscious information processing.

Can phenomenal selfhood be instantiated without qualia? Is embodiment necessary for selfhood?

As we saw in section 2.4. qualia (i.e., presentational content satisfying *constraints 2, 3, and 7*) are representationally atomic. Their atomicity is always relative to a readout mechanism (e.g., attention vs. cognition), and to the set of constraints sufficient for phenomenality for which we have opted on theoretical grounds. The question now is if we can conceive of a transparent PSM that is not made out of representational atoms. This would have to be a self-model which, although itself a representational structure active in some conscious system's information-processing mechanism, would not possess any *atoms* out of which it is constituted, for example, by binding them into an integrated gestalt-like whole. Are phenomenal primitives necessary for the special case of self-consciousness?

I can imagine two situations in which they are not. First, there could be an integrated self-model but no readout mechanism that *creates* primitives through its limited resolving power. For instance, primitive organisms could have a very simple self-model possessing no subformats whatsoever and no attentional or cognitive mechanisms by which, through metarepresentation, they could create such special subregions in their phenomenal self. Their low-level integration mechanisms would simply make them self-conscious, without turning them into attentional or cognitive subjects. They could not attend to or think about themselves. There would never be a second-order PMIR directed at a first-order self-model. Yet they could be self-conscious. If their little PSM is maximally simple and does not change over time—that is, if it does not satisfy *constraints 4* and *5*—then it could not actually exhibit any introspectively discriminable atoms or subregions. There would be no individual and distinguishable sensations, and no modalities. In a way it would be one singular self-quale or one homogeneous self-presentatum, but its singularity and its simplicity would not be equivalent to the representational atomicity that can be created by a top-down mechanism such as attention. It would be an integrated self-model resulting entirely from the dynamical self-organization of unconscious bottom-up mechanisms.

Maybe such a phenomenal self even resembles the one a human patient suffering from akinetic mutism is left with.

Then there is a second possibility. We can certainly imagine truly introspective systems possessing a second-order PMIR directed at a first-order self-model. For example, they could attend to the content of their self-model. However, if this content would change in a strictly continuous manner, if it were *grainless* on the only level of organization on which attentional processing can operate, then there would be no self-representational atoms as well. No discernible internal boundaries would exist. The content of such a self-model would smoothly change, and blend from one form of, for example, interoceptive content into another in a way that would make it impossible to introspectively$_3$ discriminate *steps* within this process. Phenomenologically, there would be a differentiated and changing, yet atomless phenomenal self. However, it could still be a *presentational* self in possessing a strongly stimulus-correlated component, functionally anchored in the physical brain.

Very interestingly, this second conceptual possibility may actually be a good way of describing human self-awareness on the proprioceptive level, on the level of gut feelings, subtle background emotions, or motion perception. We are *holistically embodied* beings. This is to say that there likely are important and interesting layers in the human PSM not even exhibiting anything in terms of Lewis qualia or Raffman qualia (see section 2.4), layers which are not only inaccessible to categorical perception and gestalt-forming grouping operations caused by attentional processing but which form a continuous multimodal mélange. Phenomenologically, isn't it true that there are aspects of the bodily and emotional self which are not only ineffable but—pardon the metaphor—so *liquid* that there is no way of holding them, fixating them (even for a brief period of time), or "zooming in" on them? You can only *be* them. If this phenomenological point is not misguided, it might be exactly those levels of phenomenal content in which the mind is closest to its body. Taking the phenomenology of embodiment seriously may help in discovering the microfunctional level of description on which we can eventually *give up* the vehicle-content distinction for self-consciousness. One might want to term this the "principle of liquid linkage." There would then be a level of phenomenal embodiment, which is below, and more holistic than, anything we could describe using the traditional terminological machinery of "first-order phenomenal properties," "structureless qualia," or "simple sensations." Given the current theory, in standard situations functional embodiment certainly is a prerequisite of phenomenal embodiment and strong first-person phenomena (e.g., see sections 5.4, 6.2.8, and 6.5.3). But I would submit the idea that carefully describing its low-level phenomenal correlates would entail creating completely *new* conceptual instruments, instruments which may be extremely hard to develop. However, it may be precisely such instruments that may bring us much closer to a solution of the self-body problem.

*What is a phenomenally represented first-person perspective? How does it contribute to
other notions of perspectivalness, for example, to logical or epistemic subjectivity?*

The content of a consciously experienced first-person perspective is the content of a PMIR.
Phenomenologically subjective states are either, in a narrow sense, states that currently
form the object component of the PMIR (the "focus" of awareness), or, more generally,
states that are integrated into an internal model of reality structured by a PMIR. On the
representational level of description, a PMIR can have two forms of content: *phenomenal*
content and *intentional* content. Please recall that I have not given an explicit theory about
intentional content in this book, or about what actually makes a mental or phenomenal
state a carrier of information, or about the conditions under which it can embody knowledge (e.g., because it can also *misrepresent* the current state of affairs). Depending on the
shape of such a theory of mental representation we could say the following: *Epistemic*
subjectivity is a phenomenon that appears whenever a fact is represented under a PMIR.
A PMIR is a functional mode of presentation. If a given PMIR has not only phenomenal
but also intentional, that is, *representational* content, then it transforms the system not only
into a subject of experience but into a subject of knowledge at the same time. This still
leaves many options open to us. Such subjective knowledge could be conceptual or nonconceptual, explicit or implicit; it could be a classic mental symbol à la Fodor or a trajectory through some suitable state space à la Churchland. What counts is the contribution
the notion of a phenomenal first-person perspective can make to the concept of an epistemic state. *Subjective* epistemic states are now characterized by an extremely rich set
of constraints (see chapter 3); they are one way—and indeed a very *special* way—out of
countless other ways, to process information, to generate intentional content, to model
reality. An epistemic first-person perspective emerges whenever a phenomenal first-person
perspective is not completely empty in terms of intentional content.

Could there be strong epistemic subjectivity that is completely devoid of *phenomenal*
content? There certainly could, if the present theory was false. For instance, the double
satisfaction of the globality constraint and the presentationality constraint could yield only
necessary, but not sufficient conditions for the appearance of what we termed "minimal
consciousness" in section 3.2.11. In order to realize first-person knowledge without first-
person phenomenal experience, there would have to be an unconscious system which possesses an integrated model of reality plus a virtual window of presence (*constraints 2* and
3), and which at the same time has a system-model (which now is not a *PSM*) and an
internal model of the intentionality relation as such (which now is not a *PMIR*). All of
these structures, like all unconscious states, would be neither transparent nor opaque,
because transparency and opacity are properties of phenomenal states. Because selfhood
emerges through the phenomenal transparency of the system model, the unconscious MIR

could only portray a *system* in the act of knowing, but never a *self* in the act of knowing. But how could that be a strong version of epistemic subjectivity? It could at best be only a weak, functional form of internally modeled knowledge acquisition. The act of knowledge acquisition would be represented, but the "perspective" it generated would be *no one's* perspective. In addition, neither the world nor the present nor the system's epistemic perspective could be portrayed as *real*, as *actually being present right now*. What would the "first-person" component in a concept like "unconscious first-person knowledge" mean in this case? Ultimately, it seems, epistemic subjectivity is anchored in the phenomenal property of selfhood as well. If we ask for a better understanding of epistemic subjectivity, we always ask for a better understanding of the *phenomenal self* as subject.

Of course, as the general concept of consciousness is still devoid of empirical content today, many absurd scenarios may still strike us as conceivable. But the set of logically possible worlds is not identical with the set of metaphysically possible worlds and as science moves on and fills the notion of consciousness with empirical content, many of these scenarios will gradually become *less* conceivable. Still, today one may, for instance, ask: Couldn't there be zombie transparency? In order to follow this line of thought, we would have to assume some kind of purely functional, but strictly nonphenomenal, notion of availability or unavailability of earlier processing stages plus the empirically unlikely possibility of an entirely unconscious form of focal attention to which it could be relative (see section 3.2.7). If any kind of introspection is at all possible—and the existence of an unconscious MIR necessarily *implies* at least introspection$_1$, that is, *some* kind of metarepresentational capacity directed at *some* aspect of the internal model of reality—then there are only two possibilities. Either earlier processing stages for this aspect are not unconsciously attentionally available or they are. Either they are (nonphenomenally, purely functionally) transparent or they are (nonphenomenally, purely functionally) opaque.

In the first case, the system *almost* exhibits the minimal degree of constraint satisfaction in order to speak about the phenomenon of "appearance," the phenomenon of consciousness at all (see section 3.2.11). It involves *constraints 2* (presentationality), *3* (globality), and *7* (transparency, but only in the weaker, now purely functional variant), that is, the activation of a coherent and functionally transparent world-model within a window of presence. *Ex hypothesi* it would be unconscious, but it would still represent *a world as now being present to this very system while it is simultaneously embedded in and directed at it*. Could one say that a reality "appears" to this system or not? In the second case, the reality-model of the system, including the purportedly unconscious MIR, is functionally opaque. Earlier processing stages are globally available for unconscious attention. Could one say that this system is not a naive realist anymore? If it would self-ascribe the property of not being a naive realist to itself, what would fill the subject-argument place in the expressions it formed? I think the central lesson to be learned is that the target property of our investigation is the property of a knowing phenomenal *self* and how it would make little sense to claim of an unconscious system that "it" had overcome naive realism.

This leaves us with two interesting borderline cases. First, the empirically unlikely class of systems just described, of course, is conceivable from a purely logical point of view: There could be systems satisfying at least *constraints 2, 3,* and *6 without* strongly satisfying *constraint 7,* the transparency constraint. Let us say they would have a model of the present, a world-model, a nonphenomenally transparent system-model, and an accordingly impoverished model of the first-person perspective as such. *All* of these models would be completely unconscious. Of course, such a state could be an epistemic state too; and arguably we could also opt for it to be called *epistemically* subjective without being called *phenomenally* subjective. The system could have knowledge, because it could potentially correctly represent facts under an unconscious MIR. This now seems to be entirely a point of terminological convention. The present theory would have to describe it as unconscious, because the transparency constraint was interpreted as a necessary condition in the conceptual ascription of phenomenality—but please remember that at the same time I have always warned against any attempts to draw absolute lines in a domain as complex as that of conscious experience. There could possibly be a conscious mirror image of the same configuration.

For the case of global opacity, and in the conscious mirror image, the expected phenomenology of this system class would involve neither selfhood nor any form of naive realism about subject-object relations, and it could probably be best described as a mixture of an enduring lucid dream (see section 7.2.5) and a prolonged mystical experience of ego dissolution (or "system consciousness," to use our new conceptual tool). It would also be nonsubjective in that, epistemically, it could constitute *selfless knowledge*, that is, an at least partially correct representation of reality, but again there would be no representation of the *subject as self.* If it would self-ascribe phenomenal properties, what would fill the subject-argument place in the expressions it formed? Many people would certainly opt for a terminological convention describing this type of system as unconscious. The "subject as self" clearly seems to be the intuitive target property we wanted to understand at the outset. This is why I would at the same time not count any possible scenarios of nonphenomenal epistemic states as subjective in any interesting sense. There is no entity which is *subjected* to the evolution of these states. Therefore, coming back to our initial question, the contribution the phenomenal first-person perspective makes to epistemic and logical notions of subjectivity is that they are inevitably anchored in an implicit notion of phenomenal selfhood. The second part of our answer is a note of caution: We may have to make domain-specific revisions in our catalogue of constraints. But this is good news, because this is precisely what this catalogue was introduced *for.*

There is a second possible borderline case. A system could fail to satisfy the transparency constraint simply because it had no attentional processing mechanisms. It follows that its representational states would be neither phenomenally opaque *nor* phenomenally transparent. It could have an internal model of the present, a world-model, a self-model, and some sort of *nonattentional* model of the first-person perspective as such, but neither content properties nor vehicle properties would be available for introspective attention. By the definition introduced in section 3.2.11 this system would not be minimally conscious. However, please note how this scenario does not exclude the possibility that this system possesses some sort of *cognitive* introspection. If something doesn't have an attentional PMIR, at least from the conceptual point of view this doesn't exclude the possible existence of a *cognitive* PMIR or a *volitional* PMIR.

Imagine nonbiological information processing characterized by a truly classicist architecture: Only GOFAI-type symbolic representations would exist in its internal ecology of epistemic states and all there was would be rule-based operations on syntactically specified tokens—and let us just grant that it could under these conditions *actually* have some kind of knowledge about the world and itself. Our artificial demon would have a symbolic world-model, a symbolic self-model, and a symbolic model of the intentionality relation as well. Their content would be cognitively available to the classicist demon, as it could in some sense *think* about it, by forming concept-like mental structures. In particular, it would only have an impoverished and purely cognitive first-person perspective, but not an attentional first-person perspective. In generating it, it could link some demonstrative self-symbol to, say, an object-symbol, forming a more complex internal expression of the sort ⟨THIS system is currently being affected by a perceptual object belonging to category X in manner Y⟩. It could be an epistemic agent, even a superb autonomous agent, a truly *cognitive* robot marching through the world, while continuously extracting information through its sensors and generating a nonbiological kind of purely symbolic knowledge. If its model of reality were a good representation of reality, then it would have intentional content. But would it have *phenomenal* content? It seems easy to dream up a possible world in which it would be an epistemic subject, but not an attentional subject. Again, this seems to be a matter of terminology. The present theory excludes the possibility that this system could be a conscious subject, because, for reasons of empirical and phenomenological plausibility, the SMT puts a strong emphasis on *subsymbolic* information processing. It is hard to see how something like our classicist demon could have *evolved*. And in this case, I would like to point out, our intuitions in favor of the thesis that the artificial demon is definitely *not* conscious are much stronger. But then again, intuitions only reflect what was phenomenally possible and necessary in our lives and the lives of our ancestors. Phenomenality comes in theory-relative degrees of constraint satisfaction. And intuitions can be chauvinistic.

Can one have a conscious first-person perspective without having a conscious self? Can one have a conscious self without having a conscious first-person perspective?

By definition, there can be no PMIR without a subject component. However, as pointed out in section 6.2.6, it is conceivable that this subject component is entirely *opaque*, and for this reason would not serve to instantiate the phenomenal property of selfhood. In such a case there could be consciousness, plus a PMIR, but one originating from what phenomenologically would be an opaque *system-model* only. So the first part of our answer is that on the level of conscious experience there would be no one *having* the respective perspective. We can describe the possibility of this type of neurophenomenological configuration in a way that involves no logical contradictions. It is an open empirical question whether the class of systems described by this configuration is *functionally* possible. It is an open philosophical question if in such cases we would still want to speak of a first-*person* perspective.

By definition, a PSM is a theoretical entity distinct from a PMIR on all levels of description. Therefore, it should be possible for a PSM to exist without a PMIR. Empirically, examples like the case of akinetic mutism discussed above constitute plausible evidence that neurophenomenological configurations of this type actually exist. Philosophically, it is a much more difficult question if the existence of a stable PMIR should be treated as a logical condition for actualized personhood, or if an impoverished, but stable, PSM is enough to ascribe personhood. Fortunately, since many patients suffering from akinetic mutism recover after some time, they certainly all possess the *potential* to regain phenomenal subjectivity all by themselves. In this sense they certainly are persons. But given the conceptual instruments now at hand, it easy to see that much more difficult cases may exist. Such cases could be constituted by people still possessing a phenomenal self, in whatever rudimentary way, but having lost all potential of regaining rationality, a cognitive or a volitional PMIR.

In which way does a phenomenal first-person perspective contribute to the emergence of a second-person perspective and to the emergence of a first-person plural perspective? What forms of social cognition are inevitably mediated by phenomenal self-awareness. Which are not?

Neurophenomenologically, a second-person perspective consists of the brain activating a PMIR with the object component being *another* person or self-as-subject. Neurophenomenologically, a first-person plural perspective corresponds to a PMIR with the subject component being represented as a *group* of persons or selves. However, this locally reductive approach only helps in understanding the conscious experience of different aspects of intersubjectivity, its phenomenal content (i.e., precisely that aspect which could also be a hallucination taking place in an isolated individual). If we want to understand what the functional foundations of real-world, successfully unfolding social cognition are, then we have to assume a more complex situation: Two individuals currently "coherencing" their PMIRs by mutually making each other their object components while at the same time also consciously representing the fact that the other self-as-subject-as-the-object-I-am-currently-directed-at also has conscious knowledge about what is currently taking place; or a group of individuals "orchestrating" their PMIRs by making a mental representation of their group an element of their individual subject components, again paradigmatically knowing that it is exactly this that is now taking place. In this type of situation, we have not only the conscious experience of an "I-Thou relationship" or of (let's say) group solidarity but also the necessary functional properties underlying *social* neurophenomenology. A dynamical functional equivalence holding across individuals is established. What forms of social cognition are necessarily mediated by conscious self-representation? We can now give a rather abstract, but straightforward answer: All forms of social cognition that make the additional functional demand for a successful transmission of globally available system-related information on both sides, or in all interacting participants. More concretely, a PSM and a PMIR are needed in all those cases where selectivity and flexibility are important: if social interaction necessarily involves the fast and flexible adaptation of your own behavior to that of another human being (global availability for action control), constant metacognitive monitoring of your own thoughts (global availability for cognition), or a permanent introspective observation of your ongoing emotional responses (global availability for self-directed attentional processing). And, of course, what we have called the virtual window of presence (*constraint 3*) is necessary for you and the other to be able to represent each other as continuously interacting *at the same time*.

Please recall a point touched upon earlier: Coherent representational structures can function as unifying windows allowing parts of a system to communicate *as wholes*, with causal forces in the environment, or with other functional subcomponents internal to the system. This well-established principle now has an interesting extension into the domain of social environments. A PSM is a representational structure creating a functional window through which a system can interact and communicate with other agents, with other self-conscious systems, with those aspects of its environment that are exclusively formed by other systems also acting and internally representing themselves *as wholes*. Therefore, a PSM is a necessary functional window onto more flexible and selective forms of agent-agent interaction. It creates a new macrolevel of information flow and causal interaction. It must have been at the heart of the process of forming more complex, evolvable, and yet stable societies. The new level of information flow is also a new level of functional granularity for *intrasocial* self-representation.

This point can now be made clearer if we consider the two examples of specifically social kinds of PMIRs just discussed, namely, the second-person perspective and the first-person plural perspective. Given our new conceptual tools, we can consider the evolution not of individuals, but of *groups* of conscious systems and say the following: PMIRs of the sort described above—made coherent and orchestrated—are unified functional windows that emerge in *groups* of biological systems. They are new causal properties. Of course, societies are information-processing and representational systems as well, and although they do not exhibit any mysterious kind of "group consciousness" they certainly come in degrees of intelligence. They also create self-models. If new functional windows—new units of transindividual representation—appear in such societies, they can in principle greatly increase their overall intelligence and adaptivity (their degree of "self-reflexivity," if readers will permit this metaphor). My proposal is that phenomenally represented I-Thou relationships and the functionally orchestrated conscious representation of the we-as-a-group emerging in groups of biological individuals are in the same way to be understood as a superbly elegant strategy in which parts of the *group* can now form transient, but stable functional windows through which the *group* can now causally and informationally interact with itself and other groups. The point is that the essential neurocomputational feature within the brains of individuals in order to achieve this step on more interesting levels of complexity must have been the human PSM.

Finally, a last question concerns the status of *phenomenal universals*. Can we define a notion of consciousness and subjectivity, which is hardware and species independent? This issue has a distinct philosophical flavor, because it amounts to an attempt to give an analysis of consciousness, the phenomenal self, and the first-person perspective that operates on the representational and functional levels of description alone, maximizing generality and aiming at a liberation from any kind of physical domain-specificity. Can there be a *universal* theory of consciousness? Today, we usually put it in other words:

Is artificial subjectivity possible? Could there be nonbiological phenomenal selves?

To actually create a *technical model* of full-blown, perspectivally organized conscious experience seems to be the ultimate technological utopian dream. It would transpose the evolution of mind onto an entirely new level—not only in terms of the physical properties on which mind now supervenes but also with regard to functional constraints and optimality conditions operative during its future development from this point onward. It would be a historical phase transition. And indeed, the project of realizing ever-stronger forms of intelligence, of coherent and content-bearing mentality, and possibly even phenomenal *selfhood* on artificial carrier systems is a fascinating one. But is this at all possible? It certainly is *conceivable*. But can it happen, given the natural laws governing this universe and the technical resources at hand? Let us here distinguish conceptual, nomological, and technological possibility (Birnbacher 1995). If an exhaustive representationalist and functionalist analysis of phenomenal content is possible, then conscious experience will be multirealizable. It may, however, be the case that in our own physical universe there is only one type of hardware—the human brain—which can *actually* realize precisely the human kind of consciousness, phenomenal selfhood, and perspectivalness. We simply don't know this. What would be needed is a physical substrate possessing a topologically equivalent phase space to the phenomenal state space of human beings. To create an artificial PSM plus PMIR, a consistent functional equivalence would have to be achieved, and on just the right level of granularity. But please note that such a system would not yet have to be intelligent, or even embodied: An appropriately stimulated chunk of nervous tissue could in principle exhibit the right kind of topological or microfunctional equivalence, without possessing any kind of *intentional* content. As its internal states would neither be grounded in the environment nor in its history in a way that could endow them with meaning, it would not have any form of knowledge. In particular, this chunk of nervous tissue would not possess self-knowledge, but only self-experience.

Cognitive robotics may soon change this situation. Just as Mother Nature first created unconscious forms of information processing and representation, and phenomenal experience only recently, it might plausibly be argued that the second evolution of minds will have to repeat an unconscious bottom-up phase as well. Embodiment, sensorimotor integration, and unconscious self-models will have to come first. On the other hand, one thing seems safe to say: The smooth and reliable type of ultrafine-grained self-presentation based on *molecular-level* dynamics—which, in human beings, drives the incessant self-stabilizing activity in the homeostatic system of the brainstem and hypothalamus—will be out of reach for a long time. The subtlety of bodily and emotional selfhood, the qualitative wealth and dynamic elegance of the *human* variety of having a conscious self, will not be available to any machine for a long time. The reason is that the microfunctional structure of our emotional self-model simply is much too fine-grained, and possibly even mathematically intractable. And, for the same reason, in terms of what is *technologically* possible, the portability of human PSMs is extremely low. Self-models emerge from elementary forms of bioregulation, from complex chemical and immunological loops—and this is simply something machines don't possess. The time when robots come to have body fluids and something even remotely resembling the complex homeodynamics of the human brain certainly is far distant. Or is it?

The new discipline of hybrid biorobotics may soon change this situation, by *taking* the hardware from what Mother Nature has to offer. Please remember our more extensive discussion of the strength or weakness concerning conscious systems not—or differently—satisfying *constraint 11* (the adaptivity constraint) in section 3.2.11: the distinction between natural and artificial systems is not an exhaustive and exclusive distinction.

Postbiotic systems fall into neither category. They might be hybrid biorobots using organic, genetically engineered hardware, or semiartificial information-processing systems employing biomorphic architectures. At the same time they could be submitted to a quasi-evolutionary optimization process of individual development and group evolution. If their PSM is actually anchored in biological hardware, things might be different. Presently, we have to admit that both of our questions concerning the nomological and technological possibility of nonbiological consciousness, and of postbiotic PSMs and PMIRs in particular, are simply open. They constitute empirical, not philosophical, issues. However, please also recall how one of the central lessons to be learned in the course of this investigation was that consciousness and self-consciousness are *graded* phenomena. There are degrees of constraint satisfaction and degrees of phenomenality. There will be degrees of phenomenal selfhood too. Therefore, just as with animals and many primitive organisms surrounding us on this planet, it is rather likely that there will soon be artificial or postbiotic systems possessing simple self-models and weaker forms of conscious experience in our environment. One aspect that these simple, nonbiological subjects will have in common with us is the capacity to *suffer*.

It is time to lay my cards on the table. There is a philosophical issue that has been neglected and which cannot simply be naturalized by gradually handing it over to the empirical mind sciences. In the end, a theory of mind has to be rationally integrated with *normative* considerations. Philosophy of mind must be supplemented by moral and eventually even by political philosophy. Above, I pointed out that the actual creation of a technical model of a full-blown, perspectivally organized conscious experience seems to be the ultimate technological Utopian dream. It might be a nightmare too. As a philosopher I am strictly against attempting to realize the Big Technological Dream, but on *ethical* grounds. Why? Put very simply, we might dramatically increase the amount of suffering, misery, and confusion on the planet. And we might do so without at the same time increasing the amount of pleasure and joy. An even deeper and more general point is that upon more careful inspection it is not at all clear if the biological form of consciousness, as so far brought about by evolution on our planet, is a *desirable* form of experience, an actual *good in itself*, something that one should simply keep on multiplying without further thought. Let me explain.

Perhaps *the* theoretical blind spot of current philosophy of mind is the issue of conscious suffering. Thousands of pages are being written about color qualia or the contents of thought, but almost no theoretical work is devoted to ubiquitous phenomenal states like physical pain or simple everyday sadness ("subclinical depression"), or to the phenomenal content associated with panic, despair, and melancholy, let alone the conscious experience of mortality or of losing one's dignity. There may be deeper evolutionary reasons behind this cognitive scotoma, but I am not going to pursue this point here. The ethical issue is of greater relevance. If one dares to take a closer look at the actual phenomenology of biological systems on our planet, the many different kinds of conscious suffering are *at least* as dominant a feature as are color vision or conscious thought, both of which appeared only very recently. Evolution is not something to be glorified. One way—out of countless others—to look at biological evolution on our planet is as a process that has created an expanding ocean of suffering and confusion where there previously was none. As not only the simple number of individual conscious subjects but also the dimensionality of their phenomenal state spaces is continuously increasing, this ocean is also *deepening*. Obviously, the process as a whole is something that has not yet ended. We should not accelerate it without need.

As this is not the place to enter into an extended ethical discussion of artificial phenomenality, let me just give two concrete examples. What would you say if someone came along and said, "Hey, we want to genetically engineer mentally retarded human infants! For reasons of scientific progress we need infants with certain cognitive and emotional deficits in order to study their postnatal psychological development—we urgently need some funding for this important and innovative kind of research!" You would certainly think this was not only an absurd and appalling but also a dangerous idea. It would hopefully not pass any ethics committee in the democratic world. However, what today's ethics committees *don't* see is how the first machines satisfying a minimally sufficient set of constraints for conscious experience could be just *like* such mentally retarded infants. They would suffer from all kinds of functional and representational deficits too. But they would now also subjectively experience those deficits. In addition, they would have no political lobby—no representatives in *any* ethics committee.

If they had a transparent world-model embedded in a virtual window of presence, then a reality would appear to them. They would be minimally conscious. If, as advanced robots, they even had a stable *bodily* self-model, then they could feel sensory pain as their *own* pain, including all the consequences resulting from bad human engineering. But particularly if their postbiotic PSM were actually anchored in biological hardware, things might be much worse. If they had an *emotional* self-model, then they could truly suffer—possibly even in degrees of intensity or qualitative richness that we as their creators cannot imagine, because it is entirely alien to us. If, in addition, they possessed a *cognitive* self-model, they could potentially not only conceive of their bizarre situation but also intellectually suffer from the fact that they never had anything like the "dignity" so important to their creators. They might be able to consciously represent the obvious fact that they are only second-rate subjects, used as exchangeable experimental tools by some other type of self-modeling system, which obviously doesn't know what it is doing and which must have lost control of its own actions long ago. Can you imagine what it would be like to *be* such a mentally retarded phenomenal clone of the first generation? Alternatively, can you imagine what it would be like to "come to" as a more advanced artificial subject, only to discover that, although possessing a distinct sense of self, you are just a *commodity*, a scientific tool never created and certainly not to be treated as an end in itself?

A lot more would have to be said at this point. Let me just highlight what seems to be the central issue: Suffering starts on the level of PSMs. You cannot consciously suffer without having a globally available self-model. The PSM is the decisive neurocomputational instrument not only in developing a host of new cognitive and social skills but also in *forcing* any strongly conscious system to functionally and representationally appropriate its own disintegration, its own failures and internal conflicts. Phenomenal appropriation goes along with functional appropriation. Evolution is not only marvellously efficient but also ruthless and cruel to the individual organism. Pain and any other nonphysical kind of suffering, generally any representational state characterized by a "negative valence" and integrated into the PSM, are now phenomenally *owned*. Now it inevitably, and transparently, is *my own* suffering. The melodrama, but also the potential tragedy of the ego both start on the level of transparent self-modeling. Therefore, we should ban all attempts to create (or even risk the creation of) artificial and postbiotic PSMs from serious academic research.

People differ widely in their *positive* moral intuitions, as well as in their explicit theories about what we should actively strive for. But in terms of a fundamental solidarity of all suffering beings against suffering, something that almost all of us should be able to agree on is what I will term the "principle of negative utilitarianism": Whatever else our exact ethical commitments and specific positive goals are, we can and should certainly all agree that, in principle, and whenever possible, the overall amount of conscious suffering in all beings capable of conscious suffering should be minimized. I know that it is impossible to give any truly conclusive argument in favor of this principle. And, of course, there exist all kinds of theoretical complications—for example, individual rights, long-term preferences, and epistemic indeterminacy. But the underlying intuition is something that can be shared by almost everybody: We can all agree that no additional suffering should be created without need. Albert Camus once spoke about the solidarity of all finite beings against death, and in just the same sense there should be a solidarity of all sentient beings capable of suffering against suffering. Out of this solidarity we should not do anything that would increase the overall amount of suffering and confusion in the universe—let alone something that highly *likely* will have this effect right from the beginning.

To put it very carefully, one obvious fact about phenomenal experience as it has developed on our planet until now is that one of its strikingly dominant features is suffering and confusion. Phenomenal experience is not something to be unconditionally glorified. Among many other new properties, biological self-consciousness has brought an enormous amount of misery and confusion into the physical world, an ocean of phenomenal suffering, which simply was not there before. As one of my students once put it: The universe may be a good place for evolution, but not such a good place for individuals. If this is true, individuals with conscious self-models will automatically reflect this fact on the level of their own phenomenal experience. It is hard for beings like us to really face this fact, because this is not the kind of fact Mother Nature *wanted* us to face. But in theoretically and technologically modeling fascinating phenomena like phenomenal selfhood and the first-person perspective we now have nothing much to go by other than our own, biological form of consciousness—simply because it is the only form of consciousness we can scientifically investigate. We are therefore in great danger of multiplying all its negative aspects on artificial carrier systems *before* we have understood where all these negative aspects come from, in exactly what properties of our biological history, of our bodies, and of our brains they are rooted, and if or how they can at all be neutralized. For this reason we should first focus all our energy—in philosophy as well as in the neuro- and cognitive sciences—on achieving a deeper understanding of our *own* consciousness and the structure of our *own* suffering. We should orient ourselves in accordance with the classical philosophical ideal of self-knowledge and the minimal ethical rule of the minimization of suffering rather than risk the triggering of a second-order evolution of post-biotic minds, which could then slip from our control and eventually contribute to a further increase in the overall amount of suffering in the universe.

Before closing by briefly considering more general and normative issues in the final section, let us stop to ask: What are the most urgent goals for future research? Where do we go from here? The beauty of the current phase of interdisciplinary research lies in the fact that the new image of the conscious mind that is now slowly emerging is the first image in the history of mankind that is anchored in a firm empirical foundation. Therefore, on our way toward a new theory of mind, this is also the first image justifying serious hopes for clearly nameable steps of progress. It is hard to underestimate the relevance of this fact for the old philosophical project of a comprehensive and unified theory of consciousness. What are rational next steps? On the level of neuroscience we should first focus on the minimally sufficient neural correlate for the PSM and the PMIR:

· Which content layers of the PSM covary with which *types of neural processing*?

· How is a *dynamic binding* of these layers achieved?

· How are we to imagine the way in which the PSM is anchored in *unconscious* processes of self-representation? What is the most simple neural structure in the brain that can still be said to represent *the system as a whole*?

· In terms of neural correlates for the PMIR, what are candidates for *object-components* in different domains (e.g., in perceptual attention, the selection of motor patterns, or in conscious concept formation)?

• At any given point in time, how is the dynamic *binding of subject and object component* into a single PMIR achieved?

• What are the unconscious processing stages necessarily *preceding* the activation of a PMIR?

• What exactly is the *minimal set of neurobiological properties* that will bring about a conscious self and a consciously experienced first-person perspective in humans?

• How does this set contribute to the set enabling *intersubjectivity* and social cognition?

On various functional levels of analysis we need more detailed descriptions of the causal and informational fine structure for given physical correlates. On the level of fine-grained functional mapping and computational modeling we need more abstract descriptions of the PSM, as well as of the PMIR:

• What is the *functional* neuroanatomy of the PSM?

• In terms of an extended teleofunctionalist analysis, is there something like a distinct biological *proper function* of self-consciousness and phenomenal perspectivity?

• What, precisely, is the *computational role* of the phenomenal self and the first-person perspective under a more abstract, mathematical description?

• How is this computational role integrated into the *behavioral ecology* of the system, for example, into sensorimotor loops, into the ongoing generation of more complex motor output, and into other-agent modeling and social cognition?

• Ontogenetic development: We certainly need to know more about the stages and the general *developmental trajectory* through which individual self-models unfold in individual human beings and other animals.

• Phylogenetic history: If my claim is true that the PSM and the PMIR are "virtual organs" that have been developed in the course of biological evolution, then it must be possible to tell an *evolutionary story* for individual species and the way in which they developed these organs in order to adapt to their specific inner and outer environment. How did PSMs *propagate* through biological populations?

There a number of important and largely unresolved *conceptual* issues as well. They begin on the representationalist level of analysis, expanding into phenomenology and ethics. These future goals mainly fall into the field of philosophy. Most pressing may be the relationship between phenomenal and epistemic subjectivity:

• Which aspects of the contents of self-consciousness can be *epistemically justified*?

• What is the difference between a *phenomenal* and an *epistemic* first-person perspective — can one exist without the other; in what way do they depend on each other?

· More generally, we urgently need an overarching *theory of mental content* that explains the relationship between intentional and phenomenal content while at the same time satisfying empirical constraints as they are, for instance, given by the best current theories in connectionist/dynamicist cognitive science. What is needed is an empirically plausible theory of mental content, which is open to future changes.

· On the phenomenological level of analysis new tools have to be developed. As ultimately they are always *phenomenological descriptions* that function as input for the method of representational analysis, these descriptions have to be optimized beyond the terminologies of classic philosophical phenomenology developed in the tradition of Brentano and Husserl. Even if nothing like "first-person data" in any stronger epistemological or methodological sense exist, the heuristic power of first-person reports has been underestimated. Careful introspective reports, particularly *in combination with real-time third-person access* through neuroimaging, transcranial magnetic stimulation, and so forth, are an important source of information in correlation studies. Therefore, innovative methods for arriving at more precise first-person descriptions of the target phenomenon are of highest relevance.

· The preliminary *catalogue of constraints* offered in chapter 3 needs to be critically assessed, continuously differentiated, and expanded. Further domains and more fine-grained levels of description have to be added.

· *Normative issues* and *cultural ramifications* have to become topics of a permanent discussion accompanying progress in the cognitive neuroscience of consciousness and selfhood. Because it has obvious *political aspects*, this discussion can not exclusively remain an expert discussion, but eventually has to include the general public. If the current proposal points in the right direction, then it is an obvious fact that we are facing a major shift in our general image of humankind and that a host of new ethical issues will eventually result. In the face of rising time pressure an important task of academic philosophy lies in offering a service to society as a whole by initiating critical and rational debates on these issues.

8.3 Being No One

What does it mean to *be someone*? "Being someone" is not a well-defined technical term, neither in philosophy nor in any other discipline. Therefore, it simultaneously means many different things to different people. We all use the idea of "being someone" in many different ways, and in many different contexts—as citizens of a state or as psychological laymen, in ethical and political discourse, or even in religious matters. As this is only a book about consciousness, the phenomenal self, and the first-person perspective, I have been mostly interested in the *phenomenological* aspects of this question: What exactly does it mean to have the *conscious experience* of being someone? In this limited sense, the folk-phenomenological notion of "being someone" denotes a phenomenal property like many others, a property like the scent of mixed amber and sandalwood or the gustatory experience of cinnamon, a property like the emotional experience of elation, or the sense of surprise going along with a sudden cognitive insight. It is just a way of experiencing reality: currently, you *are* someone. What makes consciously experienced selfhood special, and different from all the other forms of experiential content, is the fact that—in nonpathological standard situations and in beings like ourselves—it is highly invariant. It is *always* there.

This phenomenally transparent representation of invariance and continuity constitutes the intuitions that underlie many traditional philosophical fallacies concerning the existence of selves as process-independent individual entities, as ontological substances that could in principle exist all by themselves, and as mysteriously unchanging essences that generate a sharp transtemporal identity for persons. But at the end of this investigation we can clearly see how individuality (in terms of simplicity and indivisibility), substantiality (in terms of ontological autonomy), and essentiality (in terms of transtemporal sameness) are not properties of selves at all. At best, they are folk-phenomenological constructs, inadequately described conscious *simulations* of individuality, substantiality, and essentiality. And in *this* sense we truly are no one. We now arrive at a maximally simple metaphysical position with regard to selves: No such things as selves exist in the world. At least their existence does not have to be presupposed in any rational and truly explanatory theory. Metaphysically speaking, what we called "the self" in the past is neither an individual nor a substance, but the content of a transparent PSM. There is no unchanging essence, but a complex self-representational process that can be interestingly described on many different levels of analysis at the same time. For ontological purposes, "self" can therefore be substituted by "PSM." However, this first reading of the concept of "being no one" is only an answer to the crude traditional metaphysics of selfhood, and I think as such it is a rather trivial one.

On a somewhat deeper level the question arises if the dominant structural characteristic of our phenomenal space—the fact that it almost inevitably satisfies *constraint 6*, the perspectivalness constraint—makes us constitutionally unable to see certain obvious truths. Could the fact that we always operate not only under a transparent PSM but also under a PMIR *impede* epistemic progress? There is one obvious field of research at which this question is aimed: the now strongly expanding domain of the mind sciences— scientific psychology, cognitive neuroscience, AI and robotics, philosophy of mind, and the like. More specifically, could it be that the conscious experience of *being someone* itself hinders growth of knowledge in these disciplines, by making certain theoretical positions or solutions of problems look utterly implausible, dangerously provocative, absurdly humiliating, or simply *inconceivable* to beings like ourselves? A lot of today's physics, for example, describes the world in a way that is extremely counterintuitive, and certainly hard to conceive of. Yet most of us believe that these theories are among the best mankind has so far created. Basically, we trust those physicists. In the mind sciences things are different, and in an interesting way.

Take as an example the sketch of an interdisciplinary, representationalist theory of consciousness, the phenomenal self, and the first-person perspective I have offered in this book. Even if you should think that at least some of the ideas involved are potentially worthy of discussion, you could never really *believe* that the SMT, the self-model theory of subjectivity, actually is true. *You* cannot believe in it. Take what may be the central idea, the idea that metaphysically speaking no such things as selves exist in the world; that the conscious experience of self*hood* is brought about by the phenomenal transparency of the system-model; and that what philosophers call the epistemic irreducibility of conscious experience—the fact that it is tied to a first-person perspective—can be exhaustively analyzed as a *representational* phenomenon, which in the future will likely be fully explained on functional and neurobiological levels of description. *You* cannot believe in the truth of this idea. "Being convinced," like smelling mixed amber and sandalwood or *being someone*, is here interpreted as a phenomenal property. But for the current theory you cannot in principle have that property, because phenomenally simulating the truth of the SMT would involve a cognitively lucid, nonpathological way of dissolving your sense of self. It would involve being convinced and phenomenally *being no one* at the same time.

My second conclusion in this final section therefore is that the SMT is a theory of which *you cannot be convinced*, in principle. I would also claim that this fact is the true essence and the deepest core of what we *actually* mean when speaking about the "puzzle"—or sometimes even about the "mystery"—of consciousness. Furthermore, this second conclusion is another possible answer to the question which many readers may have silently been asking themselves for quite a while: Why is the title of this book *Being No One*? After all, isn't it precisely a book about the neurophenomenological conditions of personhood, a book that tells a new story about what it means to *Be Someone?* The problem is this: If the current story is true, there is no way in which it could be *intuitively* true. It could never *feel* true, because it creates a dilemma. There seem to be two alternatives: Either you see it as actually describing a set of possibilities that may be nomologically likely (i.e., empirically plausible) and conceptually coherent (i.e., philosophically plausible) at the same time. Then you *cannot be convinced.* Call this the "scientific horn of the dilemma." You cannot be convinced, because the idea that there are no such things as selves—including your own self—in the world remains strictly counterintuitive, a phenomenal impossibility. Now you might turn to the other alternative. Let us call this the "spiritual horn of the dilemma." You might change your global phenomenal model of the world in a way that *makes* it a possibility. For instance, you could do so by making it a phenomenal reality, that is, by developing a stable and cognitively lucid state of consciousness that does not satisfy *constraint 6*. Phenomenal selfhood would not be instantiated. Your new neurophenomenological configuration would then correspond to what was earlier termed "system consciousness," namely, a phenomenally *nonsubjective* state of consciousness. In this case you could not truthfully form the corresponding I*-sentences (see section 6.4.4), and therefore you could not even self-ascribe your new neurophenomenological configuration to yourself. In this case, *you* could not be convinced of the truth of the SMT, in principle. In conclusion, no one can be convinced of the current theory. And this is another one of the reasons this book has the title it has: "Being no one" in this sense describes an *epistemological stance* we would have to take toward our own minds in scientifically and philosophically investigating them, an *attitude* that is necessary to really solve the puzzle of consciousness at a deeper and more comprehensive level, an attitude of research that integrates first-person and third-person approaches in a new way and that, perhaps unfortunately, appears to be strictly impossible and absolutely necessary at the same time. It goes beyond the classic research strategy of methodological solipsism in cognitive science in a new way, because it acknowledges the need for a shift in perspective that we could call "methodological nemocentrism."

Is all of this a problem? Yes and no. It is a problem if—as opposed to other, for example, physical, theories about the nature of reality—we impose the additional constraint of intuitive plausibility on theories of consciousness, the phenomenal self, and the first-person perspective. It certainly is an absurd claim that simply listening to a theoretical description of the underlying causal reality should *create* the respective form of phenomenal content in our minds (recall Frank Jackson's Mary). One and the same fact can be given via two different modes of presentation. I would submit that a PMIR may just be such a mode of presentation. The fact that, in standard situations, you are a single and unified physical system operating in its behavioral space under a functionally centered model of reality is made globally available through a highly specific *phenomenal* mode of presentation. This is an entirely new epistemic possibility, which, however, does not entail the corresponding metaphysical possibility. There are no new and irreducible phenomenal facts—all there is is a rather complex new way of accessing an internal physical fact *under a phenomenal model*, under the PMIR mode of presentation.

The phenomenal first-person perspective described in chapter 6 is just this mode of presentation. For the more analytically inclined, we might even call it an "indexical ego mode of presentation."[6] But what is the fact that is given under a PMIR? Strictly speaking, the fact presented is that there currently is a certain brain state, the state on which the PMIR locally supervenes. This brain state can additionally be given under a different mode of presentation, for instance, one involving theories developed by the cognitive neurosciences. The same fact would then also be given under a nonphenomenal, third-person, propositionally structured description. And, of course, it is absurd to demand that reading this description *as such* could by sheer magic turn you (or a self-less machine) into a specific phenomenal self, tied to a specific phenomenal first-person perspective. Actually implementing a computational model of this theory, however, might be a different matter. So the radically counterintuitive nature of the SMT only poses a problem if we want to extend the usual criteria for the goodness of a theory (such as logical coherence, parsimony, predictive power, etc.) by additionally demanding that it be *phenomenally possible*. As you may recall, a theory is phenomenally possible relative to a given class of representational systems if and only if these systems are able to emulate its ontology. The selfless metaphysics of the SMT is not an ontology human beings can emulate. As such, this is not a problem, just as it is not a problem that we are unable to consciously emulate the ontology of quantum chromodynamics. The yet deeper question lurking in the background, of course, is if we would ever *want* to emulate—or even instantiate—this kind of ontology. "Being no one," therefore, could not only refer to the serious and sustained theoretical effort of *thinking* the unthinkable but also of the ideal of phenomenally *living* it.

6. I will not go into analytic details at this point, but just inform my readers that Albert Newen (1997) has introduced the idea of an "indexical ego-mode of presentation," which may be closely related to the more general idea I am sketching here. For instance, Newen writes: "Even though the ego-mode of presentation is not based on any identification, I claim that it nevertheless is a real cognitive structure: a representation that relates one to oneself. To characterize this cognitive structure we have to introduce the distinction between object representations and subject representations. . . . A mode of presentation is subject representational if it constitutes a mental representation that, first, one could not have if the object the thinker is related to does not exist and, second, that does not allow for misidentifications" (Newen 1997, p. 127). I propose that the PSM and the PMIR are just the "real cognitive structures" posited by Newen. However, as we have seen in chapter 7, consistent misidentification of otherwise rational subjects actually does occur. Also, given the current theory, it cannot be assumed that there are possible information-processing systems which, as opposed to the cases of Christina and Ian Waterman discussed in the same chapter, have *never* had any proprioceptive information to construct their fundamental bodily self-model and are still able to have thoughts *de se*. But Newen certainly makes a good point when writing, "Neither the kind of information nor the way the information is acquired, but rather the way the information is handled in a information-processing system is the essential feature that makes it subject representational. . . . the self is a person who is related to himself/herself in the ego-mode of presentation, i.e., this person has a special repository for indexical information that plays a characteristic role in perception, action, and thinking" (p. 128*f*.). The PSM, in particular its self-presentational layer described in chapters 5 and 6, *is* this "special repository" for indexical information. In order to anchor the philosophy of self-consciousness in scientific, third-person approaches to the mind via empirical constraints, it is therefore of great importance not to stop here, but to begin describing the representational deep structure and the functional architecture of this neurocomputational tool.

In closing, let us now once again return to our original question of what it could mean to *be no one*. The third potential reading I want to explicitly mention relates to the *ethics* of consciousness: Do we want to phenomenally emulate the ontology of our own scientific theories about the mind? Do we want to *instantiate* them? My third interim conclusion in this final section is that the cognitive neuroscience of self-consciousness will soon confront us with an extremely interesting set of *normative* challenges. Some of them are obvious and rather concrete practical issues like, for example, defining an applied ethics for medical neurotechnology, for animal experiments, or the question of rejecting military funding in consciousness research. But some of them possess an even more distinct philosophical flavor, because they are much deeper and of a more general type. Unfortunately, an in-depth discussion of such wider normative issues clearly is outside the scope of this work (but see Metzinger 2000b, p. 6*ff.*). However, let us at least take a brief look at some examples.

As we have already seen, there is more than one answer to the question of why this book has the title it has. If it is true that we are neurophenomenological cavemen, then it is also true that mankind is still in a prehistoric stage—not in terms of theoretical knowledge and technology, but in terms of *phenomenological* knowledge and technology. One more general question is if, in the long run, we want to use our new insights into the nature of consciousness, the phenomenal self, and the first-person perspective to *change* our own minds. Is it better to be *someone* or is it better to be *no one*? Is the current neurophenomenological configuration of *Homo sapiens* really a good in itself? Is this *really* something we want to perpetuate and multiply indefinitely? Or should we start to think about improving our conscious model of reality, particularly our PSM? Put crudely, we have better theories and we have better computers—why shouldn't we have better phenomenal selves as well?

In chapter 3 we made an attempt to describe the maximal as well as the minimal degree of constraint satisfaction for subjective experience to occur. Interestingly, one can now also define a notion of *optimal* constraint satisfaction: If it is true that phenomenal experience comes in many different grades and that human beings possibly possess the highest *degree* of conscious awareness (at least relative to the preliminary catalogue discussed above), then it is only natural to conclude that human beings could also possess a *higher* degree of consciousness. There is nothing mysterious about this conclusion, which can be formulated in a conceptually clear way: A stronger form of phenomenality simply comes about by a given class of systems satisfying new and *additional* constraints. Or, as we might decide on normative grounds, less could be more. Of course, there could be *other* sets of constraints as well, in extraterrestrial beings, in conscious machines, or possibly even in some animals on our planet. Such systems might simply have a very different form of phenomenal experience altogether by satisfying a rather distinct set of constraints, one only loosely overlapping with the one sketched here. The space of possible phenomenal minds is vast. Yet it is interesting to pose the following question: What could additional or different constraints for ourselves actually be?

Normative neurophenomenological considerations could yield such additional constraints. For example, they could do so in terms of maximizing intelligence or minimizing suffering in human beings. Another idea, already alluded to above, and slightly more complex, is to assimilate the implicit ontology underlying our phenomenal model of reality into the ontology of our scientific theories. One might carefully investigate the normative ideal of slowly developing a gradual *convergence* between human neurophenomenology and the metaphysics implied by our best objective theories about the deeper structure of physical reality. Call this notion "first-person–third-person convergence." A third logical possibility lies in that we could also opt for *decreasing* the degree of constraint satisfaction for one or more of our already existing constraints. We could, for example, choose to decrease phenomenal transparency. This candidate for a normative orientation—call it "minimization of transparency"—would consist in making the fundamentally *representational* character of conscious experience globally available. We could attempt to make more information about earlier processing stages available for introspective attention, thereby also gradually making more and more layers in our own self-model phenomenally opaque. This type of strategy would certainly create an additional computational load for attentional systems in the brain, but it could at the same time serve to weaken the naive-realistic self-misunderstanding characterizing our present state of consciousness.

So much for first examples. Of course, the number of options open to us is much larger than the three proposals sketched above—from a purely theoretical perspective it is as vast as the space of possible minds itself, although in present-day human beings it is much smaller due to the contigent neurofunctional constraints resulting from the physical structure of our brain. For all these proposals, the underlying principle would always consist in combining an ongoing scientific discussion of our *actual* constraint landscape with a normative discussion of what an *optimal* constraint landscape for human beings could be. In doing so we might, perhaps, eventually arrive at new and more precise answers to ancient philosophical questions like what a good life is and how we can suffer less, about how we can be more intelligent or, more generally, how we can become bearers of a *stronger* form of conscious experience.

This may also be the point where old-fashioned philosophy reenters the stage. In terms of specific normative aspects concerning potential future changes in the PSM itself, one could, for example, discuss the maximization of its internal *coherence*. Perhaps (if in a hedonist mood) we could simply set this goal as relative to ever-higher intensities of pleasant self-presentational content: How much physical pleasure can you experience without going insane? How can you use scientific knowledge to optimize sensory stimulation without forcing the self-model to disintegrate? Then there is a related, but already slightly different interpretation of the coherence ideal: The classical notion of "virtue" can now be interestingly reinterpreted, namely, in terms of increasing the internal and social consistency of the self-model, for example, in terms of functionally integrating cognitive insight, emotional self-modeling, and actual behavioral profile. Traditional notions like "intellectual integrity" and "moral integrity" now suddenly possess new and obvious interpretations, namely, in terms of a person having a highly consistent self-model. Ethical behavior may simply be the most direct way of maximizing the internal coherence of the self-model. It could therefore be directly related to the concept of mental health. And it may even be compatible with an intelligent, neurophenomenologically optimized form of rational hedonism.

But we may actually be able to go further than this. Obviously, from a more traditional philosophical point of view, the *third* logical possibility briefly sketched above—minimizing phenomenal transparency—is of greatest interest. Once the principle of auto-epistemic closure has been clearly understood on the neurocognitive level, one can define the goal of continuously minimizing the transparency of the PSM. This is in good keeping with the classical philosophical ideal of self-knowledge: To truly accept this ideal means to dissolve any form of autoepistemic closure, on theoretical *as well* as on phenomenal levels of representation—even if this implies deliberately violating the adaptivity-constraint Mother Nature so cruelly imposed on our biological ancestors. Self-knowledge never was a purely theoretical enterprise; it also involves practical neurophenomenology—the sustained effort to epistemically optimize phenomenal self-consciousness *itself*. It is interesting to note how this traditional principle also unites Eastern and Western philosophy. My prediction is that, in the centuries to come, the cognitive neuroscience of consciousness will eventually support this old philosophical project of integrating theoretical progress and individual psychological development in a much stronger way than most of us may expect today. The contribution cognitive neuroscience finally makes to the *philosophical* projects of humanity will be a significant one, because, at its core, cognitive neuroscience *is* the project of self-knowledge. As I have tried to show in this book, phenomenal selfhood originates in a *lack* of attentional, subsymbolic self-knowledge. Phenomenal transparency is a special kind of darkness. From a biological point of view this kind of darkness has been enormously successful, because it creates what I have called the "naive-realistic self-misunderstanding." But clearly, from a normative philosophical point of view, representations should always be recognizable *as* representations and naive realism is something to be abhorred. Eventually, appearance has to be transformed into knowledge.

Perhaps unfortunately, the responsibility of academic philosophy also consists in telling people what they *don't* want to hear. Biological evolution is not something to be glorified. It is blind, driven by chance, and it has no mercy. In particular, it is a process that exploits and sacrifices individuals. As soon as individual organisms start to consciously represent themselves *as* individuals, this fact will inevitably be reflected in countless facets on the level of phenomenal experience itself. Therefore, defining our own goals involves emancipating ourselves from this evolutionary process, which, over millions of years, has shaped the microfunctional landscape of our brains and the representational architecture of our conscious minds. For millions of years, Mother Nature has talked to us, through our reward system and through the emotional layers of our PSM. We have to learn to take a critical stance toward this process, and to view our own phenomenal experience as a direct result of it.[7] We have to stop glorifying our own neurophenomenological status quo, face the facts, and find the courage to think about positive alternatives in a rational way. In the end, taking responsibility for the future development of our own conscious minds also is an obvious implication of the project of Enlightenment.

Do you recall how, in the first paragraph of the first chapter, I claimed that as you read these lines you constantly *confuse* yourself with the content of the self-model currently

7. Let me give one last example to illustrate the issue: Mother Nature, self-deception, and the emotional self-model. The SMT clearly shows how—from a teleofunctionalist perspective—false beliefs about oneself can be functionally adequate relative to a certain environment. Evolution will always have favored those who, until the very last moment, stubbornly *believed in themselves*. Therefore, the transparency of our PSM may not only be a source of sensory pleasure and self-certainty but a dangerous affair, something frequently depriving us of insight and functional autonomy. To briefly return to an earlier example, the most effective way to deceive others is to deceive yourself as well. In an evolutionary context the causal effect is what counts, not the degree of actual self-knowledge. Consistent self-deception may optimize the genetic success of an organism. Of course, all this will be particularly true of the nonconceptual, for example, the emotional, layers of our self-model as well. Our emotional self-model—one of the central semantic elements in our traditional folk-psychological notion of the "soul"—may actually be more of a weapon than an instrument to accurately represent reality. It may be something that has arisen from a fundamentally competitive situation, in which cooperation was just one special case of competing in a more intelligent way. In some aspects, having an emotional self-model can even be interpreted as a way of being *possessed*, possessed by the historical reality that mercilessly burned itself into the inner motivational landscape of our biological ancestors. And the emotional self-model, including all its beautiful aspects, is what *drives* us. It is a virtual organ ultimately developed to spread genes more efficiently, and not a tool for maximizing self-knowledge. It may therefore make it difficult for us to grasp the true state of affairs, or put already existing insights into action. Any theory about consciousness and the phenomenal self that was maladaptive would immediately be intuitively implausible and emotionally unattractive. For millions of years, Mother Nature has continuously spoken to us through our conscious, emotional self-model. Whenever it is fully transparent, we don't only hear what she says, but we also have the subjective experience of *knowing that we know*. She says simple things like, "This does not feel right—and you know it doesn't!" or more complicated things like, "Ethical behavior may be the most direct way to make your self-model coherent, yes; but in many situations it will at the same time be the most direct way to end your own existence, conscious self and all—and you know this is true!" But now we know that the cave is empty. Strictly speaking, there is no one *in* the cave who could die. The little red arrow is just a representational device and the pilot is part of the simulator. Strictly speaking, no one was ever born and no one ever dies. The interesting question is whether purely theoretical points like this one can help us in the situation we now find ourselves in.

activated by your brain? We now know that this was only an introductory metaphor, because we can now see that this metaphor, if taken too literally, contains a logical mistake: There is no one *whose* illusion the conscious self could be, no one *who* is confusing herself with anything. As soon as the basic point has been grasped—the point that the phenomenal self as such is not an epistemically justified form of mental content and that the phenomenal characteristic of self*hood* involved results from the transparency of the system model—a new dimension opens. At least in principle, one can wake up from one's biological history. One can grow up, define one's own goals, and become autonomous. And one can start talking back to Mother Nature, elevating her self-conversation to a new level.

References

Adelmann, G., ed. (1987). *Encyclopedia of Neuroscience*. Vols. I and II. Basel: Birkhäuser.

Adolphs, R. (1999). Social cognition and the human brain. *Trends in Cognitive Sciences* 3: 469–79.

Adolphs, R., Damasio, H., Tranel, D., Cooper, G., and Damasio, A. R. (2000). A role for somatosensory cortices in the visual recognition of emotion as revealed by three-dimensional lesion mapping. *Journal of Neuroscience* 20: 2683–90.

Aghajanian, G. K. (1994). Serotonin and the action of LSD in the brain. *Psychiatric Annals* 24: 137–41.

Aghajanian, G. K., Foot, W. F., and Sheard, M. H. (1968). Lysergic acid diethylamide: Sensitive neuronal units in the midbrain raphe. *Science* 161: 706–8.

Aghajanian, G. K., Foot, W. F., and Sheard, M. H. (1970). Action of psychotogenic drugs on midbrain raphe neurons. *Journal of Pharmacology and Experimental Therapeutics* 171: 178–87.

Aghajanian, G. K., Haigler, H. J., and Bennett, J. L. (1975). Amine receptors in the CNS. III. 5-Hydroxytryptamine in brain. In L. L. Iversen et al., eds., *Handbook of Psychopharmacology*. Vol. 6. New York: Plenum.

Ahleid, A. (1968). Considerazioni sull'esperienza nichilistica e sulla syndrome di Cotard nelle psicosi organiche e sintomatiche. *Il Laboro neuropsichiatrico* 43: 927–45.

Allen, T. F. H., and Starr, T. B. (1982). *Hierarchies—Perspectives for Ecological Complexity*. New York: University of Columbia Press.

Altschuler, E. L., Wisdom, S. B., Stone, L., Foster, C., Galasko, D., Llewellyn, D. M. E., and Ramachandran, V. S. (1999). Rehabilitation of hemiparesis after stroke with a mirror. *Lancet* 353: 2035–6.

Alvarado, C. S. (1986). Research on spontaneous out-of-body experiences: A review of modern developments, 1960–1984. In B. Shapin and L. Coly, eds., *Current Trends in PSI Research*. New York: Parapsychology Foundation.

Alvarado, C. S. (1989). Trends in the study of out-of-body-experiences: An overview of developments since the nineteenth century. *Journal of Scientific Exploration* 3: 27–42.

Alvarado, C. S. (1992). The psychological approach to out-of-body-experiences: A review of early and modern developments. *Journal of Psychology* 12: 237–50.

Alvarado, C. S. (1997). Mapping the characteristics of out-of-body experiences. *Journal of the American Society for Psychical Research* 91: 13–30.

Alvarado, C. S. (2000). Out-of-body experiences. In E. Cardeña, S. J. Lynn, and S. Krippner, eds., *Varieties of Anomalous Experience: Examining the Scientific Evidence*. Washington, D.C.: American Psychological Association.

Anderson, E. W. (1964). *Psychiatry*, 1st edition. London: Baillière, Tindall & Cox.

Andrade, J. (2000). Using anesthetics to assess the role of conscious processes in learning. In T. Metzinger, ed., *Neural Correlates of Consciousness—Empirical and Conceptual Questions*. Cambridge, MA: MIT Press.

Anton, G. (1898). Ueber die Herderkrankungen des Gehirns, welche vom Patienten selbst nicht wahrgenommen werden. *Wiener klinische Wochenschrift* 11 (March 10, 1898): 227–9.

Anton, G. (1899). Über die Selbstwahrnehmungen der Herderkrankungen des Gehirns durch den Kranken bei Rindenblindheit und Rindentaubheit. *Archiv für Psychiatrie und Nervenkrankheiten* 32: 86–127.

Atkinson, A. P., Thomas, M. S. C., and Cleeremans, A. (2000). Consciousness: Mapping the theoretical landscape. *Trends in Cognitive Sciences* 4: 372–82.

Avant, L. (1965). Vision in the Ganzfeld. *Psychological Bulletin* 64: 246–58.

Azzopardi, P., and Cowey, A. (1998). Blindsight and visual consciousness. *Consciousness and Cognition* 7: 292–311.

Azzopardi, P., and Cowey, A. (2001). Motion discrimination in cortically blind patients. *Brain* 124: 30–46.

Baars, B. J. (1988). *A Cognitive Theory of Consciousness*. Cambridge: Cambridge University Press.

Baars, B. J. (1997). *In the Theater of Consciousness: The Workspace of the Mind*. Oxford: Oxford University Press.

Baars, B. J., and Newman, J. (1994). A neurobiological interpretation of the global workspace theory of consciousness. In A. Revonsuo and M. Kamppinen, eds., *Consciousness in Philosophy and Cognitive Neuroscience.* Hillsdale, NJ: Lawrence Erlbaum Associates.

Babinski, J. (1914). Contribution à l'étude des troubles mentaux dans l'hémiplégie organique cérébrale (anosognosie). *Revue Neurologique (Paris)* 27: 845–8.

Baddeley, A. D. (1986). *Working Memory.* Oxford: Oxford University Press.

Bailey, A. A., and Moersch, F. P. (1941). Phantom limb. *Canadian Medical Association Journal* 45: 37–42.

Baker, L. R. (1998). The first-person perspective: A test for naturalism. *American Philosophical Quarterly* 35: 327–46.

Baldissera, F., Cavallari, P., Craighereo, L., and Fadiga, L. (2001). Modulation of spinal excitability durino observation of hand actions in humans. *European Journal of Neuroscience* 13: 190–4.

Banks, G., Short, P., Martinez, A. J., Latchaw, R., Ratcliff, G., and Boller, F. (1989). The alien hand syndrome—clinical and post-mortem findings. *Archives of Neurology* 46: 456–9.

Barbur, J. L., Harlow, J. A., Sahraie, A., Stoerig, P., and Weiskrantz, L. (1994). Responses to chromatic stimuli in the absence of V1: Pupillometric and psychophysical studies. *Optical Society of America Technical Digest* 2: 312–5.

Barfield, W., and Furness III, T. A., eds. (1995). *Virtual Environments and Advanced Interface Design.* New York: Oxford University Press.

Barfield, W., Zeltzer, D., Sheridan, T., and Slater, M. (1995). Presence and performance within virtual environments. In W. Barfield and T. A. Furness III, eds., *Virtual Environments and Advanced Interface Design.* New York: Oxford University Press.

Barlow, H. (1994). What is the computational goal of the neocortex? In C. Koch and J. Davies, eds., *Large-Scale Neuronal Theories of the Brain.* Cambridge, MA: MIT Press.

Barrett, J. L. (2000). Exploring the natural foundations of religion. *Trends in Cognitive Sciences* 4: 29–34.

Basar, E., and Bullock, T., eds. (1992). *Induced Rhythms in the Brain.* Boston: Birkhäuser.

Bechtel, W. (1998). Representations and cognitive explanations: Assessing the dynamicist challenge in cognitive science. *Cognitive Science* 22: 295–318.

Bechtel, W., and Abrahamsen, A. (1991). *Connectionism and the Mind—An Introduction to Parallel Processing in Networks.* Cambridge, MA: Blackwell.

Beckermann, A. (1977). *Gründe und Ursachen.* Kronberg: Scriptor.

Beckermann, A. (1979). Intentionale vs. kausale Handlungserklärungen. In H. Lenk, ed., *Handlungstheorien—interdisziplinär. Band 2. Zweiter Halbband.* München: Fink.

Beckermann, A. (1996). Is there a problem about intentionality? *Erkenntnis* 45: 1–23.

Beer, R. D. (2000). Dynamical approaches to cognitive science. *Trends in Cognitive Sciences* 4: 91–9.

Benson, D. F., and Greenberg, J. P. (1969). Visual Form Agnosia. *Archives of Neurology* 20: 82–9.

Berlucchi, G., and Aglioti, S. (1997). The body in the brain: neural bases of corporeal awareness. *Trends in Neurosciences* 20: 560–4.

Bermúdez, J. L. (1997). Reduction and the self. *Journal of Consciousness Studies* 4: 458–66.

Bermúdez, J. L. (1998). *The Paradox of Self-Consciousness.* Cambridge, MA: MIT Press.

Bermúdez, J. L., Marcel, A., and Eilan, N., eds. (1995). *The Body and the Self.* Cambridge, MA: MIT Press.

Berrios, G. E., and Luque, R. (1995). Cotard's syndrome: Analysis of 100 cases. *Acta Psychiatrica Scandinavica* 91: 185–8.

Bieri, P. (1995). Why is consciousness puzzling? In Metzinger 1995a.

Bieri, P., ed. (1981). *Analytische Philosophie des Geistes.* Königstein: Hain.

Binkofski, F., Buccino, G., Dohle, C., Seitz, R. J., and Freund, H.-J. (1999). Mirror agnosia and mirror ataxia constitute different parietal lobe disorders. *Annals of Neurology* 46: 51–61.

Birnbacher, D. (1995). Artificial consciousness. In T. Metzinger, ed., *Conscious Experience*. Thorverton, UK: Imprint Academic.

Bisiach, E. (1988). The (haunted) brain and consciousness. In A. Marcel, and E. Bisiach, eds., *Consciousness in Contemporary Science*. Oxford: Oxford University Press.

Bisiach, E., and Luzzatti, C. (1978). Unilateral neglect, representational schema, and consciousness. *Cortex* 14: 129–33.

Bisiach, E., and Vallar, G. (1988). Hemineglect in humans. In F. Boller and J. Grafman, eds., *Handbook of Neuropsycology*. Vol. 1. New York: Elsevier.

Bisiach, E., Capitani, E. Luzzatti, C., and Perani, D. (1981). Brain and conscious representation of outside reality. *Neuropsychologia* 19: 543–52.

Bisiach, E., Luzatti, C., and Perani, D. (1979). Unilateral neglect, representational schema and consciousness. *Brain* 102: 609–18.

Bisiach, E., Rusconi, M. L., and Vallar, G. (1992). Remission of somatophrenic delusion through vestibular stimulation *Neuropsychologia* 29. 1029–31.

Blackmore, S. (1982a). *Beyond the Body: An Investigation of Out-of-the-Body-Experiences*. London: Granada.

Blackmore, S. (1982b). Out-of-body experiences, lucid dreams, and imagery: two surveys. *Journal of the American Society for Psychical Research* 4: 301–17.

Blackmore, S. (1984). A psychological theory of the out-of-body-experience. *Journal of Parapsychology* 48: 201–18.

Blackmore, S. J. (1986). Spontaneous and deliberate OBEs: A questionnaire survey. *Journal of the Society for Psychical Research*. 53: 218–24.

Blackmore, S. J. (1987). Where am I? Perspectives in imagery and the out-of-body experience. *Journal of Mental Imagery* 11: 53–66.

Blau, U. (1986). Die Paradoxie des Selbst. *Erkenntnis* 25: 177–96.

Block, N. (1978). Troubles with Functionalism. In Savage 1978, reprinted in N. Block, ed., *Readings in Philosophy of Psychology*. Vol. 1. Cambridge, MA: Methuen.

Block, N., ed. (1980). *Readings in Philosophy of Psychology*, Vol. 1. Cambridge, MA: Methuen.

Block, N. (1995). On a confusion about the function of consciousness. *Behavioral and Brain Sciences* 18: 227–87. Reprinted in Block et al. 1997.

Block, N. (1998). How not to find the neural correlate of consciousness. In S. Hameroff, A. Kaszniak, and A. Scott eds., *Toward a Science of Consciousness II*. Cambridge, MA: MIT Press.

Block, N., and Fodor, J. (1972). What psychological states are not. In N. Block, ed., *Readings in Philosophy of Psychology*. Vol. 1. Cambridge, MA: Harvard University Press.

Block, N., Flanagan, O., and Güzeldere, G., eds. (1997). *The Nature of Consciousness: Philosophical Debates*. Cambridge, MA: MIT Press.

Bodis-Wollner, I. (1977). Recovery from cerebral blindness: Evoked potential and psychophysical measurement. *Electroencephalography and Clinical Neurophysiology* 42: 178.

Boller, F., and Grafman, J., eds. (1988). *Handbook of Neuropsychology*. Vol. 1. New York: Elsevier.

Bonda, E., Petrides, M., Frey, S., and Evans, A. (1995). Neural correlates of mental transformations of the body in space. *Proceedings of the National Academy of Sciences U S A* 92: 11180–4.

Bonnet, C. (1769). *Essai Analytique sur les Facultés de l'Âme*. Vol. 11. Copenhagen/Geneva: Cl. Philibert.

Bovet, P., and Parnas, J. (1993). Schizophrenic delusions: A phenomenological approach. *Schizophrenia Bulletin* 19: 579–97.

Braude, S. E. (1991). *First Person Plural: Multiple Personality and the Philosophy of Mind*. London: Routledge.

Breen, N., Caine, D., Coltheart, M., Hendy, J., and Roberts, C. (2000) Towards an understanding of delusions of misidentification: Four case studies. In M. Coltheart and M. Davies, eds., *Pathologies of Belief*. Oxford: Blackwell.

Brent, P. J., Kennard, C., and Ruddock, K. H. (1994). Residual colour vision in a human hemianope: Spectral responses and colour discrimination. *Proceedings of the Royal Society of London. Series B: Biological Sciences* 256: 219–25.

Brentano, F. [1874](1973). *Psychology from an Empirical Standpoint*. Edited by Oskar Kraus. English edition edited by Linda McAlister. Translated by Antos, C. Rancurello, D. B. Terrell and Linda McAlister. London: Routledge & Kegan Paul / New York: Humanities Press.

Bressloff, P. C., Cowan, J. D., Golubitsky, M., Thomas, P. J., and Wiener, M. C. (2001). Geometric visual hallucinations, Euclidean symmetry and the functional architecture of striate cortex. *Philosophical Transactions of the Royal Society of London. Series B: Biological Sciences* 356: 299–330.

Brinck, I., and Gärdenfors, P. (1999). Representation and self-awareness in intentional agents. *Synthese* 118: 89–104.

Brion, S., and Jedynak, C.-P. (1972). Troubles du transfert interhémisphérique (callosal disconnection). A propos de trois observations de tumeurs du corps calleux. Le signe de la main étrangère. *Revue Neurologique* (Paris) 126: 257–66.

Brugger, P. (2000). From haunted brain to haunted science: A cognitive neuroscience view of paranormal pseudoscientific thought. In J. Houran and R. Lange, eds., *Spirited Exchanges: Multidisciplinary Perspectives on Hauntings and Poltergeists*. Jefferson, N. C.: McFarland.

Brugger, P., Agosti, R., Regard, M., Wieser, H.-G., and Landis, T. (1994). Heautoscopy, epilepsy, and suicide. *Journal of Neurology, Neurosurgery, and Psychiatry* 57: 838–9.

Brugger, P., Kollias, S. K., Müri, R. M., Crelier, G., Hepp-Reymond, M.-C., and Regard, M. (2000). Beyond remembering: Phantoms sensations of congenitally absent limbs. *Proceedings of the National Academy of Sciences U S A* 97: 6167–72.

Brugger, P., Regard, M., and Shiffrar, M. (2001). Hand movement observation in a person born without hands: Is body scheme innate? *Journal of Neurology, Neurosurgery, and Psychiatry* 70: 276.

Buccino, G., Binkofski, F., Fink, G. R., Fadiga, L., Fogassi, L, Gallese, V., Seitz, R. J., Zilles, K., Rizzolatti, G., and Freund, H.-J. (2001). Action observation activates premotor and parietal areas in a somatotopic manner: an fMIRI study. *European Journal of Neuroscience* 13: 400–4.

Burge, T. (1979). Individualism and the mental. *Midwest Studies in Philosophy* 4: 73–121.

Burge, T. (1995). Zwei Arten von Bewußtsein. In T. Metzinger, ed., *Bewußtsein-Beiträge ans der Gegenwartsphilosophie*. Paderborn: mentis.

Cahill, C., and Frith, C. (1996). False perceptions or false beliefs? Hallucinations or delusions in schizophrenia. In P. W. Halligan and J. C. Marshall, eds., *Method in Madness*: Case studies in cognitive neuropsychiatry. Hove, UK: Psychology Press.

Campbell, J. (1999). Schizophrenia, the space of reasons, and thinking as a motor process. *The Monist* 82: 609–25.

Campbell, K. K. (1971). *Body and Mind*. New York: Doubleday Anchor.

Carpenter, W. B. (1875). *Principles of Mental Physiology*. London: Routledge.

Castañeda, H. N. (1966). »He«: A study on the logic of self-consciousness. *Ratio* 8: 130–57.

Chalmers, D. J. (1995a). Facing up to the problem of consciousness. *Journal of Consciousness Studies*. 2: 200–19.

Chalmers, D. J. (1995b). Absent qualia, fading qualia, dancing qualia. In T. Metzinger, ed., *Conscious Experience*. Thorverton, UK: Imprint Academic.

Chalmers, D. J. (1997). Availability: The cognitive basis of experience? In N. Block, O. Flanagan, and G. Güzeldere, eds., *The Nature of Consciousness: Philosophical Debates*. Cambridge, MA: MIT Press.

Chalmers, D. J. (1998). On the search for the neural correlate of consciousness. In S. Hameroff, A. Kaszniak, and A. Scott, eds., *Toward a Science of Consciousness II*. Cambridge, MA: MIT Press.

Chalmers, D. J. (2000).What is a neural correlate of consciousness? In T. Metzinger, ed., *Neural Correlates of Consciousness—Empirical and Conceptual Questions*. Cambridge, MA: MIT Press.

Chiel, H. J., and Beer, R. D. (1997). The brain has a body: Adaptive behavior emerges from interactions of nervous system, body and environment. *Trends in Neurosciences* 20: 553–7.

Chisholm, R. (1981). *The First Person*. Minneapolis: University of Minnesota Press.

Chugani, H. T. (1999). Metabolic imaging: A window on brain development and plasticity. *Neuroscientist* 5: 29–40.

Churchland, P. M. (1981). Eliminative materialism and the propositional attitudes. *Journal of Philosophy* 78: 67–90.

Churchland, P. M. (1986). Some reductive strategies in cognitive neurobiology. *Mind* 95: 279–309.

Churchland, P. M. (1989). *A Neurocomputational Perspective*. Cambridge, MA: MIT Press.

Churchland, P. M. (1995). *The Engine of Reason, the Seat of the Soul: A Philosophical Journey into the Brain*. Cambridge, MA: MIT Press.

Churchland, P. M. (1996). The rediscovery of light. *Journal of Philosophy* 1993: 211–28.

Churchland, P. M. (1998), Conceptual similarity across sensory and neural diversity: The Fodor/Lepore challenge answered. *Journal of Philosophy* 65: 5–32.

Churchland, P. M. Neurosemantics: On the mapping of minds and the portrayal of worlds. Unpublished manuscript.

Churchland, P. S. (1986). *Neurophilosophy: Toward a Unified Understanding of the Mind-Brain*. Cambridge, MA: MIT Press.

Churchland, P. S. (1988). Reduction and the neurobiological basis of consciousness. In A. Marcel and E. Bisiach, eds., *Consciousness in Contemporary Science*. Oxford: Oxford University Press.

Clark, A. (1989). *Microcognition—Philosophy, Cognitive Science, and Parallel Distributed Processing*. Cambridge, MA: MIT Press.

Clark, A. (1993). *Associative Engines*. Cambridge, MA: MIT Press.

Clark, A. (1997a). The dynamical challenge. *Cognitive Science* 21: 461–81.

Clark, A. (1997b). *Being There*. Cambridge, MA: MIT Press.

Clark, A. (1999). An embodied cognitive science? *Trends in Cognitive Sciences* 3: 345–51.

Clark, Austen. (1993). *Sensory Qualities*. Oxford: Oxford University Press.

Clark, Austen. (2000). *A Theory of Sentience*. Oxford: Oxford University Press.

Clark, A., and Chalmers, D. (1998). The extended mind. *Analysis* 58: 7–19.

Clark, S. R. L. (1993). Minds, memes, and rhetoric. *Inquiry* 36: 3–16.

Cleeremans, A., ed. (2002). *The Unity of Consciousness: Binding, Integration, and Dissociations*. Oxford: Oxford University Press.

Cleeremans, A. (forthcoming). *Mechanisms of Implicit Learning: Connectionist Models of Sequence Processing*. Cambridge, MA: MIT Press.

Cohen, W. (1957). Spatial and textural characteristics of the Ganzfeld. *American Journal of Psychology* 70: 403–10.

Cohen, W. (1958). Color perception in the chromatic Ganzfeld. *American Journal of Psychology* 71: 390–4.

Cole, J. (1995). *Pride and a Daily Marathon*. Cambridge, MA: MIT Press.

Cole, J. (1997). On "being faceless": Selfhood and facial embodiment. *Journal of Consciousness Studies* 4: 467–84.

Cole, J. (1998). *About Face*. Cambridge, MA: MIT Press.

Cole, J., and Paillard, J. (1995). Living without touch and peripheral information about body position and movement: Studies with deafferented subjects. In J. L. Bermúdez, A. Marcel, and N. Eilan, eds., *The Body and the Self*. Cambridge, MA: MIT Press.

Coltheart, M., and Davies, M., eds. (2000). *Pathologies of Belief*. Oxford: Blackwell.

Conant, R. C., and Ashby, W. R. (1970). Every good regulator of a system must be a model of that system. *International Journal of Systems Science* 2: 89–97. Reprinted in G. J. Klir, ed. (1991), *Facets of System Science*. New York: Plenum Press.

Cooney, B. (1979). The neural basis of self-consciousness. *Nature and System*, 1: 16–31.

Cotard, J. (1880). Du délire hypocondriaque dans une form grave de la mélancolie anxieuse. *Annales Médico-Psychologiques* 38: 168–70.

Cotard, J. (1882). Du délire des négations. *Archives de Neurologie* 4: 152–70, 282–95.

Courtney, S. M., Petit, L., Haxby, J. V., and Ungerleider L. G. (1998). The role of prefrontal cortex in working memory: Examining the contents of consciousness. *Philosophical Transactions of the Royal Society of London B* 353: 1819–28.

Cowey, A. (1979). Cortical maps and visual perception. *Quarterly Journal of Experimental Psychology* 31: 1.

Cowey, A., and Heywood, A. H. (1997). Cerebral achromatopsia: Colour blindness despite wavelength processing. *Trends in Cognitive Sciences*, 1: 133–9.

Craik, F. I. M., Moroz, T. M., Moscovitch, M., Stuss, D. T., Winocur, G., Tulving, E., and Kapur, S. (1999). In search of the self: A positron emision tomography study. *Psychological Science* 10: 26–34.

Craik, K. J. W. (1943). *The Nature of Explanation*. Cambridge: Cambridge University Press.

Crane, H., and Piantanida, T. P. (1983). On seeing reddish green and yellowish blue. *Science* 221: 1078–80.

Crick, F., and Mitchison, G. (1983). The function of dream sleep. *Nature* 304: 111–4.

Crick, F. H. C., and Koch, C. (1990). Toward a neurobiological theory of consciousness. *Seminars in the Neurosciences* 2: 263–75.

Crick, F. H. C., and Koch, C. (2000). The unconscious homunculus. In T. Metzinger, ed., *Neural Correlates of Consciousness—Empirical and Conceptual Questions*. Cambridge, MA: MIT Press.

Critchley, M. (1953). *The Parietal Lobes*. New York: Hafner Press.

Cruse, H. (1999). Feeling our body—The basis of cognition? *Evolution and Cognition* 5: 162–73.

Cruse, H., Dean, J., and Ritter, H. (1998). *Die Entdeckung der Intelligenz oder Können Ameisen denken?* Munich: Beck.

Cummins, R. (1989). *Meaning and Mental Representation*. Cambridge, MA: MIT Press.

Damasio, A. R. (1987). Agnosia. In G. Adelmann, ed., *Encyclopedia of Neuroscience*. Vol. 1. Bos Birkhäser.

Damasio, A. R. (1994). *Descartes' Error*. New York: Putnam/Grosset.

Damasio, A. R. (1999). *The Feeling of What Happens: Body and Emotion in the Making of Consciousness*. New York: Harcourt Brace.

Damasio, A. R. (2000). A neurobiology for consciousness. In T. Metzinger, ed., *Neural Correlates of Consciousness—Empirical and Conceptual Questions*. Cambridge, MA: MIT Press.

Damasio, A. R., and Damasio, H. (1996a). Images and subjectivity: Neurobiological trials and tribulations. In R. N. McCauley, ed., *The Churchlands and their Critics*. Cambridge, MA: Blackwell.

Damasio, A. R., and Damasio, H. (1996b). Making images and creating subjectivity. In R. Llinás and S. Churchland, eds., *The Mind-Brain Continuum*. Cambridge, MA: MIT Press.

Damasio, A. R., Damasio, H., and van Hoesen, G. B. (1982). Prosopagnosia: Anatomic basis at behavioral mechanisms. *Neurology* 32: 331–41.

Damasio, A. R., Grabowski, T. J., Bechara, A., Damasio, H., Ponto, L. L. B., Parvizi, J., and Hichwa, R. D. (2000). Subcortical and cortical brain activity during the feeling of self-generated emotions. *Nature Neuroscience* 3: 1–8.

Daprati, E., Franck, N., Georgieff, N., Proust, J., Pacherie, E., Dalery, J., and Jeannerod, M. (1997). Looking for the agent: An investigation into consciousness of action and self-consciousness in schizophrenic patients. *Cognition* 65: 71–86.

Davidson, D. (1970). Mental events. In L. Forster and J. W. Swanson, eds., *Experience and Theory*. Amherst: University of Massachusetts Press.

Davidson, D. (1987). Knowing one's own mind. *In Proceedings and Addresses of the American Philosophical Association* 60: p. 46.

Davies, M., and Humphreys, G., eds. (1993) *Consciousness: Psychological and Philosophical Essays*. Oxford: Basil Blackwell.

Davies, M., Coltheart, M., Langdon, R., and Breen, N. (2001). Monothematic delusions: Towards a two-factor account. In C. Hoerl, ed., *On Understanding and Explaining Schizophrenia*. Special issue 8, *Philosophy, Psychiatry and Psychology*.

Davis, K. D., Kiss, Z. H. T., Luo, L., Tasker, R. R., Lozano, A. M., and Dostrovsky, J. O. (1998). Phantom sensations generated by thalamic microstimulation. *Nature* 391: 385–7.

de Morsier, G. (1967). Le syndrome de Charles Bonnet. Hallucinations visuelles sans déficience mentale. *Annales Médico-Psychologiques* 125: 677–702.

Decety, J., Grèzes, J., Costes, N., Perani, D., Jeannerod, M., Procyk, E., Grassi, E., and Fazio, F. (1997). Brain activity during observation of actions. Influence of action content and subject's strategy. *Brain* 120: 1763–77.

Dehaene, S., and Naccache, L. (2001). Towards a cognitive neuroscience of consciousness: Basic evidence and a workspace framework. *Cognition* 79: 1–37.

Delacour, J. (1997). Neurobiology of consciousness: An overview. *Behavioural Brain Research* 85: 127–41.

Della Sala, S., Marchetti, C., and Spinnler, H. (1991). Right sided anarchic (alien) hand: A longitudinal study. *Neuropsychologia* 29: 1113–27.

Della Sala, S., Marchetti, C., and Spinnler, H. (1994). The anarchic hand: A fronto-mesial sign. In F. Boller and J. Grafman, eds., *Handbook of Neuropsychology*. Vol. 9. Amsterdam: Elsevier.

Dennett, D. C. (1969). *Content and Consciousness*. London: Routledge & Kegan Paul.

Dennett, D. C. (1976). Are Dreams Experiences? *Philosophical Review* 73: 151–71.

Dennett, D. C. (1978a). *Brainstorms: Philosophical Essays on Mind and Psychology*. Montgomery, VT: Bradford Books.

Dennett, D. C. (1978b). Conditions of personhood. In D. C. Dennett, ed., *Brainstorms: Philosophical Essays on Mind and Psychology*. Montgomery, VT: Bradford Books. Reprinted from A. O. Rorty, ed. (1976), *The Identities of Persons*. University of California Press.

Dennett, D. C. (1987a). Intentional systems in cognitive ethology: The "Panglossian paradigm" defended. In D. C. Dennett, *The Intertional Stance*. Cambridge, MA: MIT Press.

Dennett, D. C. (1987b). *The Intentional Stance*. Cambridge, MA: MIT Press.

Dennett, D. C. (1988). Quining qualia. In A. Marcel and E. Bisiach, eds., *Consciousness in Contemporary Science*. Oxford: Oxford University Press.

Dennett, D. C. (1991). *Consciousness Explained*. Boston: Little, Brown.

Dennett, D. C. (1995). *Darwin's Dangerous Idea*. New York: Simon & Schuster.

Dennett, D. C. (1998). Postscript. In D. C. Dennett, ed., *Brainchildren—Essays on Designing Minds*. Cambridge MA: MIT Press.

Dennett, D. C. (2001). Are we explaining consciousness yet? *Cognition* 79: 221–37.

Dennett, D. C., and Humphrey, N. (1989). Speaking for ourselves: An assessment of multiple personality disorder. *Raritan: A Quarterly Review*, 9: 68–98.

Descartes, R. ([1642]1911). *Meditations on a First Philosophy*. (Translated by E. S. Haldane and G. R. T. Ross) Cambridge: Cambridge University Press.

Devinsky, O., Feldmann, E., Burrowes, K., and Bromfield, E. (1989). Autoscopic phenomena with seizures. *Archives of Neurology* 46: 1080–8.

Dierks, T., Linden, D. E. J., Jandl, M., Formisano, E., Goebel, R., Lanfermann, H., and Singer, W. (1999). Activation of Heschl's gyrus during auditory hallucinations. *Neuron* 22: 615–21.

di Pellegrino, G., Fadiga, L., Fogassi, L., Gallese V., and Rizzolatti G. (1992) Understanding motor events: A neurophysiological study. *Experimental Brain Research* 91: 176–180.

Dominy, N. C., and Lucas, P. W. (2001). Ecological importance of trichromatic vision to primates. *Nature* 410: 363–6.

Dreisbach, C. (2000). Dreams in the history of philosophy. *Dreaming* 10: 31–41.

Dretske, F. (1969). *Seeing and Knowing*. Chicago: Chicago University Press.

Dretske, F. (1986). Misrepresentation. In R. Bodgan, ed. *Belief*. Oxford: Oxford University Press.

Dretske, F. (1988). *Explaining Behavior—Reasons in a World of Causes*. Cambridge, MA: London: MIT Press.

Dretske, F. (1995). *Naturalizing the Mind*. Cambridge, MA: MIT Press.

Driver, J., and Mattingley, J. B. (1998). Parietal neglect and visual awareness. *Nature Neuroscience* 1: 17–22.

Driver, J., and Vuilleumier, P. (2001). Perceptual awareness and its loss in unilateral neglect and extinction. *Cognition* 79: 39–88.

Düzel, E., Yonelinas, A. P., Mangun, G. R., Heinze, H.-J., and Tulving, E. (1997). Event-related brain potential correlates of two states of conscious awareness in memory. *Proceedings of the National Academy of Sciences U S A* 94: 5973–8.

Dyken, M. E., Lin-Dyken, D. C., Seaba, P., and Yamada, T. (1995). Violent sleep-related behavior leading to subdural hemorrhage. *Archives of Neurology* 52: 318–21.

Edelman, G. M. (1989). *The Remembered Present—A Biological Theory of Consciousness*. New York: Basic Books.

Edelman, G. M., and Tononi, G. (2000a). Reentry and the dynamic core: Neural correlates of conscious experience. In T. Metzinger, ed., *Neural Correlates of Consciousness—Empirical and Conceptual Questions*. Cambridge, MA: MIT Press.

Edelman, G. M., and Tononi, G. (2000b). *A Universe of Consciousness. How Matter Becomes Imagination*. New York: Basic Books.

Eliasmith, C. (2000). How Neurons Mean: A Neurocomputational Theory of Representational Content. Ph. D. dissn., Washington University in St. Louis.

Ellis, S. R. (1995). Origins and elements of virtual environments. In W. Barfield and T. A. Furness III, eds., *Virtual Environments and Advance Interface Design*. New York: Oxford University Press.

Engel, A. K., and Singer, W. (2000). Binding and the neural correlates of consciousness. *Trends in Cognitive Sciences* 5: 16–25.

Enoch, M. D., and Trethowan, W. H. (1991). *Uncommon Psychiatric Syndromes*. Third edition. Oxford: Butterworth-Heinemann.

Ermentrout, G. B., and Cowan, J. D. (1979). A mathematical theory of visual hallucination patterns. *Biological Cybernetics* 34: 137–50.

Esken, F., and Heckmann, H.-D., eds. (1998). *Bewußtsein und Repräsentation*. Paderborn, Germany: Schöningh.

Fadiga, L., Fogassi, L., Pavesi, G., and Rizzolatti, G. (1995). Motor facilitation during action observation: A magnetic stimulation study. *Journal of Neurophysiology* 73: 2608–11.

Fahay, T. A. (1988). The diagnosis of multiple personality disorder: A critical review. *British Journal of Psychiatry* 153: 597–606.

Farah, M. (1990). *Visual Agnosia: Disorders of Object Recognition and What They Tell Us about Normal Vision*. Cambridge, MA: MIT Press.

Feinberg, I. (1978). Efference copy and corollary discharge: Implications for thinking and its disorders. *Schizophrenia Bulletin* 4: 636–40.

Feinberg, T. E. (1997). The irreducible perspectives of consciousness. *Seminars in Neurology* 17: 85–93.

Feinberg, T. E. (2001). *Altered Egos—How the Brain Creates the Self*. Oxford: Oxford University Press.

ffytche, D. H. (2000). Imaging conscious vision. In T. Metzinger, ed., *Neural Correlates of Consciousness—Empirical and Conceptual Questions*. Cambridge, MA: MIT Press.

ffytche, D. H., and Howard, R. J. (1999). The perceptual consequences of visual loss: "Positive" pathologies of vision. *Brain* 122: 1247–60.

ffytche, D. H., Howard, R. J., Brammer, M. J., David, A., Woodruff, P., and Williams, S. (1998). The anatomy of conscious vision: An fMRI study of visual hallucinations. *Nature Neuroscience* 1: 738–42.

Flanagan, O. (1992). *Consciousness Reconsidered*. Cambridge, MA: MIT Press.

Flanagan, O. (1994). Multiple identity, character transformation, and self-reclamation. In G. Graham and G. L. Stephens, eds., *Philosophical Psychopathology*. Cambridge, MA: MIT Press.

Flanagan, O. (1995). Deconstructing dreams: The spandrels of sleep. *Journal of Philosophy* 112: 5–27.

Flanagan, O. (1997). Prospects for a unified theory of consciousness or, What dreams are made of. In J. D. Cohen and J. W. Schooler, eds., *Scientific Approaches to Consciousness*. Mahwah, NJ: Lawrence Erlbaum.

Flohr, H. (2000). NMDA-receptor-complex–mediated computational processes as a candidate for the NCC. In T. Metzinger, ed., *Neural Correlates of Consciousness—Empirical and Conceptual Questions*. Cambridge, MA: MIT Press.

Fluornoy, T. (1902). Le cas de Charles Bonnet. Hallucinations visuelles chéz a un vieillard operé de la cataracte. *Archives of Psychology* (Geneva) 1: 1–23.

Fodor, J. A. (1975). *The Language of Thought*. Cambridge, MA: Harvard University Press.

Fodor, J. A. (1983). *The Modularity of Mind*. Cambridge, MA: MIT Press.

Fodor, J. A. (1984). Semantics, Wisconsin Style. *Synthese* 59: 231–50.

Fodor, J. A., and LePore, E. (1996). Paul Churchland and state-space semantics. In R. N. McCauley, ed., *The Churchlands and Their Critics*. Oxford: Basil Blackwell.

Förstl, H., Almeida, O. P., Owen, A., Burns, A., and Howard, R. (1991). Psychiatric, neurological and medical aspects of misidentifications syndromes: A review of 260 cases. *Psychological Medicine* 21: 905–10.

Fourneret, P., Paillard, J., Lamarre, Y., Cole, J., and Jeannerod, M. (2002). Lack of conscious recognition of one's own actions in a haptically deafferented patient. *Neuroreport* 13: 541–7.

Fox, O. (1962). *Astral Projection*. New Hyde Park, NY: University Books.

Frank, M. (1991). *Selbstbewußtsein und Selbsterkenntnis*. Stuttgart: Reclam.

Frankfurt, H. (1971). Freedom of the will and the concept of a person. *Journal of Philosophy* 68: 5–20.

Franks, N. P., and Lieb, W. R. (2000). An assessment of the role of NMDA receptor function in consciousness: What can we learn from the mechanisms of general anesthesia? In T. Metzinger, ed., *Neural Correlates of Consciousness—Empirical and Conceptual Questions*. Cambridge, MA: MIT Press.

Freud, S. (1947). *Eine Schwierigkeit der Psychoanalyse*. In Gesammelte Werke. Vol. 12 (*Werke aus den Jahren 1917–1920*). Frankfurt: Fischer.

Fries, P., Neuenschwander, S., Engel, A. K., Goebel, R., and Singer W. (2001). Rapid feature selective neuronal synchronization through correlated latency shifting. *Nature Neuroscience* 4: 194–200.

Frith, C. D. (1992). Consciousness, information processing, and the brain. *Journal of Psychopharmacology* 6: 436–40.

Frith, C. D. (1996). The role of prefrontal cortex in self-consciousness: The case of auditory hallucinations. *Philosophical Transactions of the Royal Society of London. Series B: Biological Sciences* 351: 1505–12.

Frith, C. D., Blakemore, S.-J., and Wolpert, D. M. (2000). Abnormalities in the awareness and control of action. *Philosophical Transactions of the Royal Society of London. Series B: Biological Sciences* 355: 1771–88.

Frith, C. D., Perry, R., and Lumer, E. (1999). The neural correlates of conscious experience: An experimental framework. *Trends in Cognitive Sciences* 3: 105–14.

Furness, T. A., III, and Barfield, W. (1995). Introduction to virtual environments and advanced interface design. In W. Barfield and T. A. Furness, eds., *Virtual Environments and Advanced Interface Design*. New York: Oxford University Press.

Gackenbach, J. (1978). A Personality and Cognitive Style Analysis of Lucid Dreaming. Abstract in *Dissertation Abstracts International*, 39: 3487B, University Microfilms No. 79-01560.

Gackenbach, J. (1988). The psychological content of lucid dreams. In J. Gackenbach and S. LaBerge, eds., *Conscious Mind, Sleeping Brain*. New York: Plenum Press.

Gackenbach, J., and LaBerge, S., eds. (1988). *Conscious Mind, Sleeping Brain*. New York: Plenum Press.

Gackenbach, J., Curren, R., and Cutler, G. (1983). Presleep determinants and postsleep results of lucid versus vivid dreams. *Lucidity Letter* 2: 55.

Gallagher, S. (1986). Body image and body schema: A conceptual clarification. *Journal of Mind and Behavior* 7: 541–54.

Gallagher, S. (1995). Body schema and intentionality. In J. L. Bermúdez, A. Marcel, and N. Eilan, eds., *The Body and the Self* Cambridge, MA: MIT Press.

Gallagher, S., and Cole, J. (1995). Body schema and body image in a deafferented subject. *Journal of Mind and Behavior* 16: 369–90.

Gallagher, S., and Meltzoff, A. N. (1996). The earliest sense of self and others: Merleau-Ponty and recent developmental studies. *Philosophical Psychology* 9: 211–33.

Gallagher, S., Butterworth, G. E., Lew, A., and Cole, J. (1998). Hand-mouth coordination, congenital absence of limb, and evidence for innate body schemas. *Brain and Cognition* 38: 53–65.

Gallese, V. (2000). The inner *sense* of action: Agency and motor-representations. *Journal of Consciousness Studies* 7: 23–40.

Gallese, V. (2001). The "shared manifold" hypothesis: From mirror neurons to empathy. *Journal of Consciousness Studies* 8: 33–50.

Gallese, V., and Goldman, A. (1998). Mirror neurons and the simulation theory of mind-reading. *Trends in Cognitive Sciences* 2: 493–501.

Gallese, V., Ferrari, P. F., Kohler, E., and Fogassi, L. (2002). The eyes, the hand, and the mind: behavioral and neurophysiological aspects of social cognition. In C. Allen and M. Bekoff, eds., *The Cognitive Animal*. Cambridge, MA: MIT Press.

Gallese, V., Fogassi, L., Fadiga, L., and Rizzolatti, G. (2001). Action representation and the inferior parietal lobule. In W. Prinz and B. Hommel, eds., *Attention and Performance XIX*. Oxford: Oxford University Press.

Gallup, G. G., Jr. (1970). Chimpanzees: Self-recognition. *Science* 167: 86–7.

Gallup, G. G., Jr. (1991). Toward a comparative psychology of self-awareness: Species limitations and cognitive consequences. In J. Strauss and G. R. Goethals, eds., *The Self: Interdisciplinary Approaches*. New York: Springer-Verlag.

Gallup, G. G., Jr. (1997). On the rise and fall of self-conception in primates. In J. G. Snodgrass and R. L. Thompson, eds., *The Self across Psychology—Self-Recognition, Self-Awareness, and the Self Concept. Annals of the New York Academy of Sciences* 818: 4–17.

Gärdenfors, P. (1995). Konzeptuelle Räume. *Kognitionswissenschaft* 4: 185–8.

Gärdenfors, P. (2000). *Conceptual Spaces. The Geometry of Thought*. Cambridge, MA: MIT Press.

Garfield, P. (1975). Psychological concomitants of the lucid dream state. *Sleep Research* 4: 183.

Georgieff, N., and Jeannerod, M. (1998). Beyond consciousness of external reality: A "who" system for consciousness and action and self-consciousness. *Consciousness and Cognition* 7: 465–77.

Gerrans, P. (1999). Delusional misidentification as subpersonal disintegration. *The Monist* 82: 590–608.

Gerrans, P. (2000). Refining the explanation of Cotard's delusion. In M. Coltheart and M. Davies, eds., *Pathologies of Belief*. Oxford: Blackwell.

Geschwind, D. H., Iacoboni, M., Mega, M. S., Zaidel, D. W., Clughesy, T. and Zaidel, E. (1995). Alien hand syndrome: Interhemispheric disconnection due to lesion in the midbody of the corpus callosum. *Neurology* 45: 802–8.

Gold, I., and Hohwy, J. (2000). Rationality and schizophrenic delusion. In M. Coltheart and M. Davies, eds., *Pathologies of Belief*. Oxford: Blackwell.

Goldberg, G., Mayer, N. H., and Toglia, U. T. (1981). Medial frontal cortex infarction and the alien hand sign. *Archives of Neurology* 38: 683–6.

Goldstein, K. (1908). Zur Lehre der motorischen Apraxie. *Journal für Psychologie und Neurologie* 11: 169–87.

Goodale, M. A., and Milner, A. D. (1992). Separate visual pathways for perception and action. *Trends in Neuroscience* 15: 20–5.

Görnitz, T., Ruhnau, E., and Weizsacker, C. F. (1992). Temporal asymmetry as precondition of experience. The foundation of the arrow of time. *International Journal of Theoretical Physics* 31: 37–46.

Goschke, T., and Koppelberg, D. (1990). Connectionist representation, semantic compositionality, and the instability of concept structure. *Psychological Research* 52: 253–70.

Grafton, S. T., Arbib, M. A., Fadiga, L., and Rizzolatti, G. (1996). Localization of grasp representations in humans by positron emission tomography. 2. Observation compared with imagination. *Experimental Brain Research* 112: 103–11.

Gray, C. M. (1994). Synchronous oscillations in neuronal systems: Mechanisms and functions. *Journal of Computational Neuroscience* 1: 11–38.

Green, C. (1968). *Lucid Dreams*. Oxford: Institute of Psychophysical Research.

Green, M. B. (1979). The grain objection. *Philosophy of Science* 46: 559–89.

Gregory, R. L. (1997). Visual illusions classified. *Trends in Cognitive Sciences* 1: 190–4.

Grèzes, J., Costes, N., and Decety, J. (1998). Top-down effect of the strategy on the perception of biological motion: A PET investigation. *Cognitive Neuropsychology* 15: 553–82.

Grush, R. (1997). The architecture of representation. *Philosophical Psychology* 10: 5–23.

Grush, R. (1998). Wahrnehmung, Vorstellung, und die sensomotorische Schleife. In F. Esken and H.-D. Heckmann, eds., Bewußtsein und Repräsentation. Paderborn, Germany: Schöningh.

Grush, R. (2000). Self, world and space: The meaning and mechanisms of ego- and allocentric spatial representation. *Brain and Mind* 1: 59–92.

Grush, R. (2002). Manifolds, coordination, imagination, objectivity. UCSD Philosophy Department Tech Report UCSDPHI-2002-03.

Gunderson, K. (1974). The texture of mentality. In R. Bambrough, ed., *Wisdom—Twelve Essays*. Oxford: Oxford University Press.

Gur, M. (1989). Color and brightness fade-out in the Ganzfeld is wavelength dependent. *Vision Research* 29: 1335–41.

Gustafson, D. F., and Tapscott, B. L., eds. (1979). *Body, Mind, and Method*. Dordrecht, Netherlands: D. Reidel.

Güzeldere, G. (1995). Is consciousness the perception of what passes in one's own mind? In T. Metzinger, ed., *Conscious Experience*. Thorverten, UK: Imprint Academic.

Gybels, J. M., and Sweet, W. H. (1989). Stereotactic mesencephalotomy. In J. M. Gybels and W. H. Sweet, eds., *Neurosurgical Treatment of Persistent Pain*. Basel: Karger.

Haggard, P., and Eimer, M. (1999). On the relation between brain potentials and the awareness of voluntary movements. *Experimental Brain Research* 126: 128–33.

Haggard, P., and Magno, E. (1999). Localising awareness of action with transcranial magnetic stimulation. *Experimental Brain Research* 127: 102–7.

Haggard, P., Clark, S., and Kalogeras, J. (2002). Voluntary action and conscious awareness. *Nature Neuroscience* 5: 382–5.

Haggard, P., Newman, C., and Magno, E. (1999). On the perceived time of voluntary actions. *British Journal of Psychology* 90: 291–303.

Halligan, P. W., and Marshall, J. C. (1995). Supernumerary phantom limb after right hemispheric stroke [letter]. *Journal of Neurology, Neurosurgery, and Psychiatry* 59: 341–2.

Halligan, P. W., and Marshall, J. C. (1996). The wise prophet makes sure of the event first: Hallucinations, amnesia, and delusions. In P. W. Halligan and J. C. Marshall, eds., *Method in Madness: Case Studies in Cognitive Neuropsychiatry*. Hove, UK: Psychology Press, an imprint of Erlbaum (UK) Tailor & Franciys Ltd.

Halligan, P. W., and Marshall, J. C. (1998). Neglect of awareness. *Consciousness and Cognition* 7: 356–80.

Halsey, R. M., and Chapanis, A. (1951). Number of absolutely identifiable hues. *Journal of the Optical Society of America* 41: 1057–8.

Hardcastle, V. G. (2000). How to understand the N in NCC. In T. Metzinger, ed., *Neural Correlates of Consciousness—Empirical and Conceptual Questions*. Cambridge, MA: MIT Press.

Hari, R., Hänninen, R., Mäkinen, T., Jousmäki, V., Forss, N., Seppä, M., and Salonen, O. (1998). Three hands: Fragmentation of human bodily awareness. *Neuroscience Letters* 240: 131–4.

Harman, G. (1990). The intrinsic quality of experience. In J. Tomberlin, ed., *Philosophical Perspectives*. Vol. 4. *Action Theory and Philosophy of Mind*. Atascadero, CA: Ridgeview.

Hartmann, J. A., and Wolz, W. A. (1991). Denial of visual perception. *Brain and Cognition* 16: 29–40.

Hecaen, H., and Albert, M. L. (1978). *Human Neuropsychology*. New York: Wiley.

Heeter, C. (1992). *Being* there: The subjective experience of presence. *Presence* 1: 262–71.

Heil, J., and Mele, A., eds. (1993). *Mental Causation*. Oxford: Clarendon Press.

Heilman, K. M., Barrett, A. M., and Adair, J. C. (1998). Possible mechanisms of anosognosia: A defect in self-awareness. *Philosophical Transactions of the Royal Society of London, Series B: Biological Sciences* 353: 1903–9.

Heimann, H. (1989). Zerfall des Bewußtseins in der Psychose. In E. Pöppel, ed., *Gehirn und Bewußtsein*. Weinheim Germany: VCH Verlagssesellschaft.

Helm, G. (1991). *Symbolische und konnektionistische Modelle der menschlichen Informationsverarbeitung*. Berlin: Springer-Verlag.

Helmholtz, H. von (1925). *Physiological Optics*. Vol. 3. Edited by J. P. C. Southall. Menasha, WI: Banta.

Herrmann, T. (1988). *Mentale Repräsentation—ein erklärungsbedürftiger Begriff*. Arbeiten der Forschungs-gruppe Kognition am Lehrstuhl III der Universität Mannheim. Report No. 42.

Hill, A. (1999). Phantom limb pain: A review of the literature on attributes and potential mechanisms. *Journal of Pain and Symptom Management* 17: 125–42.

Hirstein, W., and Ramachandran, V. S. (1997). Capgras syndrome: A novel probe for understanding the neural representation of the identity and familiarity of persons. *Proceedings of the Royal Society of London. Series B: Biological Sciences* 264: 437–44.

Hobson, J. A. (1988). *The Dreaming Brain*. New York: Basic Books.

Hobson, J. A. (1997). Consciousness as a state-dependent phenomenon. In J. D. Cohen and J. W. Schooler, eds., *Scientific Approaches to Consciousness*. Mahwah, NJ: Lawrence Erlbaum.

Hobson, J. A. (1999). *Dreaming as Delirium—How the Brain Goes out of Its Mind*. Cambridge MA: MIT Press. Originally published in 1994 as *The Chemistry of Conscious states: How the Brain Changes Its Mind*. Boston: Little, Brown.

Hobson, J. A., and McCarley, R. W. (1977). The brain as a dream-state generator: An activation-synthesis hypothesis of the dream process. *American Journal of Psychiatry* 134: 1335–48.

Hobson, J. A., Pace-Schott, E., and Stickgold, R. (2000). Dreaming and the brain: Toward a cognitive neuroscience of conscious states. *Behavioral and Brain Sciences* 23: 793–842.

Hochberg, J., Triebel, W., and Seaman, G. (1951). Color adaptation under conditions of homogeneous visual stimulation (Ganzfeld). *Journal of Experimental Psychology* 41: 153–9.

Holst, E. von, and Mittelstaedt, H. (1950). Das Reafferenzprinzip. *Naturwissenschaften* 37: 464–76.

Honderich, T. (1994). Seeing things. *Synthese* 98: 51–71.

Horgan, T., ed. (1983). Spindel Conference: Supervenience. *The Southern Journal of Philosophy* 22(Suppl).

Hull, J. (1992). *Touching the Rock*. New York: Random House.

Humphrey, N. (1992). *A History of the Mind. Evolution and the Birth of Consciousness*. New York: Simon & Schuster.

Hurvich, L. M. (1981). *Color Vision*. Sunderland, MA: Sinauer.

Iacoboni, M., Woods, R. P., Brass, M., Bekkering, H., Mazziotta, J. C., and Rizzolatti, G. (1999). Cortical mechanisms of imitation. *Science* 286: 2526–8.

Iriki, A., Tanaka, M., Obayashi, S., and Iwamura, Y. (2001). Self-images in the video monitor coded by monkey intraparietal neurons. *Neuroscience Research* 40: 163–73.

Irwin, H. (1985). *Flight of Mind*. Metuchen, NJ: Scarecrow Press.

Jack, A. I., and Shallice, T. (2001). Introspective physicalism as an approach to the science of consciousness. *Cognition* 79: 161–96.

Jackendoff, R. (1987). *Consciousness and the Computational Mind*. Cambridge, MA: MIT Press.

Jackson, F. (1982). Epiphenomenal qualia. *Philosophical Quarterly* 32: 127–36.

Jaeger, H. (1996). Dynamische Systeme in der Kognitionswissenschaft. *Kognitionswissenschaft* 5: 151–74.

Jakab, Z. (2000). The ineffability of qualia. *Consciousness and Cognition* 9: 329–51. (doi:10.1006/ccog.2000.0430)

Jeannerod, M. (1999). The 25th Bartlett Lecture. To act of not to act: Perspectives on the representation of action. *The Quarterly Journal of Experimental Psychology* 52A: 1–29.

Jennett, B., and Plum, F. (1972). Persistent vegetative state after brain damage. A syndrome in search of a name. *Lancet* 1: 734–7.

Johnson-Laird, P. N. (1983). *Mental Models: Towards a Cognitive Science of Language, Inference and Consciousness*. Cambridge: Cambridge University Press.

Johnson-Laird, P. N. (1988). A computational analysis of consciousness. In A. Marcel and E. Bisiach, eds., *Consciousness in Contemporary Science*. Oxford: Oxford University Press.

Johnson-Laird, P. N. (1989). Mental models. In M. L. Posner, ed., *Foundations of Cognitive Science*. Cambridge, MA: MIT Press.

Johnson-Laird, P. N. (1990). *Modelling the Mind*. Oxford: Clarendon Press.

Johnson-Laird, P. N. (1995). Mental models, deductive reasoning, and the brain. In M. Gazzaniga, ed., *The Cognitive Neurosciences*. Cambridge, MA: MIT Press.

Jouvet, M. (1999). *The Paradox of Sleep—The Story of Dreaming*. Cambridge: MIT Press.

Kahan, T. L., and LaBerge, S. (1994). Lucid dreaming as metacognition: Implications for cognitive science. *Consciousness and Cognition* 3: 246–64.

Kahn, D., and Hobson, J. A. (1993). Self-organization theory of dreaming. *Dreaming* 3: 151–78.

Kahn, D., Pace-Schott, E. F., and Hobson, J. A. (1997). Consciousness in waking and dreaming: The roles of neuronal oscillation and neuromodulation in determining similarities and differences. *Neuroscience* 78: 13–38.

Kamitami, Y., and Shimojo, S. (1999). Manifestation of scotomas created by transcranial magnetic stimulation of human visual cortex. *Nature Neuroscience* 2: 767–71.

Katz, J., and Melzack, R. (1990). Pain "memories" in phantom limbs: Review and clinical observations. *Pain* 43: 319–36.

Kelso, J. A. S. (1995). *Dynamic Patterns: The Self-Organization of Brain and Behavior.* Cambridge, MA: MIT Press.

Khurana, B. (2000). Face representation without conscious processing. In T. Metzinger, ed., *Neural Correlates of Consciousness—Empirical and Conceptual Questions.* Cambridge, MA: MIT Press.

Kilmer, W. (2001). A thalamo-cortical model of the executive attention system. *Biological Cybernetics* 84: 279–89.

Kim, J. (1978). Supervenience and nomological incommensurables. *American Philosophical Quarterly* 15: 149–56.

Kim, J. (1979). Causality, identity, and supervenience in the mind-body problem. *Midwest Studies in Philosophy* 4: 31–49.

Kim, J. (1982). Psychophysical supervenience. *Philosophical Studies* 41: 51–70.

Kim, J. (1984). Epiphenomenal and supervenient causation. *Midwest Studies in Philosophy* 9: 257–70.

Kim, J. (1985). Supervenience, determination and reduction. *Journal of Philosophy* 82: 616–8.

Kim, J. (1993). *Supervenience and Mind.* Cambridge: Cambridge University Press.

Kinsbourne, M. (1995). Awareness of one's own body: An attentional theory of its nature, development, and brain basis. In J. L. Bermúdez, A. Marcel, and N. Eilan, eds., *The Body and the Self.* Cambridge, MA: MIT Press.

Kircher, T., Senior, C., Phillips, M. L., Rabe-Hesketh, S., Benson, P. J., Bullmore, E. T., Brammer, M., Simmons, S., Bartels, M., and David, A. S. (2001). Recognizing one's own face. *Cognition* 78: B1–B5.

Kistler, W. M., Seitz, R., and van Hemmen, J. L. (1998). Modeling excitations in cortical tissue. *Physica D* 114: 273–95.

Kitchen, A., Denton, D., and Brent, L. (1996). Self-recognition and abstractional abilities in the common chimpanzee studied with distorting mirrors. *Proceedings of the National Academy of Sciences U S A* 93: 7405–8.

Klüver, H. (1967). *Mescal and the Mechanisms of Hallucination.* Chicago: University of Chicago Press.

Knauff, M. (1997). *Räumliches Wissen und Gedächtnis.* Wiesbaden, Germany: Deutscher Universitäts-Verlag.

Koestler, A. (1967). *The Ghost in the Machine.* New York: Macmillan.

Koffka, K. (1935). *Principles of Gestalt Psychology.* London: Lund Humphries.

Kolb, F. C., and Braun, J. (1995). Blindsight in normal observers. *Nature* 377: 336–8.

Kremer, S., Chassagnon, S., Hoffmann, D., Benabid, A. L., and Kahane, P. (2001). The cingulate hidden hand [letter]. *Journal of Neurology, Neurosurgery and Psychiatry* 70: 264–8.

Krill, A. E., Alpert, H. J., and Ostfield, A. M. (1963). Effects of a hallucinogenic agent in totally blind subjects. *Archives of Ophtalmology* 69: 180–5.

Kukla, R. (1992). Cognitive models and representation. *British Journal of Philosophy of Science* 43: 219–32.

Kurthen, M. (1990). Qualia, Sensa und absolute Prozesse. Zu W. Sellars' Kritik des psychocerebralen Reduktionismus. *Journal for General Philosophy of Science* 21: 25–46.

Laakso, A., and Cottrell, G. (1998). How can I know what you think?: Assessing representational similarity in neural systems. In *Proceedings of the Twentieth Annual Cognitive Science Conference*, Madison, WI. Mahwah, NJ: Lawrence Erlbaum.

LaBerge, D. (1995). *Attentional Processing: The Brain's Art of Mindfulness.* Cambridge, MA: Harvard University Press.

LaBerge, D. (1997). Attention, awareness, and the triangular circuit. *Consciousness and Cognition* 6: 149–81.

LaBerge, S. (1980a). Induction of lucid dreams. *Sleep Research* 9: 138.

LaBerge, S. (1980b). Lucid dreaming as a learnable skill: A case study. *Perceptual and Motor Skills* 51: 1039–41.

LaBerge, S. (1980c). Lucid Dreaming: An Exploratory Study of Consciousness during Sleep. Abstract in *Dissertation Abstracts International* 41: 1966B, University Microfilms No. 80-24691.

LaBerge, S. (1985). *Lucid Dreaming*. Los Angeles: Jeremy Tarcher.

LaBerge, S. (1988). Lucid dreaming in Western literature. In J. Gackenbach and S. LaBerge, eds., *Conscious Mind, Sleeping Brain*. New York: Plenum Press.

LaBerge, S. (1990). Psychophysiological studies of consciousness during sleep. In R. R. Bootzen, J. F. Kihlstrom, and D. L. Schacter, eds., *Sleep and Cognition*. Washington, DC: American Psychological Association.

LaBerge, S., and Gackenbach, J. (2000). Lucid dreaming. In E. Cardeña, S. J. Lynne and S. Krippner, eds., *Varieties of Anomalous Experience: Examining the Scientific Evidence*. Washington, DC: American Psychological Association.

LaBerge, S., and Rheingold, H. (1990). *Exploring the World of Lucid Dreaming*. New York: Ballantine.

LaBerge, S., Nagel, L., Dement, W., and Zarcone, V. (1981a). Lucid dreaming verified by volitional communication during REM sleep. *Perceptual and Motor Skills* 52: 727–32.

LaBerge, S., Nagel, L., Taylor, W., Dement, W., and Zarcone, V. (1981b). Psychophysiological correlates of the initiation of lucid dreaming. *Sleep Research* 10: 149.

Lacroix, R., Melzack, R., Smith, D., and Mitchell N. (1992). Multiple phantom limbs in a child. *Cortex* 28: 503–7.

Lanz, P. (1996). *Das phänomenale Bewußtsein: Eine Verteidigung*. Frankfurt: Vittorio Klostermann.

Leopold, D. A., and Logothetis, N. K. (1999). Multistable phenomena: Changing views in perception. *Trends in Cognitive Sciences* 3: 254–64.

Leuner, H.-C. (1981). *Halluzinogene*. Bern: Hans Huber.

Levine, J. (1995). Qualia: Intrinsic, relational, or what? In T. Metzinger, ed., *Conscious Experience*. Thorverton, UK: Imprint Academic.

Levine, M. (1984). The placement and misplacement of you-are-here maps. *Environment and Behavior* 16: 139–57.

Lewis, C. I. (1929). *Mind and the World Order*. New York: Scribner's.

Lewis, D. K. (1979). Attitudes de dicto and de se. *Philosophical Review* 88: 513–43.

Lewis, D. K. (1988). What experience teaches. In *Proceedings of the Russelian Society*. Sydney, Australia: University of Sydney. Reprinted in N. Block, O. Flanagan, and G. Güzeldere, eds., *The Nature Consciousness: Philosophical Debates*. Cambridge, MA: MIT Press.

Libermann, A. M., and Mattingly, I. G. (1985). The motor theory of speech perception revised. *Cognition* 21: 1–36.

Libet, B., Gleason, C. A., Wright, E. W., and Pearl, D. K. (1983). Time of conscious intention to act in relation to onset of cerebral activity (readiness-potential): The unconscious initiation of a freely voluntary act. *Brain* 106: 623–42.

Lipps, T. (1903). Einfühlung, innere Nachahmung und Organempfindung. *Archive der Psychologie* 1: 185–204.

Lishman, J. R., and Lee, D. N. (1973). The autonomy of visual kinaesthesis. *Perception* 2: 287–94.

Llinás, R., and Ribary, U. (1998). Temporal conjunction in thalamocortical transactions. In H. H. Jasper, L. Descarries, V. F. Castellucci, and S. Rossignol, eds., *Consciousness: At the Frontiers of Neuroscience. Advances in Neurology*. Vol. 77. Philadelphia: Lippincott-Raven. 95–103.

Llinás, R., Ribary, U., Contreras, D., and Pedroarena, C. (1998). The neuronal basis for consciousness. *Philosophical Transactions of the Royal Society of London, Series B: Biological Sciences* 353: 1841–9.

Llinás, R., Ribary, U., Joliot, M., and Wang, X.-J. (1994). Content and context in temporal thalamocortical binding. In G. Buzaki, R. Llinás, W. Singer, A. Berthoz, and Y. Christen, eds., *Temporal Coding in the Brain*. Berlin: Springer-Verlag. pp. 251–272.

Llinás, R. R., and Paré, D. (1991). Of dreaming and wakefulness. *Neuroscience* 44: 521–35.

Llinás, R. R., and Ribary, U. (1992). Rostrocaudal scan in human brain: A global characteristic of the 40-Hz response during input. In E. Basar and T. Bullock, eds., *Induced Rhythms in the Brain*. Boston: Birkhäuser.

Llinás, R. R., and Ribary, U. (1993). Coherent 40 Hz oscillation characterizes dream state in humans. *Proceedings of the National Academy of Sciences U S A* 90: 2078–81.

Llinás, R. R., and Ribary, U. (1994). Perception as an oneiric-like state modulated by the senses. In C. Koch and J. L. Davies eds., *Large-Scale Neuronal Theories of the Brain*. Cambridge, MA: MIT Press.

Loar, B. (1990). Phenomenal states. Revised version reprinted in N. Block, O. Flonagan, and G. Güzeldere, eds., *The Nature of Consciousness: Philosophical Debates*. Cambridge, MA: MIT Press.

Loar, B. (2003). Phenomenal intentionality as the basis of mental content. In M. Hahn and B. T. Ramberg, eds., *Reflections and Replies: Essays on Tyler Burge*. Cambridge, MA: MIT Press. Pp. 564–633.

Lockwood, M. (1993). The grain problem. In H. Robinson, ed., *Objections to Physicalism*. Oxford: Oxford University Press.

Lycan, W. G. (1987). *Consciousness*. Cambridge, MA: MIT Press.

Lycan, W. G., ed. (1990). *Mind and Cognition*. Cambridge, MA: Blackwell.

Lycan, W. G. (1996). *Consciousness and Experience*. Cambridge, MA: MIT Press.

Mack, A., and Rock, I. (1998). *Inattentional Blindness*. Cambridge, MA: MIT Press.

Mahowald, M. W., and Schenck, C. H. (1999). Dissociated states of wakefulness and sleep. In R. Lydic and H. A. Baghdoyan, eds., *Handbook of Behavioral State Control*: *Molecular and Cellular Mechanisms*. Boca Raton, FL: CRC Press.

Malcolm, N. (1956). Dreaming and skecpticism. *The Philosophical Review* 65: 14–37.

Malcolm, N. (1959). *Dreaming*. New York: Humanities Press.

Malcolm, N. (1988). Subjectivity. *Philosophy* 63: 147–60.

Malsburg, C. von der (1981). The correlation theory of brain functioning. Internal Report 81-2. Göttingen: Max-Planck-Institut für Biophysikalische Chemie. Reprinted in K. Schulten and J. von Hemmen, eds., (1994), *Models of Neural Networks*. Vol. 2. Berlin: Springer-Verlag.

Malsburg, C. von der (1997). The coherence definition of consciousness. In M. Ito, Y. Miyashita and E. T. Rolls, eds., *Cognition, Computation, and Consciousness*. Oxford: Oxford University Press.

Mamelak, A. N., and Hobson, J. A. (1989). Dream bizarreness as the cognitive correlate of altered neuronal behavior in REM sleep. *Journal of Cognitive Neuroscience* 1: 201–22.

Manford, M., and Andermann, F. (1998). Complex hallucinations: Clinical and neurobiological insights. *Brain* 121: 1819–40.

Mangan, B. (1993). Taking phenomenology seriously: The "fringe" and its implications for cognitive research. *Consciousness and Cognition* 2: 89–108.

Marcel, A. (1983). Conscious and unconscious perception: An approach to the relations between phenomenal experience and perceptual processes. *Cognitive Psychology* 15: 238–300.

Marchetti, C., and Della Sala, S. (1998). Disentangling the alien and the anarchic hand. *Cognitive Neuropsychiatry* 3: 191–207.

Martin, M. G. F. (1995). Bodily awareness: A sense of ownership. In J. L. Bermúdez, A. Marcel, and N. Eilan, eds., *The Body and the Self*. Cambridge, MA: MIT Press.

Matelli, M., Luppino, G., and Rizzolatti, G. (1985). Patterns of cytochrome oxidase activity in the frontal agranular cortex of the macaque monkey. *Behavioral Brain Research* 18: 125–37.

Mausfeld, R. (1998). Color perception: From Grassmann codes to a dual code for object and illumination colors. In W. Backhaus, R. Kliegl, and J. S. Werner, eds., *Color Vision—Perspectives from Different Disciplines*. New York: de Gruyter.

Mausfeld, R. (2002). Attributes of color and the physicalistic trap in color theory. In B. Saunders and J. van Brakel, eds., *Color*: *Theory, Technologies, Instrumentalities*. Washington: University Press of America.

Maxwell, G. (1978). Rigid designators and mind-body identity. In C. W. Savage, ed., *Perception and Cognition: Issues in the Foundations of Psychology. Minnesota Studies in the Philosophy of Science, IX*. Minneapolis: University of Minnesota Press.

Maxwell, S. (submitted). Intrinsically structureless qualia: A constraint on explanations of consciousness.

McClelland, J. L., Rumelhart, D. E., and the PDP Research Group, eds. (1986). *Parallel Distributed Processing. Explorations in the Microstructure of Cognition*. Vol. 2. Cambridge, MA: MIT Press.

McGinn, C. (1989a). *Mental Content*. Oxford: Oxford University Press.

McGinn, C. (1989b). Can we solve the mind-body problem? *Mind* 98: 349–66. Reprinted in Block et al. 1997.

McGinn, C. (1991). *The Problem of Consciousness: Essays toward a Resolution*. Oxford: Basil Blackwell.

McGinn, C. (1995). Consciousness and space. In T. Metzinger, ed., *Conscious Experience*. Thorverton, UK: Imprint Academic.

McGlynn, S., and Schacter, D. L. (1989). Unawareness of deficits in neuropsychological syndromes. *Journal of Clinical and Experimental Neuropsychology* 11: 143–205.

McKay, A. P., McKenna, P. J., and Laws, K. (1996). Severe schizophrenia: What is it like? In P. W. Halligan and J. C. Marshall, eds., *Method in Madness: Case Studies in cognitive Neuropsychiatry*. Hove, UK; Psychology Press/Erlbaurn (UK) Tailor & Francis Ltd.

Mead, E. R. S. (1919). *The Doctrine of the Subtle Body in Western Tradition*. London: John M. Watkins.

Meehl, P. E. (1966). The compleat autocerebroscopist: A thought experiment on Professor Feigl's mind-body identity thesis. In P. K. Feyerabend, and G. Maxwell, eds., *Mind, Matter and Method*. Minneapolis: University of Minnesota Press.

Mellor, D. H. (1977–8). Conscious belief. *Proceedings of the Aristotelian Society* 78: 87–101.

Mellor, D. H. (1980). Consciousness and degrees of belief. In D. H. Mellor, ed., *Prospects for Pragmatism*. Cambridge: Cambridge University Press.

Meltzoff, A., and Moore, M. K. (1977). Imitation of facial and manual gestures by human neonates. *Science* 198: 75–78.

Meltzoff, A. N., and Moore, M. K. (1983). Newborn infants imitate adult facial gestures. *Child Development* 54: 702–9.

Meltzoff, A. N., and Moore, M. K. (1989). Imitation in newborn infants: Exploring the range of gestures imitated and underlying mechanisms. *Developmental Psychology* 25: 954–62.

Melzack, R. (1989). Phantom limbs, the self and the brain. The D.O. Hebb Memorial Lecture. *Canadian Psychology* 30: 1–16.

Melzack, R. (1992). Phantom limbs. *Scientific American* 266(4): 90–6.

Melzack, R., and Bromage, P. R. (1973). Experimental phantom limbs. *Experimental Neurology* 39: 261–9.

Melzack, R., Israel, R., Lacroix, R., and Schultz, G. (1997). Phantom limbs in people with congenital limb-deficiency or amputation in early childhood. *Brain* 120 (Pt. 9): 1603–20.

Merikle, P. M., Smilek, D., and Eastwood, J. D. (2001). Perception without awareness; Perspectives from cognitive psychology. *Cognition* 79: 115–34.

Merleau-Ponty, M. (1962). *Phenomenology of Perception*. Translated by Colin Smith. London: Routledge & Kegan Paul.

Mesulam, M.-M. (1987). Neglect (selective inattention). In G. Adelmann, ed., *Encylopedin of Neuroscience*. Boston: Birkhäser.

Metzinger, T. (1990). Kriterien für eine Theorie zur Lösung des Leib-Seele-Problems. *Erkenntnis* 32: 127–45.

Metzinger, T. (1993/1999). *Subjekt und Selbstmodell*. Paderborn: mentis.

Metzinger, T. (1994). Schimpansen, Spiegelbilder, Selbstmodelle und Subjekte. In S. Krämer, ed., *Geist-Gehirn-Künstliche Intelligenz, Zeitgenössische Modelle des Denkens*. Berlin: de Gruyter.

Metzinger, T., ed. (1995a). *Conscious Experience*. Thorverton, UK: Imprint Academic.

Metzinger, T. (1995b). Faster than thought: Holism, homogeneity, and temproal coding. In T. Metzinger, ed., *Conscious Experience*. Thorverton, UK: Imprint Academic.

Metzinger, T. (1995c). Perspektivische Fakten? Die Naturalisierung des "Blick von nirgendwo." In Meggle, G. and Nida-Rümelin, J., eds. (1997). *Analyomen 2—Perspektiven der analytischen Philosophie*. New York: de Gruyter.

Metzinger, T. (1995d). Phänomenale mentale Modelle. In K. Sachs-Hombach, ed., *Bilder im Geiste: Zur kognitiven und erkenntnistheoretischen Funktion piktorialer Repräsentationen*. Series "Philosophie and Repräsentation." Atlanta: Rodopi.

Metzinger, T. (1995e). The problem of consciousness. In T. Metzinger, ed., *Conscious Experience*. Thorverton, UK: Imprint Academic.

Metzinger, T. (1997). Präsentationaler Gehalt. In F. Esken and H.-D. Heckmann, eds., *Bewußtsein und Repräsentation*. Paderborn: mentis.

Metzinger, T. (1998). Anthropologie und Kognitionswissenschaft. In T. Gold and A. K. Engel, eds., *Der Mensch in der Perspektive der Kognitionswissenschaften*. Frankfurt: Suhrkamp.

Metzinger, T., ed. (2000a). *Neural Correlates of Consciousness—Empirical and Conceptual Questions*. Cambridge, MA: MIT Press.

Metzinger, T. (2000b). Introduction: Consciousness research at the end of the twentieth century. In T. Metzinger, ed., *Neural Correlates of Consciousness—Empirical and Conceptual Questions*. Cambridge, MA: MIT Press.

Metzinger, T. (2000c). The *subjectivity* of subjective experience: A representationalist analysis of the first-person perspective. In T. Metzinger, ed., *Neural Correlates of Consciousness—Empirical and Conceptual Questions*. Cambridge, MA: MIT Press.

Metzinger, T. (2000d). "Selected Bibliography—Consciousness in Philosophy, Cognitive Science and Neuroscience: 1970–2000." Available from
http://www.philosophie.uni-mainz.de/metzinger/publikationen/ConsciousnessBib.pdf.

Metzinger, T. (2001). Postbiotisches Bewusstsein: Wie man ein künstliches Subjekt baut und warum wir es nicht tun sollten. In Heinz Nixdorf MuseumsForum (Hrsg.), *Computer. Gehirn. Was kann der Mensch? Was können die Computer?* Begleitpublikation zur Sonderausstellung "Computer.Gehirn" im Heinz Nixdorf MuseumsForum. Paderborn: Schöningh.

Metzinger, T. (2004). Conscious volition and mental representation: Towards a more fine-grained analysis. In N. Sebanz and W. Prinz (eds.), *Disorders of Volition*. Cambridge, MA: MIT Press.

Metzinger, T., and Chalmers, D. J. (1995). Selected bibliography—Consciousness in philosophy, cognitive science and neuroscience: 1970–1995. In T. Metzinger, ed., *Conscious Experience*. Thorverton, UK: Imprint Academic.

Metzinger, T., and Gallese, V. (2003). *The emergence of a shared action ontology: Building blocks for a theory*. In G. Knoblich, B. Elsner, G. von Aschersleben, and T. Metzinger, eds., *Grounding Selves in Action*. Special issue of *Consciousness & Cognition*, December 2003.

Metzinger, T., and Schumacher, R. (1999). Bewußtsein. In H.-J. Sandkühler, ed., *Enzyklopädie der Philosophie*. Hamburg: Meiner.

Metzinger, T., and Walde, B. (2000). Commentary on Jakab's "Ineffability of qualia." *Consciousness and Cognition* 9: 352–62 (doi:10.1006/ccog.2000.0463).

Michel, F., and Peronnet, F. (1980). A case of cortical deafness: Clinical and electrical physiological data. *Brain and Language* 10: 367–77.

Miller, S. D., and Triggiano, P. J. (1992). The psychophysiological investigation of multiple personality disorder: Review and update. *American Journal of Clinical Hypnosis* 35: 47–61.

Millikan, R. G. (1984). *Language, Thought, and Other Biological Categories*. Cambridge, MA: MIT Press.

Millikan, R. G. (1989). Biosemantics. *Journal of Philosophy* 86: 281–97.

Millikan, R. G. (1993). *White Queen Psychology and Other Essays for Alice*. Cambridge, MA: MIT Press.

Millikan, R. G. (1997). Images of identity: In search of modes of presentation. *Mind* 106: 499–519.

Milner, A. D., and Goodale, M. A. (1995). *The Visual Brain in Action*. Oxford: Oxford University Press.

Mitchell, S. W. (1871). Phantom limbs. *Lippincott's Magazine of Popular Literature and Science* 8: 563–69.

Mohr, G. (1997). Bewußtseinsphänomene in der Neuropsychologie und der experimentellen allgemeinen Psychologie. *Psychologische Rundschau* 48: 125–40.

Moore, G. E. (1903). The refutation of idealism. *Mind* 12: 433–53.

Morgan, M. (1999). Making holes in the visual world. *Nature Neuroscience* 2: 685–6.

Muldoon, S., and Carrington, H. (1929). *The Projection of the Astral Body*. London: Rider & Co.

Nagel, T. (1974). What is it like to be a bat? *Philosophical Review* 83: 435–50.

Nagel, T. (1986). *The View from Nowhere*. New York: Oxford University Press.

Nagel, T. (1991). What we have in mind when we say we're thinking. [Review of D. C. Dennett, *Consciousness Explained*.] *Wall Street Journal* Nov. 7, 1991.

Neander, K. (1998). The division of phenomenal labor: A problem for representational theories of consciousness. In J. Tomberlin, ed., *Philosophical Perspectives*. Vol. 12: *Language, Mind, and Ontology*. Malden, MA: Blackwell.

Newell, A., and Simon, H. (1961). GPS, a program that simulates human thought. Reprinted in E. Feigenbaum and J. Feldman, eds. (1963), *Computers and Thought*. New York: McGraw-Hill.

Newen, A. (1997). The logic of indexical thoughts and the metaphysics of the "self." In W. Künne, A. Newen, and M. Anduschus, eds., *Direct Reference, Indexicality and Propositional Attitudes*. Stanford, CA: CSLI.

Nida-Rümelin, M. (1995). What Mary couldn't know: Belief about phenomenal states. In T. Metzinger, ed., *Conscious Experience*. Thorverton, UK: Imprint Academic.

Nida-Rümelin, M. (1997). Subjekte von Erfahrung und die Zuschreibung mentaler Eigenschaften. *Logos* N.F. 4: 59–81.

Nielsen, T. A. (2000). A review of mentation in REM and NREM sleep: "Covert" REM sleep as a possible reconciliation of two opposing models. *Behavioral and Brain Sciences* 23: 851–66.

Nijhawan, R., and Khurana, B. (2000). Conscious registration of continuous and discrete visual events. In T. Metzinger, ed., *Neural Correlates of Consciousness—Empirical and Conceptual Questions*. Cambridge, MA: MIT Press.

Oatley, K. (1988). On changing one's mind: A possible function of consciousness. In A. Marcel and E. Bisiach, eds., *Consciousness in Contemporary Science*. Oxford: Oxford University Press.

O'Brien, E., and Opie, J. (1999). A connectionist theory of phenomenal experience. *Behavioral and Brain Sciences* 22: 127–48.

Opie, J., and O'Brien, G. (2001). Connectionist Vehicles, Structural Resemblance, and the Phenomenal Mind. In J. Veldeman, ed., *Naturalism and the Phenomenal Mind*. Special issue of *Communication and Cognition* 34: 13–38.

Paillard, J., Michel, F., Stelmach, G. (1983). Localization without content: A tactile analogue of "blindsight". *Archives of Neurology* 40: 548–51.

Palmer, J. (1978). The out-of-body-experience: A psychological theory. *Parapsychology Review* 9: 19–22.

Palmer, S. E. (1978). Fundamental aspects of cognitive representation. In E. Rosch and B. B. Lloyd, eds., *Cognition and Categorization*. Hillsdale, NJ: Erlbaum.

Palmer, S. E. (1999). *Vision Science—Photons to Phenomenology*. Cambridge, MA: MIT Press.

Panksepp, J. (1998). *Affective Neuroscience—The Foundations of Human and Animal Emotions*. New York: Oxford University Press.

Papineau, D. (1987). *Reality and Representation*. Oxford: Blackwell.

Papineau, D. (1993). Physicalism, consciousness and the antipathetic fallacy. *Australasian Journal of Philosophy* 71: 169–83.

Parnia, S., Waller, D. G., Yeates, R., and Fenwick, P. (2001). A qualitative and quantitative study of the incidence, features and aetiology of near death experiences in cardiac arrest survivors. *Resuscitation* 48: 149–56.

Parvizi, J., and Damasio, A. (2001). Consciousness and the brainstem. *Cognition* 79: 135–59.

Pasemann, F. (1996). Repräsentation ohne Repräsentation: Überlegungen zu einer Neurodynamik modularer kognitiver Systeme. In G. Rusch, S. J. Schmidt and O. Breidbach, eds., *Interne Repräsentationen*. Frankfurt: Suhrkamp.

Pashler, H. (1994). Divided attention: Storing and classifying briefly presented objects. *Psychonomic Bulletin and Review* 1: 115–8.

Perner, J., and Lang, B. (1999). Development of theory of mind and executive control. *Trends in Cognitive Sciences* 3: 337–44.

Perry, E., Walker, M., Grace, J., and Perry, R. (1999). Acetylcholine in mind: A neurotransmitter correlate of consciousness. *Trends in Neurosciences* 22: 273–80.

Perry, J. (1979). The problem of the essential indexical. *Noûs* 13: 3–22.

Picton, T. W., and Stuss, D. T. (1994) Neurobiology of conscious experience. *Current Opinion in Neurobiology* 4: 256–65.

Place, U. T. (1956). Is consciousness a brain process? *British Journal of Psychology* 47: 44–50.

Plato (2000). *The Republic. Books VI–X.* 10th ed. Translation by Paul Shorey. Cambridge, MA: Harvard University Press.

Plum, F., Schiff, N., Ribary, U., and Llinás, R. (1998). Coordinated expression in chronically unconscious persons. *Philosophical Transactions of the Royal Society of London. Series B, Biological Science* 353: 1929–33.

Podlech, A. (1984). Repräsentation. In O. Brunner, W. Conze, and R. Koseleck, eds., *Geschichtliche Grundbegriffe*, Vol. 5. Stuttgart: Klett-Cotta.

Poeck, K. (1964). Phantoms following amputation in early childhood and in congenital absence of limbs. *Cortex* 1: 269–75.

Pollen, D. A. (1999). On the neural correlates of visual perception. *Cerebral Cortex* 9: 4–19.

Pöppel, E. (1972). Oscillations as possible basis for time perception. In J. T. Fraser, ed., *The Study of Time*. Berlin: Springer-Verlag.

Pöppel, E. (1978). Time perception. In R. Held, H. W. Leibowitz, and H. L. Teuber, eds., *Handbook of Sensory Physiology*, Vol. 8. New York: Springer-Verlag.

Pöppel, E. (1985). *Grenzen des Bewußtseins*. Munich: DTV.

Pöppel, E. (1987). Blindsight, residual vision. In G. Adelmann, ed., *Encylopedia of Neuroscience*. Vol 1. Boston: Birkhäuser.

Pöppel, E. (1988). *Mindworks: Time and Conscious Experience*. New York: Hartcourt Brace Jovanovich.

Pöppel, E., ed. (1989). *Gehirn und Bewußtsein*. Weinheim, Germany: VCH Verlagsgesellschaft.

Pöppel, E. (1994). Temporal mechanisms in perception. *International Review of Neurobiology* 37: 185–202.

Pöppel, E., Held, R., and Frost, D. (1973). Residual vision function after brain wounds involving the central visual pathways in man. *Nature* 243: 295f.

Port, R. F., and van Gelder, T., eds., (1995). *Mind as Motion: Explorations in the Dynamics of Cognition*. Cambridge, MA: MIT Press.

Posner, M. I., and Rothbart, K. (1998). Attention, self regulation and consciousness. *Philosophical Transactions of the Royal Society of London* B 353: 1915–27.

Povinelli, D. J. (1993). Reconstrucing the evolution of mind. *American Psychologist* 48: 493–509.

Povinelli, D. J., and Cant, J. G. H. (1995). Arboreal clambering and the evolution of self-conception. *Quarterly Review of Biology* 70: 393–421.

Povinelli, D. J., and Prince, C. G. (1998) When self met other. In M. Ferrari and R. J. Sternberg, eds., *Self-Awareness: Its Nature and Development*. New York: Guilford Press.

Proust, J. (2000). Awareness of being the actor of one's actions: Three levels of analysis. In T. Metzinger, ed., *Neural Correlates of Consciousness—Empirical and Conceptual Questions*. Cambridge, MA: MIT Press.

Putnam, F. W. (1984). The psychophysiological investigation of multiple personality disorder. In J. Quen, ed., *Split Minds–Split Brains*. New York: New York University Press.

Putnam, F. W. (1989). *Diagnosis and Treatment of Multiple Personality Disorder*. New York: Guilford Press.

Putnam, H. (1967). Psychological predicates. In W. H. Capitan and D. D. Merrill, eds., *Art, Mind, and Religion*. Reprinted as "The nature of mental states" in H. Putnam (1975), *Mind, Language, and Reality—Philosophical Papers Vol. 2*. Cambridge, MA: Cambridge University Press.

Putnam, H. (1975a). The meaning of "meaning." In K. Gunderson, ed., *Language, Mind, and Knowledge*. Minneapolis: University of Minnesota Press. Reprinted in Putnam 1975b.

Putnam, H. (1975b). *Mind, Language and Reality. Philosophical Papers*. Vol. 2. Cambridge: Cambridge University Press.

Putnam, H. (1991). *Repräsentation und Realität*. Frankfurt: Suhrkamp.

Putnam, H. (1999). *The Threefold Cord—Mind, Body, and World*. New York and Chichester, West Sussex: Columbia University Press.

Quine, W. V. (1969). Propositional objects. In *Ontological Relativity and Other Essays*. New York: Columbia University Press.

Radden, J. (1996). *Divided Minds and Successive Selves: Philosophical Issues in Disorders of Identity and Personality*. Cambridge, MA: MIT Press.

Radden, J. (1999). Pathologically divided minds—Synchronic unity and models of self. In S. Gallagher and J. Shear, eds., *Models of the Self*. Thorverton, UK: Imprint Academic.

Raffman, D. (1993). Qualms about Quining qualia. In *Language, Music, and Mind*. Cambridge, MA: MIT Press.

Raffman, D. (1995). On the persistence of phenomenology. In T. Metzinger, ed., *Conscious Experience*. Thorverton, UK: Imprint Academic.

Raffman, D. (in preparation). The long and short of perceptual memory: A new argument for qualia.

Raichle, M. E. (1998). The neural correlates of consciousness: an analysis of cognitive skill learning. *Philosophical Transactions of the Royal Society of London* B 353: 1889–901.

Ramachandran, V. S. (1993). Behavioral and magnetoencephalographic correlates of plasticity in the adult human brain. *Proceedings of the National Academy of the Sciences U S A* 90: 10413–20.

Ramachandran, V. S. (1994). Phantom limbs, neglect syndromes, repressed memories and Freudian psychology. *International Revue of Neurobiology* 37: 291–333.

Ramachandran, V. S. (1995). Anosognosia in parietal lobe syndrome. *Consciousness and Cognition* 4: 22–51.

Ramachandran, V. S. (1998). Consciousness and body image: lessons from phantom limbs, Capgras syndrome and pain asymbolia. *Philosophical Transactions of the Royal Society of London. Series B: Biological Sciences* 353: 1851–9.

Ramachandran, V. S., and Blakeslee, S. (1998). *Phantoms in the Brain*. New York: William Morrow.

Ramachandran, V. S., and Hirstein, W. (1997). Three laws of qualia: What neurology tells us about the biological functions of consciousness. *Journal of Consciousness Studies* 4: 429–57.

Ramachandran, V. S., and Hirstein, B. (1998). The perception of phantom limbs. The D.O. Hebb Lecture. *Brain* 121: 1603–30.

Ramachandran, V. S., and Rogers-Ramachandran, D. (1996). Synaestesia in phantom limbs induced with mirrors. *Proceedings of the Royal Society of London. Series B: Biological Sciences* 377–86.

Ramachandran, V. S., Altschuler, E. L., and Hillyer, S. (1997). Mirror agnosia. *Proceedings of the Royal Society London* 264: 645–647.

Ramachandran, V. S., Rogers-Ramachandran, D., and Cobb, S. (1995). Scientific correspondence: Touching the phantom limb. *Nature* 377: 489–90.

Ramachandran, V. S., Rogers-Ramachandran, D., and Stewart, M. (1992a). Perceptual correlates of massive cortical reorganization. *Science* 258: 1159–60.

Ramachandran, V. S., Stewart, M., and Rogers-Ramachandran, D. (1992b). Perceptual correlates of massive cortical reorganization. *Neuroreport* 3: 583–6.

Ramsey, W., Stich, S., and Garon, J. (1991). Connectionism, eliminativism, and the future of folk psychology. In W. Ramsey, S. Stich, and D. E. Rumelhart, eds., *Philosophy and Connectionist Theory*. Hillsdale, NY: Lawrence Erlbaum.

Raney, A. A., and Nielsen, J. M. (1942). Denial of blindness (Anton's symptom). *Feuilleton of the Los Angeles Neurological Society* 7: 150–1.

Rauh, R., Schlieder, C., and Knauff, M. (1997). Präferierte mentale Modelle beim räumlich-relationalen Schließen: Empirie und kognitive Modellierung. *Kognitionswissenschaft* 6: 21–34.

Rees, G. (2001). Neuroimaging of visual awareness in patients and normal subjects. *Current Opinion in Neurobiology* 11: 150–6.

Reiss, D., and Marino, L. (2001). Mirror self-recognition in the bottlenose dolphin: A case of cognitive convergence. *Proceedings of the National Academy of Sciences U S A* 98: 5937–42.

Revonsuo, A. (1995). Consciousness, dreams, and virtual realities. *Philosophical Psychology* 8: 35–58.

Revonsuo, A. (1997). How to take consciousness seriously in cognitive neuroscience. *Communication and Cognition* 30: 185–296.

Revonsuo, A. (1999). Binding and the phenomenal unity of consciousness. *Consciousness and Cognition* 8: 173–85.

Revonsuo, A. (2000a). Prospects for a scientific research program on consciousness. In T. Metzinger, ed., *Neural Correlates of Consciousness—Empirical and Conceptual Questions*. Cambridge, MA: MIT Press.

Revonsuo, A. (2000b). The reinterpretation of dreams: An evolutionary hypothesis of the function of dreaming. *Behavioral and Brain Sciences* 23: 877–901.

Revonsuo, A., and Salmivalli, C. (1995). A content analysis of bizarre elements in dreams. *Dreaming* 5: 169–87.

Rey, G. (1993). Sensational sentences. In M. Davies and G. Humphreys, eds., *Consciousness: Psychological and Philosophical Essays*. Oxford: Blackwell.

Rey, G. (1998). A narrow representationalist account of qualitative experience. In J. Tomberlin, ed., *Philosophical Perspectives*. Vol. 12: *Language, Mind, and Ontology*. Malden, MA: Blackwell.

Richardson, R. C., and Muilenburg, G. (1982). Sellars and sense impressions. *Erkenntnis* 17: 171–211.

Richter, H. (1957). Zum Problem der ideomotorischen Phänomene. *Zeitschrift für Psychologie* 71: 161–254.

Rizzolatti, G., and Arbib, M. A. (1998). Language within our grasp. *Trends in Neurosciences* 21: 188–94.

Rizzolatti, G., and Gentilucci, M. (1988). Motor and visual-motor functions of the premotor cortex. In P. Rakic and W. Singer, eds., *Neurobiology of Neocortex*. New York: Wiley.

Rizzolatti, G., Fadiga, L., Fogassi, L., and Gallese, V. (2002). From mirror neurons to imitation: facts and speculations. In W. Prinz and A. Meltzoff, eds., *The Imitative Mind: Development, Evolution and Brain Bases*. Cambridge: Cambridge University Press.

Rizzolatti, G., Fadiga, L., Gallese, V., and Fogassi, L. (1996). Premotor cortex and the recognition of motor actions. *Cognitive Brain Research* 3: 131–41.

Rorty, R. (1965). Mind-body identity, privacy, and categories. *Review of Metaphysics* 19: 24–54.

Rorty, R. (1970). Incorrigibility as the mark of the mental. *Journal of Philosophy* 67: 406–24.

Rorty, R. (1981a). Leib-Seele Identität, Privatheit und Kategorien. In P. Bieri, ed., *Analytische Philosophie des Geistes*. Königstein, Germany: Hain.

Rorty, R. (1981b). Unkorrigierbarkeit als Merkmal des Mentalen. In P. Bieri, ed., *Analytische Philosophie des Geistes*. Königstein, Germany: Hain.

Rosenthal, D. (1986). Two concepts of consciousness. *Philosophical Studies* 49: 329–59.

Rosenthal, D. M. (2003). *Consciousness and Mind*. Oxford: Clarendon Press.

Rossetti, Y. (2001). Implicit perception in action: Short-lived motor representation of space. In P. Grossenbacher, ed., *Finding Consciousness in the Brain*. Philadelphia: John Benjamins.

Rossetti, Y., Rode, G., and Boisson, G. (1995). Implicit processing of somaesthetic information: A dissociation between where and how? *Neuroreport* 6: 506–10.

Roth, G. (2000). The evolution and ontogeny of consciousness. In T. Metzinger, ed., *Neural Correlates of Consciousness—Empirical and Conceptual Questions*. Cambridge, MA: MIT Press.

Ruhnau, E. (1992). Zeit—das verborgene Fenster der Kognition. *Kognitionswissenschafte*, 2: 171–9.

Ruhnau, E. (1994a). The Now—A hidden window to dynamics. In A. Atmanspacher and G. J. Dalenoort, eds., *Inside versus Outside. Endo- and Exo-Concepts of Observation and Knowledge in Physics, Philosophy and Cognitive Science*. Berlin: Springer.

Ruhnau, E. (1994b). The Now—The missing link between matter and mind. In M. Bitbol and E. Ruhnau, eds., *The Now, Time and the Quantum*. Gif-sur-Yvette: Editions Frontières.

Ruhnau, E. (1995). Time-Gestalt and the observer. In T. Metzinger, ed., *Conscious Experience*. Thorverton, UK: Imprint Academic.

Ruhnau, E., and Pöppel, E. (1991). Adirectional temporal zones in quantum physics and brain physiology. *International Journal of Theoretical Physics* 30: 1083–90.

Rumelhart, D. E., McClelland, J. L., and The PDP Research Group. (1986). Parallel distributed processing. *Explorations in the Microstructure of Cognition*. Vol. 1. Cambridge, MA: MIT Press.

Saadah, E. S., and Melzack, R. (1994). Phantom limb experiences in congenital limb-deficient adults. *Cortex* 30: 479–85.

Sacks, O. (1998). *The Man Who Mistook his Wife for a Hat*. New York: Simon & Schuster.

Salthe, S. N. (1985). *Evolving Hierarchical Systems*. New York: Columbia University Press.

Śamkara (1966). Vivekacūdāmani, 2nd ed. Edited and translated by Swami Madhavananda. Almora, India: Advaita Ashram.

Scheerer, E. (1990a). *Mental Representation: Its History and Present Status—1. "Representatio" from Cicero to Suarez*. Report No. 27 and 1990 of the Research Group on MIND AND BRAIN, Perspectives in Theoretical Psychology and the Philosophy of Mind, ZiF, Universität Bielefeld, Germany.

Scheerer, E. (1990b). *Mental Representation: Its History and Present Status—2. Descartes, His Followers and His Opponents*. Report No. 43 and 1990 of the Research Group on MIND AND BRAIN, Perspectives in Theoretical Psychology and the Philosophy of Mind, ZiF, Universität Bielefeld, Germany.

Scheerer, E. (1991). Artikel "Repräsentation I.1, I.2, 1.4 (Antike, Mittelalter, 17. und 18. Jahrhundert)." In J. Ritter and K. Gründer, eds., *Historisches Wörterbuch der Philosophie*. Vol. 8. Basel: Schwabe.

Schenck, C. H., and Mahowald, M. W. (1996). REM sleep parasomnias. *Neurological Clinics* 14: 697–720.

Schmidt, T. (2000). Visual perception without awareness: Priming responses by color. In T. Metzinger, ed., *Neural Correlates of Consciousness—Empirical and Conceptual Questions*. Cambridge, MA: MIT Press.

Scholz, O. (1991a). *Bild, Darstellung, Zeichen—Philosophische Theorien bildhafter Darstellung*. Freiburg im Breisgau, Germany: Alber.

Scholz, O. (1991b). Article "Repräsentation III (19. und 20. Jahrhundert). In J. Ritter and K. Gründer, eds., *Historisches Wörterbuch der Philosophie*. Vol. 8. Basel: Schwabe, p. 826*ff.*

Schultz, G., and Melzack, R. (1991). The Charles Bonnet syndrome: Phantom visual images. *Perception* 20: 809–25.

Schumacher, R. (1996). Mentale Präsentationen, Wissenstransfer und Wahrnehmung. In C. Hubig and H. Poser, eds., *Cognitio humana—Dynamik des Wissens und der Werte*. Vol. 2. Leipzig: Allgemeine Gesellschaft für Philosophie in Deutschland.

Schumacher, R. (1998). Visual perception and blindsight: The role of the phenomenal qualities. *Acta Analytica* 20: 71–82.

Searle, J. R. (1983). *Intentionality*. Cambridge: Cambridge University Press.

Séglas, J. (1897). *Le Délire des Négations* : *Séméiologie et Diagnostic*. Paris: Masson, Gauthier-Villars.

Sellars, W. (1963). *Science, Perception and Reality*. London: Routledge & Kegan Paul.

Sellars, W. (1965). The identity approach to the mind-body problem. *Review of Metaphysics* 18: 430–51.

Shannon, B. (1993). *The Representational and the Presentational. An Essay on Cognition and the Study of Mind*. New York: Harvester Wheatsheaf (Prentice Hall)/Hempe Hempstead.

Shoemaker, S. (1968). Self-reference and self-awareness. *Journal of Philosophy* 65: 555–67. Reprinted in S. Shoemaker, *The First-Person Perspective and Other Essays*. Cambridge: Cambridge University Press.

Shoemaker, S. (1990). Qualities and qualia: What's in the mind? *Philosophy and Phenomenological Research Supplement* 50: 109–31.

Shoemaker, S. (1996). *The First-Person Perspective and Other Essays*. Cambridge: Cambridge University Press.

Siegel, R. K. (1992). *Fire in the Brain: Clinical Tales of Hallucinations*. New York: Dutton.

Siegel, R. K., and Jarvik, M. E. (1975). Drug-induced hallucinations in animals and man. In R. K. Siegel and L. J. West, eds., *Hallucinations. Behavior, Experience, and Theory*. New York: Wiley.

Siegel, R. K., and West, L. J., eds. (1975). *Hallucinations, Behavior, Experience, and Theory*. New York: Wiley.

Silbersweig, D. A., and Stern, E. (1998). Towards a functional neuroanatomy of conscious perception and its modulation by volition: Implications of human auditory neuroimaging studies. *Philosophical Transactions of the Royal Society of London. Series B: Biological Sciences* 353: 1883–8.

Singer, W. (1994). Putative functions of temporal correlations in neocortical processing. In C. Koch and J. L. Davis, eds., *Large-Scale Neuronal Theories of the Brain*. Cambridge, MA: MIT Press.

Singer, W. (2000). Phenomenal awareness and consciousness from a neurobiological perspective. In T. Metzinger, ed., *Neural Correlates of Consciousness—Empirical and Conceptual Questions*. Cambridge, MA: MIT Press.

Skoyles, J. R. (1990). Is there a genetic component to the body schema? *Trends in Neurosciences* 13: 409.

Slade, P. D., and Bentall, R. P. (1988). *Sensory Deception: A Scientific Analysis of Hallucination*. London: Crom Helm.

Smith, L. B., and Thelen, E., eds. (1993). *A Dynamic Systems Approach to Development—Applications*. Cambridge, MA: MIT Press.

Sobel, N., Prabhakaran, V., Hartley, C. A., Desmond, J. E., Glover, G. H., Sullivan, E. V., and Gabrieli, J. D. E. (1999). Blind smell: Brain activation induced by an undetected air-borne chemical. *Brain* 122: 209–17.

Solms, M. (2000). Dreaming and REM sleep are controlled by different brain mechanisms. *Behavioral and Brain Sciences* 23: 843–50.

Sparrow, G. S. (1976). Effects of meditation on dreams. *Sundance Community Dream Journal* 1: 48–9.

Spence, S. A., Brooks, D. J., Hirsch, S. R., Liddle, P. F., Meehan, J., and Grasby, P. M. (1997). A PET study of voluntary movement in schizophrenic patients experiencing passivity phenomena (delusions of alien control). *Brain* 120: 1997–2011.

Sperry, R. W. (1950). Neural basis of the spontaneous optokinetic response produced by visual inversion. *Journal of Comparative and Physiological Psychology* 43: 482–9.

Stephan, A. (1999). *Emergenz—Von der Unvorhersagbarkeit zu Selbstorganisation*. Dresden: Dresden University Press.

Sternman, A. B., Schaumberg, H. H., and Asbury, A. K. (1980). The acute sensory neuropathy syndrome: A distinct clinical entity. *Annals of Neurology* 7: 354–8.

Stich, S. (1983). *From Folk Psychology to Cognitive Science*. Cambridge, MA: MIT Press.

Stich, S. (1992). What is a theory of mental representation? *Mind* 402: 241–61.

Stich, S. P. (1978) Beliefs and subdoxastic states. *Philosophy of Science* 45: 499–518.

Stoerig, P., and Cowey, A. (1990). Wavelength sensitivity in blindsight. *Nature* 342: 916–18.

Stoerig, P., and Cowey, A. (1992). Wavelength discrimination in blindsight. *Brain* 115: 425–44.

Stoerig, P., Hubner, M., and Pöppel, E. (1985). Signal detection analysis of residual vision in a field defect due to a post-geniculate lesion. *Neuropsychologia* 23: 589–9.

Stuss, D. T. (1991). Self, awareness, and the frontal lobes: A neuropsychological perspective. In J. Strauss and G. R. Goethals, eds., *The Self: Interdisciplinary Approaches*. New York: Springer-Verlag.

Stuss, D. T., and Benson, D. F. (1986). *The Frontal Lobes*. New York: Raven Press.

Sweet, W. H. (1941). Seeping intracranial anuerysm simulating neoplasm. *Archives of Neurology and Psychiatry* 194: 86–104.

Szechtmann, H., Woody, E., Bowers, K. S., and Nahmias, C. (1998). Where the imaginal appears real? A positron emission tomography study of auditory hallucinations. *Proceedings of the National Academy of Sciences U S A*, 95: 1956–60.

Tani, J. (1999). An interpretation of the "self" from the dynamical systems perspective—A constructivist approach. In S. Gallagher and J. Shear, eds., *Models of the Self*. Thorverton, UK: Imprint Academic.

Tart, C. (1972a). The "high" dream: a new state of consciousness. In C. Tart, ed., *Altered States of Consciousness: A Book of Readings*. New York: Doubleday Anchor.

Tart, C. (1972b). States of consciousness and state-specific sciences. *Science* 174: 1203–10.

Tart, C. (1988). From spontaneous event to lucidity—A review of attempts to consciously control nocturnal dreaming. In J. Gackenbach and S. LaBerge, eds., *Conscious Mind, Sleeping Brain*. New York: Plenum Press.

Taylor, J., ed. (1958). *Selected Writings of John Hughlings Jackson*. Vol. 1. New York: Basic Books.

Teuber, H. (1965). Postscript: Some needed revisions of the classical views of agnosias. *Neuropsychologia* 3: 371–8.

Teunisse, R. J., Cruysberg, J. R., Hoefnagles, W. H., Verbeek, A. L., and Zitman, F. G. (1996). Visual hallucinations in psychologically normal people: Charles Bonnet's syndrome. *Lancet* 347: 794–7.

Thelen, E., and L. B. Smith. (1994). *A Dynamic Systems Approach to the Development of Cognition and Action*. Cambridge, MA: MIT Press.

Tholey, P. (1983). Techniques for inducing and manipulating dreams. *Perceptual and Motor Skills* 59: 875–8.

Tholey, P. (1984). Der Klartraum—Hohe Schule des Traums. In K. Schnelting, ed., *Hilfe ich träume!* Munich: Goldmann.

Tholey, P. (1987). *Schöpferisch träumen*. Niedernhausen Germany: Falken Verlag.

Tholey, P. (1988). A model for lucidity training as a means of self-healing and psychological growth. In J. Gackenbach and S. LaBerge, eds., *Conscious Mind, Sleeping Brain*. New York: Plenum Press.

Thompson, E., and Varela, F. (2001). Radical embodiment: Neural dynamics and consciousness. *Trends in Cognitive Sciences* 5: 418–25.

Titchener, E. B. (1911). A note on the consciousness of self. *American Journal of Psychology* 22: 540–52.

Tononi, G., and Edelman, G. M. (1998a). Consciousness and complexity. *Science* 282: 1846–51.

Tononi, G., and Edelman, G. M. (1998b). Consciousness and the integration of information in the brain. In H. H. Jasper, L. Descarries, V. F. Castellucci and S. Rossignol, eds., *Consciousness: At the Frontiers of Neuroscience. Advances in Neurology*. Vol. 77. Philadelphia: Lippincott-Raven.

Tononi, G., Edelman, G. M., and Sporns, O. (1998). Complexity and the integration of information in the brain. *Trends in Cognitive Sciences* 2: 44–52.

Tononi, G., McIntosh, A. R., Russell, D. P., and Edelman, G. M. (1998). Functional clustering: Identifying strongly interactive brain regions in neuroimaging data. *Neuroimage* 7: 133–49.

Tononi, G., Sporns, O., and Edelman, G. M. (1996). A complexity measure for selective matching of signals by the brain. *Proceedings of the National Academy of Sciences U S A* 93: 3422–7.

Tranel, D., and Damasio, A. R. (1985). Knowledge without awareness: An autonomic index of facial recognition by prosopagnosics. *Science* 228: 1453–4.

Tranel, D., and Damasio, A. R. (1988). Nonconscious face recognition in patients with prosopagnosia. *Behavioral Brain Research* 30: 235–49.

Treede, R. D. (2001). Neural basis of pain. In N. J. Smelser and P. B. Baltes, eds., *Encyclopedia of the Social and Behavioral Sciences*. Vol. 16, Amsterdam: Elsevier.

Turing, A. M. (1950). Computing machinery and intelligence. *Mind* 59: 433–60.

Tye, M. (1991). *The Imagery Debate*. Cambridge, MA: MIT Press.

Tye, M. (1994). Blindsight, the absent qualia hypothesis, and the mystery of consciousness. In C. Hookway and D. Peterson, eds., *Philosophy and the Cognitive Sciences*. Royal Institute of Philosophy Supplement 34. Cambridge: Cambridge University Press.

Tye, M. (1995). *Ten Problems of Consciousness*. Cambridge, MA: MIT Press.

Tye, M. (1998). Inverted earth, swampman, and representationism. In J. Tomberlin, ed., *Philosophical Perspectives*. Vol. 12: *Language, Mind, and Ontology*. Malden, MA: Blackwell.

Tye, M. (1999). Phenomenal consciousness: the explanatory gap as a cognitive illusion. *Mind* 108: 705–25.

Tye, M. (2000). *Consciousness, Color, and Content*. Cambridge, MA: MIT Press.

Ure, J., Faccio, E., Videla, H., Caccuri, R., Giudice, F., Ollari, J., and Diez, M. (1998). Akinetic mutism: A report of three cases. *Acta Neurologica Scandinavica* 98: 439–44.

Valentin, G. (1836). Über die subjectiven Gefühle von Personen, welche mit mangelhaften Extremitäten geboren sind. *Reprium Antomicum Physiologicum* 1: 328–37.

Valentin, G. (1844). *Lehrbuch der Physiologie des Menschen für Aerzte und Studirende*. Vol. 2. Braunschweig, Germany: Verlag Friedrich Vieweg und Sohn.

van Eeden, F. (1913). A study of dreams. *Proceedings of the Society for Psychical Research* 26: 431–61.

Van Gelder, T. (1999). Wooden iron? Husserlian phenomenology meets cognitive science. In J. Petito, F. Varela, B. Pachoud, and J. M. Roy, eds., *Naturalizing Phenomenology: Current Issues in Contemporary Phenomenology and Cognitive Science*. Stanford CA: Stanford University Press.

Van Gulick, R. (1988a). A functionalist plea for self-consciousness. *The Philosophical Review* 97: 149–81.

Van Gulick, R. (1988b). Consciousness, intrinsic intentionality, and self-understanding machines. In A. Marcel and E. Bisiach, eds., *Consciousness in Contemporary Science*. Oxford: Oxford University Press.

Varela, F. (1999). The specious present: A neurophenomenology of time consciousness. In J. Petito, F. Varela, B. Pachoud, and J. M. Roy, eds., *Naturalizing Phenomenology: Current Issues in Contemporary Phenomenology and Cognitive Science*. Stanford, CA: Stanford University Press.

Varela, F., Lachaux, J.-P., Rodriguez, E., and Martinerie, J. (2001). The brainweb: Phase synchronization and large-scale integration. *Nature Neuroscience* 2: 229–39.

Vecera, S. P., and Behrmann, M. (1997). Spatial attention does not require preattentive grouping. *Neural Psychology* 11: 30–43.

Vecera, S. P., and Gilds, K. S. (1997). What is it like to be a patient with apperceptive agnosia? *Consciousness and Cognition* 6: 237–66.

Vertes, R. P., and Eastman, K. E. (2000). The case against memory consolidation in REM sleep. *Behavioral and Brain Sciences* 23: 867–76.

Vetter, R. J., and Weinstein, S. (1967). The history of the phantom in congenitally absent limbs. *Neuropsychologia* 5: 335–8.

Vogeley, K. (2000). Selbstkonstrukt und präfrontaler Cortex. In A. Newen and K. Vogeley, eds., *Selbst und Gehirn*. Paderborn: mentis.

Vogeley, K., Kurthen, M, Falkai, B., and Maier, B. (1999). Essential features of the human self-model are implemented in the prefrontal cortex. *Consciousness and Cognition* 8: 343–63.

Von Bonin, G., and Bailey, P. (1947). *The Neocortex of Macaca Mulatta*. Urbana, IL: University of Illinois Press.

Von Eckardt, B. (1993). *What Is Cognitive Science?* Cambridge, MA: MIT Press.

Vuilleumier, P., Reverdin, A., and Landis, T. (1997). Four legs: Illusory reduplication of the lower limbs after bilateral parietal lobe damage. *Archives of Neurology* 54: 1543–7.

Waelti, E. (1983). *Der dritte Kreis des Wissens*. Interlaken: Ansata.

Walde, B. (2002). *Metaphysik des Bewusstseins*. Paderborn, Germany: mentis.

Walsh, F. B., and Hoyt, W. F. (1969). *Clinical Neuro-Ophtalmology*, 3rd ed. Baltimore: Williams & Wilkins.

Walter, H. (1998). Emergence and the cognitive neuroscience approach to psychiatry. *Zeitschrift für Naturforschung* 53c: 723–37.

Walter, H. (1999). Emotionales Denken statt kalter Vernunft: Das Konzept des Selbst in der Neurophilosophie der Willensfreiheit. In A. Newen and K. Vogeley, eds., *Selbst und Gehirn*. Paderborn: mentis.

Walter, H. (2001). *Neurophilosophy of Free Will. From Libertarian Illusions to a Concept of Natural Autonomy*. Cambridge, MA: MIT Press.

Wegner, D. M. (1997). Why the mind wanders. In J. D. Cohen and J. W. Schooler, eds., *Scientific Approaches to Consciousness*. Mahwah, NJ: Lawrence Erlbaum.

Wegner, D. M. (2002). *The Illusion of Conscious Will*. Cambridge, MA: MIT Press.

Wegner, D. M., and Wheatley, T. P. (1999). Apparent mental causation: Sources of the experience of will. *American Psychologist* 54: 480–92.

Weinstein, S., and Sersen, E. A. (1961). Phantoms in cases of congenital absence of limbs. *Neurology* 11: 905–11.

Weinstein, S., Sersen, E. A., and Vetter, R. J. (1964). Phantoms and somatic sensation in cases of congenital aplasia. *Cortex* 1: 276–90.

Weiskrantz, L. (1986). *Blindsight: A Case Study and Implications*. Oxford: Oxford University Press.

Weiskrantz, L. (1988). Some contributions of neuropsychology of vision and memory to the problem of consciousness. In A. Marcel and E. Bisiach, eds., *Consciousness in Contemporary Science*. Oxford: Oxford University Press.

Weiskrantz, L. (1997). *Consciousness Lost and Found. A Neuropsychological Exploration*. Oxford: Oxford University Press.

Weiskrantz, L., Warrington, E. K., Sanders, M. D., and Marshall, J. (1974). Visual capacity in the hemianopic field following a restricted occipital ablation. *Brain* 97: 709 ff.

Werth, R. (1983). *Bewußtsein—Psychologische, neurobiologische und wissenschaftstheoretische Aspekte*. Berlin: Springer-Verlag.

Werth, R. (1998). *Hirnwelten. Berichte vom Rande des Bewußtseins*. Munich: C.H. Beck.

Wilkes, K. V. (1988a). *Real People—Personal Identity without Thought Experiments*. Oxford: Clarendon Press.

Wilkes, K. V. (1988b). —, yishi, duh, um, and consciousness. In A. Marcel and E. Bisiach, eds., *Consciousness in Contemporary Science*. Oxford: Oxford University Press.

Williams, D. (1992). *Nobody Nowhere*. New York: Random House.

Williams, D. (1994). *Somebody Somewhere*. New York: Random House.

Winson, J. (1991). Neurobiologie des Träumens. *Spektrum der Wissenschaft* 1: 126–34.

Wittgenstein, L. (1953). *Philosophical Investigations*. Translated by G. E. M. Anscombe. London: Macmillan.

Wittgenstein, L. (1958a). *The Blue and Brown Books*. Oxford: Oxford University Press.

Wittgenstein, L. (1958b). *Philosophical Investigations*, trans. G. E. M. Anscombe. The English Text of the Third Edition. Upper Saddle River, NJ: Prentice Hall.

Wolfradt, U., and Watzke, S. (1999). Out-of-body-experiences, depersonalization and schizotypal traits. *Journal of the American Society for Psychical Research* 93: 249–57.

Wolpert, D., Ghahramani, Z., and Jordan, M. (1995). An internal model for sensorimotor integration. *Science* 269: 1880–2.

Wolpert, D. M., and Ghahramani, Z. (2000). Computational principles of movement neuroscience. *Nature Neuroscience Supplement* 3: 1212–7.

Yates, J. (1985). The content of awareness is a model of the world. *Psychological Review* 92: 249–84.

Young, A. W. (1999). Delusions. *Monist* 82: 571–90.

Young, A. W., and de Haan, E. H. F. (1993). Impairments of visual awareness. In M. Davies and G. W. Humphreys, eds., *Consciousness—Psychological and Philosophical Essay*. Oxford: Blackwell.

Young, A. W., and Leafhead, K. M. (1996). Betwixt of life and death: Case studies of the Cotard delusion. In P. W. Halligan and J. C. Marshall, eds., *Method in Madness: Case Studies in Cognitive Neuropsychiatry*. Hove, UK: Psychology Press.

Young, A. W., Robertson, I. H., Hellawell, D. J., de Pauw, K. W., and Pentland, B. (1992). Cotard delusion after brain injury. *Psychological Medicine* 22: 799–804.

Zeki, S. M. (1990). A century of cerebral achromatopsy. *Brain* 113: 1721–77.

Zeki, S., and Bartels, A. (1998). The autonomy of the visual systems and the modularity of conscious vision. *Philosophical Transactions of the Royal Society of London* B 353: 1911–4.

Zihl, J. (1980). "Blindsight": Improvement of visually guided eye movements by systematic practice in patients with cerebral blindness. *Neuropsychologia* 18: 71–7.

Zihl, J., von Cramon, D., and Mai, N. (1983). Selective disturbance of movement vision after bilateral brain damage. *Brain* 106: 313–40.

Zihl, J., von Cramon, D., Mai, N., and Schmid, C. (1991). Disturbance of movement vision after bilateral posterior brain damage. *Brain* 114: 2235–52.

Name Index

Subject Index

A priori impossibility, 455
A priori necessity, 598
Ability to predict one's own behavior, 327
Absence automatism, 419–420
Absence seizures, 495. *See also* Epilepsy
Absent-qualia argument, 235
Absolute dimension, 104
Absorption, 500
Abstract organ, 522. *See also* Virtual organs
Abstract properties, 300
Access consciousness, 229
 types of, 124–125
Achromatic field, 101
Achromatic level of luminance, 185
Achromatopsia, 217
Acknowledging each other as persons, 601
Acquisition history, 603
Act of reference, 177
Acting subject, 151
Action, 450
Action control, 31, 372
 selective, 121
Action goals, 184, 418
Action observation, 367
Action representation, 366, 372
 abstract, 515
 allocentric, 511
 supramodal, 378
Active externalism (AE), 112, 274
Active intermodal matching, 378
Actor model, 368
Actuality, 25
Adaptation process, 101
Adaptive value, 60
Adaptivity, 346, 597
Affective arousal, 536
Affective dissolution of the self, 603
Affective profile, 528
Affective tone, 199, 288
Affordances, 366, 425
Afunctional
 artifacts, 249
 simulata, 472
 simulation, 335
Agency, 40, 150, 180, 275, 277, 283, 325, 327, 358,
 377, 472, 532, 609
 attentional, 151, 252, 307, 326, 391, 394, 406, 499,
 502
 cognitive, 151, 326, 397, 404, 406, 444, 499, 607,
 609
 experience of, 507
 first-person, 609
 flow of, 512
 internal, 391, 506
 judgments, 410

moment of, 423
motor, 406
phenomenal, 276, 349, 406
phenomenal property of, 531
subjective experience of, 391
volitional, 151, 422
Agent, 296, 325, 348, 367, 376, 497
 action representations without an, 451
 artificial, 292
 autonomous, 552, 558
 cognitive, 119, 172, 201, 342
 epistemic agent, 172, 615
 hallucinogenic, 45
 mental, 181
 moral, 41
 virtual, 416
Agent-agent interaction
 selective forms of, 617
Agent-detection device, 371
Agnosia
 apperceptive, 219
 associative, 219
 color, 217
 for drawing, 217
 object, 217
 visuospatial, 217
Aha experiences, 385
Ahistoric character, 191
Akinetic mutism, 418, 420, 568, 570, 571, 608, 616
Alien control, delusions of, 451
Alien hand syndrome, 424, 426, 473
Allocation of computational resources, 475. *See also*
 Attention
Allocentric coding, 319
Allocentric goal simulation, 406. *See also* Action
 representation
Ambiguity minimization, 239
Amnesia, 252, 262, 531
Amusia, 218
Analogue indicator, 188, 295
Analysanda, 3
 and explananda, catalogue, 204
Anarchic hand syndrome, 424, 426
Anesthesia, 439, 573
Animal emotions, 207
Anosodiaphoria, 218, 431
Anosognosia, 218, 235, 260, 463
 remission from, 434
Anschauung, 78
Antihallucinogenic drugs, 543
Antireductionist reply, 330
Anton's syndrome, 234, 258, 429, 588
 inverse, 431
Anwesenheit, 400
Aplasia, 478